Advances in Pulmonary Physiology and Drug Delivery

Advances in Pulmonary Physiology and Drug Delivery

Editor: Laurence Booth

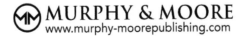
MURPHY & MOORE
www.murphy-moorepublishing.com

www.murphy-moorepublishing.com

MURPHY & MOORE

Cataloging-in-Publication Data

Advances in pulmonary physiology and drug delivery / edited by Laurence Booth.
   p. cm.
Includes bibliographical references and index.
ISBN 978-1-63987-769-0
1. Lungs--Physiology. 2. Respiratory organs--Physiology. 3. Pulmonary pharmacology.
I. Booth, Laurence.
QP121 .A38 2023
612.2--dc23

Murphy & Moore Publishing
1 Rockefeller Plaza,
New York City,
NY 10020, USA

ISBN 978-1-63987-769-0

Contents

Permissions

List of Contributors

Index

Preface

Pulmonary drug delivery refers to all the techniques used to deliver drugs and aerosols to the respiratory epithelium and epithelial cells directly through inhalation. It is used as a targeted therapy for the treatment of respiratory diseases such as chronic obstructive pulmonary disease, asthma and lung cancer. Drug delivery through the pulmonary route offers the distinct advantages of high bioavailability and no first-pass effect, which makes it an important means of delivering therapeutics directly to lung lesions. The benefits of pulmonary delivery include increased efficiency, a faster onset of delivery, decreased side effects, self-administration of non-invasive delivery, and localized action. The inherent properties of lungs such as their low enzymatic environment and high surface area make pulmonary delivery even more effective. This book provides significant information to help develop a good understanding of pulmonary physiology and drug delivery in respiratory diseases. Its extensive content will provide the readers with a thorough understanding of the subject.

The researches compiled throughout the book are authentic and of high quality, combining several disciplines and from very diverse regions from around the world. Drawing on the contributions of many researchers from diverse countries, the book's objective is to provide the readers with the latest achievements in the area of research. This book will surely be a source of knowledge to all interested and researching the field.

In the end, I would like to express my deep sense of gratitude to all the authors for meeting the set deadlines in completing and submitting their research chapters. I would also like to thank the publisher for the support offered to us throughout the course of the book. Finally, I extend my sincere thanks to my family for being a constant source of inspiration and encouragement.

Editor

1

Tobacco Smoke and Inhaled Drugs Alter Expression and Activity of Multidrug Resistance-Associated Protein-1 (MRP1) in Human Distal Lung Epithelial Cells *in vitro*

Mohammed Ali Selo[1,2]*, Anne-Sophie Delmas[1], Lisa Springer[1], Viktoria Zoufal[1,3],
Johannes A. Sake[1], Caoimhe G. Clerkin[1], Hanno Huwer[4], Nicole Schneider-Daum[5],
Claus-Michael Lehr[5,6], Sabrina Nickel[1], Oliver Langer[3,7,8] and Carsten Ehrhardt[1]*

[1] School of Pharmacy and Pharmaceutical Sciences and Trinity Biomedical Sciences Institute, Trinity College Dublin, Dublin, Ireland, [2] Faculty of Pharmacy, University of Kufa, Al-Najaf, Iraq, [3] Preclinical Molecular Imaging, AIT Austrian Institute of Technology GmbH, Seibersdorf, Austria, [4] Department of Cardiothoracic Surgery, Völklingen Heart Centre, Völklingen, Germany, [5] Helmholtz Institute for Pharmaceutical Research Saarland, Helmholtz Centre for Infection Research, Saarbrücken, Germany, [6] Department of Pharmacy, Saarland University, Saarbrücken, Germany, [7] Department of Clinical Pharmacology, Medical University of Vienna, Vienna, Austria, [8] Division of Nuclear Medicine, Department of Biomedical Imaging and Image-guided Therapy, Medical University of Vienna, Vienna, Austria

*Correspondence:
Mohammed Ali Selo
mohammeda.mohsin@uokufa.edu.iq;
selom@tcd.ie
Carsten Ehrhardt
ehrhardc@tcd.ie

Multidrug resistance-associated protein-1 (MRP1/*ABCC1*) is highly expressed in human lung tissues. Recent studies suggest that it significantly affects the pulmonary disposition of its substrates, both after pulmonary and systemic administration. To better understand the molecular mechanisms involved, we studied the expression, subcellular localization and activity of MRP1 in freshly isolated human alveolar epithelial type 2 (AT2) and type 1-like (AT1-like) cells in primary culture, and in the NCI-H441 cell line. Moreover, the effect of cigarette smoke extract (CSE) and a series of inhaled drugs on MRP1 abundance and activity was investigated *in vitro*. MRP1 expression levels were measured by q-PCR and immunoblot in AT2 and AT1-like cells from different donors and in several passages of the NCI-H441 cell line. The subcellular localization of the transporter was studied by confocal laser scanning microscopy and cell surface protein biotinylation. MRP1 activity was assessed by bidirectional transport and efflux experiments using the MRP1 substrate, 5(6)-carboxyfluorescein [CF; formed intracellularly from 5(6)-carboxyfluorescein-diacetate (CFDA)] in AT1-like and NCI-H441 cell monolayers. Furthermore, the effect of CSE as well as several bronchodilators and inhaled corticosteroids on MRP1 abundance and CF efflux was investigated. MRP1 protein abundance increased upon differentiation from AT2 to AT1-like phenotype, however, *ABCC1* gene levels remained unchanged. MRP1 abundance in NCI-H441 cells were comparable to those found in AT1-like cells. The transporter was detected primarily in basolateral membranes of both cell types which was consistent with net basolateral efflux of CF. Likewise, bidirectional transport studies showed net apical-to-basolateral transport of CF which was sensitive to the MRP1 inhibitor MK-571. Budesonide, beclomethasone dipropionate, salbutamol sulfate, and CSE decreased

CF efflux in a concentration-dependent manner. Interestingly, CSE increased MRP1 abundance, whereas budesonide, beclomethasone dipropionate, salbutamol sulfate did not have such effect. CSE and inhaled drugs can reduce MRP1 activity *in vitro*, which implies the transporter being a potential drug target in the treatment of chronic obstructive pulmonary disease (COPD). Moreover, MRP1 expression level, localization and activity were comparable in human AT1-like and NCI-H441 cells. Therefore, the cell line can be a useful alternative *in vitro* model to study MRP1 in distal lung epithelium.

Keywords: COPD, ABC transporters, pulmonary drug disposition, inhalation biopharmaceutics, efflux transporters

INTRODUCTION

Multidrug resistance-associated protein-1 (MRP1, 190 kDa), a member of the ATP binding cassette (ABC) superfamily of transporters, is encoded by the *ABCC1* gene (Cole, 2014a). As an efflux transporter, MRP1 plays a pivotal role in physiological detoxification. Its substrates include glutathione, glucuronate, and sulfate conjugates of drugs and endogenous molecules (Cole, 2014a,b). The transporter is highly expressed in the human lung, including bronchial, bronchiolar and alveolar epithelial cells (Flens et al., 1996; Scheffer et al., 2002).

We have become interested in pulmonary MRP1 for two reasons, its impact on inhaled drugs disposition and its potential role as a target in the treatment of chronic obstructive pulmonary disease (COPD).

It has been hypothesized that MRP1 protects lung cells against toxic insults of xenobiotics and from damage induced by oxidative stress by maintaining intracellular glutathione-glutathione disulfide homeostasis (Cole and Deeley, 2006; Cole, 2014b; Nickel et al., 2016). Inhibition of MRP1 was observed to worsen cigarette smoke extract (CSE)-induced cytotoxicity *in vitro* (van der Deen et al., 2007) and pre-clinical and clinical data suggest that changes in abundance (van der Deen et al., 2006; Wu et al., 2019) or function (Budulac et al., 2010) of the transporter are associated with occurrence and severity of COPD. Moreover, recent *in vivo* data from our group showed that pulmonary distribution and clearance of the MRP1 substrate S-(6-(7-[^{11}C] methylpurinyl)) glutathione ([^{11}C]MPG), measured with positron emission tomography (PET), was significantly dependent on MRP1 abundance (Mairinger et al., 2020).

On a molecular level, the expression and activity of MRP1 in distal lung epithelium, however, remains poorly investigated. Thus, the aims of this study were to determine the expression, cellular localization and activity of MRP1 in freshly isolated human alveolar epithelial cells in primary culture and to compare these data to the human adenocarcinoma cell line NCI-H441, which present several features of human distal lung epithelium, such as an ability to form electrically tight monolayers of polarized cells. Further it has been previously proposed to be the most promising continuously growing *in vitro* surrogate of human distal lung epithelial cells (Salomon et al., 2014; Salomon et al., 2019). In addition, the influence of CSE and commonly prescribed inhaled drugs on the abundance and activity of MRP1 *in vitro* was studied.

MATERIALS AND METHODS

Cell Culture

NCI-H441 human distal lung epithelial cells (ATCC HTB-174) were purchased from LGC Standards (Teddington, United Kingdom). Human alveolar type 2 epithelial (AT2) cells were isolated from non-tumor lung tissue obtained from patients undergoing lung surgery according to a previously published protocol (Daum et al., 2012). The freshly isolated AT2 cells were either used directly for RNA and protein isolation or left for 2 days to attach on collagen/fibronectin coated surfaces. Alternatively, cells were cultured for 8–10 days to undergo transdifferentiation into an alveolar type 1-like (AT1-like) phenotype. Primary cell culture was performed using small airways growth medium (SAGM, Lonza, Verviers, Belgium) supplemented with penicillin (100 U/ml), streptomycin (100 µg/ml), and 1% fetal bovine serum (all purchased from Sigma-Aldrich, Dublin, Ireland). Where indicated, 10 ng/ml keratinocyte growth factor (KGF, ProSpec-Tany TechnoGene, Ltd., Rehovot, Israel) was added to the culture medium to inhibit differentiation of AT2 cells into an AT1-like phenotype. The use of human tissue specimens was approved by Saarland State Medical Board (Saarbrücken, Germany). All cell types were cultured in a humidified atmosphere at 37°C in 5% CO_2 as described in more detail by Nickel et al. (2017).

Preparation of CSE

The smoke of two University of Kentucky research cigarettes (3R4F) was bubbled into 20 ml of RPMI 1640 medium (Biosciences, Dublin, Ireland) using a vacuum pump to generate 100% CSE. The latter was sterile filtered to remove any particulate matter and further diluted with RPMI medium to prepare 5 and 10% CSE which was used for exposure studies. Human AT1-like and NCI-H441 cells were exposed to either freshly prepared or aged CSE, which was prepared and stored at room temperature for 14 days, to investigate their effect on MRP1 abundance and activity.

Isolation of RNA and Real-Time Polymerase Chain Reaction (q-PCR)

RNA was isolated from freshly isolated AT2 cells, which were cultured for 8–10 days to transdifferentiate into the AT1-like phenotype and NCI-H441 cells grown in six-well plates

(Greiner Bio-One GmbH, Frickenhausen, Germany) using Tri-Reagent (Sigma-Aldrich) according to the manufacturer's instructions and as described in a previously published protocol (Nickel et al., 2017). Semi-quantitative, one-step real time PCR (q-PCR) was carried out on a 7500 Real-Time PCR System (Applied Biosystems, Inc., Foster City, CA, United States) as described previously (Nickel et al., 2017) using KiCqStart predesigned primers [(Sigma-Aldrich) for *ACTB* (forward GACGACATGGAGAAAATCTG; reverse ATGATCTGGGTCATCTTCTC) and *ABCC1* (forward AGC AGAAAAATGTGTTAGGG; reverse TACCCACTGGTAATA CTTGG)].

Immunoblot

Western blotting was carried out to investigate MRP1 abundance in AT2, AT1-like and in NCI-H441 cells. It was also used to assess the influence of different cell culture conditions [i.e., whether growing cells under air-interfaced culture (AIC) or liquid-covered culture (LCC)] on MRP1 protein level in NCI-H441 cells. In addition, the analysis was used to determine the effect of CSE, budesonide and salbutamol sulfate on MRP1 abundance in NCI-H441 cells. Cells were grown in presence of 5 or 10 µM budesonide (Mundipharma Pharmaceuticals Limited, Dublin, Ireland) or 100 µM salbutamol sulfate (Sigma-Aldrich) for up to 6 days and compared with the negative control (medium alone) or incubated with the solvent [i.e., dimethyl sulfoxide (DMSO)] when appropriate.

Confluent cell monolayers were washed twice with ice cold phosphate buffered saline (PBS) and lysed with cell extraction buffer (Life Technologies, Eugene, OR, United States) supplemented with protease inhibitor cocktail (Roche, Mannheim, Germany). Subsequently, samples were sonicated and centrifuged at $12,000 \times g$ for 15 min at 4°C. The total protein amount was determined by Pierce BCA protein assay kit (Thermo Fisher Scientific, Waltham, MA, United States) according to the manufacturer's instructions. Polyacrylamide gel electrophoresis was carried out as described previously (Nickel et al., 2017). Following transfer onto immunoblot polyvinylidine fluoride membranes, blots were blocked with washing buffer [PBS containing 0.05% Tween 20 (PBST)] supplemented with 3% (w/v) bovine serum albumin (BSA) for at least 1 h at room temperature before being incubated overnight at 4°C with rat monoclonal anti-MRP1 Ab (clone MRPr1, GTX13368, GeneTex, Inc., Irvine, CA, United States, 1:50) in PBST supplemented with 1% (w/v) BSA. The following day, membranes were washed three times and incubated with secondary anti-rat antibody (1:5000; Santa Cruz, Dallas, TX, United States) for 1 h at room temperature. Peroxidase activity was detected with Immobilon Western Chemiluminescent HRP substrate (Millipore, Carrigtwohill, Ireland). Signals were documented using a ChemiDoc system (Bio-Rad Laboratories, Hercules, CA, United States).

Biotinylation of Cell Surface Proteins

Cell surface protein biotinylation was carried out to determine whether MRP1 is localized at the apical or basolateral membranes of polarized AT1-like and NCI-H441 cells. The analysis was not carried out in freshly isolated AT2 cells due to their unpolarized phenotype. Apical or basolateral membrane proteins of confluent, Transwell-grown cell monolayers were labeled with sulpho-NHS-biotin (Thermo Fisher Scientific), isolated and analyzed as described in a previously published protocol (Schwagerus et al., 2015).

Immunohistochemistry and Confocal Laser Scanning Microscopy (CLSM)

NCI-H441, AT2, and AT1-like cells cultured in Lab-Tek chamber slides (Nunc A/S, Roskilde, Denmark) or on Transwell Clear inserts (either 12 mm or 6.5 mm in diameter, 0.4 µm pore size, Corning, Bedford, MA, United States) were used and processed for immunocytochemistry, as described previously (Nickel et al., 2017). Cells were fixed with 2% paraformaldehyde, incubated with 50 mM aqueous NH_4Cl and then permeabilized with 0.1% Triton X-100. Monolayers were blocked with 2% BSA in PBS and incubated overnight with rat monoclonal anti-MRP1 Ab (1:50 dilution). The following day, cell monolayers were washed twice and incubated with Alexa Fluor 488-conjugated goat anti-rat secondary antibody (ab150165, abcam, Cambridge, United Kingdom, 1:100) for 1 h at room temperature, followed by 5 min incubation with a Hoechst 33342 solution (1 µg/ml) to counterstain nuclei. Samples were visualized on a Leica SP8 confocal laser scanning microscope (Leica Microsystems, Wetzlar, Germany) with a 63× oil immersion objective, a 488 nm diode laser and 520 nm Alexa Fluor 488 detection filter (green antibody signal) and a 405 nm diode laser in combination with a Hoechst 33342 detection filter (blue nucleic signal).

Bidirectional 5(6)-Carboxyfluorescein Transport Studies

Multidrug resistance-associated protein-1 activity *in vitro* was determined by carrying out bidirectional transport studies of the MRP1 substrate 5(6)-carboxyfluorescein (CF) across polarized monolayers of AT1-like and NCI-H441 cells as described by Salomon et al. (2014). CF is formed intracellularly from the cleavage of its non-fluorescent diacetate conjugate (CFDA) which diffuses passively into the cells. Due to their unpolarized phenotype, transport studies could not be carried out in freshly isolated AT2 cells. Cells were grown in Transwell Clear inserts and studies were carried out only across monolayers with transepithelial electrical resistance (TEER) values exceeding $500 \ \Omega \times cm^2$. Monolayers were washed twice with pre-warmed Krebs-Ringer buffer (KRB; 116.4 mM NaCl, 5.4 mM KCl, 0.78 mM NaH_2PO_4, 25 mM $NaHCO_3$, 5.55 mM glucose, 15 mM HEPES, 1.8 mM $CaCl_2$, and 0.81 mM $MgSO_4$; pH 7.4) and then pre-equilibrated with the buffer solution for 1 h in the presence or absence of the MRP1 inhibitor MK-571 (20 µM, Santa Cruz). Permeation studies were initiated by replacing the buffer solution in the donor chambers with 100 µM CFDA solution (Applied BioProbes, Rockville, MD, United States) with or without the inhibitor compound. Cells were maintained at 37°C and 200 µl samples were collected from the receptor chambers after 0, 15, 30, 45, 60, 75, and 90 min and replaced with the same volume of buffer solution. Fluorescence intensity was analyzed using an automated plate reader (FLUOstar Optima, BMG LABTECH, Offenburg, Germany) at excitation and emission wavelengths of 485 and 520 nm, respectively. TEER values were measured before and after the study to verify cell monolayer integrity. The apparent permeability coefficient (P_{app}) was calculated using the following equation:

$$P_{app} = \frac{\Delta Q/\Delta t}{A \times C_0} \qquad (1)$$

where ΔQ is the change in the amount of CF over the designated period of time (Δt), A is the nominal surface area of the growth supports (i.e., 1.13 and 0.33 cm^2 in case of 3460 and 3470 Transwell inserts, respectively), and C_0 is the initial concentration of CFDA in the donor fluid.

CF Efflux Studies

Bidirectional CF efflux studies were carried out on polarized AT1-like and NCI-H441 cell monolayers grown in Transwell Clear inserts. Cell monolayers were washed twice and then incubated with KRB alone or supplemented with MK-571 (20 μM) for 1 h. Afterward, cells were loaded with 100 μM CFDA solutions (± MK-571) by adding 0.5 and 1.5 ml into the apical and basolateral chambers, respectively. Following 1 h incubation, monolayers were washed twice, and the donor solutions were replaced with the same volumes of fresh KRB alone or supplemented with the inhibitor compound. Afterward, 200 μl samples were collected from both apical and basolateral chambers every 15 min and up to 90 min and replaced with the same volumes of fresh KRB. At the end of experiments, TEER values were measured to confirm cell monolayers integrity.

Carboxyfluorescein efflux studies from AT-like and NCI-H441 cell monolayers grown in 24-well plates (Greiner Bio-One) were carried out to determine the effect of a series of inhaled drugs and CSE on MRP1 activity *in vitro*. As described above, cell monolayers were loaded with CFDA solution alone or containing either budesonide (5 or 10 μM), beclomethasone dipropionate (50 μM, Sigma-Aldrich), salbutamol sulfate (100 μM), salbutamol base (100 μM, Sigma-Aldrich), R-salbutamol HCl (100 μM, Sunovion Pharmaceuticals, Marlborough, MA, United States), S-salbutamol HCl, (100 μM, Sunovion Pharmaceuticals), terbutaline (100 μM, Sunovion Pharmaceuticals), formoterol fumarate (100 μM, Santa Cruz), L-sulforaphane (10 μM, Cayman Chemical, Ann Arbor, MI, United States), 5 or 10% CSE or the solvent [i.e., dimethyl sulfoxide (DMSO)] when appropriate. Following 1 h incubation, CFDA solutions were replaced with fresh KRB alone or supplemented with one of the above compounds and CF efflux was assessed by collecting 200 μl samples every 15 min. After 90 min, cell monolayers were washed twice with ice cold KRB and lysed in cell extraction buffer and fluorescence intensity was analyzed as described above. For standardization, the total protein concentration of whole cell lysate was determined by Pierce BCA assay (Thermo Fischer Scientific) according to the manufacturer's instructions and the amount of CF effluxed per μg of protein was calculated.

Data Analysis

Results are expressed as means ± SD. The significance of differences between mean values was determined either by unpaired, two-tailed Student's *t*-test or one-way ANOVA followed by Bonferroni's *post hoc* comparisons test. $P \leq 0.05$ was considered significant. All experiments were carried out at least in triplicate using cells from three different passages or donors.

RESULTS

Expression Analysis of MRP1/*ABCC1* in Human Alveolar Epithelial Cells

Semi-quantitative real-time PCR analysis revealed *ABCC1* mRNA expression at similar levels in freshly isolated AT2 cells and cells differentiated into an AT1-like phenotype (**Figure 1A**). Analysis of immunoblot data, however, revealed significantly ($P \leq 0.01$) lower MRP1 protein abundance in freshly isolated AT2 cells than in AT1-like cells from the same donors (**Figures 1B,C**). To exclude the probability that the lower protein levels observed in freshly isolated AT2 cells was an artifact due to cleavage of MRP1 protein by enzymes used for cell isolation, AT2 cells from the same donors were cultured in the presence or absence of 10 ng/ml KGF for at least 8 days. The growth factor has been shown to inhibit differentiation of AT2 cells into AT-like phenotype in primary culture (Demling et al., 2006). MRP1 abundance was, again, significantly ($P \leq 0.01$) lower in cells which retained their AT2 characteristics than in cells differentiated into an AT1-like phenotype (**Figures 1D,E**). CLSM analysis was inconclusive in terms of MRP1 localization in unpolarized AT2 cells (**Figure 1F**), but MRP1 signals were primarily localized to the basolateral cell membranes of AT1-like cells grown to monolayers for at least 8 days (**Figure 1G**). The localization of MRP1 in the basolateral membranes of AT1-like cells was further confirmed by cell surface protein biotinylation and subsequent analysis by Western blotting (**Figure 2A**).

Expression Analysis of MRP1/*ABCC1* in NCI-H441 Cells

Semi-quantitative real-time PCR and Western blot analyses showed stable MRP1/*ABCC1* expression across several passages of NCI-H441 cells. Neither passage number nor cell culture conditions (i.e., whether cells were grown in LCC or AIC conditions) had an influence on MRP1 abundance (**Figures 3A–C**). Protein levels of the transporter in the NCI-H441 cell line were comparable to AT1-like cells (**Figures 3D,E**). CLSM analysis of MRP1 in NCI-H441 cells grown under AIC (**Figure 3F**) and LCC (**Figure 3G**) conditions showed MRP1 signals mainly along the basolateral membranes. Cell surface protein biotinylation of Transwell-grown NCI-H441 monolayers further confirmed the basolateral localization of the protein (**Figure 2A**).

MRP1 Activity in Distal Lung Epithelial Cells

Multidrug resistance-associated protein-1 activity was studied *in vitro* by bidirectional transport and efflux studies of

Tobacco Smoke and Inhaled Drugs Alter Expression and Activity of Multidrug Resistance-Associated Protein-1...

5

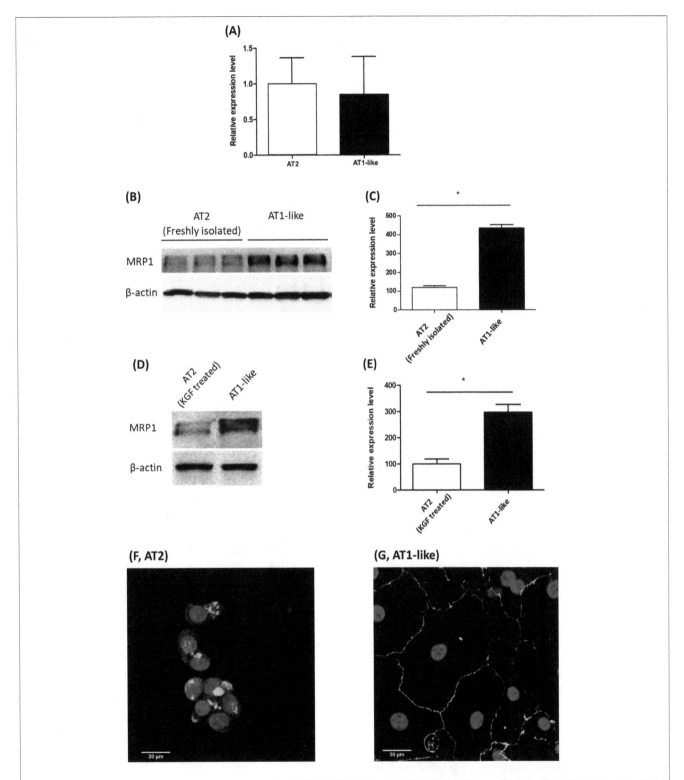

FIGURE 1 | Expression of multidrug resistance-associated protein-1 (MRP1)/*ABCC1* during transdifferentiation of human primary alveolar epithelial cells. **(A)** q-PCR analysis of *ABCC1* mRNA from three donors shows stable expression upon differentiation of alveolar type 2 epithelial (AT2) cells into an alveolar type 1-like (AT1-like) phenotype. **(B,C)** Representative Western blot and corresponding densitometric analyses of MRP1 protein in alveolar cells isolated from three donors show significantly lower levels in freshly isolated AT2 cells than cells differentiated into AT1-like phenotype. **(D,E)** show lower MRP1 abundance observed in cells cultured in the presence of KGF and thus retaining their AT2 properties than in cells differentiated into AT1-like cells in the absence of the growth factor. Data are represented as means + SD, $n \geq 3$, *$P \leq 0.01$. Unpaired, two-tailed Student's *t*-test was used. Confocal laser scanning microscopic analysis of MRP1 (green signals) in AT2 cells cultured for 2 days **(F)** was inconclusive because of the non-polarized phenotype of the cells. **(G)** In AT1-like cells, the signals detected were mainly at the basolateral cell membranes. Cell nuclei were counterstained with Hoechst 33342 (blue signals).

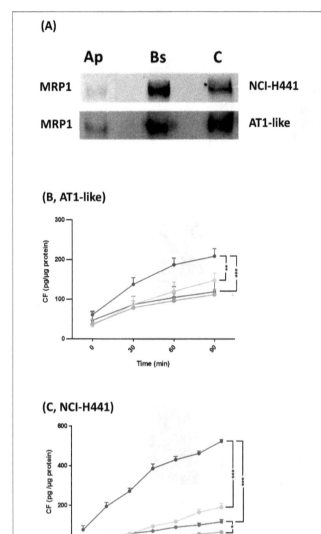

(A)

(B, AT1-like)

(C, NCI-H441)

- Basolateral efflux
- Basolateral efflux + MK-571 (20 µM)
- Apical efflux
- Apical efflux + MK-571 (20 µM)

FIGURE 2 | Multidrug resistance-associated protein-1 is localized to the basolateral membranes of alveolar type 1-like (AT1-like) and NCI-H441 cells. **(A)** Apical or basolateral membranes proteins of polarized, Transwell-grown NCI-H441 **(upper)** and human AT1-like **(lower)** cell monolayers were biotinylated, isolated and detected by immunoblot. Immunoblots clearly show MRP1 localization in the basolateral membranes of both cell models. Ap and Bs, indicate apically and basolaterally sulfo-NHS-biotin treated cells, respectively, and C indicates whole cell lysate. **(B,C)** show bidirectional carboxyfluorescein (CF) efflux studies from AT1-like **(B)** and NCI-H441 **(C)** cell monolayers. Consistent with the basolateral localization of the transporter, MK-571 sensitive, net basolateral efflux of CF from both cell models was observed. Data are represented as means + SD, $n = 9$, *P (0.05, **P (0.01, ***P (0.001. One-way ANOVA followed by Bonferroni's post hocpost-hoc comparisons test was used.

CF in polarized, Transwell-grown AT1-like and NCI-H441 monolayers, respectively. Data obtained were consistent with a basolateral localization of the transporter. A significantly ($P = 0.001$) higher amount of CF was effluxed into the basolateral receiver chamber than the apical receiver chamber from human AT1-like (**Figure 2B**) as well as NCI-H441 (**Figure 2C**) monolayers. The CF efflux was sensitive to inhibition by MK-571. Likewise, bidirectional transport studies showed MK-571-sensitive, net apical-to-basolateral transport of CF across both cell types (**Figures 4A,B**).

Effect of Inhaled Drugs on MRP1 Activity and Abundance

Carboxyfluorescein efflux studies were carried out to assess the effect of a set of commonly prescribed inhaled drugs on MRP1 activity *in vitro*. Budesonide (5 or 10 µM) decreased CF efflux from AT1-like and NCI-H441 cell monolayers in a dose-dependent manner (**Figure 5A** and **Table 1**). Similarly, beclomethasone dipropionate (50 µM) and salbutamol sulfate (100 µM) resulted in a significant reduction of CF efflux from NCI-H441 cells. Other tested bronchodilator compounds had no such effect (**Table 1**).

Immunoblot analysis of NCI-H441 cells grown in the presence of either 5 or 10 µM budesonide or 100 µM salbutamol sulfate for up to 6 days showed no influence of the drugs on MRP1 abundance (**Figure 5B**).

Effect of CSE and Sulforaphane on MRP1 Activity and Abundance

Carboxyfluorescein efflux studies and immunoblot analysis were used to determine the influence of CSE on MRP1 activity and abundance in AT1-like and NCI-H441 cells. Twenty-four hours exposure to freshly prepared 10% CSE caused a significant ($P \leq 0.01$) reduction in CF efflux from AT1-like and NCI-H441 cell monolayers (**Figures 6A,B**). The effect of the freshly prepared CSE was dose-dependent and more pronounced than that of aged CSE in NCI-H441 cells (**Figure 6A**). Interestingly, CSE exposure resulted in a significant increase in MRP1 abundance in NCI-H441 cells (**Figures 6C,D**).

The nuclear factor erythroid 2 related factor 2 (Nrf2)-antioxidant response elements (ARE) pathway has been previously suggested to be involved in the regulation of MRP1 expression (Ji et al., 2013). CF efflux studies were, therefore, carried out in the presence of the Nrf2 activator, sulforaphane to determine if it can improve MRP1 activity. The compound increased CF efflux from AT1-like cell monolayers (**Figure 6B**) but it had no influence on MRP1 activity in NCI-H441 cells (data not shown).

DISCUSSION

Multidrug resistance-associated protein-1 has previously been found to be the most abundant ABC transporter in human lung tissue in a study using liquid chromatography-tandem mass spectrometry for protein quantification (Sakamoto et al., 2013). The protein has also been detected in bronchial and

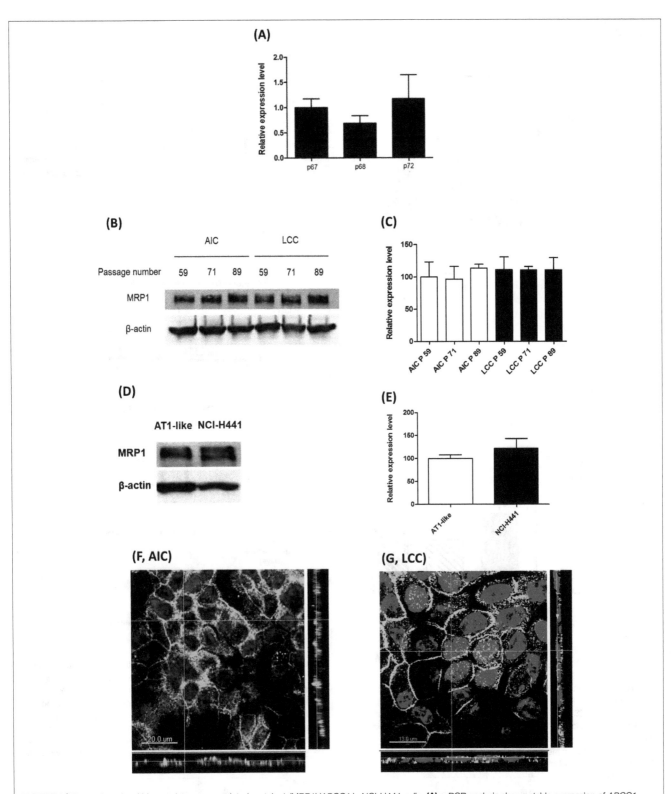

FIGURE 3 | Expression of multidrug resistance-associated protein-1 (MRP1)/*ABCC1* in NCI-H441 cells. **(A)** q-PCR analysis shows stable expression of *ABCC1* mRNA across several passages, p67, p68, and p72 indicate 67th, 68th, and 72th passage numbers, respectively. **(B,C)** Western blot and densitometric analyses of MRP1 in NCI-H441 cells grown either under air-interfaced culture (AIC) or liquid-covered culture (LCC) conditions for at least 7 days show similar abundance across different passage numbers and culture conditions. **(D,E)** Western blot and densitometric analysis showing similar protein levels of MRP1 in alveolar type 1-like (AT1-like) and NCI-H441 cells. Data are represented as means + SD, $n \geq 3$. Confocal laser scanning microscopy (CLSM) analysis of MRP1 (green signals) in NCI-H441 cells grown under AIC **(F)** and LCC **(G)** conditions show MRP1 signals primarily along the basolateral cell membranes. Cell nuclei were counterstained with Hoechst 33342 (blue signals).

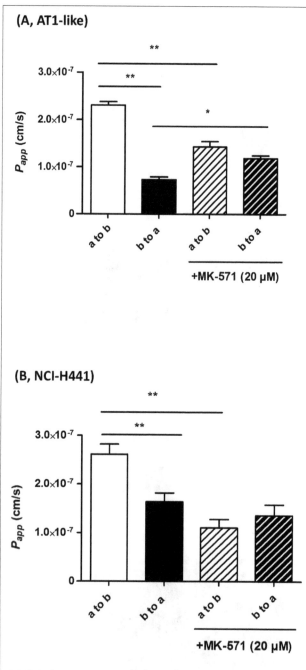

(A, AT1-like)

(B, NCI-H441)

+MK-571 (20 µM)

FIGURE 4 | Bidirectional transport studies of carboxyfluorescein (CF) across Transwell-grown confluent monolayers of human alveolar type 1-like (AT1-like) **(A)** and NCI-H441 **(B)** cells show significant net absorption of CF, consistent with the basolateral localization of multidrug resistance-associated protein-1 (MRP1). This net apical-to-basolateral transport can be attenuated by MK-571. Data represent means + SD, n = 9, *P ≤ 0.05, **P ≤ 0.01. One-way ANOVA followed by Bonferroni *post hoc* comparisons test was used.

(A)

(B)

Control   DMSO   Budesonide (5 µM)

Exposure time (Days)   1   3   6

MRP1   190 kDa
β-actin   42 kDa

Control   DMSO   Budesonide (10 µM)

Exposure time (Days)   1   3   6

MRP1   190 kDa
β-actin   42 kDa

Control   Salbutamol sulphate (100 µM)

Exposure time (Days)   1   3   6

MRP1   190 kDa
β-actin   42 kDa

FIGURE 5 | Effect of several inhaled drugs on multidrug resistance-associated protein-1 (MRP1) activity and expression. **(A)** Efflux studies from alveolar type 1-like (AT1-like) cell monolayers show significant and dose-dependent reduction of carboxyfluorescein (CF) efflux in the presence of budesonide. **(B)** Immunoblot analysis shows that treatment of NCI-H441 cells with budesonide (5 or 10 µM) or salbutamol sulfate (100 µM) for up to 6 days has no effect on MRP1 abundance. Data are represented as means + SD, n ≥ 6, **P ≤ 0.01, ***P ≤ 0.001. One-way ANOVA followed by Bonferroni's *post hoc* comparisons test was used.

bronchiolar epithelial cells, alveolar macrophages, seromucinous glands and nasal epithelium (Flens et al., 1996; Bréchot et al., 1998; Wioland et al., 2000). The transporter has also been detected in normal human bronchial epithelial cells in primary culture with substantial variations in the expression levels in

cells obtained from different donors (Lehmann et al., 2001). However, the expression, subcellular localization, and activity of the transporter are poorly investigated in distal lung epithelial cells. Previous reports have shown differences in mRNA and protein expression levels of several membrane transporters

TABLE 1 | Influence of Inhaled drugs on multidrug resistance-associated protein-1 (MRP1) activity in NCI-H441 cells.

Treatment	CF effluxed after 60 min (% of intracellular conc. at T_0)
KRB	45.4 ± 11.2
KRB + DMSO	47.2 ± 7.5
Budesonide 5 μM	36.5 ± 4.3
Budesonide 10 μM	34.2 ± 7.4*
Beclomethasone dipropionate 50 μM	20.4 ± 3.04***
Salbutamol sulfate 100 μM	35.1 ± 5.9*
Salbutamol base 100 μM	41.6 ± 2.3
R-Salbutamol HCl 100 μM	41.8 ± 2.5
S-Salbutamol HCl 100 μM	37.8 ± 6.2
Formoterol fumarate 100 μM	45.3 ± 3.6
Terbutaline 100 μM	43.7 ± 1.1

*Carboxyfluorescein (CF) efflux studies from NCI-H441 cells were carried out in presence of a set of beta-agonists and inhaled corticosteroids and compared with controls to assess their effect on MRP1 activity. Cells treated with transport buffer alone served as control. Data are represented as means ± SD, n ≥ 9. *$P \leq 0.05$, ***$P \leq 0.001$. One-way ANOVA followed by Bonferroni's post hoc comparisons test was used.*

both regarding spatial expression in different lung regions and regarding immortalized vs. primary cells (Endter et al., 2009; Salomon et al., 2012). To our knowledge, this is the first study in which the expression, subcellular localization, and activity of MRP1 is comprehensively investigated in human alveolar epithelial cells in primary culture and in the distal lung epithelial cell line NCI-H441. Data obtained revealed MRP1 to be expressed at high levels and functionally active in human distal lung epithelial cells. Immunoblots followed by densitometric analysis of samples from three donors showed a significant increase in MRP1 protein abundance upon differentiation of freshly isolated human AT2 cells into an AT1-like phenotype (**Figures 1B,C**). Likewise, MRP1 abundance was significantly lower in cells cultured in the presence of KGF and retaining their AT2 characteristics than in cells differentiated into AT1-like phenotype in the absence of the growth factor (**Figures 1D,E**). Similar results have previously been reported by Patel et al. (2008) in rat alveolar epithelial cells in primary culture. However, q-PCR analysis of *ABCC1* mRNA showed similar expression levels in AT2 cells and those differentiated into an AT1-like phenotype (**Figure 1A**). In fact, mRNA levels do not always strongly correlate with protein abundance due to distinct regulation controls at different stages and existence of numerous biological mechanisms that decouples gene level from protein level (Vogel and Marcotte, 2012; Fortelny et al., 2017).

Consistent with data previously reported in other lung epithelial cells (Bréchot et al., 1998; Hamilton et al., 2001), the subcellular localization experiments confirmed the transporter to be expressed primarily in the basolateral membranes of polarized AT1-like cells (**Figure 1G**, **2A** lower panel). In NCI-H441 cells, MRP1/*ABCC1* expression was stable across several passage numbers. Moreover, the protein level and the subcellular localization of the transporter were comparable to human primary AT1-like cells (**Figures 3A–G**, **2A** upper panel).

On a functional level, *in vitro* MRP1 activity data were also comparable between NCI-H441 cells and human AT1-like cells. Bidirectional CF efflux studies were consistent with a basolateral localization of the transporter in both cell types and the majority of substrate was effluxed into the basolateral receiver compartment. This efflux was sensitive to inhibition by MK-571 (**Figures 2B,C**). Small amounts of CF were also found in the apical compartment in both cell models, which may be due to paracellular transport of CF from the basolateral to the apical compartment. In addition, CF is a pan-MRP substrate and therefore a contribution of apically localized MRP2 and/or MRP4 to substrate efflux is conceivable as low *ABCC2* and *ABCC4* mRNA levels were reported previously in AT1-like cells (Endter et al., 2009). Bidirectional CF transport data were, again, comparable between human AT1-like and NCI-H441 cells. Consistent with basolateral localization of MRP1, MK-571 sensitive, net absorption of CF was observed in both cell models (**Figure 4**).

Multidrug resistance-associated protein-1, among other ABC transporters, plays a key role in the disposition of a wide variety of chemically unrelated drugs across various cellular and tissue barriers (Szakács et al., 2008). The transporter can, therefore, influence the pharmacokinetic profile and result in drug–drug interactions and modulation of pharmacologic activity of its drug substrates (Szakács et al., 2008; Marquez and Van Bambeke, 2011). The broad substrate spectrum together with the high abundance and functional activity of MRP1 observed at the alveolar epithelial barrier in our study suggest a potential role for the transporter in the pulmonary disposition of inhaled drug substrates. This is further supported by a recent *in vivo* study from our group in which profound differences in the pulmonary distribution and elimination kinetics of the MRP1 substrate [^{11}C]MPG were observed with PET imaging between wild type and $Abcc1^{(-/-)}$ rats following intratracheal aerosolisation of the radiotracer (Mairinger et al., 2020). In addition, a number of inhaled drugs have previously been reported to modulate MRP1 activity in the immortalized 16HBE14o- human bronchial cell line *in vitro* (van der Deen et al., 2008). Thus, we studied the potential interaction of a set of inhaled drugs with MRP1 in distal lung epithelial cells. Experiments carried out in human AT1-like and NCI-H441 monolayers showed a significant decrease of CF efflux in the presence of budesonide, beclomethasone dipropionate and salbutamol sulfate (**Table 1** and **Figure 5A**). Similar findings were reported with budesonide in previous studies performed on the 16HBE14o- (van der Deen et al., 2008) and the Calu-1 (Bandi and Kompella, 2002) epithelial cell lines. To determine whether the observed effect is attributed to a reduction of MRP1 protein levels, NCI-H441 cells were grown in the presence or absence of budesonide and salbutamol sulfate for up to 6 days. Immunoblot analysis showed no change in the transporter protein level suggesting that inhaled drugs above are either inhibitors or substrates of MRP1 (i.e., competing with CF). Due to complexity of lung anatomy, determination of clinically achievable concentrations of inhaled drugs in the lung fluid and epithelial cells is extremely challenging (van der Deen et al., 2008; Mukherjee et al., 2012). Thus, the concentrations applied in our study were mainly based on

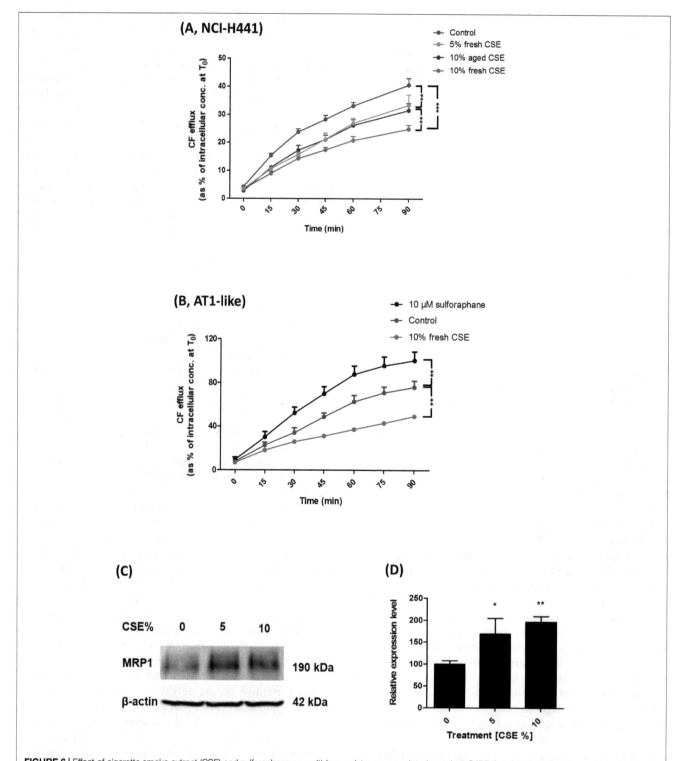

FIGURE 6 | Effect of cigarette smoke extract (CSE) and sulforaphane on multidrug resistance-associated protein-1 (MRP1) activity and abundance. Exposing NCI-H441 **(A)** and alveolar type 1-like (AT1-like) **(B)** cells to CSE for 24 h results in a significant and dose-dependent reduction of MRP1-mediated carboxyfluorescein (CF) efflux from both cell types. **(C,D)** Immunoblot analysis of NCI-H441 cells exposed to CSE show a dose-dependent increase in MRP1 abundance. Data are represented as means + SD, $n \geq 3$, $*P \leq 0.05$, $**P \leq 0.01$, $***P \leq 0.001$. One-way ANOVA followed by Bonferroni's *post hoc* comparisons test was used.

previous *in vitro* studies (van der Deen et al., 2008; Mukherjee et al., 2012; Salomon et al., 2012). Reduced MRP1 activity observed with inhaled drug substrates may be a source of

drug–drug interaction and variability in drug pharmacokinetics and could ultimately influence the safety and therapeutic efficacy of inhaled drugs.

Previous reports have suggested a potential role for MRP1 in smoking-related lung function loss and development of COPD. Reduced MRP1 protein levels were observed in lung tissue of COPD patients (van der Deen et al., 2006) and in an experimental rat model of COPD (Wu et al., 2019) using immunohistochemistry analysis. Moreover, the pulmonary clearance of inhaled [^{99m}Tc] methoxyisobutyl isonitrile ([^{99m}Tc] sestamibi), a radiolabeled MRP1 substrate, has been recorded to decrease in smokers and the decrement was attributed to modulation in MRP1 activity and expression profile (Mohan et al., 2019). The distal lung epithelium has been reported to be the initial site of development of tobacco smoke-induced diseases such as COPD (Baskoro et al., 2018). Thus, we investigated the potential impact of CSE on MRP1 activity and/or abundance in human AT1-like and NCI-H441 cells. Results showed a dose dependent reduction in CF efflux from monolayers of both cell types (**Figures 6A,B**). Immunoblot analysis, however, showed a dose dependent increase in MRP1 protein level upon exposure to CSE (**Figures 6C,D**). Given the protective role of MRP1 by extruding a variety of toxic xenobiotics out of lung epithelial cells, reduced MRP1 activity induced by CSE itself or inhaled drugs could further worsen the damage induced by tobacco smoke and may have a negative impact on the incidence and/or progression of COPD. The Nrf2-ARE pathway has been previously suggested to play a role in regulation of MRP1 expression (Ji et al., 2013). Therefore, we investigated whether the Nrf2 stimulator, sulforaphane, can improve MRP1 activity in distal lung epithelial cells. The compound had a positive impact on MRP1 activity in human AT1-like cells but not in NCI-H441 cells implying a possible beneficial effect in reversing the negative effect of CSE on MRP1 activity. The difference in response between both cell types

could be, theoretically, attributed to differences in Nrf2-ARE pathway activity which requires further investigations.

CONCLUSION

Multidrug resistance-associated protein-1 is functionally expressed at high levels to the basolateral membranes of human alveolar AT1-like cells in primary culture. The expression and activity profile of the transporter in NCI-H441 cells and AT1-like cells are similar and thus the cell line can be used as an *in vitro* model to study MRP1 in the distal lung epithelial barrier. Furthermore, tobacco smoke, inhaled drugs and sulforaphane can modulate MRP1 activity and/or abundance in distal lung epithelial cells *in vitro*, implying the transporter could be a novel therapeutic target of COPD.

AUTHOR CONTRIBUTIONS

CE, MS, OL, and SN: conceptualization. MS, JS, SN, and CE: data analysis. OL, CE, CC, and MS: funding acquisition. MS, A-SD, LS, VZ, JS, CC, HH, NS-D, and SN: investigation. MS and CE: project administration. HH, NS-D, and C-ML: resources. MS, SN, and CE: supervision. MS and CE: original draft. MS, A-SD, LS, VZ, JS, CC, C-ML, SN, OL, and CE: manuscript review and editing. All authors contributed to the article and approved the submitted version.

ACKNOWLEDGMENTS

The authors would like to acknowledge the contribution of the COST Actions BM1201 and MP1404.

REFERENCES

Bandi, N., and Kompella, U. B. (2002). Budesonide reduces multidrug resistance-associated protein 1 expression in an airway epithelial cell line (Calu-1). *Eur. J. Pharmacol.* 437, 9–17. doi: 10.1016/s0014-2999(02)01267-0

Baskoro, H., Sato, T., Karasutani, K., Suzuki, Y., Mitsui, A., Arano, N., et al. (2018). Regional heterogeneity in response of airway epithelial cells to cigarette smoke. *BMC Pulm. Med.* 18:148. doi: 10.1186/s12890-018-0715-714

Bréchot, J. M., Hurbain, I., Fajac, A., Daty, N., and Bernaudin, J. F. (1998). Different pattern of MRP localization in ciliated and basal cells from human bronchial epithelium. *J. Histochem. Cytochem.* 46, 513–517. doi: 10.1177/002215549804600411

Budulac, S. E., Postma, D. S., Hiemstra, P. S., Kunz, L. I., Siedlinski, M., Smit, H. A., et al. (2010). Multidrug resistance-associated protein-1 (MRP1) genetic variants, MRP1 protein levels and severity of COPD. *Respir. Res.* 11:60. doi: 10.1186/1465-9921-11-60

Cole, S. P. (2014a). Multidrug resistance protein 1 (MRP1, ABCC1), a "multitasking". ATP-binding cassette (ABC) transporter. *J. Biol. Chem.* 289, 30880–30888. doi: 10.1074/jbc.R114.609248

Cole, S. P. (2014b). Targeting multidrug resistance protein 1 (MRP1, ABCC1): past, present, and future. *Annu. Rev. Pharmacol. Toxicol.* 54, 95–117. doi: 10.1146/annurev-pharmtox-011613-135959

Cole, S. P., and Deeley, R. G. (2006). Transport of glutathione and glutathione conjugates by MRP1. *Trends Pharmacol. Sci.* 27, 438–446. doi: 10.1016/j.tips.2006.06.008

Daum, N., Kuehn, A., Hein, S., Schaefer, U. F., Huwer, H., and Lehr, C. M. (2012). Isolation, cultivation, and application of human alveolar epithelial cells. *Methods Mol. Biol.* 806, 31–42. doi: 10.1007/978-1-61779-367-7_3

Demling, N., Ehrhardt, C., Kasper, M., Laue, M., Knels, L., and Rieber, E. P. (2006). Promotion of cell adherence and spreading: a novel function of RAGE, the highly selective differentiation marker of human alveolar epithelial type I cells. *Cell Tissue Res.* 323, 475–488. doi: 10.1007/s00441-005-0069-60

Endter, S., Francombe, D., Ehrhardt, C., and Gumbleton, M. (2009). RT-PCR analysis of ABC, SLC and SLCO drug transporters in human lung epithelial cell models. *J. Pharm. Pharmacol.* 61, 583–591. doi: 10.1211/jpp/61.05.0006

Flens, M. J., Zaman, G. J., van der Valk, P., Izquierdo, M. A., Schroeijers, A. B., Scheffer, G. L., et al. (1996). Tissue distribution of the multidrug resistance protein. *Am. J. Pathol.* 148, 1237–1247.

Fortelny, N., Overall, C. M., Pavlidis, P., and Freue, G. V. C. (2017). Can we predict protein from mRNA levels? *Nature* 547, E19–E20. doi: 10.1038/nature22293

Hamilton, K. O., Topp, E., Makagiansar, I., Siahaan, T., Yazdanian, M., and Audus, K. L. (2001). Multidrug resistance-associated protein-1 functional activity in Calu-3 cells. *J. Pharmacol. Exp. Ther.* 298, 1199–1205.

Ji, L., Li, H., Gao, P., Shang, G., Zhang, D. D., Zhang, N., et al. (2013). Nrf2 pathway regulates multidrug-resistance-associated protein 1 in small cell lung cancer. *PLoS One* 8:e63404. doi: 10.1371/journal.pone.0063404

Lehmann, T., Köhler, C., Weidauer, E., Taege, C., and Foth, H. (2001).). Expression of MRP1 and related transporters in human lung cells in culture. *Toxicology* 167, 59–72. doi: 10.1016/s0300-483x(01)00458-9

Mairinger, S., Sake, J. A., Hernandez Lozano, I., Filip, T., Sauberer, M., Stanek, J., et al. (2020). Assessing the activity of multidrug resistance-associated protein 1 at the lung epithelial barrier. *J. Nucl. Med.* (in press). doi: 10.2967/jnumed.120.244038

Marquez, B., and Van Bambeke, F. (2011). ABC multidrug transporters: target for modulation of drug pharmacokinetics and drug-drug interactions. *Curr. Drug Targets* 12, 600–620. doi: 10.2174/138945011795378504

Mohan, H. K., Livieratos, L., and Peters, A. M. (2019). Lung clearance of inhaled aerosol of Tc-99m-methoxyisobutyl isonitrile: relationships with cigarette smoking, age and gender. *Clin. Physiol. Funct. Imaging* 39, 236–239. doi: 10.1111/cpf.12562

Mukherjee, M., Pritchard, D. I., and Bosquillon, C. (2012). Evaluation of air-interfaced Calu-3 cell layers for investigation of inhaled drug interactions with organic cation transporters in vitro. *Int. J. Pharm.* 426, 7–14. doi: 10.1016/j.ijpharm.2011.12.036

Nickel, S., Clerkin, C. G., Selo, M. A., and Ehrhardt, C. (2016). Transport mechanisms at the pulmonary mucosa: implications for drug delivery. *Expert Opin. Drug Deliv.* 13, 667–690. doi: 10.1517/17425247.2016.1140144

Nickel, S., Selo, M. A., Fallack, J., Clerkin, C. G., Huwer, H., Schneider-Daum, N., et al. (2017). Expression and activity of breast cancer resistance protein (BCRP/ABCG2) in human distal lung epithelial cells in vitro. *Pharm. Res.* 34, 2477–2487. doi: 10.1007/s11095-017-2172-9

Patel, L. N., Uchiyama, T., Kim, K. J., Borok, Z., Crandall, E. D., Shen, W. C., et al. (2008). Molecular and functional expression of multidrug resistance-associated protein-1 in primary cultured rat alveolar epithelial cells. *J. Pharm. Sci.* 97, 2340–2349. doi: 10.1002/jps.21134

Sakamoto, A., Matsumaru, T., Yamamura, N., Uchida, Y., Tachikawa, M., Ohtsuki, S., et al. (2013). Quantitative expression of human drug transporter proteins in lung tissues: analysis of regional, gender, and interindividual differences by liquid chromatography-tandem mass spectrometry. *J. Pharm. Sci.* 102, 3395–3406. doi: 10.1002/jps.23606

Salomon, J. J., Endter, S., Tachon, G., Falson, F., Buckley, S. T., and Ehrhardt, C. (2012). Transport of the fluorescent organic cation 4-(4-(dimethylamino)styryl)-N-methylpyridinium iodide (ASP+) in human respiratory epithelial cells. *Eur. J. Pharm. Biopharm.* 81, 351–359. doi: 10.1016/j.ejpb.2012.03.001

Salomon, J. J., Gausterer, J. C., Selo, M. A., Hosoya, K. I., Huwer, H., Schneider-Daum, N., et al. (2019). OCTN2-mediated acetyl-l-carnitine transport in human pulmonary epithelial cells in vitro. *Pharmaceutics* 11:396. doi: 10.3390/pharmaceutics11080396

Salomon, J. J., Muchitsch, V. E., Gausterer, J. C., Schwagerus, E., Huwer, H., Daum, N., et al. (2014). The cell line NCl-H441 is a useful in vitro model for transport studies of human distal lung epithelial barrier. *Mol. Pharm.* 11, 995–1006. doi: 10.1021/mp4006535

Scheffer, G. L., Pijnenborg, A. C., Smit, E. F., Muller, M., Postma, D. S., Timens, W., et al. (2002). Multidrug resistance related molecules in human and murine lung. *J. Clin. Pathol.* 55, 332–339. doi: 10.1136/jcp.55.5.332

Schwagerus, E., Sladek, S., Buckley, S. T., Armas-Capote, N., Alvarez de la Rosa, D., Harvey, B. J., et al. (2015). Expression and function of the epithelial sodium channel delta-subunit in human respiratory epithelial cells in vitro. *Pflugers. Arch.* 467, 2257–2273. doi: 10.1007/s00424-015-1693-1695

Szakács, G., Váradi, A., Ozvegy-Laczka, C., and Sarkadi, B. (2008). The role of ABC transporters in drug absorption, distribution, metabolism, excretion and toxicity (ADME-Tox). *Drug Discov. Today* 13, 379–393. doi: 10.1016/j.drudis.2007.12.010

van der Deen, M., de Vries, E. G., Visserman, H., Zandbergen, W., Postma, D. S., Timens, W., et al. (2007). Cigarette smoke extract affects functional activity of MRP1 in bronchial epithelial cells. *J. Biochem. Mol. Toxicol.* 21, 243–251. doi: 10.1002/jbt.20187

van der Deen, M., Homan, S., Timmer-Bosscha, H., Scheper, R. J., Timens, W., Postma, D. S., et al. (2008). Effect of COPD treatments on MRP1-mediated transport in bronchial epithelial cells. *Int. J. Chron. Obstruct. Pulmon. Dis.* 3, 469–475. doi: 10.2147/copd.s2817

van der Deen, M., Marks, H., Willemse, B. W., Postma, D. S., Muller, M., Smit, E. F., et al. (2006). Diminished expression of multidrug resistance-associated protein 1 (MRP1) in bronchial epithelium of COPD patients. *Virchows Arch.* 449, 682–688. doi: 10.1007/s00428-006-0240-243

Vogel, C., and Marcotte, E. M. (2012). Insights into the regulation of protein abundance from proteomic and transcriptomic analyses. *Nat. Rev. Genet.* 13, 227–232. doi: 10.1038/nrg3185

Wioland, M. A., Fleury-Feith, J., Corlieu, P., Commo, F., Monceaux, G., Lacau-St-Guily, J., et al. (2000). CFTR, MDR1, and MRP1 immunolocalization in normal human nasal respiratory mucosa. *J. Histochem. Cytochem.* 48, 1215–1222. doi: 10.1177/002215540004800905

Wu, J., Wang, X., Yao, Z., Wu, Q., Fang, W., Li, Z., et al. (2019). Allyl isothiocyanate may reverse the expression of MRP1 in COPD rats via the Notch1 signaling pathway. *Arch. Pharm. Res* 42, 1000–1011. doi: 10.1007/s12272-019-01183-1184

2

Pulmonary Surfactant and Drug Delivery: An Interface-Assisted Carrier to Deliver Surfactant Protein SP-D into the Airways

Cristina García-Mouton[†], Alberto Hidalgo[†‡], Raquel Arroyo[‡], Mercedes Echaide, Antonio Cruz and Jesús Pérez-Gil[*]

Department of Biochemistry and Molecular Biology, Faculty of Biology, Research Institute "Hospital 12 de Octubre (imas12)," Complutense University, Madrid, Spain

*Correspondence:
Jesús Pérez-Gil
jperezgil@bio.ucm.es

[†] *These authors have contributed equally to this work*

This work is focused on the potential use of pulmonary surfactant to deliver full-length recombinant human surfactant protein SP-D (rhSP-D) using the respiratory air-liquid interface as a shuttle. Surfactant protein D (SP-D) is a collectin protein present in the pulmonary surfactant (PS) system, involved in innate immune defense and surfactant homeostasis. It has been recently suggested as a potential therapeutic to alleviate inflammatory responses and lung diseases in preterm infants suffering from respiratory distress syndrome (RDS) or bronchopulmonary dysplasia (BPD). However, none of the current clinical surfactants used for surfactant replacement therapy (SRT) to treat RDS contain SP-D. The interaction of SP-D with surfactant components, the potential of PS as a respiratory drug delivery system and the possibility to produce recombinant versions of human SP-D, brings the possibility of delivering clinical surfactants supplemented with SP-D. Here, we used an *in vitro* setup that somehow emulates the respiratory air-liquid interface to explore this novel approach. It consists in two different compartments connected with a hydrated paper bridge forming a continuous interface. We firstly analyzed the adsorption and spreading of rhSP-D alone from one compartment to another over the air-liquid interface, observing low interfacial activity. Then, we studied the interfacial spreading of the protein co-administered with PS, both at different time periods or as a mixed formulation, and which oligomeric forms of rhSP-D better traveled associated with PS. The results presented here demonstrated that PS may transport rhSP-D long distances over air-liquid interfaces, either as a mixed formulation or separately in a close window time, opening the doors to empower the current clinical surfactants and SRT.

Keywords: pulmonary surfactant, interfacial delivery, respiratory drug delivery, air-liquid interface, lipid-protein interaction

INTRODUCTION

Surfactant protein D (SP-D) is a C-type calcium-dependent lectin that belongs to the collectin family. It is involved in the innate immune properties of pulmonary surfactant (PS) (Crouch et al., 1994; Crouch, 2000) and contributes to alveolar and surfactant homeostasis (Korfhagen et al., 1998). PS is a lipid-protein material essential for the process of breathing that has been proposed as potent drug delivery system (Van't Veen et al., 1996; De Backer et al., 2013; Banaschewski et al., 2015; Hidalgo et al., 2015, 2017). PS is mainly composed by lipids (90% by mass), mainly phospholipids, and four different proteins (6–8% by mass): two hydrophobic (SP-B and SP-C) and two hydrophilic (SP-A and SP-D) (Pérez-Gil, 2008; Parra and Pérez-Gil, 2015). SP-B and SP-C are essential for the maintenance and organization of PS at the air-liquid interface, while SP-A and SP-D are mostly involved in innate immune defense (Perez-Gil and Weaver, 2010). PS enables the process of breathing by lowering the surface tension of the layer of water covering the whole respiratory surface, minimizing the work of breathing and avoiding the alveolar collapse. Apart from the interfacial and immune defense functions, its composition and interfacial properties confers PS the possibility to spread efficiently over air-liquid interfaces and transport therapeutic molecules by surfing the respiratory surface, what has been called an interfacial delivery (Hidalgo et al., 2020).

As the rest of collectins, SP-D monomers (43 kDa) contain four different structural domains: a short N-terminal region enriched in cysteines, a collagen-like domain of Gly-X-Y repetitions, a neck region with α-helical structure and a C-terminal carbohydrate recognition domain (CRD), which constitutes the key structure for most of the protein functions and interactions (Orgeig et al., 2011; Casals et al., 2018). Monomers may associate into trimers (130 kDa), constituting the minimal functional unit to allow the recognition of specific molecules through the CRD. Trimers can also associate forming hexamers, dodecamers (520 kDa) and the so-called "fuzzy balls," which have been recently considered as the most potent oligomeric form of SP-D in bacterial aggregation (Arroyo et al., 2018, 2020). By recognizing a wide range of pathogens and foreign particles mostly through the CRD, SP-D promotes opsonization and aggregation and further clearance by phagocytic alveolar cells (Orgeig et al., 2011; Watson et al., 2019). Additionally, it also modulates the release of pro- and anti-inflammatory mediators via toll-like receptors and calreticulin/CD91 (Kingma and Whitsett, 2006; Sorensen, 2018).

Due to the immuno-modulatory and anti-inflammatory potential of SP-D, its delivery through the airways has been proposed in recent years as a potential therapeutic approach to alleviate inflammatory processes in the lungs. Since Clark and Reid highlighted in 2003 the potential benefits of delivering recombinant fragments of human SP-D (rfhSP-D) as a potential therapy to reduce inflammation in neonatal chronic lung disease, cystic fibrosis and emphysema (Clark and Reid, 2003), few works have explored this anti-inflammatory strategy and how this protein can be delivered through the airways. The instillation of rfhSP-D alone showed a reduction of inflammation derived from allergy in mice (Strong et al., 2003; Liu et al., 2005) or LPS in lambs (Ikegami et al., 2006) using recombinant fragments or full length recombinant human SP-D (rhSP-D), respectively. A recent study demonstrated the benefits of encapsulating SP-D in PLGA nanoparticles as a sustained release approach during several days from the administration (Cohen et al., 2020). In spite of the therapeutic effects of SP-D, the current commercially available clinical surfactants are all still lacking SP-D. However,

since SP-D interacts with pulmonary surfactant components (Korfhagen et al., 1998), preferentially with phosphatidylinositol (PI) (Ogasawara et al., 1992), the possibility of delivering clinical surfactants supplemented with rhSP-D has also been explored showing enhanced anti-inflammatory effects of PS/SP-D formulations on ventilation- (Sato et al., 2010) and LPS-derived (Ikegami et al., 2007) inflammation in lambs and mice, respectively. However, to the best of our knowledge, the capability of PS to transport SP-D interfacially to optimize PS/SP-D formulations and delivery has not been studied.

Therefore, in the present study we have evaluated for the first time (1) the possibility of SP-D to adsorb into and spread over air-liquid interfaces, (2) whether PS enhances this process, and (3) the influence of PS structures to interact with the different oligomeric forms of SP-D (i.e., trimers, hexamers and "fuzzy balls"). To do so, we used self-designed vehiculization setups consisting in two aqueous compartments connected by an interfacial bridge, and different PS/SP-D preparations and modes of administration were tested.

MATERIALS AND METHODS

Unless otherwise indicated, all chemicals and reagents were purchased from commercial suppliers (i.e., Sigma-Aldrich®, Merck KGaA or Macron Fine Chemicals™). Water was filtered and treated with a Merck-Millipore Direct-Q3 purification system and further distilled for the surface balance experiments.

Pulmonary Surfactant Preparations
Native Surfactant
Native pulmonary surfactant (NS) was isolated from bronchoalveolar lavage (BAL) of fresh slaughtered porcine lungs as previously described (Taeusch et al., 2005). Briefly, BAL was centrifuged at 1,000 g for 5 min to eliminate cells and tissue debris. Then, it was subsequently ultracentrifuged for 1 h at 100,000 g and 4°C. Pellets, containing the surfactant complexes, were resuspended in 16% NaBr 0.9% NaCl to perform a discontinuous NaBr density gradient at 120,000 g for 2 h at 4°C to purify the surfactant complexes from other cell membranes. After the gradient, pulmonary surfactant complexes, concentrated between the lighter (0.9% NaCl) and the medium dense solution (13% NaBr 0.9% NaCl), were homogenized with 0.9% NaCl and stored at −80°C until used.

Surfactant Organic Extract
Surfactant organic extract (OE), containing all the lipids plus the hydrophobic proteins SP-B and SP-C, was obtained following the organic extraction protocol established by Blight and Dyer (Bligh and Dyer, 1959). A mixture of chloroform/methanol/water (1:2:1 v/v/v) was added to the NS and incubated during 30 min at 37°C to allow protein flocculation. An additional volume of water and chloroform were added to the mixture and centrifuged 5 min at 3,000 g and 4°C. The fraction at the bottom containing the hydrophobic components of NS (organic phase) was collected. The upper fraction (aqueous phase) was subjected to two successive lavages by adding two volumes of chloroform

and centrifuged 5 min at 3,000 g and 4°C. Finally, the material recovered was stored at −20°C until used.

To prepare aqueous suspensions from OE, proper amounts of the material were dried under a nitrogen stream and further vacuum for 2 h to form a dry film without organic solvent traces. The dried films were reconstituted by hydration with a buffer solution (5 mM Tris, 150 mM NaCl, pH 7.4) during 1 h at 45°C, shacking vigorously every 10 min. When needed, the aqueous solution was sonicated in ice during 2 min (burst for 0.6, and 0.4 s between bursts) at 65% amplitude for 7 cycles in a UP 200S sonifier, with a 2 mm microtip.

Poractant α

Poractant α, commercially available as Curosurf®, was obtained from Chiesi Farmaceutici S.p.A. (Parma, Italy) at a concentration of 80 mg/mL.

Recombinant Human SP-D (rhSP-D)

rhSP-D was provided by Airway Therapeutics Inc. It has been produced and purified as previously described by Arroyo et al. (2018). All the different clones used have been previously analyzed by atomic force microscopy (AFM) to qualitatively and quantitatively characterize the oligomeric forms of the protein.

Fluorescent Labeling of rhSP-D

rhSP-D was conjugated with the amine-reactive fluorescent dye Alexa Fluor 488. First, the protein was exchanged to Hepes buffer (10 mM Hepes, 200 mM NaCl, 1 mM EDTA, pH 7.4) by dialysis at 4°C, in which the labeling reaction would take place. The proper amount of the probe, dissolved in methanol, to get a 1:20 (mol/mol) protein/probe ratio was dried under a nitrogen stream and under vacuum for 30 min and further dissolved in water. To shift the pH to values near 9 and activate amines, $NaHCO_3$ was added to the solution. Then, the labeling reaction was performed for 1 h at room temperature with continuous stirring. Finally, to separate fluorescently labeled protein (F-rhSP-D) from the free probe, the solution was dialyzed against Histidine buffer (5 mM His, 200 mM NaCl, 1 mM EDTA, pH 6).

Interfacial Assays

In the present study, the adsorption and spreading properties of rhSP-D by itself and the delivery capabilities of PS were characterized in Wilhelmy and vehiculization troughs.

Adsorption Tests

To evaluate the interfacial adsorption of the protein, experiments were performed using a single Wilhelmy trough (NIMA technologies, Coventry, UK). To do so, 1.8 mL of a buffered solution (5 mM Tris, 150 mM NaCl, pH 7.4) was placed in the Wilhelmy trough and an aqueous aliquot of 10 μL at 0.34 mg/mL (3.4 μg) of rhSP-D was injected into the subphase close to the surface, before monitoring the changes in surface pressure during 100 min with a pressure sensor (NIMA technologies, Coventry, UK). The subphase was constantly stirred to reduce diffusion limitation and thermostated at 25 ± 1°C.

Spreading and Vehiculization Assays

In order to explore the interfacial spreading capabilities of SP-D and its potential interface-assisted vehiculization by PS, an in vitro vehiculization setup was used (Yu and Possmayer, 2003; Hidalgo et al., 2017). Briefly, it consists in two different troughs containing a buffered solution (5 mM Tris, 150 mM NaCl, pH 7.4) connected by an interfacial bridge. One of the troughs is used as a donor (surface area: 315 mm^2; subphase volume: 1.8 mL), somehow mimicking delivery at the upper airways, and the other as the recipient, which emulates the target surfaces at the distal airways and may vary depending on the experiment. Both troughs are connected by an interfacial bridge (6 cm length × 1 cm width), made of a hydrated filter paper (No. 1 Whatman filter paper), which creates a continuous air-liquid interface between both compartments, somehow recreating the conductive airways (**Supplementary Figure 1**). The filter paper was hydrated by submersion into the same buffer solution during 5 min before connecting both compartments. The samples were added directly onto the donor interface by drop deposition. This should simulate the arrival of surfactant or surfactant/drug drops, either upon nebulization or direct bolus deposition, into the upper airways. Changes in surface pressure were simultaneously monitored in both donor and recipient compartments (pressure sensors from NIMA technologies, Coventry, UK). An increase of surface pressure at the donor trough indicates that the sample adsorbs into the air-liquid interface. The increase of surface pressure at the recipient trough is a signal indicating that the sample can interfacially spread over the air-liquid interface. This interfacial spreading of material is likely governed by Marangoni convection. The surface tension gradient between both connected compartments leads to the spread of material from the donor, where the surface tension is lower (higher surface pressure) and near the equilibrium, to the recipient trough, where the surface tension is initially high (low surface pressure) (Borgas and Grotberg, 1988; Grotberg and Gaver III, 1996; Halpern et al., 1998). To determine whether PS can transport SP-D, the recipient interface was measured by fluorescence or visualized under transmission electron microscopy (TEM) or atomic force microscopy (AFM) as detailed in the next sections. The experimental temperature was maintained constant at 25 ± 1°C. Different vehiculization setups and samples were used for each assay:

Spreading Properties of rhSP-D Alone

An aliquot of 20 μL at 0.6 mg/mL (12 μg) of rhSP-D, an amount enough to have an excess of protein, was added by drop deposition onto the donor interface connected to a recipient trough with a surface area of 25 cm^2 and 25 mL subphase volume. To determine the fluorescence of F-shSP-D, a smaller version of the recipient trough (surface area: 315 mm^2; subphase volume: 1.8 mL) was used in order to collect the whole volume.

Interfacial Vehiculization of a Combined PS/rhSP-D Formulation

An aqueous suspension of OE was incubated with rhSP-D (1% by mass with respect to lipids) at 37°C for 30 min. In these experiments, a rhSP-D clone enriched with higher amounts of fuzzy ball oligomers (82% by weight of total protein mass) compared with the average quantity [29% weight (Arroyo et al., 2018)] was used to facilitate its detection and recognition under the microscopes. Then, an aqueous aliquot of 15 μL at 50 mg/mL (750 μg) of OE was added by drop deposition onto the donor interface connected to the recipient trough (surface area: 25 cm²; subphase volume: 25 mL). To visualize the protein under TEM and AFM, the interfacial films were transferred to carbon-coated cupper grids and mica plates, respectively, as explained in the next sections. In addition, to evaluate the differential vehiculization of the oligomeric forms of rhSP-D, the aqueous suspension of OE was sonicated or not prior incubation with 1% rhSP-D by mass. In this case, a Langmuir-Blodgett trough (surface area: 60–184 cm²; subphase volume: 350 mL) was used as recipient to transfer the interfacial film onto mica plates.

Co-administration of PS and rhSP-D

In an attempt to strategize a sequential co-administration of PS and rhSP-D and understand the mechanisms of the interaction and interfacial spreading of PS and rhSP-D, we added both materials sequentially instead of as a combined formulation to the donor compartment connected to the recipient trough (surface area: 25 cm²; subphase volume: 25 mL). The clinical surfactant Curosurf (50 μL at 80 mg/mL; 4 mg) and the fluorescent derivative of rhSP-D (15 μL at 1 mg/mL; 15 μg) were used for these experiments. In a first scenario, Curosurf was firstly added by drop deposition onto the donor interface and F-rhSP-D 70 s later. This favors the interaction of the protein with a previously-formed surfactant interfacial film at the donor compartment and allows to analyze whether, in the case of interactions with Curosurf, the interfacial spreading driving forces promote the interfacial vehiculization of F-rhSP-D. In a second scenario, F-rhSP-D was first added onto the donor interface by drop deposition and Curosurf 70 s later to evaluate whether the surfactant can somehow take the SP-D that potentially diffuses through the aqueous subphase and transport it interfacially. The interface from the recipient trough was collected after 30 min to measure the fluorescence spectra. Additionally, experiments applying OE in organic solvent (Chloroform/Methanol 2:1 v/v) were performed to avoid the formation of surface-associated structures. To do so, 20 μL of OE at 18 μg/μL (360 μg) were added by drop deposition onto the donor interface and, 10 min later for letting the organic solvents evaporate, 2.5% (9 μg; data not shown) and 5% (18 μg) of rhSP-D by mass with respect to lipids was also added on top of the donor surfactant-occupied interface by drop deposition. A Langmuir-Blodgett trough (surface area: 60–184 cm²; subphase volume: 350 mL) was used as recipient to transfer the interfacial film onto mica plates for AFM analysis.

Fluorescence Spectroscopy

The vehiculization of the fluorescently-labeled F-rhSP-D by PS was detected by collecting the interface of the recipient trough and measuring the fluorescence of the covalently attached Alexa Fluor 488 ($\lambda_{excitation} = 490$ nm; $\lambda_{emission} = 525$ nm) in an Aminco Browman Series 2 spectrofluorometer. The emission spectra were measured at 25°C.

Atomic Force Microscopy (AFM)

This technique was used to visualize the oligomers of rhSP-D that were transported by PS over the air-liquid interface. The transference of the interfacial film at the target recipient surface to mica supports was performed following two different methods: (1) by direct deposition of the mica plate on top of the interface of the recipient trough, or (2) by forming Blodgett films using a Langmuir-Blodgett trough as the recipient compartment. In the latter method, the mica plate was cleaved and submerged into the buffered subphase prior sample addition. At the end of each experiment, the mica plate was progressively raised maintaining the surface pressure constant at 20 mN/m (barrier speed: 25 cm²/min; dipper speed: 5 mm/min). We selected that transfer pressure in order to avoid the potential exclusion of some components and the formation of three-dimensional structures that would hinder the acquisition of images under AFM. Images were acquired using an AFM from Nanotec (Nanotec Electrónica, Madrid, Spain) with PointProbePlus tips (Nanosensors, Neuchâtel, Switzerland), or a NanoScope IIIa scanning probe microscope (Bruker, Billerica, USA) with TESP-SS tips (Bruker, Billerica, USA), in the Centro Nacional de Biotecnología (CNB, CSIC) and ICTS Centro Nacional de Microscopía Electrónica (Universidad Complutense de Madrid). Samples were imaged in tapping mode in air, at room temperature and low humidity. The images were processed using the WSxM freeware and the NanoScope Analysis software.

Transmission Electron Microscopy

To observe the surfactant structures and confirm that PS can transport rhSP-D over air-liquid interfaces, carbon-coated cupper grids (EMS400-Cu, Gilder grids) were deposited on the interface of the recipient troughs and incubated for 30 s. Then, the grids were directly incubated for 1 min with 2% uranyl acetate (w/v) to perform negative staining. Samples were observed under a JEOL JEM-1010 transmission electron microscope (ICTS Centro Nacional de Microscopía Electrónica, Universidad Complutense de Madrid) at a magnification of 40,000x and 120,000x.

Dynamic Light Scattering (DLS)

In order to characterize the OE samples after sonication, the hydrodynamic radius (R_H) of aqueous suspensions in the presence or the absence of 1% rhSP-D by mass were determined using a DynaPro MS/X DLS detector equipped with a 824.7 nm-laser (Wyatt Inc). R_H was calculated by the Stokes-Einstein equation (Equation 1):

$$D = \frac{k_B \cdot T}{6\pi \eta R_H} \quad (1)$$

where D is the translational diffusion coefficient, k_B the Boltzman constant, T the temperature, and η the viscosity. Water used to dilute the samples was 10 times filtered using filters of 0.22 μm (Q-Pod, Merck). Polydispersity values smaller than 15% were considered to correspond to monodisperse samples.

RESULTS

Interfacial Properties and Spreading of rhSP-D Alone

As shown in **Figure 1A**, the surface pressure does not increase during the first 40 min. Then, it raises to values around 5 mN/m. It indicates that the protein slowly adsorbs into the air-liquid interface, but long periods of time are required to have enough amount of protein at the interface to cause a slight increase of surface pressure.

Figure 1B shows the interfacial spreading of rhSP-D by means of changes in surface pressure during 40 min both in donor and recipient compartments. Surface pressure at donor compartment increases until stabilizing at a limited surface pressure of ∼3 mN/m. Then, it slightly decreases as the surface pressure at the recipient compartment increases. The stabilization of the pressure at the donor trough and its subsequent decrease could indicate a transient adsorption of the protein into the interface and further diffusion to the recipient trough. However, once the surface pressure at the recipient equals the pressure at the donor compartment, the latter increases as well, indicating a continuous adsorption of rhSP-D at the donor interface until the interface stabilizes. To confirm the presence of the protein in the recipient trough, interfacial films were transferred to carbon-coated cupper grids and observed by TEM (**Supplementary Figure 2**), but no traces of SP-D were observed. Therefore, we also performed the vehiculization assays using the fluorescent derivative of rhSP-D. In this case, the smallest recipient trough was used to collect the whole volume (1.8 mL) and also measure the F-rhSP-D that might diffuse and dilute away from the interface into the subphase. As observed in **Figure 1C**, fluorescence was detected in the recipient compartment, suggesting that rhSP-D may actually cross the bridge alone from the donor to the recipient trough. However, the fluorescent signal was very low and maximal sensitivity in the fluorometer was required to detect it.

Interfacial Delivery of rhSP-D in the Presence of Pulmonary Surfactant

Once analyzed the adsorption and spreading properties of the rhSP-D alone confirming low interfacial adsorption and spreading capabilities, the next step was to analyze how the presence of PS influences the interface-assisted vehiculization process. To do so, different strategies were followed including a PS/rhSP-D combined formulation and the addition of PS and rhSP-D separately.

Interfacial Vehiculization of a Combined PS/rhSP-D Formulation

Figure 2A shows that right after addition of OE/rhSP-D mixture, the surface pressure at the donor compartment increases sharply above 30 mN/m, indicating a proper interfacial adsorption of the formulation. After 10 min, the surface pressure in the recipient trough starts increasing as well, though this increase seems to be lower than the one observed in the donor compartment. This, together with the high error bars could indicate that rhSP-D could somehow affect or modulate the adsorption and spreading

capabilities of pulmonary surfactant, something that needs further exploration to elucidate the relevant factors involved in this potential effect. In spite of the donor-to-recipient diffusion of OE/rhSP-D, the surface pressure at the donor trough always remained stable, indicating a rapid and continuous adsorption and spreading of new material from the surface-associated reservoirs at the donor compartment.

To confirm the potential of OE to transport rhSP-D over the air-liquid interface, the material placed at the recipient interface was transferred onto carbon-coated cupper grids and mica plates for TEM and AFM visualization, respectively. The micrographs obtained by TEM (**Figure 2B**) shows accumulation at the interface of fuzzy-ball-like structures, recognizable by the higher electron density of the central N-terminal collagenous stem. These structures are similar to the ones observed somewhere else (Holmskov, 2000). The AFM phase images (**Figure 2C**) demonstrated the presence of rhSP-D fuzzy balls at the air-liquid interface, appearing both grouped and isolated.

Understanding the Mechanisms Behind the Interaction and Interfacial Spreading of PS and rhSP-D

Figures 3A,B show $\prod$-time isotherms adding first Curosurf or F-rhSP-D, respectively. In both scenarios, Curosurf reaches the equilibrium surface pressure (around 40 mN/m) in the donor compartment right after injection, and subsequently the surface pressure in the recipient trough also increased. The injection of F-rhSP-D after 70 s in the presence of the preformed surfactant film does not induce further changes in surface pressure either in the donor neither in the recipient. This indicates that the protein does not affect the interfacial and spreading properties of Curosurf. After 30 min, the recipient interface was collected to measure the fluorescence of F-rhSP-D. As shown in **Figure 3C**, F-rhSP-D was detected at the recipient trough in both scenarios. Although no statistically significant differences were observed ($p = 0.078$), the injection of Curosurf prior to the protein seems to show a tendency to enhance the vehiculization, which could indicate a more extensive interaction with rhSP-D at the air-liquid interface when surfactant structures are already adsorbed at the interface.

To avoid formation of surface-associated reservoirs and to have both donor and recipient interfaces saturated with surfactant and stable prior to the addition of rhSP-D, OE in organic solvent was firstly applied onto the donor air-liquid interface. **Figure 4A** shows that OE rapidly spreads over the interface, reaching and stabilizing at the equilibrium surface pressure. Then, to allow organic solvent to evaporate, rhSP-D was applied at the donor interface 10 min later. At the end of the experiment, the recipient interface was transferred onto a mica plate for detecting the presence of rhSP-D by AFM analysis. As observed in the images shown in **Figure 4B**, rhSP-D was not detectable at the recipient interface.

Differential Vehiculization of Oligomeric Forms of rhSP-D by Pulmonary Surfactant

In an attempt to elucidate whether the different oligomers are transported differently and whether surfactant structure

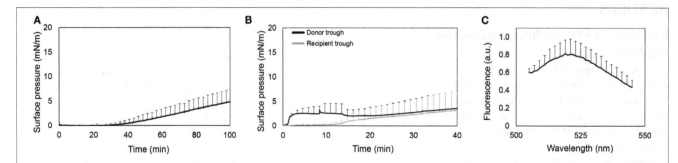

FIGURE 1 | Interfacial activity of rhSP-D. **(A)** Recording of surface pressure as a function of time for the adsorption of an aliquot of 10 µL at 0.34 mg/mL (3.4 µg) of rhSP-D injected into the subphase of a Wilhelmy balance. **(B)** Adsorption and spreading isotherms of rhSP-D upon injection of an aliquot of 20 µL at 0.6 mg/mL (12 µg) of the protein at the air-liquid interface in a double-Wilhelmy balance. Surface pressure measured in the donor (black line) and recipient troughs (gray line). **(C)** Fluorescence emission spectra of the F-rhSP-D detected in the whole volume taken from the recipient trough at the end of the experiments. Data represented by the mean and standard deviations of three different replicates.

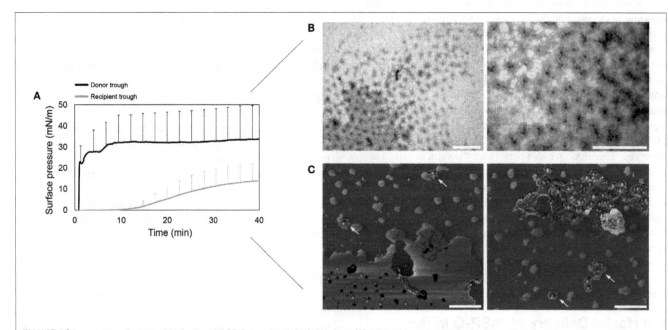

FIGURE 2 | Pulmonary surfactant vehiculization of rhSP-D over the air-liquid interface. **(A)** Adsorption and spreading isotherm of a suspension of the organic extract from native surfactant (OE) reconstituted and mixed with rhSP-D at 1% protein/lipid (w/w) ratio. An aqueous aliquot of 15 µL (50 mg/mL; 750 µg) of the material were deposited dropwise at the donor interface in the double-Wilhelmy balance and changes in surface pressure were measured in both troughs. Mean and standard deviations were obtained from three replicates. **(B)** Transmission electron microscopy (TEM) micrographs of the rhSP-D fuzzy balls detected at the recipient air-liquid interface upon surfactant-promoted interfacial vehiculization. **(C)** rhSP-D vehiculized by surfactant detected at the recipient air-liquid interface by atomic force microscopy (AFM) phase images. Some examples of fuzzy balls are pointed with white arrows. Scale bar: 400 nm.

could influence this process, vehiculization of the OE/rhSP-D combination was assessed with sonicated and non-sonicated OE suspensions. The sonication process favors the formation of smaller surfactant vesiculated structures with higher curvature (García-Fojeda et al., 2019), which has been proposed to promote interaction of amphiphilic proteins. As observed in **Supplementary Figure 3**, sonication induced fragmentation of OE vesicles observable by means of more monodispersed population of smaller vesicles. The presence of rhSP-D caused a shift in the peak to larger sizes in both sonicated and non-sonicated surfactant, indicating an interaction of rhSP-D with surfactant membranes.

Figure 5A compares the $\prod$-time isotherms of both donor and recipient compartments upon application of sonicated or non-sonicated samples. After 30 min, the interfacial film at the recipient trough was transferred onto a mica plate at a constant surface pressure of 20 mN/m to avoid the formation of multilayered structures and the exclusion of material from the interface once higher pressures are reached. The surfactant vehiculization of rhSP-D by both approaches was demonstrated by observing the presence of rhSP-D oligomers under the AFM (see **Figure 5B**). Coexistence of liquid-condensed (L_c) and liquid-expanded (L_e) lipid phases are differentiable in **Figure 5B**, where L_c domains exhibit round-shaped areas with an average

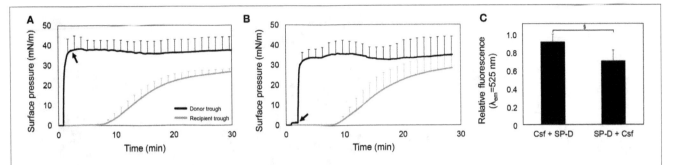

FIGURE 3 | rhSP-D conjugated with Alexa Fluor 488 transported over the interface by the association with Curosurf (Csf). **(A)** Adsorption and spreading isotherm obtained from the interfacial injection of 50 μL (80 mg/mL; 4 mg) of Curosurf and, 70 s after, 15 μL (1 mg/mL; 15 μg) of F-rhSP-D (black arrow), measured in the double-Langmuir balance. **(B)** Pressure-time isotherm upon injection of, first, F-rhSP-D and, 70 s after, Curosurf (black arrow), in a double-Langmuir balance. **(C)** Relative fluorescence emission at $\lambda_{em} = 525$ nm of the material collected from the recipient interface by aspiration at the end of each experiment. Data represent mean and standard deviation calculated from three different experiments. Pair t-test: (§) $p = 0.078$.

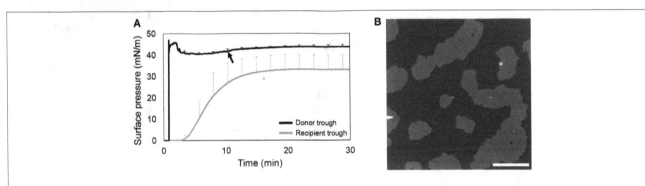

FIGURE 4 | rhSP-D association to the interface in the absence of surfactant-associated reservoirs. **(A)** Spreading isotherm of OE in organic solvent in a double-Langmuir balance and **(B)** AFM height image obtained from the transference of the recipient interfacial film after the spreading of 360 μg of OE in organic solvent and the injection of 5% w/w rhSP-D 10 min after (black arrow in **A**). Three replicates were performed to obtain mean and standard deviation data.

difference in height of 5.5 ± 0.89 Å (mean ± SD) surrounded by more extended L_e phases (see **Supplementary Figure 4A**), consistent with previous observations (Yuan and Johnston, 2002; Blanco et al., 2012). The percentage of area that occupied big (>200 nm) or small (<200 nm) L_c domains was also analyzed, but no differences were observed between the films formed by sonicated or non-sonicated samples (**Supplementary Figure 4B**). SP-D molecules are predominantly distributed associated with the L_e phase compared with the fraction of the protein seen associated with L_c-L_e boundaries (**Figure 5C**). Interestingly, the protein seems to present a closed configuration of their collagenic arms, and seems to be at least partly buried into the lipid film, observed as protein molecules with similar height but shorter in length than previously described (Arroyo et al., 2018) (**Supplementary Figure 4C**). This particular configuration makes difficult to identify the number of trimers taking part of each oligomer. To assess whether smaller or larger oligomeric forms were preferentially transported by interfacial films assembled from smaller or larger surfactant vesicles, we quantified the oligomers including trimers or hexamers on one group and higher ordered dodecamers and fuzzy balls on the other (see **Figures 5D,E**). In both cases, when using sonicated or non-sonicated surfactant suspensions, an apparently larger number of trimers/hexamers were transported

from the donor to the recipient trough in comparison with the proportion of dodecamers and fuzzy balls vehiculized and with the proportion of smaller and larger oligomers in this preparation when examined on plain mica (roughly 50% of each). No significant differences were observed when comparing sonicated and non-sonicated samples, although the intrinsic variability of the few replicas examined prevents a clear conclusion at this stage. The proportion of SP-D trimers and hexamers observed as associated with the interfacial film seems to be higher when smaller surfactant vesicles were accessible to the protein, possibly indicating a trend of the smaller oligomers to interact better with highly curved membranes.

DISCUSSION

Pulmonary surfactant protein SP-D plays essential roles in alveolar immunity and surfactant metabolism (Clark and Reid, 2003). However, the current clinical surfactants used for surfactant replacement therapy (SRT) to treat infant respiratory distress syndrome (RDS), a common cause of morbidity and mortality in preterm neonates characterized by pulmonary immaturity and lack of PS, lack the hydrophilic collectins SP-A and SP-D (Johansson and Curstedt, 2019; Hentschel et al., 2020). Therefore, in this study we have investigated the possibility that

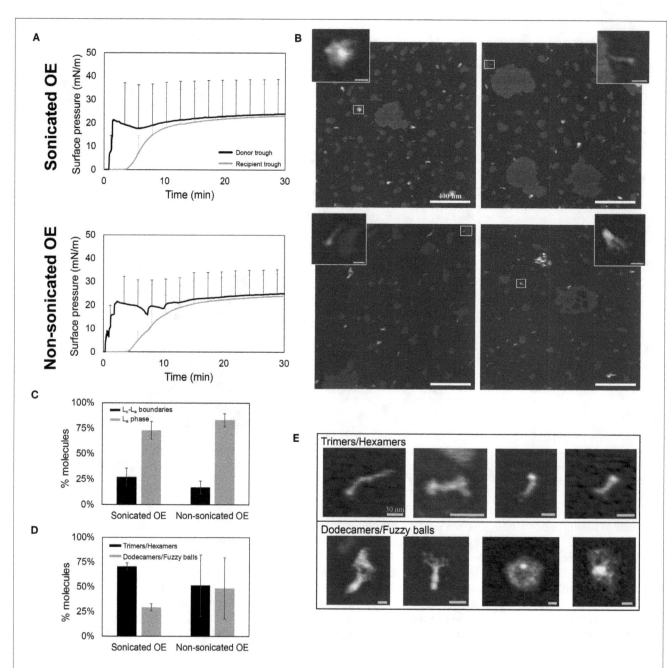

FIGURE 5 | Analysis of rhSP-D oligomers transported over the air-liquid interface associated to surfactant complexes. An aqueous aliquot of OE/rhSP-D at 50 mg/mL (750 μg) and 1% rhSP-D by mass (7.5 μg) was applied at the donor interface. **(A)** Adsorption and spreading isotherms performed in the double-Langmuir balance. **(B)** AFM height images taken after transference onto mica surface of the recipient interfacial film. Data obtained by the vehiculization of sonicated (top) or non-sonicated (bottom) OE before mixing with 1% w/w rhSP-D. Scale bar: 400 nm. Zoom regions show examples of rhSP-D oligomers corresponding to the areas highlighted with white rectangles. Scale bar: 30 nm. **(C)** Percentage of rhSP-D oligomers found at the L_c-L_e boundaries (black) or distributed into the L_e phase (gray) upon vehiculization by sonicated or non-sonicated surfactant. **(D)** Quantitative distribution of smaller and larger rhSP-D oligomers observed in surfactant films, upon association of the protein with sonicated or non-sonicated surfactant structures. **(E)** Representative AFM images of the different SP-D oligomers grouped into trimers/hexamers and dodecamers/fuzzy balls. Scale bar: 30 nm.

protein SP-D could interact with interfacial surfactant films and, through the interface, diffuse over the whole respiratory surface, which could facilitate its function to encounter, interact and label for clearance potential harmful entities impinging the surfactant film, the first barrier exposed to the outer environment in the lungs. In the study, we have used a recombinant form of human SP-D. Our experiments are therefore also useful to show how the combination of the protein with PS could be a useful strategy to facilitate an efficient delivery of the protein through the airways as a therapeutic option, using PS as a shuttle. The use of PS as a drug delivery system to carry and distribute different therapeutic molecules over the respiratory surfaces have been studied in the recent years both *in vitro* and *in vivo* (Van't Veen et al., 1996; Hidalgo et al., 2017, 2020; Baer et al., 2018). The combination of exogenous PS with rhSP-D could have the potential to serve as a preventive or therapeutic approach to treat inflammatory responses and lung diseases in preterm infants such as RDS or bronchopulmonary dysplasia (BPD) (Ikegami et al., 2007; Sato et al., 2010).

The research about SP-D has been focused around its immune roles and anti-inflammatory properties (Crouch et al., 1995; Cai et al., 1999; Liu et al., 2005; Ikegami et al., 2006; Cohen et al., 2020), but little is known about its interfacial properties and its potential combination with PS to complement anti-inflammatory actions, or to define novel therapeutic approaches through the airways. In this work, we report a low interfacial adsorption and spreading properties of rhSP-D by itself on clean air-water interfaces. However, in the presence of pulmonary surfactant, either delivered as a PS/rhSP-D combined formulation or co-administered one right after the other, rhSP-D efficiently traveled associated to air-liquid interfaces. Although the combination of rhSP-D with PS seems to slightly affect the interfacial performance of PS revealed by lower surfaces pressures reached at the recipient compartment and larger experimental variability, it is clear that the mixed formulation favors the interaction and permanence of the protein at the interface and, consequently, its spreading over it (**Figure 2**). When rhSP-D was applied with the donor interface already occupied by PS, it was also detected in the recipient compartment, indicating that the protein is able to interact with pre-existing surfactant films at the interface and used them as a sort of shuttle to rapidly spread long distances via the interface. Similarly, the fact that adding PS right after rhSP-D also promoted the interfacial vehiculization of the protein, in contrast to the poor interfacial spreading of rhSP-D alone (**Figures 1, 3**), suggests that the protein can shift from a free form in the aqueous bulk phase to a lipid-associated state that is competent to diffuse over the interface. We propose that SP-D/lipid complexes, or alternatively, the interaction of SP-D with any of the hydrophobic surfactant proteins present in the film, converts SP-D into a form that is stably associated with the interface and facilitates its "surfing" capabilities. The injection of rhSP-D on top of a pre-formed surfactant film that had reached surface pressure values of around 15 mN/m, produced an instantaneous and visible increase in surface pressure, confirming the rapid adsorption of the protein into the interface and its insertion into the surfactant film (data not shown). These observations are consistent with the effect on the initial surface pressure as a consequence of SP-D adsorption that was described by Taneva et al. (1997). At surface pressures above $\sim$30 mN/m, SP-D, as occurring with other hydrophilic proteins, cannot penetrate into the lipid films. Thus, rhSP-D may somehow attach to either PS at the interface or the PS reservoirs at the subphase, most likely through the interaction of its CRD with PS phospholipids (Ogasawara et al., 1992; Persson et al., 1992), and leverage the interfacial spreading forces even without their previous combination. This opens the possibility to deliver rhSP-D as a mixed formulation together with PS or administered

in a close time window but separately one after the other, without the necessity to develop *de-novo* PS/rhSP-D combined formulations, which could reduce time and costs associated with the design and implementation of clinical trials *ad hoc*.

Nonetheless, when rhSP-D was applied with both donor and recipient interfaces completely saturated with PS to emulate the physiological conditions, the protein was not detected in the recipient compartment (**Figure 4**). This could indicate that SP-D could be able to interact and spread mainly in physiological contexts where surfactant has been depleted from the interface for some reason. However, the absence of breathing-like interfacial compression/expansion dynamics in the current experiments could limit the behavior of SP-D compared with the potential action of the protein *in vivo*. We have recently demonstrated that breathing dynamics could be essential to understand the interfacial behavior of surfactant, particularly with respect to potential interface-assisted spreading capabilities and release processes (Hidalgo et al., 2020), as a consequence of surface tension-driven interfacial flows and the potential progressive exclusion of material from the interface (Borgas and Grotberg, 1988; Pastrana-Rios et al., 1994; Grotberg and Gaver III, 1996; Halpern et al., 1998; Keating et al., 2012; Hidalgo et al., 2020). These effects could be important to promote the spreading of new material coming from upstream reservoirs and better distribute the therapeutics over the respiratory surface (Hidalgo et al., 2020). Thus, further experiments are needed to explore the interfacial delivery of rhSP-D in saturated interfaces subjected to breathing-like dynamic conditions.

The structures of SP-D identified in the images taken by TEM and AFM (**Figures 2, 5**) are consistent with those obtained in previous studies (Holmskov, 2000; Arroyo et al., 2018), though the association/vehiculization with PS seem to modulate their conformation slightly. All the oligomers analyzed presented a closed conformation, with the collagen domains and the CRD heads less defined. This is likely a consequence of their association with phospholipid surfaces, as it occurs with other hydrophilic proteins (Maget-Dana and Ptak, 1995), something that should be investigated in more detail. We also found a differential vehiculization of the different rhSP-D oligomers over the air-liquid interface. Trimers and hexamers are apparently better transported associated to pulmonary surfactant than dodecamers and fuzzy balls (**Figure 5**). This can be related with their smaller size and a facilitated diffusion associated with the interfacial film. This effect could have some consequences on the role of SP-D in PS homeostasis. SP-D seems to be involved in the regulation of surfactant lipid pool sizes, contributing somehow to the transformation of surfactant large aggregates into small aggregates, preferentially taken up by alveolar type II pneumocytes but not macrophages (Horowitz et al., 1997; Ikegami et al., 2000). Still, when higher order oligomers-enriched batches, the most active oligomers in bacterial aggregation (Arroyo et al., 2020), were used (**Figure 2**), PS was also able to transport them efficiently.

Although our data suggests that PS improves the travel of SP-D across air-liquid interfaces, the Wilhelmy balance results may not be identical to the properties of the alveolar air-liquid interface. In addition, it is uncertain how much PS is needed to facilitate SP-D movement. It is possible that PS levels may be sufficient to achieve maximum SP-D distribution even in surfactant depleted conditions such as RDS.

The above limitations notwithstanding, altogether, this work points out the potential synergistic effect that PS/rhSP-D formulations could have to empower surfactant replacement therapy (SRT) to treat infants with RDS or BPD. It could also offer new possibilities to use SRT in acute lung injuries such as acute respiratory distress syndrome (ARDS) or lung infections in both children and adults. The administration of exogenous surfactants either animal-derived (Kesecioglu et al., 2009) or synthetic (Spragg et al., 2004) has failed so far for treating ARDS, possibly, at least in part, due to the presence in the airways of surfactant inhibitors such as serum components or phospholipases (Autilio et al., 2020) derived from severe inflammation processes and the damage of alveolar epithelium. The incorporation of recombinant forms of human SP-D could contribute to mitigate the inflammation process at the distal airways and enhance the efficacy of SRT. Interestingly, SP-D has also demonstrated different anti-infective activities including antifungal actions (Madan et al., 2001; Ordonez et al., 2019), abilities to recognize and promote virus and bacterial killing and clearance (Crouch, 2000; Hillaire et al., 2013) and specifically binding to the highly glycosylated S-protein of coronavirus inhibiting their replication (Leth-Larsen et al., 2007). Thus, an efficient administration of SP-D could also be beneficial for the treatment of diseases associated with lung infection such as the current COVID-19 pandemic caused by the SARS-CoV-2 virus. The administration of SP-D combined with PS to patients suffering from severe ARDS could help to mitigate lung inflammation and counteract the secondary bacterial and

viral infection. In summary, the optimization of PS/rhSP-D formulations could be interesting to empower the current clinical surfactants increasing their potential to replace the lack or damaged endogenous surfactant, to open damaged and poorly-aerated areas in the lungs and to act as a carrier distributing rhSP-D over the respiratory surface. A similar principle could be explored to optimize surfactant-promoted vehiculization of other therapeutic proteins along the interface, including versions of the proteins that could be modified to facilitate their association with surfactant and a efficient interface-driven vehiculization through the airways.

AUTHOR CONTRIBUTIONS

CG-M and AH designed the study, acquired data by performing most of laboratory experiments, interpreted data, and drafted the manuscript. RA acquired data by performing some experiments. ME and AC supervised some data analyses. JP-G conceptualized the study, supervised the whole work, and interpreted all the data. All authors critically revised the paper for important intellectual content and finally approved the paper in the present form. All authors agreed to be accountable for all aspects of the work in ensuring that questions related to the accuracy or integrity of any part of the work were appropriately investigated and resolved.

ACKNOWLEDGMENTS

Authors are indebted to Dr. Fernando Moreno-Herrero and his team, at the National Center of Biotechnology (CNB-CSIC) for their technical assistance with the AFM experiments.

REFERENCES

Arroyo, R., Echaide, M., Moreno-Herrero, F., Perez-Gil, J., and Kingma, P. S. (2020). Functional characterization of the different oligomeric forms of human surfactant protein SP-D. Biochim. Biophys. Acta Prot. Proteom. 1868:140436. doi: 10.1016/j.bbapap.2020.140436

Arroyo, R., Martin-Gonzalez, A., Echaide, M., Jain, A., Brondyk, W., Rosenbaum, J., et al. (2018). Supramolecular assembly of human pulmonary surfactant protein SP-D. J. Mol. Biol. 430, 1495–1509. doi: 10.1016/j.jmb.2018.03.027

Autilio, C., Echaide, M., Shankar-Aguilera, S., Bragado, R., Amidani, D., Salomone, F., et al. (2020). Surfactant injury in the early phase of severe meconium aspiration syndrome. Am. J. Respir. Cell Mol. Biol. 63, 327–337. doi: 10.1165/rcmb.2019-0413OC

Baer, B., Veldhuizen, E. J., Possmayer, F., Yamashita, C., and Veldhuizen, R. (2018). The wet bridge transfer system: a novel tool to assess exogenous surfactant as a vehicle for intrapulmonary drug delivery. Discov. Med. 26, 207–218. Available online at: https://www.discoverymedicine.com/Brandon-Baer/2018/11/wet-bridge-transfer-exogenous-surfactant-intrapulmonary-drug-delivery/

Banaschewski, B. J. H., Veldhuizen, E. J. A., Keating, E., Haagsman, H. P., Zuo, Y. Y., Yamashita, C. M., et al. (2015). Antimicrobial and biophysical properties of surfactant supplemented with an antimicrobial peptide for treatment of bacterial pneumonia. Antimicrob. Agents Chemother. 59, 3075–3083. doi: 10.1128/AAC.04937-14

Blanco, O., Cruz, A., Ospina, O. L., López-Rodriguez, E., Vázquez, L., and Pérez-Gil, J. (2012). Interfacial behavior and structural properties of a clinical lung surfactant from porcine source. Biochim. Biophys. Acta 1818, 2756–2766. doi: 10.1016/j.bbamem.2012.06.023

Bligh, E., and Dyer, W. (1959). A rapid method of lipid extraction and purification. Can. J. Biochem. Physiol. 37, 911–917. doi: 10.1139/y59-099

Borgas, M. S., and Grotberg, J. B. (1988). Monolayer flow on a thin film. J. Fluid Mech. 193, 151–170. doi: 10.1017/S0022112088002095

Cai, G.-Z., Griffin, G. L., Senior, R. M., Longmore, W. J., and Moxley, M. A. (1999). Recombinant SP-D carbohydrate recognition domain is a chemoattractant for human neutrophils. Am. J. Physiol. Lung Cell. Mol. Physiol. 276, L131–L136. doi: 10.1152/ajplung.1999.276.1.L131

Casals, C., Campanero-Rhodes, M. A., García-Fojeda, B., and Solís, D. (2018). The role of collectins and galectins in lung innate immune defense. Front. Immunol. 9:1998. doi: 10.3389/fimmu.2018.01998

Clark, H., and Reid, K. (2003). The potential of recombinant surfactant protein D therapy to reduce inflammation in neonatal chronic lung disease, cystic fibrosis, and emphysema. Arch. Dis. Child 88, 981–984. doi: 10.1136/adc.88.11.981

Cohen, S. A., Kingma, P. S., Whitsett, J., Goldbart, R., Traitel, T., and Kost, J. (2020). SP-D loaded PLGA nanoparticles as drug delivery system for prevention and treatment of premature infant's lung diseases. Int. J. Pharm. 585:119387. doi: 10.1016/j.ijpharm.2020.119387

Crouch, E., Persson, A., Chang, D., and Heuser, J. (1994). Molecular structure of pulmonary surfactant protein D (SP-D). *J. Biol. Chem.* 269, 17311–17319.

Crouch, E. C. (2000). Surfactant protein-D and pulmonary host defense. *Respir. Res.* 1:6. doi: 10.1186/rr19

Crouch, E. C., Persson, A., Griffin, G. L., Chang, D., and Senior, R. M. (1995). Interactions of pulmonary surfactant protein D (SP-D) with human blood leukocytes. *Am. J. Respir. Cell Mol. Biol.* 12, 410–415. doi: 10.1165/ajrcmb.12.4.7695920

De Backer, L., Braeckmans, K., Demeester, J., De Smedt, S. C., and Raemdonck, K. (2013). The influence of natural pulmonary surfactant on the efficacy of siRNA-loaded dextran nanogels. *Nanomedicine* 8, 1625–1638. doi: 10.2217/nnm.12.203

García-Fojeda, B., González-Carnicero, Z., De Lorenzo, A., Minutti, C. M., De Tapia, L., Euba, B., et al. (2019). Lung surfactant lipids provide immune protection against Haemophilus influenzae respiratory infection. *Front. Immunol.* 10:458. doi: 10.3389/fimmu.2019.00458

Grotberg, J. B., and Gaver III, D. P. (1996). A synopsis of surfactant spreading research. *J. Coll. Interf. Sci.* 178, 377–378. doi: 10.1006/jcis.1996.0130

Halpern, D., Jensen, O., and Grotberg, J. (1998). A theoretical study of surfactant and liquid delivery into the lung. *J. Appl. Physiol.* 85, 333–352. doi: 10.1152/jappl.1998.85.1.333

Hentschel, R., Bohlin, K., Van Kaam, A., Fuchs, H., and Danhaive, O. (2020). Surfactant replacement therapy: from biological basis to current clinical practice. *Pediatr. Res.* 88, 176–183. doi: 10.1038/s41390-020-0750-8

Hidalgo, A., Cruz, A., and Pérez-Gil, J. (2015). Barrier or carrier? Pulmonary surfactant and drug delivery. *Eur. J. Pharm Biopharm.* 95, 117–127. doi: 10.1016/j.ejpb.2015.02.014

Hidalgo, A., Garcia-Mouton, C., Autilio, C., Carravilla, P., Orellana, G., Islam, M. N., et al. (2020). Pulmonary surfactant and drug delivery: vehiculization, release and targeting of surfactant/tacrolimus formulations. *J. Control. Release* 329, 205–222. doi: 10.1016/j.jconrel.2020.11.042

Hidalgo, A., Salomone, F., Fresno, N., Orellana, G., Cruz, A., and Perez-Gil, J. (2017). Efficient interfacially driven vehiculization of corticosteroids by pulmonary surfactant. *Langmuir* 33, 7929–7939. doi: 10.1021/acs.langmuir.7b01177

Hillaire, M. L., Haagsman, H. P., Osterhaus, A. D., Rimmelzwaan, G. F., and Van Eijk, M. (2013). Pulmonary surfactant protein D in first-line innate defence against influenza A virus infections. *J. Innate Immun.* 5, 197–208. doi: 10.1159/000346374

Holmskov, U. (2000). Collectins and collectin receptors in innate immunity [based on 9 publications]. *APMIS Suppl.* 100, 1–59. doi: 10.1111/j.1600-0463.2000.tb05694.x

Horowitz, A., Kurak, K., Moussavian, B., Whitsett, J., Wert, S., Hull, W., et al. (1997). Preferential uptake of small-aggregate fraction of pulmonary surfactant *in vitro*. *Am. J. Physiol. Lung Cell. Mol. Physiol.* 273, L468–L477. doi: 10.1152/ajplung.1997.273.2.L468

Ikegami, M., Carter, K., Bishop, K., Yadav, A., Masterjohn, E., Brondyk, W., et al. (2006). Intratracheal recombinant surfactant protein D prevents endotoxin shock in the newborn preterm lamb. *Am. J. Respir. Crit. Care Med.* 173, 1342–1347. doi: 10.1164/rccm.200509-1485OC

Ikegami, M., Scoville, E. A., Grant, S., Korfhagen, T., Brondyk, W., Scheule, R. K., et al. (2007). Surfactant protein-D and surfactant inhibit endotoxin-induced pulmonary inflammation. *Chest* 132, 1447–1454. doi: 10.1378/chest.07-0864

Ikegami, M., Whitsett, J. A., Jobe, A., Ross, G., Fisher, J., and Korfhagen, T. (2000). Surfactant metabolism in SP-D gene-targeted mice. *Am. J. Physiol. Lung Cell. Mol. Physiol.* 279, L468–L476. doi: 10.1152/ajplung.2000.279.3.L468

Johansson, J., and Curstedt, T. (2019). Synthetic surfactants with SP-B and SP-C analogues to enable worldwide treatment of neonatal respiratory distress syndrome and other lung diseases. *J. Intern. Med.* 285, 165–186. doi: 10.1111/joim.12845

Keating, E., Zuo, Y. Y., Tadayyon, S. M., Petersen, N. O., Possmayer, F., and Veldhuizen, R. A. (2012). A modified squeeze-out mechanism for generating high surface pressures with pulmonary surfactant. *Biochim. Biophys. Acta* 1818, 1225–1234. doi: 10.1016/j.bbamem.2011.12.007

Kesecioglu, J., Beale, R., Stewart, T. E., Findlay, G. P., Rouby, J.-J., Holzapfel, L., et al. (2009). Exogenous natural surfactant for treatment of acute lung injury and the acute respiratory distress syndrome. *Am. J. Respir. Crit. Care Med.* 180,

989–994. doi: 10.1164/rccm.200812-1955OC

Kingma, P. S., and Whitsett, J. A. (2006). In defense of the lung: surfactant protein A and surfactant protein D. *Curr. Opin. Pharmacol.* 6, 277–283. doi: 10.1016/j.coph.2006.02.003

Korfhagen, T. R., Sheftelyevich, V., Burhans, M. S., Bruno, M. D., Ross, G. F., Wert, S. E., et al. (1998). Surfactant protein-D regulates surfactant phospholipid homeostasis *in vivo*. *J. Biol. Chem.* 273, 28438–28443. doi: 10.1074/jbc.273.43.28438

Leth-Larsen, R., Zhong, F., Chow, V. T., Holmskov, U., and Lu, J. (2007). The SARS coronavirus spike glycoprotein is selectively recognized by lung surfactant protein D and activates macrophages. *Immunobiology* 212, 201–211. doi: 10.1016/j.imbio.2006.12.001

Liu, C. F., Chen, Y. L., Shieh, C. C., Yu, C. K., Reid, K., and Wang, J. Y. (2005). Therapeutic effect of surfactant protein D in allergic inflammation of mite-sensitized mice. *Clin. Exp. Allergy* 35, 515–521. doi: 10.1111/j.1365-2222.2005.02205.x

Madan, T., Kishore, U., Singh, M., Strong, P., Clark, H., Hussain, E. M., et al. (2001). Surfactant proteins A and D protect mice against pulmonary hypersensitivity induced by Aspergillus fumigatus antigens and allergens. *J. Clin. Invest.* 107, 467–475. doi: 10.1172/JCI10124

Maget-Dana, R., and Ptak, M. (1995). Interactions of surfactin with membrane models. *Biophys. J.* 68, 1937–1943. doi: 10.1016/S0006-3495(95)80370-X

Ogasawara, Y., Kuroki, Y., and Akino, T. (1992). Pulmonary surfactant protein D specifically binds to phosphatidylinositol. *J. Biol. Chem.* 267, 21244–21249.

Ordonez, S. R., Van Eijk, M., Salazar, N. E., De Cock, H., Veldhuizen, E. J., and Haagsman, H. P. (2019). Antifungal activities of surfactant protein D in an environment closely mimicking the lung lining. *Mol. Immunol.* 105, 260–269. doi: 10.1016/j.molimm.2018.12.003

Orgeig, S., Morrison, J. L., and Daniels, C. B. (2011). Evolution, development, and function of the pulmonary surfactant system in normal and perturbed environments. *Compr. Physiol.* 6, 363–422. doi: 10.1002/cphy.c150003

Parra, E., and Pérez-Gil, J. (2015). Composition, structure and mechanical properties define performance of pulmonary surfactant membranes and films. *Chem. Phys. Lipids* 185, 153–175. doi: 10.1016/j.chemphyslip.2014.09.002

Pastrana-Rios, B., Flach, C. R., Brauner, J. W., Mautone, A. J., and Mendelsohn, R. (1994). A direct test of the "Squeeze-Out" hypothesis of lung surfactant function. external reflection FT-IR at the air/wave interface. *Biochemistry* 33, 5121–5127. doi: 10.1021/bi00183a016

Pérez-Gil, J. (2008). Structure of pulmonary surfactant membranes and films: the role of proteins and lipid–protein interactions. *Biochim. Biophys. Acta* 1778, 1676–1695. doi: 10.1016/j.bbamem.2008.05.003

Perez-Gil, J., and Weaver, T. E. (2010). Pulmonary surfactant pathophysiology: current models and open questions. *Physiology* 25, 132–141. doi: 10.1152/physiol.00006.2010

Persson, A. V., Gibbons, B. J., Shoemaker, J. D., Moxley, M. A., and Longmore, W. J. (1992). The major glycolipid recognized by SP-D in surfactant is phosphatidylinositol. *Biochemistry* 31, 12183–12189. doi: 10.1021/bi00163a030

Sato, A., Whitsett, J. A., Scheule, R. K., and Ikegami, M. (2010). Surfactant protein-d inhibits lung inflammation caused by ventilation in premature newborn lambs. *Am. J. Respir. Crit. Care Med.* 181, 1098–1105. doi: 10.1164/rccm.200912-1818OC

Sorensen, G. L. (2018). Surfactant protein D in respiratory and non-respiratory diseases. *Front. Med.* 5:18. doi: 10.3389/fmed.2018.00018

Spragg, R. G., Lewis, J. F., Walmrath, H.-D., Johannigman, J., Bellingan, G., Laterre, P.-F., et al. (2004). Effect of recombinant surfactant protein C–based surfactant on the acute respiratory distress syndrome. *New Eng. J. Med.* 351, 884–892. doi: 10.1056/NEJMoa033181

Strong, P., Townsend, P., Mackay, R., Reid, K., and Clark, H. (2003). A recombinant fragment of human SP-D reduces allergic responses in mice sensitized to house dust mite allergens. *Clin. Exp. Immunol.* 134, 181–187. doi: 10.1046/j.1365-2249.2003.02281.x

Taeusch, H. W., De La Serna, J. B., Perez-Gil, J., Alonso, C., and Zasadzinski, J. A. (2005). Inactivation of pulmonary surfactant due to serum-inhibited adsorption and reversal by hydrophilic polymers: experimental. *Biophys. J.* 89, 1769–1779. doi: 10.1529/biophysj.105.062620

Taneva, S., Voelker, D. R., and Keough, K. M. (1997). Adsorption of pulmonary surfactant protein D to phospholipid monolayers at the air- water interface. *Biochemistry* 36, 8173–8179. doi: 10.1021/bi9 63040h

Van't Veen, A., Mouton, J. W., Gommers, D., and Lachmann, B. (1996). Pulmonary surfactant as vehicle for intratracheally instilled tobramycin in mice infected with Klebsiella pneumoniae. *Br. J. Pharmacol.* 119, 1145–1148. doi: 10.1111/j.1476-5381.1996.tb 16016.x

Watson, A., Phipps, M. J., Clark, H. W., Skylaris, C.-K., and Madsen, J. (2019). Surfactant proteins A and D: trimerized innate immunity proteins with an affinity for viral fusion proteins. *J. Innate Immun.* 11, 13–28. doi: 10.1159/000492974

Yu, S.-H., and Possmayer, F. (2003). Lipid compositional analysis of pulmonary surfactant monolayers and monolayer-associated reservoirs. *J. Lipid Res.* 44, 621–629. doi: 10.1194/jlr.M200380-JLR200

Yuan, C., and Johnston, L. (2002). Phase evolution in cholesterol/DPPC monolayers: atomic force microscopy and near field scanning optical microscopy studies. *J. Microsc.* 205, 136–146. doi: 10.1046/j.0022-2720.2001.00982.x

3

A Custom-Made Device for Reproducibly Depositing Pre-Metered Doses of Nebulized Drugs on Pulmonary Cells *in vitro*

Justus C. Horstmann[1,2], Chelsea R. Thorn[3], Patrick Carius[1,2], Florian Graef[1†],
Xabier Murgia[1*†], Cristiane de Souza Carvalho-Wodarz[1*] and Claus-Michael Lehr[1,2]

[1] Helmholtz Institute for Pharmaceutical Research Saarland (HIPS), Saarbrücken, Germany, [2] Department of Pharmacy, Saarland University, Saarbrücken, Germany, [3] Clinical and Health Science, University of South Australia, Adelaide, SA, Australia

*Correspondence:
Xabier Murgia
xabi_murgia@hotmail.com
Cristiane de Souza Carvalho-Wodarz
cristiane.carvalho@helmholtz-hips.de

The deposition of pre-metered doses (i.e., defined before and not after exposition) at the air–liquid interface of viable pulmonary epithelial cells remains an important but challenging task for developing aerosol medicines. While some devices allow quantification of the deposited dose after or during the experiment, e.g., gravimetrically, there is still no generally accepted way to deposit small pre-metered doses of aerosolized drugs or pharmaceutical formulations, e.g., nanomedicines. Here, we describe a straightforward custom-made device, allowing connection to commercially available nebulizers with standard cell culture plates. Designed to tightly fit into the approximately 12-mm opening of either a 12-well Transwell® insert or a single 24-well plate, a defined dose of an aerosolized liquid can be directly deposited precisely and reproducibly (4.8% deviation) at the air–liquid interface (ALI) of pulmonary cell cultures. The deposited dose can be controlled by the volume of the nebulized solution, which may vary in a range from 20 to 200 μl. The entire nebulization-deposition maneuver is completed after 30 s and is spatially homogenous. After phosphate-buffered saline (PBS) deposition, the viability and barrier properties transepithelial electrical resistance (TEER) of human bronchial epithelial Calu-3 cells were not negatively affected. Straightforward in manufacture and use, the device enables reproducible deposition of metered doses of aerosolized drugs to study the interactions with pulmonary cell cultures grown at ALI conditions.

Keywords: inhalation, aerosol, pulmonary drug delivery, epithelial cells, air–liquid interface

INTRODUCTION

The development of drugs against pulmonary diseases requires testing of both safety and efficacy. In this context there recently has been a growing interest in using *in vitro* cell culture models to replace, reduce, and refine animal experiments (Tannenbaum and Bennett, 2015; Ehrmann et al., 2020). Initially, such tests were and still are performed with submerged cell culture models (Pulskamp et al., 2007; Rothen-Rutishauser et al., 2007; Metz et al., 2020). However, as patients inhale drugs as an aerosol, air–liquid interface

(ALI) models are more physiologically relevant (Lacroix et al., 2018). It has been shown that testing of aerosolized excipients under ALI conditions is, in many ways, different from testing under liquid-covered conditions (LCCs) (Brandenberger et al., 2010; Paur et al., 2011; Upadhyay and Palmberg, 2018). For instance, drug transport rates across *in vitro* cell culture inserts depend on the donor compartment concentrations and are, therefore, dramatically increased when drugs are applied as dry particles without any additional liquid at the ALI (Bur et al., 2010). Vice versa, adverse effects could be shown at lower doses in ALI conditions compared with LCC, albeit only the nominal—not the cell-delivered dose—would be obtained for submerged culture conditions (Loret et al., 2016). On the contrary, there is also evidence that the culture conditions do not affect the dose-specific efficacy of certain drugs (e.g., bortezomib) in A549 lung epithelial cells (Lenz et al., 2014). Once inhaled *in vivo*, particles tend to land on a layer of mucus or thin lining fluid (e.g., pulmonary surfactant) that is only 1/10 of the particles' size (Bastacky et al., 1995). Modeling physiological situations when developing models and protocols for meaningful *in vitro* tests is, therefore, pivotal (Bastacky et al., 1995; Hiemstra et al., 2018).

To date, several laboratory methods have already been described to deposit aerosolized drugs on epithelial cells, such as modified impactors or impingers (Cooney et al., 2004; Bur et al., 2009), using electrostatic attraction forces (Jeannet et al., 2016; Frijns et al., 2017) or insufflator devices developed initially for animals (Blank et al., 2006; Bur et al., 2010). Vibrating mesh nebulizers (i.e., Omron NE-U22) have been used to deposit pH-sensitive archeosomes onto macrophages covered with pulmonary surfactant in classic 24-well plates (Altube et al., 2017). While depositing a fine mist onto cell cultures seems trivial, ALI conditions are hardly used, adding complexity to the application. There has also been considerable interest in the pharmaceutical application of dry powders. To study the deposition of metered aerosols from commercially available dry powder inhaler (DPI) devices, systems such as the Pharmaceutical Aerosol Deposition Device on Cell Cultures (PADDOCC) (Hein et al., 2010, 2011) or the Vitrocell® Dry Powder Chamber (Hittinger et al., 2017) have been developed. Other commercially available devices, including the Cultex Devices (Cultex® Technology, 2020), the PreciseInhale®, and XposeALI® (Inhalation Sciences, 2020), and the PRIT® System (Fraunhofer P.R.I.T® Systems, 2020), have emerged; and more details are described in recent review articles (Schneider-Daum et al., 2019; Ehrmann et al., 2020). However, the Vitrocell® Cloud systems—originally called Air-liquid Interface Cell Exposure-Cloud (ALICE-Cloud) (Lenz et al., 2014), have become quite popular, as seen in the number of recent publications in both the field of (nano-)particle toxicity (Chortarea et al., 2017; He et al., 2020) and preclinical drug testing (Röhm et al., 2017; D'Angelo et al., 2018). The available standard device consists of a polycarbonate chamber connected to a vibrating mesh nebulizer (Aeroneb® Lab nebulizer unit), generating a cloud of liquid aerosol settling down on multiple Transwell® inserts at the same time. These wells sit in a base module that controls the temperature of the cell medium, and the cell-delivered dose can be determined with a quartz crystal microbalance (Lenz et al., 2009, 2014). Only recently, the Vitrocell® Cloud MAX has been introduced (Vitrocell® Cloud Systems, 2020), which was designed for metered-dose delivery to one Transwell® insert at a time (Cei et al., 2020).

Nevertheless, experimental setups enabling the controlled deposition of predetermined aerosol doses onto one Transwell® insert at a time for exposure of pulmonary epithelial cells under ALI conditions are seldomly available. To close this gap, we here present an easy-to-make and easy-to-use device, consisting of a machined polyoxymethylene (POM) cylinder, which directs a single aerosol dose generated by a vibrating mesh nebulizer (Aeroneb® Lab nebulizer unit) to the bottom of individual wells or inserts of standard multi-well plates. The data presented here demonstrate its suitability to reproducibly deposit pre-metered doses by nebulizing between 20 and 200 µl of an aqueous drug solution and a nanoparticle pharmaceutical drug formulation. Apart from cleaning the device after use, no further maintenance is needed, making it easy to handle under sterile conditions. A proof-of-concept experiment with Transwell® insert-grown Calu-3 cells revealed no signs of cytotoxicity, and the epithelial barrier function as measured by the transepithelial electrical resistance (TEER) was the same as for untreated cells. The system has already been successfully employed earlier by our group for other tasks (Graef et al., 2018) but was so far not further described in detail concerning its construction or application to deposit single doses of drugs on cells.

MATERIALS AND METHODS

Manufacturing of the Chamber and Setup of the System

The deposition device is made of POM and was produced at the workshop of Saarland University (Saarbrücken, Germany). With a standard (computerized numerical control)-milling machine, the cylinder is made from a rod following the dimensions shown in **Figure 1A**. The cylindrical device has a wider opening to fit on the nebulizer and a smaller opening to fit in a 12-well Transwell® insert, Cat. No. 3460, with a pore size of 0.4 µm (Corning™ Costar™, Lowell, MA, United States, **Figure 1B**). An Aeroneb® Lab nebulizer unit (standard VMAD, 4.0–6.0 µm droplet diameter) plugged into the deposition device was used and is connected to an Aerogen® USB controller (both Aerogen®, Galway, Ireland). The device's wider opening contains a rim to fit the nebulizer, which stops at the edge of the rim after an 8-mm distance from the entrance (**Figure 1A**). The rim contains a circular cavity to fit a rubber ring to connect the device in the nebulizing process and prevent aerosol loss. The cylinder itself tapers conically to the opening leading outside to the smaller protruding outlet. This part at the bottom opening is designed precisely to fit the dimensions of a 12-well Transwell® insert (**Figure 1B**). It does not touch the Transwell® membrane or the well's walls and leads the aerosol exactly on the apical side of the membrane and not to the basolateral side. Alternatively, the system can also be placed on 24-well plates instead of Transwell® inserts.

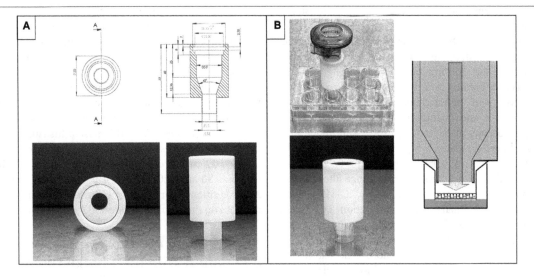

FIGURE 1 | Design and dimensions of the deposition system. **(A)** Technical drawing and images of the device alone. **(B)** Nebulizer connected to deposition device on top of Transwell® inserts ready for nebulization on cells (top image) and details of placement in an insert (bottom). On the right side, schematic view of the process of nebulization in a Transwell® insert.

Aerosol Generation and Deposition Protocol

In aerosol deposition studies, sodium fluorescein salt (Sigma-Aldrich) was used at various concentrations (as indicated, 2.5, 25, 100, or 250 µg/ml) diluted in phosphate-buffered saline (PBS; without calcium and magnesium, Sigma-Aldrich, D8537) or loaded into lipid liquid crystalline nanoparticles (LCNPs) as a model pharmaceutical formulation described below. To deposit aerosols, the system is assembled as described. To initialize the nebulization process, 100 µl of PBS was aerosolized three times in the whole system (nebulizer + device). The system is then placed on the respective wells. A volume of 20–200 µl from the desired liquid (or particle suspension) is added to the nebulizer mesh. Once the nebulization process is finished (shown by a small puff of a cloud above the mesh), the nebulizer is kept over the well for another 30 s (or as indicated) to allow the cloud to settle. The nebulizer and the device are separated again, and the remaining solution drops are removed from the downstream side of the mesh membrane by gently wiping with a (sterile) tissue. After the experiments were finished, the nebulizer and device are cleaned with (sterile) deionized water.

To contrast the solution, lipid nanoparticles (LCNPs) loaded with sodium fluorescein (3.5 mg/ml) or tobramycin (5 mg/ml, free base, Sigma-Aldrich) were formed with monoolein (MO; Myverol 18-99K; part number: 5D01253, Kerry Ingredients, and Flavors), as previously described (Thorn et al., 2020). The sodium fluorescein-LCNPs (250 µg/ml) were aerosolized onto Transwell® inserts at volumes of 20–200 µl, to compare with the sodium fluorescein solution. These studies were obtained in another lab as the studies done with free sodium fluorescein to compare the reproducibility of the method. For tobramycin, the aerosolization of a solution was compared with the tobramycin-LCNPs with 200 µl of varying concentrations (0.1, 0.2, 1, and 2 mg/ml) into 24-well plates.

Drug Deposition Studies in 24-Well Plates

Nebulization with sodium fluorescein (as a surrogate drug) was done as described above. First, parameters affecting drug deposition were changed in order to characterize the system. Two hundred microliters of PBS was filled into 24-well plates, and sodium fluorescein was deposited. Different invested volumes were tested under constant concentration and settling time (20, 50, 100, and 200 µl; 100 µg/ml, 30 s). Different concentrations were tested under constant volume and settling time (2.5, 25, and 250 µg/ml; 20 and 200 µl, 30 s); and different settling times were analyzed under constant volume and concentration (0, 30, and 60 s; 20 µl, 100 µg/ml, and 200 µl with 25 µg/ml). Multiple dosing of the drug was analyzed by nebulizing either 200 µl of 25 µg/ml or 20 µl of 100 µg/ml with 30-s settling time. The deposition was done two and three times in one well.

Analysis of the Deposited Amounts and Total Recovery of Aerosolized Material

The deposition system was set up as described and placed on Transwell® inserts. Two hundred microliters of PBS was filled on the apical and basolateral sides of the Transwell® inserts to analyze the deposited substance. Basolateral liquid did not touch the bottom side of the Transwell® membrane to prevent free diffusion. Sodium fluorescein or LCNPs in PBS were deposited as described (with 30-s settling time). Afterward, the nebulizer and the device were separated carefully and placed on Petri dishes. Each part was rinsed with 3 ml of PBS in the Petri dishes. One hundred microliters of the apical and basolateral sides and from either the nebulizer or device rinse fluid was withdrawn to analyze deposited mass. The drug deposition efficiency percentage was calculated by the mass of substance in the acceptor well divided by the mass invested in nebulizer times 100.

The fluorescence intensity of sodium fluorescein determined the aerosol-deposited dose measured in 96-well plates at 485-nm excitation and 550-nm emission wavelength with a plate reader (Tecan Trading AG, Infinite M200 Pro). Sodium fluorescein-LCNPs were detected via solubilizing the LCNPs with 0.05% Triton-X and quantifying sodium fluorescein via fluorescent spectroscopy plate reader (Inspire Multimode Plate reader, Perkin Elmer). Similarly, tobramycin was quantified after solubilizing the LCNPs in 0.05% Triton-X in 0.9% sodium chloride and filtration with 4-mm Millex® syringe filters. Liquid chromatography–tandem mass spectrometry (LC-MS) with a Dionex UltiMate 3000 Binary Rapid Separation LC System (Thermo Scientific) coupled with a TSQ Quantum Access Max (QQQ, Thermo Scientific) and a modified ion-pairing method was used for quantification. Trifluoroacetic acid (0.1%), heptafluorobutyric acid (0.1%), and pentafluoropropionic acid (0.1%) were added to eluent A (acetonitrile) and eluent B (water), as a mobile phase. A Zorbax Eclipse xdb C-18 column (5 μm, 50 * 4.6 mm, Agilent, Santa Clara, CA, United States) with C18 guard column was used as the analytical column. At a flow of 0.7 ml/min, samples were run with a gradient of eluents A and B, beginning at 20:80 (first minute), changing to 70:30 (1–3.5 min), and restored to 20:80 (3.5–4.5 min). Three microliters of the samples was injected and quantified by positive electrospray ionization (ESI+) and selected reaction monitoring (SRM) of the ion 468.184 → 323.960. A total of nine replicates were analyzed per concentration.

Viability Testing and Transepithelial Electrical Resistance Measurement After Aerosol Deposition on Calu-3 Cells

The Calu-3 HTB-55 cell line was received from American Type Culture Collection (ATCC®) and cultivated in minimum essential medium supplemented with Earle's salts, L-glutamine, 1% non-essential amino acids (NEAAs), 1 mM of sodium pyruvate, and 10% fetal calf serum (FCS) (all Gibco™, Thermo Fisher Scientific Inc. Waltham, MA, United States). The medium was changed every 2–3 days while using passages between 35 and 55. For experiments, cells were detached using trypsin/EDTA, and 1×10^5 cells were seeded per Transwell® insert. After 3 days, cells were switched to ALI conditions and grown for a total of 11–13 days until being used in the experiments.

Before PBS is aerosolized, the basolateral medium was changed. The controls included wells not exposed to nebulization and inserts with 1% Triton-X 100 (Sigma-Aldrich) in the basolateral medium (control consisting of dead cells). The deposition on cells was done under sterile conditions. Transwell® inserts in a 12-well plate were placed on a heating plate at 37°C. Then, one insert was transferred into a new, empty, 12-well plate with a sterile tweezer, and the aerosolization-deposition maneuver of PBS was performed, as previously described. Permeable supports were placed back to the original well plate filled with 500 μl of medium on the basolateral side. Inserts were incubated at 37°C and 5% CO_2 for 24 h. Lactate

dehydrogenase (LDH) release was assessed with a kit based on color reaction (Roche, Cytotoxicity Detection Kit) from the basolateral medium according to the manufacturer's advice. The color change was detected with a spectrophotometer (Thermo-Fisher™, Multiskan™ GO) and calculated in % viability of the respective controls. To measure TEER, cells were incubated for another hour at submerged conditions (500/1,500 μl) with the medium. Then, TEER was assessed via electrical Volt-Ohm-meter (EVOM2, World Precision Instruments) with STX2 chopstick electrodes. Values were corrected to the Transwell® insert (1.12 cm²) area and the respective value of a blank insert (between 90 and 120 Ω·cm²). After that, cells were put back to ALI conditions by replacing the medium with 500 μl of fresh medium on the basolateral side and stored in an incubator.

Nanoparticle Aerosol Deposition Evaluation With the Spatial Distribution

The deposition in the Transwell® inserts was also assessed for spatial distribution using the described method with sodium fluorescein-LCNPs. To ensure no intentional manipulation, directly after sodium fluorescein-LCNP deposition, the membranes were left to equilibrate at room temperature for 1 h. The bottom of the Transwell® insert was then attached to coverslips (#1.5) with Dako Mounting medium (Agilent Technologies). An inverted fluorescent microscope (Olympus IX53) connected to CoolLed pE-300 illuminator system was used with a 2 × objective to visualize the deposition of sodium fluorescein-LCNPs on the membranes, from the bottom side up. Sodium fluorescein was illuminated with the blue-green LED filter and adjusted according to an untreated Transwell® membrane. Three replicates at each volume tested were imaged. ImageJ extracted the fluorescent intensities per pixel across the midline of the membrane's diameter. For each membrane, four lines were systematically drawn horizontally, vertically, and diagonally in each direction, splitting the membranes into eight parts to obtain an average fluorescent intensity profile. The pixel distances were equated to a numerical distance of the membrane. The pixels' intensities were converted to a heat map, where the highest intensities were represented by a red color and the lowest intensities by blue. For quantitative analysis, the average fluorescent intensities were correlated to the mean intensity. The intensities were normalized for each volume invested with the highest value in each data equated to an arbitrary value of one and the lowest to zero and plotted against the membrane's diameter.

Statistical Analysis

Differences were tested for statistical significance by one-way ANOVA, followed by Tukey's multiple comparisons test for all solution deposition analyses. The statistical comparison between solution-LCNP formulation and Transwell®-well plate inserts were performed by a two-way ANOVA, followed by a Sidak's multiple comparisons test. $P < 0.05$ were considered statistically significant as described in the respective figure legends. Error bars indicate standard deviation (SD). All statistical tests were performed with GraphPad Prism® 8.

RESULTS

Effects of Concentration, Settling Time, and Repeated Deposition

The entire setup consisted of (1) a commercially available nebulizer (e.g., Aeroneb® Lab nebulizer and Aerogen® USB controller) plugged on the (2) custom-made deposition device (as described in the section "Materials and Methods"), which is then (3) placed on either the well of a standard 24-well plate or a 12-well Transwell® insert. The deposition system itself (**Figure 1A**) is designed not to touch the bottom of the well/Transwell® insert and forms a closed chamber together with the well/Transwell® insert, leaving 5.5-mm distance to the insert or 5.7 mm to the well plate bottom (**Figure 1B**).

To explore the reproducibility and identify critical factors for aerosol deposition with this device, we investigated the effect of different concentrations, settling times, and multiple depositions (**Figure 2**). Apart from those factors, the invested volume is the most critical factor, as the generated aerosol deposits directly in a single well. Preliminary trials revealed that invested volumes lower than 20 µl show very high SDs, discouraging the application of smaller volumes (data not shown). This is probably related to the characteristics of the nebulizer's vibrating mesh, which also propels substance to the apical side of the vibrating mesh. Beginning with 20 µl, the SD of the measured dose for repeated experiments was acceptable in our experiments (22%). At the higher end, 200 µl turned out to be the largest volume to be reproducibly deposited (4.8% SD), since higher volumes lead to condensing drops on the inside wall of the device that dropped out on the well. Notably, these volumes are much smaller than in clinical settings, where volumes of up to 5 ml are used with

similar nebulizers (Dolovich and Dhand, 2011; Acrogen® , 2020). On account of this, both 20 and 200 µl of invested volumes were further analyzed. A 10-fold change in invested substance concentration did not lead to higher deposition efficiencies at either 20 or 200 µl ($p \leq 0.6$, **Figures 2A,B**, respectively).

Regardless of the nebulized volume, longer settling times (time after complete nebulization of invested liquid) had a positive influence on the deposition efficiency, in line with the observation that the generated aerosol cloud is still settling after the end of the nebulization itself. When nebulizing 200 µl, a 30-s settling time was found to be necessary, but further increasing it to 60 s did not significantly improve deposition efficiency (**Figures 2A,B**). In the case of 20 µl, which takes only about 3 s for nebulization, the benefit of a 30-s waiting time became still more prominent and was therefore adopted as routine for the protocol.

To show that a distinct dose is precisely deposited and can even be enlarged linearly by its increment, multiple repeated depositions were performed for both small and high volumes (**Figure 2**). After each respective nebulization step, the nebulized dose was added up and reproducibly deposited multiple times to achieve the desired dose. Even so, R^2-values show a more precise deposition with 200 µl of volume than with 20 µl (0.9420 vs. 0.8482).

The Deposited Mass Linearly Depends on the Invested Volume

After identifying the range of possible volumes between 20 and 200 µl and the necessary settling time of 30 s, we asked if the volume of the nebulized solution could control the deposited amount of a dissolved compound. Hence, the system was tested with increasing volumes of sodium fluorescein (100 µg/ml)

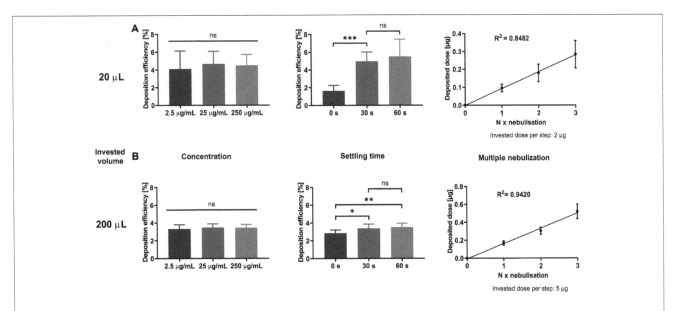

FIGURE 2 | Deposition characteristics at different concentrations, settling time, and multiple nebulization steps. Sodium fluorescein solution is deposited as described in the section "Materials and Methods." Either 20 µl **(A)** or 200 µl **(B)** was used for nebulization. From left to right, 10-fold increasing concentrations were nebulized, the efficiency of different settling times after the end of nebulization processes was assessed, and respective doses nebulized one or more times into one well at 30-s settling time were analyzed, as indicated. Error bars show standard deviation. One-way ANOVA, Tukey's multiple comparisons test, ns $p > 0.12$; *$p < 0.033$; **$p < 0.002$; ***$p < 0.001$. $N = 9$ of three experiments.

to confirm this hypothesis. Six repetitions were performed and analyzed in triplicate for each volume tested, yielding 18 observations for each data point. As shown in **Figure 3A**, the deposited dose increased linearly and thus can be controlled by the invested volume (R^2: 0.9706). Not surprisingly, calculating and plotting the deposition efficiency of the same dataset show that the smaller the invested volume, the higher the SD (1.44 for 20 µl and 0.18 for 200 µl) (**Figure 3B**). Nevertheless, the system allows to deposit a finite pre-metered dose with reasonable reproducibility, and the invested volume may control this dose.

Mass Balance Reveals the Distribution of the Deposited Substance in the System

Consistently, about 4% of the nebulized dose was deposited in the well. Therefore, the question arises where the rest of the nebulized substance goes. Besides the mass deposited on the apical side of a Transwell® insert, we also quantified the amounts deposited in the device itself and remaining in the nebulizer after loading it with 20, 100, and 200 µl of a 25 µg/ml sodium fluorescein solution (**Table 1**). With increasing volume, the relative amount of deposited mass in the device increased from 46 to 63%, as did the relative amount remaining in the nebulizer (from 21 to 27%). The respective amounts of mass deposited on the inserts remained around 4%. As calculated by the sum of the amounts collected in all three compartments (=total recovery), the total recovery was 80% after nebulization with 20 µl but increased to 93 and 94% after nebulization of 100 and 200 µl, respectively. After deposition on the apical side of the Transwell® insert, no substance was found on the basolateral side, confirming that the tapered cylinder structure restricts the deposition to the apical side (data not shown). As described, this is tested in Transwell® inserts with a pore size of 0.4 µm and without contact to basolateral medium to avoid free diffusion.

Analysis of Reproducibility of Deposition Between Free Drug and Particles and Well Plates

The deposition of sodium fluorescein as an aerosolized solution or in a pharmaceutical formulation (i.e., LCNPs) was compared

TABLE 1 | Total recovery of substance in the system after nebulization and deposition on the apical side of permeable supports.

	20 µl	100 µl	200 µl
Nebulizer	20.5 ± 12.2	34.2 ± 2.83	27.2 ± 3.64
Device	45.8 ± 9.37	55.4 ± 3.32	63.0 ± 8.77
Transwell	5.52 ± 0.84	3.31 ± 0.54	3.43 ± 0.23
Total recovery	79.7 ± 9.02	92.9 ± 2.02	93.5 ± 8.51

20, 100, and 200 µl of sodium fluorescein solution are nebulized at 25 µg/ml as described in the section "Materials and Methods." The relative abundance of deposited substance in each part of the system is displayed for each nebulized volume. "Total recovery" is the sum of the relative abundance of each invested volume. Error represents standard deviation. N = 9 of three experiments; 100 µl, N = 6 of three experiments.

to evaluate the robustness of using the device for other applications in a wider pharmaceutical field. Deposition of sodium fluorescein was performed in another lab than the deposition of sodium fluorescein formulation (Lab 1: Helmholtz Institute for Pharmaceutical Research Saarland; Lab 2: University of South Australia). When investing 20, 100, or 200 µl, sodium fluorescein's deposition efficiency as a free solution or in LCNPs was comparable (**Figure 4A**). While only the 20 µl of free sodium fluorescein showed a slight, statistically significant increase, all other groups showed a deposition efficiency that was well comparable. The same trend was observed by comparing the deposition of free sodium fluorescein into a 24-well plate and Transwell® inserts, which was essentially the same, except for the 20 µl deposition into Transwell® (**Figure 4B**). The variation in the accuracy of pipetted micro-volumes increases toward lower volumes, which may further explain the variation observed at 20 µl of invested volume. Compared with a different compound (i.e., tobramycin), the deposition efficiency remained consistent at ~4% ($p > 0.05$, **Figure 5**) across 0.1–2 mg/ml invested concentrations at 200 µl of invested volume, in both conditions of a solution and LCNPs. This is the same as sodium fluorescein deposition efficiency, proving the usability of this surrogate substance. Generally, the deposition of different formulations and drugs on different well plates demonstrates the high versatility of using this device.

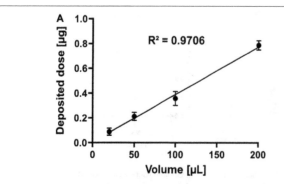
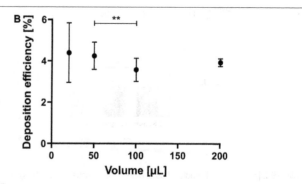

FIGURE 3 | Linearity by dose and efficiency. Sodium fluorescein solution is nebulized as described in the section "Materials and Methods." **(A)** Deposited dose of a 100 µg/ml solution at different invested volumes. **(B)** Deposition efficiency at different invested volumes. Error bars indicate standard deviation. N = 18 of six experiments (for 20 and 200 µl) and N = 21 of seven experiments (for 50 and 100 µl). One-way ANOVA, Tukey's multiple comparisons test; **p = 0.002.

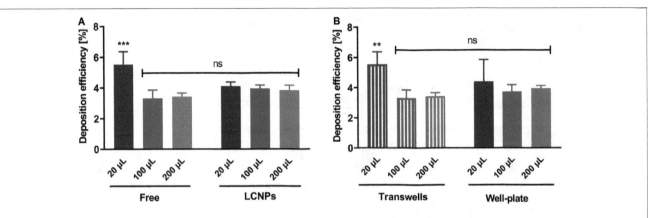

FIGURE 4 | Comparison of deposition efficiency of different volumes, substances, and wells. **(A)** Deposition efficiencies of free sodium fluorescein and LCNPs loaded with sodium fluorescein. Substance deposited on the apical side of permeable supports was analyzed (the section "Materials and Methods"), N = 9 of two experiments (for 20 μl of free and LCNP, 100 and 200 μl of LCNP); N = 6 of two experiments (for 100 μl of free); N = 8 of three experiments (for 200 μl of free). **(B)** Comparison of deposition efficiency on 24-well plates and Transwell® inserts. Sodium fluorescein was nebulized using the device as described. Either the device deposited on Transwell® inserts or 24-well plate inserts. Data show mean and standard deviation. N = 9 of three experiments; 100 μl, N = 6 of two experiments. Two-way ANOVA, Sidak's multiple comparisons test; ***p < 0.001; **p < 0.003; ns, no significant difference (p > 0.05).

Homogeneity of Deposition

Control over the amount of aerosol deposited is essential, so too is the aerosol evenly spread over the surface. The sodium fluorescein-LCNPs were aerosolized onto Transwell® insert membranes (area of 1.12 cm^2) at 20–200 μl to determine the deposition's homogeneity. Extraction of the fluorescent intensities of sodium fluorescein across each pixel of the membrane's diameter provided a quantitative analysis that was normalized for comparison (as indicated). The sub-200-nm particles are evenly spread across the Transwell® membranes, as quantified by the trend in the normalized intensity data in **Figures 6A–D**. The heat maps of each individual membrane depict the whole spatial deposition and dictate greater heat spots toward the center of the membranes that spread toward the edges.

The visual representation suggests an increase in the spread of the particles across the membrane from 20 up to 200 μl, which does not correlate to a difference in spatial homogeneity from the (normalized) quantified data. While the smaller invested volumes have overall lower proportions of red areas, this may reflect the lower dose deposited compared with the higher volumes. There was no statistical difference (p = 0.945) between the normalized mean across the diameter, indicating similarities in the homogenous spatial distribution from all four doses. The mean deposition across the diameter was consistent across all volumes invested, normalized to 1.04, 1.02, 1.08, and 1.07 AU for 20, 50, 100, and 200 μl, respectively, indicative of a consistent maximum dose of the compound that was spread homogenously across the membrane. On average, the SD between samples was 7, 12, 10, and 9%, respectively, for 20–200 μl of investment. Even though 10 × more mass is invested, the SD did not severely change and further highlighted the device's robustness depositing spatially even pre-metered doses.

Deposition on Epithelial Cells Is Well Tolerated

To demonstrate that the nebulization-deposition maneuver itself with the new device is not noxious to pulmonary epithelial cells, either 20 or 200 μl of PBS was nebulized on the widely used human bronchial epithelial cell line Calu-3, which forms tight monolayers at ALI conditions (Foster et al., 2000; Schneider-Daum et al., 2019). The cells did not show any loss of viability as measured by LDH release (**Figure 7A**). The TEER as an indicator for the epithelial barrier function remained unchanged as well (**Figure 7B**).

DISCUSSION

Here, we describe a new, custom-designed device intended for aerosol deposition into single Transwell® inserts for drug delivery

FIGURE 5 | Comparison of deposition efficiency of free and LCNP encapsulated tobramycin (TOB), either as a free solution or in LCNPs after nebulizing 200 μl with Aerogen® Pro nebulizer and nebulization chamber into 24-well plates. Data represented as mean ± standard deviation, N = 9 (of three experiments). Two-way ANOVA, Sidak's multiple comparisons test. No significant difference (p > 0.05) was found between the groups.

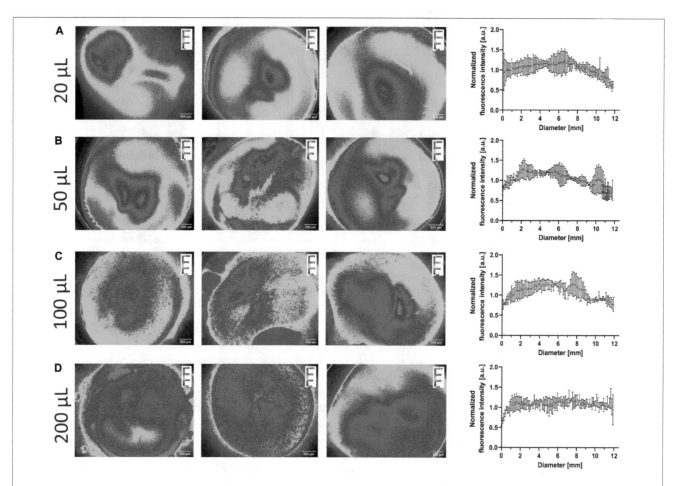

FIGURE 6 | Homogeneity of deposition. Sodium fluorescein-liquid crystalline nanoparticles (LCNPs) were nebulized onto Transwell® insert membranes as described in the section "Materials and Methods." **(A–D)** Representative fluorescent micrographs of the membranes (from the bottom up), where the highest fluorescence intensities are color-coded as red and the lowest as blue. The fluorescence intensities per pixel were extracted across the center of the membrane. The individual intensities (correlated to the mean intensity) were normalized to arbitrary 1 and plotted against the diameter of the membrane. $N = 3$, data are reported as mean with standard deviation, where every 25th data point is shown for clarity. a.u, Arbitrary units.

applications of *in vitro* cell culture models. It consists of a tapered cylinder design, which is very compact and connects to commonly used nebulizers (**Figure 1**). The Aeroneb® Lab nebulizer produces an aerosol cloud into the device that enables a precise and reproducible deposition of a pre-metered dose into the respective well (**Figure 1B**). The device can be used for single experiments nebulizing one dose on one or more inserts, or the device can be employed to deposit more than one dose on one insert. Due to its low price, many devices can be used without the necessity to clean them during time-critical experiments, as there are examples in the literature comparing many substances instead of using only single agents (Meindl et al., 2015; Röhm et al., 2017; Barosova et al., 2020).

There are two commercially available devices from Vitrocell® Systems that also allow for single insert exposure using an Aeroneb® Lab nebulizer and a cloud-settling principle for dose-controlled aerosol delivery, as comparable with the one presented here. These include 1) the Vitrocell® Cloud MAX and (2) the so-called "Starter Kit." However, both systems differ significantly from the device described here, as they offer extensive technical

features such as an integrated microbalance to determine the post-metered dose and are significantly more costly. The "Starter Kit" design is comparable with the Cloud Systems with a rectangular aerosol-cell exposure system (Lenz et al., 2014). Rather than exposing an entire well plate with several Transwell® inserts at a time, the chamber is smaller (ca. 1 L) to expose a single Transwell® insert (Di Cristo et al., 2020; Vitrocell® Cloud Systems, 2020). The former, the Vitrocell® Cloud MAX, had been introduced a few months ago, and its performance has been described for a prototype version in the literature (Cei et al., 2020). Its exposure chamber has a compact cylindrical design with roughly comparable dimensions to the device reported here (40–60 mm height, diameter ca. 20 mm) tailored toward providing just enough space for one 6-well Transwell® insert (or a smaller-sized insert), with a settling time of ca. 1 min. The bottom part of the cylindrical chamber is not tapered to a diameter of 12 mm (12-well Transwell® insert), and the Transwell® insert has to be put into a base module for exposure. The Vitrocell® Cloud MAX system comes with three or six exposure units arranged in parallel.

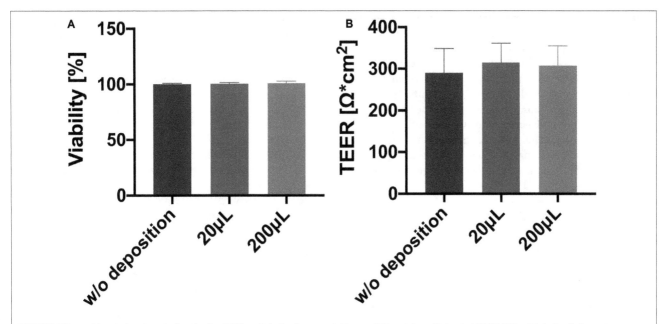

FIGURE 7 | Deposition of phosphate-buffered saline (PBS) on Calu-3 cells grown in Transwell® inserts is well tolerated. **(A)** Viability of Calu-3 cells [Lactate dehydrogenase (LDH), see section "Materials and Methods"] 24 h after deposition of PBS. **(B)** Barrier properties of Calu-3 cells 24 h after deposition. $N = 9$ of three individual experiments. No significant difference was found between the groups ($p > 0.05$).

Despite some commonalities with existing deposition systems, the crucial advantage of the cost-effective and straightforward custom-made device presented here is the precise ability to control and predetermine the exact deposited dose achieved, as would be done in the clinic (Dolovich and Dhand, 2011). The deposited dose increases linearly with the invested volume (**Figure 3A**), where micro-sized volumes can be efficiently deposited and do not differ between drugs or pharmaceutical formulations. The system also allows for consecutive dosing to the cells for any invested volume (**Figures 2A,B**). Thus, the simple design and the low-cost production of the present device allow for reproducible drug deposition as an aerosol *in vitro*.

While a deposition efficiency of about 4% may appear relatively low, it is sufficient for performing meaningful *in vitro* studies, where the amount of compound needed is much smaller than for *in vivo* studies. By increasing the settling time, higher deposition efficiencies can be achieved (**Figure 2**). Still, we recommend using only 30 s, as the deposition efficiency is not significantly higher ($p = 0.60$). It is more important that the absolute dose is well controlled, as widely observed with our device. In comparable studies with the Vitrocell® Cloud MAX system prototype version, a drug delivery efficiency of 52% was reported, albeit for a six-well Transwell® insert (Cei et al., 2020). By extrapolating these data to smaller inserts/wells, it may be expected that for 12-well Transwell® inserts, the delivery efficiency is about 4.5-fold lower (ca. 12% delivery efficiency), since the surface area of a 12-well Transwell® insert is about 4.5 times less than a six-well Transwell® insert. By using a similar nebulizer and the ALICE/Vitrocell® Cloud system, a deposition efficacy of about 17% was reported (Lenz et al., 2014), but this refers to the simultaneous deposition of an entire six-well plate and needs to be divided by the respective

number of wells, which equates to an approximate 3% deposition efficiency per well.

Moreover, Di Cristo et al. (2020) have also recently used the newer Vitrocell® Starter Kit, investing 125 µl of a 1 mg/ml particle suspension. From these data, one can calculate a deposition efficiency per well (1.12 cm²) by dividing the deposited amount by the invested amount, yielding an efficiency of 0.64% per well (1.12 cm²). This value, which is lower than what we report in the present study, is likely attributable to the larger space that the cloud is nebulized in and the larger surface area for deposition, which is the space around the insert and the walls of the device.

None of the previous studies further investigated the fraction of the lost aerosol during the nebulization process. In this study, it was hypothesized that most of the aerosol lands in the cylinder device. Indeed, with elevating the nebulized dose, more than half of the substance deposits in the cylinder [46% (20 µl) vs. 64% (200 µl)]. This finding explains the already mentioned upper limit of possible nebulized volume (see section Effects of Concentration, Settling Time, and Repeated Deposition). Nebulization of more than 200 µl leads to condensing drops to fall, foiling the intended use at ALI conditions. Regardless, as long as it remains consistent, the deposition of aerosol droplets on the device's walls is not a clinically relevant problem in practice. By gently wiping the device with (sterile) tissues, repeated nebulization-deposition maneuvers can be done in a row. According to the deposition efficiencies, the total maximum volume deposited onto the wells/inserts was never more than 8 µl, challenging to spread evenly using a pipette without touching the cells.

As could be expected, the deposition of aerosolized saline was well tolerated by commonly used Calu-3 cells, which is in concordance with comparable devices following the same principle, as there are no impaction forces or drying processes (Lenz et al., 2009). The device is usable under sterile experimental circumstances, as it is easily cleanable with ethanolic disinfectant and can be autoclaved with steam. Both LDH release and TEER values show no differences to the control that was not deposited with PBS at either 20 or 200 μl after 24 h (**Figure 7**). Epithelial cells and the biological absorption barrier formed by their tight junctions must not be harmed following deposition, especially when creating infected or inflamed models and then treated. The spatial distribution snapshot demonstrates an almost-even distribution of the aerosol, as represented in **Figure 6**, across 20–200 μl of invested dose and further suggests that cell cultures will be exposed to an even dose.

Here, we have visually shown and quantified the fluorescent intensity of nanoparticles deposited onto Transwell® membranes. The precise spatial distribution was observed on a non-wetted membrane that was not tampered with during the nebulization and imaging processes. The particles are homogeneously spread from the quantification of the normalized fluorescent intensity across the membrane's diameter. This is in agreement with other devices, such as ALICE, which produced a spatially homogenous spread of zinc oxide nanoparticles (Lenz et al., 2009), while in ALI cell culture conditions, the membrane may be wetted from the basolateral compartment and lining fluid of the cells, and this would lead to a greater spread of the aerosol over time. Our snapshot dictates that the aerosol spreads evenly on a dry membrane and does not need to rely on the surface's wettability. Comparatively, the naturally dried membrane may have resulted in small amounts of crystal formation from the deposited dose resulting in some small artifacts in the micrographs. The consistent ca. 10% SD of the deposited dose across all invested volumes tends to be higher than that of other reports from the Vitrocell® Cloud systems (Ding et al., 2020); however, it may be indicative of the fluorescent microscopy imaging technique as opposed to quartz crystal microbalance quantification. In any case, the device deposits a robust, spatially homogenous dose.

The present paper describes a straightforward device, in both manufacture and use, that enables reproducible deposition (4.8% relative SD) of pre-metered doses of aerosolized drugs on pulmonary *in vitro* cell cultures grown at ALI conditions. With this device, volume-defined amounts of solubilized drugs and pharmaceutical aerosol formulations can be deposited precisely on wells. The distribution of the deposited mass of free drug could be analyzed throughout the whole system. As expected, the deposition, when using this device on cell culture inserts, does not interfere with cell viability and epithelial barrier function. It is easy to clean, cost-efficient, and easily transferable to the bench. It can be customized to connect to any nebulizer and is the only device that could be completely produced using 3D printers, a technology that is employed universally at most universities in the world. Therefore, it can provide a valuable tool for studying the effects of aerosolized drugs and nanoscale delivery systems on *in vitro* pulmonary cell culture models.

AUTHOR CONTRIBUTIONS

JH performed the experiments and wrote the manuscript. CT performed the LCNP experiments, including the data analysis of deposition efficiency and spatial deposition of the aerosol and revising the manuscript. PC helped in the setup and design of the deposition chamber and technical questions and in revising the manuscript. XM and FG had the initial idea of producing the cylinder, planned the concept, and developed the device. CC-W advised on experiments and strategy and helped to create the manuscript and to enhance it. C-ML provided help in planning the experiments and supervised, creating, and enhancing the manuscript. All authors contributed to the article and approved the submitted version.

ACKNOWLEDGMENTS

We gratefully thank Rudolf Richter (Workshop, Department of Physical Chemistry and Didactics of Chemistry, Saarland University) for support in technical planning, construction of the device, and providing the scheme for **Figure 1A**; Pascal Paul for his help in conducting some of the deposition experiments; and Petra König and Jana Westhues for their support in cell cultures.

REFERENCES

Aerogen® (2020). *Aerogen Pro. Descubra Aerogen Pro.* Available online at: https://www.aerogen.com/de/aerogen-produkte/aerogen-pro/ (accessed September 2, 2020)

Altube, M. J., Cutro, A., Bakas, L., Morilla, M. J., Disalvo, E. A., and Romero, E. L. (2017). Nebulizing novel multifunctional nanovesicles: the impact of macrophage-targeted-pH-sensitive archaeosomes on a pulmonary surfactant. *J. Mater. Chem. B* 5, 8083–8095. doi: 10.1039/c7tb01694h

Barosova, H., Maione, A. G., Septiadi, D., Sharma, M., Haeni, L., Balog, S., et al. (2020). Use of EpiAlveolar lung model to predict fibrotic potential of multiwalled carbon nanotubes. *ACS Nano* 14, 3941–3956. doi: 10.1021/acsnano.9b06860

Bastacky, J., Lee, C. Y. C., Goerke, J., Koushafar, H., Yager, D., Kenaga, L., et al. (1995). Alveolar lining layer is thin and continuous: low-temperature scanning electron microscopy of rat lung. *J. Appl. Physiol.* 79, 1615–1628. doi: 10.1152/jappl.1995.79.5.1615

Blank, F., Rothen-Rutishauser, B. M., Schurch, S., and Gehr, P. (2006). An optimized in vitro model of the respiratory tract wall to study particle cell interactions. *J. Aerosol Med.* 19, 392–405. doi: 10.1089/jam.2006.19.392

Brandenberger, C., Mühlfeld, C., Ali, Z., Lenz, A. G., Schmid, O., Parak, W. J., et al. (2010). Quantitative evaluation of cellular uptake and trafficking of plain and polyethylene glycol-coated gold nanoparticles. *Small* 6, 1669–1678. doi: 10.1002/smll.201000528

Bur, M., Huwer, H., Muys, L., and Lehr, C.-M. (2010). Drug transport across pulmonary epithelial cell monolayers. *J. Aerosol Med. Pulm. Drug Deliv.* 23, 119–127. doi: 10.1089/jamp.2009.0757

Bur, M., Rothen-Rutishauser, B., Huwer, H., and Lehr, C. M. (2009). A novel cell compatible impingement system to study in vitro drug absorption from dry powder aerosol formulations. *Eur. J. Pharm. Biopharm.* 72, 350–357. doi: 10.1016/j.ejpb.2008.07.019

Cei, D., Doryab, A., Lenz, A., Schröppel, A., Mayer, P., Burgstaller, G., et al. (2020).

Development of a dynamic in vitro stretch model of the alveolar interface with aerosol delivery. *Biotechnol. Bioeng.* 118, 690–702. doi: 10.1002/bit.27600

Chortarea, S., Barosova, H., Clift, M. J. D., Wick, P., Petri-Fink, A., and Rothen-Rutishauser, B. (2017). Human asthmatic bronchial cells are more susceptible to subchronic repeated exposures of aerosolized carbon nanotubes at occupationally relevant doses than healthy cells. *ACS Nano* 11, 7615–7625. doi: 10.1021/acsnano.7b01992

Cooney, D. J., Kazantseva, M., and Hickey, A. J. (2004). Development of a size-dependent aerosol deposition model utilising human airway epithelial cells for evaluating aerosol drug delivery. *ATLA Altern. Lab. Anim.* 32, 581–590. doi: 10.1177/026119290403200609

Cultex® Technology (2020). *Leading the Field in Quality and Expertise.* Available online at: https://www.cultex-technology.com/products/ (accessed September 1, 2020)

D'Angelo, I., Costabile, G., Durantie, E., Brocca, P., Rondelli, V., Russo, A., et al. (2018). Hybrid lipid/polymer nanoparticles for pulmonary delivery of siRNA: development and fate upon in vitro deposition on the human epithelial airway barrier. *J. Aerosol Med. Pulm. Drug Deliv.* 31, 170–181. doi: 10.1089/jamp.2017. 1364

Di Cristo, L., Grimaldi, B., Catelani, T., Vázquez, E., Pompa, P. P., and Sabella, S. (2020). Repeated exposure to aerosolized graphene oxide mediates autophagy inhibition and inflammation in a three-dimensional human airway model. *Mater. Today Bio* 6:100050. doi: 10.1016/j.mtbio.2020.100050

Ding, Y., Weindl, P., Lenz, A. G., Mayer, P., Krebs, T., and Schmid, O. (2020). Quartz crystal microbalances (QCM) are suitable for real-time dosimetry in nanotoxicological studies using Vitrocell® Cloud cell exposure systems. *Part. Fibre Toxicol.* 17:44. doi: 10.1186/s12989-020-00376-w

Dolovich, M. B., and Dhand, R. (2011). Aerosol drug delivery: developments in device design and clinical use. *Lancet* 377, 1032–1045. doi: 10.1016/S0140-6736(10)60926-9

Ehrmann, S., Schmid, O., Darquenne, C., Rothen-Rutishauser, B., Sznitman, J., Yang, L., et al. (2020). Innovative preclinical models for pulmonary drug delivery research. *Expert Opin. Drug Deliv.* 17, 463–478. doi: 10.1080/17425247. 2020.1730807

Foster, K. A., Avery, M. L., Yazdanian, M., and Audus, K. L. (2000). Characterization of the Calu-3 cell line as a tool to screen pulmonary drug delivery. *Int. J. Pharm.* 208, 1–11. doi: 10.1016/S0378-5173(00)00452-X

Fraunhofer P.R.I.T® Systems (2020). *P.R.I.T. Professionelle In-Vitro Technologien.* Available online at: https://www.prit-systems.de/de/home.html (accessed October 27, 2020)

Frijns, E., Verstraelen, S., Stoehr, L. C., Van Laer, J., Jacobs, A., Peters, J., et al. (2017). A novel exposure system termed NAVETTA for in vitro laminar flow electrodeposition of nanoaerosol and evaluation of immune effects in human lung reporter cells. *Environ. Sci. Technol.* 51, 5259–5269. doi: 10.1021/acs.est. 7b00493

Graef, F., Richter, R., Fetz, V., Murgia, X., De Rossi, C., Schneider-Daum, N., et al. (2018). In vitro model of the gram-negative bacterial cell envelope for investigation of anti-infective permeation kinetics. *ACS Infect. Dis.* 4, 1188–1196. doi: 10.1021/acsinfecdis.7b00165

He, R. W., Gerlofs-Nijland, M. E., Boere, J., Fokkens, P., Leseman, D., Janssen, N. A. H., et al. (2020). Comparative toxicity of ultrafine particles around a major airport in human bronchial epithelial (Calu-3) cell model at the air–liquid interface. *Toxicol. In Vitro* 68:104950. doi: 10.1016/j.tiv.2020.104950

Hein, S., Bur, M., Kolb, T., Muellinger, B., Schaefer, U. F., and Lehr, C. M. (2010). The Pharmaceutical Aerosol Deposition Device on Cell Cultures (PADDOCC) in vitro system: design and experimental protocol. *ATLA Altern. Lab. Anim.* 38, 285–295. doi: 10.1177/026119291003800408

Hein, S., Bur, M., Schaefer, U. F., and Lehr, C. M. (2011). A new Pharmaceutical Aerosol Deposition Device on Cell Cultures (PADDOCC) to evaluate pulmonary drug absorption for metered dose dry powder formulations. *Eur. J. Pharm. Biopharm.* 77, 132–138. doi: 10.1016/j.ejpb.2010. 10.003

Hiemstra, P. S., Grootaers, G., van der Does, A. M., Krul, C. A. M., and Kooter, I. M. (2018). Human lung epithelial cell cultures for analysis of inhaled toxicants: lessons learned and future directions. *Toxicol. In Vitro* 47, 137–146. doi: 10. 1016/j.tiv.2017.11.005

Hittinger, M., Barthold, S., Siebenbürger, L., Zäh, K., Gress, A., Guenther, S., et al. (2017). "Proof of concept of the Vitrocell® dry powder chamber: a new in vitro test system for the controlled deposition of aerosol formulations," in *Proceedings of the Europe Respiratory Drug Delivery 2017 Scientific Conference* (Antibes),

283–288.

Inhalation Sciences (2020). *Technical Specifications.* Available online at: https://inhalation.se/products/technical-specifications/ (accessed September 1, 2020).

Jeannet, N., Fierz, M., Schneider, S., Künzi, L., Baumlin, N., Salathe, M., et al. (2016). Acute toxicity of silver and carbon nanoaerosols to normal and cystic fibrosis human bronchial epithelial cells. *Nanotoxicology* 10, 279–291. doi: 10. 3109/17435390.2015.1049233

Lacroix, G., Koch, W., Ritter, D., Gutleb, A. C., Larsen, S. T., Loret, T., et al. (2018). Air-liquid interface in vitro models for respiratory toxicology research: consensus workshop and recommendations. *Appl. In Vitro Toxicol.* 4, 91–106. doi: 10.1089/aivt.2017.0034

Lenz, A. G., Karg, E., Lentner, B., Dittrich, V., Brandenberger, C., Rothen-Rutishauser, B., et al. (2009). A dose-controlled system for air-liquid interface cell exposure and application to zinc oxide nanoparticles. *Part. Fibre Toxicol.* 6:32. doi: 10.1186/1743-8977-6-32

Lenz, A. G., Stoeger, T., Cei, D., Schmidmeir, M., Semren, N., Burgstaller, G., et al. (2014). Efficient bioactive delivery of aerosolized drugs to human pulmonary epithelial cells cultured in air-liquid interface conditions. *Am. J. Respir. Cell .Mol. Biol.* 51, 526–535. doi: 10.1165/rcmb.2013-0479OC

Loret, T., Peyret, E., Dubreuil, M., Aguerre-Chariol, O., Bressot, C., le Bihan, O., et al. (2016). Air-liquid interface exposure to aerosols of poorly soluble nanomaterials induces different biological activation levels compared to exposure to suspensions. *Part. Fibre Toxicol.* 13:58. doi: 10.1186/s12989-016-0171-3

Meindl, C., Stranzinger, S., Dzidic, N., Salar-Behzadi, S., Mohr, S., Zimmer, A., et al. (2015). Permeation of therapeutic drugs in different formulations across the airway epithelium in vitro. *PLoS One* 10:e0135690. doi: 10.1371/journal.pone. 0135690

Metz, J. K., Scharnowske, L., Hans, F., Schnur, S., Knoth, K., Zimmer, H., et al. (2020). Safety assessment of excipients (SAFE) for orally inhaled drug products. *Altex* 37, 275–286. doi: 10.14573/altex.1910231

Paur, H. R., Cassee, F. R., Teeguarden, J., Fissan, H., Diabate, S., Aufderheide, M., et al. (2011). In-vitro cell exposure studies for the assessment of nanoparticle toxicity in the lung-A dialog between aerosol science and biology. *J. Aerosol Sci.* 42, 668–692. doi: 10.1016/j.jaerosci.2011.06.005

Pulskamp, K., Diabaté, S., and Krug, H. F. (2007). Carbon nanotubes show no sign of acute toxicity but induce intracellular reactive oxygen species in dependence on contaminants. *Toxicol. Lett.* 168, 58–74. doi: 10.1016/j.toxlet.2006.11.001

Röhm, M., Carle, S., Maigler, F., Flamm, J., Kramer, V., Mavoungou, C., et al. (2017). A comprehensive screening platform for aerosolizable protein formulations for intranasal and pulmonary drug delivery. *Int. J. Pharm.* 532, 537–546. doi: 10.1016/j.ijpharm.2017.09.027

Rothen-Rutishauser, B., Mühlfeld, C., Blank, F., Musso, C., and Gehr, P. (2007). Translocation of particles and inflammatory responses after exposure to fine particles and nanoparticles in an epithelial airway model. *Part. Fibre Toxicol.* 4:9. doi: 10.1186/1743-8977-4-9

Schneider-Daum, N., Carius, P., Horstmann, J., and Lehr, C.-M. (2019). "Cell- and tissue-based (reconstituted) 2D In vitro models to study drug transport processes across the air-blood barrier," in *Pharmaceutical Inhalation Aerosol Technology*, eds A. J. Hickey and S. Da Rocha (Boca Raton, FL: CRC Press), 627–651.

Tannenbaum, J., and Bennett, B. T. (2015). Russell and Burch's 3Rs then and now: the need for clarity in definition and purpose. *J. Am. Assoc. Lab. Anim. Sci.* 54, 120–132.

Thorn, C. R., Clulow, A. J., Boyd, B. J., Prestidge, C. A., and Thomas, N. (2020). Bacterial lipase triggers the release of antibiotics from digestible liquid crystal nanoparticles. *J. Control. Release* 319, 168–182. doi: 10.1016/j.jconrel.2019. 12.037

Upadhyay, S., and Palmberg, L. (2018). Air-liquid interface: relevant in vitro models for investigating air pollutant-induced pulmonary toxicity. *Toxicol. Sci.* 164, 21–30. doi: 10.1093/toxsci/kfy053

Vitrocell® Cloud Systems (2020). *Vitrocell® Cloud For The Exposure to Liquid Aerosols.* Available online at: https://www.vitrocell.com/inhalation-toxicology/exposure-systems/vitrocell-cloud-system (accessed October 27, 2020)

4

In situ-Like Aerosol Inhalation Exposure for Cytotoxicity Assessment using *Airway-on-Chips* Platforms

Shani Elias-Kirma, Arbel Artzy-Schnirman, Prashant Das, Metar Heller-Algazi, Netanel Korin and Josué Sznitman*

Department of Biomedical Engineering, Technion – Israel Institute of Technology, Haifa, Israel

*Correspondence:
Josué Sznitman
sznitman@bm.technion.ac.il

Lung exposure to inhaled particulate matter (PM) is known to injure the airway epithelium via inflammation, a phenomenon linked to increased levels of global morbidity and mortality. To evaluate physiological outcomes following PM exposure and concurrently circumvent the use of animal experiments, *in vitro* approaches have typically relied on traditional assays with plates or well inserts. Yet, these manifest drawbacks including the inability to capture physiological inhalation conditions and aerosol deposition characteristics relative to *in vivo* human conditions. Here, we present a novel *airway-on-chip* exposure platform that emulates the epithelium of human bronchial airways with critical cellular barrier functions at an air–liquid interface (ALI). As a proof-of-concept for *in vitro* lung cytotoxicity testing, we recapitulate a well-characterized cell apoptosis pathway, induced through exposure to 2 µm airborne particles coated with αVR1 antibody that leads to significant loss in cell viability across the recapitulated airway epithelium. Notably, our *in vitro* inhalation assays enable simultaneous aerosol exposure across multiple airway chips integrated within a larger bronchial airway tree model, under physiological respiratory airflow conditions. Our findings underscore *in situ*-like aerosol deposition outcomes where patterns depend on respiratory flows across the airway tree geometry and gravitational orientation, as corroborated by concurrent numerical simulations. Our *airway-on-chips* not only highlight the prospect of realistic *in vitro* exposure assays in recapitulating characteristic local *in vivo* deposition outcomes, such platforms open opportunities toward advanced *in vitro* exposure assays for preclinical cytotoxicity and drug screening applications.

Keywords: pulmonary, airway, organ-on-chip, *in vitro*, human primary cells, inhalation, aerosol, cytotoxicity

INTRODUCTION

With a vast and highly vascularized surface optimized for gas exchange (Grotberg, 2011; Janssen et al., 2016), the lungs constitute the largest organ directly exposed to the external environment. As such, the lungs are vulnerable to a breadth of threats associated with occupational (Leggat et al., 2007) and environmental (Brulle and Pellow, 2006) hazards. In particular, exposure to inhaled airborne particulate matter (PM) represents a global health problem due to adverse cardiovascular and respiratory outcomes linked to increased morbidity and mortality (Anderson et al., 2012; Kim et al., 2015; Conibear et al., 2018; Wu et al., 2018). To protect the body from continuous exposure to foreign PM, and also pathogens and other toxic chemicals (Bals and Hiemstra, 2004), the lungs' luminal surface is populated with a confluent, uninterrupted epithelial cell carpet that exists as a continuum across the airway tree (Daniels and Orgeig, 2003). In the conducting airways specifically, epithelial cells are covered with an extracellular periciliary lining (Button et al., 2012) itself immersed under a mucus layer present at an air–liquid interface (ALI) (Fahy and Dickey, 2010). Briefly, the secretion of mucus by goblet and club cells (Barnes et al., 2003; Lai et al., 2008; Fahy and Dickey, 2010; Whitsett, 2018), in combination with ciliated cells, contributes to airway clearance (Janssen et al., 2016) by trapping (Stannard and O'Callaghan, 2006) inhaled particles and pathogens (e.g., bacteria) depositing on the pulmonary epithelium. This complex cellular environment requires a well-differentiated bronchial epithelium that constitutes the conducting airways' innate defense mechanisms and maintains pulmonary homeostasis.

In an effort to evaluate physiological outcomes following PM exposure and its association with diseases (e.g., COPD; Anderson et al., 2012), *in vivo* animal experiments have been traditionally pursued. For example, *in vivo* studies have demonstrated that pulmonary exposure to PM causes lung inflammation and oxidative stress (Inoue et al., 2006; Nemmar et al., 2009, 2011). Nemmar et al. (2009) showed that 24 h post intratracheal instillation of diesel exhaust particles, the influx of macrophages and neutrophils in broncho-alveolar mice lavages was elevated. Despite such progress, *in vivo* animal studies remain contentious due to critical differences in anatomy, immune systems, and inflammatory responses compared with humans (Benam et al., 2015), thereby raising the need for more relevant platforms for evaluation (Bueters et al., 2013). To overcome such drawbacks and uncover cellular mechanisms in which PM toxicity affects the respiratory system, *in vitro* studies with cell cultures have been actively sought (Paur et al., 2011; Nemmar et al., 2013; Drasler et al., 2017). In particular, ALI conditions can be recapitulated by culturing cells on the apical side of a porous membrane using for instance commercially available Transwell inserts; such setups are indeed critical in striving to mimic physiologically relevant characteristics of the bronchial airway lumen, including for example mucus secretion (Grainger et al., 2006; Lin et al., 2007). Furthermore, capturing biological airway responses specific to humans following PM exposure to toxins (Mustafiz et al., 2015) calls for the use of human primary cells (Skardal et al., 2016) in an effort to overcome ongoing limitations with animal studies. Although the aforementioned macroscopic *in vitro* approaches reproduce some of the cellular functions of the human pulmonary environment, both true-scale anatomical airway features and physiological (air) flow conditions are still widely absent from existing *in vitro* exposure assays. Such drawbacks continue to restrict *in vitro* setups from addressing faithfully the physical aerosol transport determinants leading to PM deposition along the inhalation route. Since direct *in vivo* human exposure studies are ethically controversial, the development of realistic *in vitro* human exposure assays is

thus desired to advance our understanding of inflammation and disease following harmful PM exposure under realistic *in situ* inhalation conditions.

Over the past decade, *organ-on-chips* have gained momentum in laying the foundations for constructing attractive *in vitro* models that mimic more realistically physiologically relevant organ functions in humans (Nesmith et al., 2014; Abaci et al., 2015; Bovard et al., 2018; Ronaldson-Bouchard and Vunjak-Novakovic, 2018; Shirure et al., 2018). Such platforms allow *in vitro* examinations within micro-devices lined with human cells, thereby fostering new physiological insights, in both health and disease, complementary to current tools available for diagnostics and conventional *in vitro* approaches (Tenenbaum-Katan et al., 2018). Specifically, lung-related models have been devised to mimic the human alveolar–capillary interface and stimulate inflammatory responses *in vitro* (Huh et al., 2010, 2012; Artzy-Schnirman et al., 2019b). For example, Huh et al. (2010) demonstrated the importance of using cyclic mechanical strain, which accentuates toxic and lung inflammatory responses to silica nanoparticles, associated with the development of vascular leakage, which leads to pulmonary edema. In parallel, Benam et al. (2015) reconstituted a human lung *small airway-on-a-chip* model by co-culturing both endothelium cells and epithelial tissue from healthy individuals and COPD patients to model human lung inflammatory disorders. In addition, using the *small airway-on-a-chip* model connected to a smoking instrument, Benam et al. (2016) established a platform to study a patient-specific response to inhaled smoke. Punde et al. (2015) showed protein-induced lung inflammation and emphasized the need of using flow, which allows reconstituting the blood vessel-tissue interface for *in vitro* assays, and by that improve pre-clinical studies. Together with other recent efforts (Douville et al., 2011; Nesmith et al., 2014; Stucki et al., 2014; Li et al., 2015; Hassell et al., 2017; Humayun et al., 2018), these studies have brought tremendous progress in lung research but are still widely limited to platforms with a single airway channel, thus short of mimicking the complexity of the conducting airway tree. This is especially critical when exploring the fate of inhaled aerosols where the coupling between respiratory airflows and lung anatomy is known to modulate particle deposition outcomes (Kleinstreuer and Zhang, 2010; Fishler et al., 2015; Koullapis P.G. et al., 2018).

Motivated by the critical need to deliver *in vitro* platforms that mimic more closely physiological inhalation conditions of human lung exposure with characteristic *in situ*-like deposition outcomes (Artzy-schnirman et al., 2019a), we have established a novel inhalation assay integrated with an *airway-on-chip* platform comprising three-generational bronchial airways cultured with a differentiated human bronchial epithelium. Specifically, such *in vitro* inhalation assay reproduces mechanistically faithful aerosol transport determinants leading to airway deposition at a functional epithelial barrier. As a proof-of-concept, we characterize PM toxicity whereby we recapitulate a well-characterized apoptosis pathway (Agopyan et al., 2003, 2004). One of the better-known pathways in which PM affects human airway cytotoxicity is mediated by receptors which induce cell apoptosis (Becker et al., 1996; Holian et al., 1998), including importantly the Vanilloid (i.e., VR1) receptor (Agopyan et al., 2003). Seminal *in vitro* studies using primary cells have shown that 48 h post PM particle stimulation the level of apoptotic cells is elevated by activation of such VR1 receptor (Agopyan et al., 2004). Here, apoptosis is induced through exposure to 2-μm airborne particles coated by αVR1 antibody; an aerosol size known to deposit in the small bronchi and bronchioles (Bair, 1989; Stahlhofen et al., 1989; Hinds, 1999). Importantly, our *in vitro* inhalation assays deliver aerosols simultaneously across four *airway-on-chips* integrated within a larger conductive airway tree model to explore *in situ*-like aerosol deposition outcomes under physiological respiratory airflows and for various gravitational orientations. Given that current cytotoxicity assays are still widely based on either non-physiological liquid installations of PM suspensions (Hittinger et al., 2017) or alternatively direct spraying at an ALI (Blank et al., 2006; Lenz et al., 2014; Röhm et al., 2017), our *airway-on-chip* exposure setup is part of steadfast efforts (Artzy-schnirman et al., 2019a) leading toward a new generation of advanced *in vitro* lung toolkits for human inhalation toxicity assays.

MATERIALS AND METHODS

Airway-on-Chip
Device Design
The design of the proposed *airway-on-chips* consists of a planar, symmetric airway tree spanning three generations (with a total of four outlets), as schematically shown in **Figure 1a**. Individual airways consist of lumens of semi-circular cross-sections (chosen as a result of the need for a porous membrane for cell culture, see below) where dimensions, summarized in **Table 1**, are based on morphometric measurements representative of a typical human adult lung, following the seminal works of Weibel et al. (1963) and Horsfield et al. (1971). Note that our *in vitro* platform broadly mimics small bronchial branches of the conducting zone, with airway diameters <2.5 mm, along with an idealized constant planar bifurcating angle of 60° across all generations (Ménache et al., 2008). In line with recent *lung-on-chip* designs limited to single airway channels, the present design allows to culture cells at ALI conditions together with access for inhalation airflows through the apical compartment using a syringe pump (see below).

Device Fabrication
The model negative is 3D printed in house via stereo-lithography (Formlabs, Form 2). The mould is used as a master template for polydimethylsiloxane (PDMS) casting. PDMS was mixed with a curing agent (Dow Corning) at a 10:1 weight ratio, poured on the template and baked for 4 h at ~65°C. Cured PDMS was subsequently pealed from the mould and punched using a biopsy punch of 1 mm size (Miltex, 3331) to create inlet and outlets. Next, a 10 μm thick polyethylene terephthalate (PET) membrane with 0.4 μm pore size (Corning, CLS3450) was bonded to the PDMS model and channels were irreversibly sealed. Upon seeding cells on the apical side of the PET membrane, the model is placed above a medium reservoir (i.e., basal side). The completed assembly of the platform is presented in **Figure 1b**.

Aerosol Exposure Experiments
Particle Preparation
Following an established protocol, 2 μm monodispersed polystyrene (PS) particles [FluoSpheres Carboxylate-Modified microspheres, Red Fluorescent (580/605), 2% solid F8826, Thermo Scientific] were coupled to αVR1 antibody (Baker et al., 2019) (Abcam, ab3487)/bovine serum albumin (BSA; MP Biomedicals, 160069) in phosphate-buffered saline (PBS; Sigma-Aldrich, D8537), respectively, using a two-step *EDC/Sulfo NHS Covalent Coupling Procedure* (Merck, 2015) (Merck Millipore). Such protocol yields 2 μm monodispersed PS particles conjugated with αVR1 antibody/BSA. Briefly, after 15 min sonication, 250 μl PS particles were suspended in 250 μl of 50 mM MES buffer solution (pH 6). The suspension was vortexed and centrifuged at 3000 × g for 5 min at 4°C. This washing procedure was repeated three times. Next, 12 μl of 200 mM EDC reagent solution and 120 μl of 200 mM Sulfo-NHS reagent solution were added to the particle suspension with 250 μl of MES buffer. The suspension was vortexed and mixed gently in a vertically rotating plate for 30 min at room temperature (RT), followed by three washes with 1 ml MES buffer. Next, 33 μl of αVR1 antibody (1 mg/ml)/100 μl of BSA (1 mg/ml), respectively, were added to the particles with 1 ml MES buffer, vortexed and mixed gently in a vertically rotating plate for 3 h at RT. The suspension was washed from the unreacted protein using a spin down centrifugation cycle (the supernatant was kept for protein content analysis), and the particles were suspended in 1 ml MES buffer and 15 μl of ethanolamine to quench the reaction. Finally, the particles were washed three times using 1 ml blocking buffer [containing 0.5% (w/v) casein in MES buffer], and three times with 1 ml of PBS. The particles were kept at 4°C until used for an experiment. To assess qualitatively the PS-VR1 conjugation, particles were incubated for 1 h at RT with secondary antibody Alexa Fluor 488 anti-rabbit, before confocal microscopy imaging of fluorescent immunostaining was performed on the conjugated particles (**Supplementary Figure S2**).

Aerosol Exposure Assay
The present *in vitro* aerosol exposure assays strive to recapitulate *in situ*-like inhalation conditions. In a first step, aerosol exposure assays were conducted in the absence of cells to characterize *in vitro* aerosol transport determinants and examine solely aerosol deposition patterns inside the devices. Subsequently, the identical protocol was implemented to explore cytotoxicity on the epithelium. Briefly, a monodispersed aerosol was produced by aerosolization (Fishler et al., 2015) of PBS-suspended 2 μm red fluorescent PS microspheres conjugated to αVR1 antibody (as described above) using an aerosol generator (TSI, 3076) with air as the gas source and subsequently drying the PBS droplets using two consecutive diffusion driers (TSI, 3062). The rationale for selecting such particle size follows as 2 μm represents a good candidate for aerosol deposition in the deep tracheobronchial (TB) regions (Bair, 1989; Stahlhofen et al., 1989; Hinds, 1999). To avoid aggregate formation prior to the

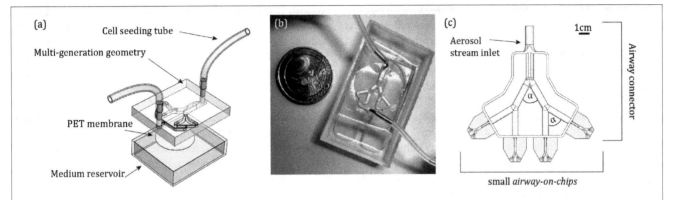

FIGURE 1 | Design of the *airway-on-chip* platform and its integration for aerosol inhalation exposure assays. **(a)** Computer-aided drawing (CAD) schematic of the device including the airway tree model (apical side), a porous PET membrane (gray circle) separating the bottom reservoir for medium (basal side). **(b)** Photograph of the assembled device. **(c)** CAD schematic of the custom-designed 3D airway tree connector which allows to simultaneously perform experiments across four individual *airway-on-chip* devices (shown in gray), and control the orientation of gravity during an exposure assay, with bifurcating angle of $\alpha = 60°$ (**Supplementary Figure S1**).

TABLE 1 | Dimensions of the *airway-on-chip* platform.

Generation	Length (mm)	Diameter (mm)
1	6.59	2.20
2	5.55	1.68
3	3.58	1.25

deposition assays, the microspheres were first sonicated in a water bath for 20 min. Next, the 2 μm PS particles were diluted in distilled water to a concentration of 1×10^7 particle/ml for aerosol exposure, while for the cell viability assay in the cultured *airway-on-chips*, particles were diluted in PBS to a concentration of 4.55×10^8 particle/ml (see the section "Results"). The aerosol flow was fed through an antistatic tube where the flow rate was controlled by a pinch valve. To deliver a physiologically relevant exposure assay, the flow rate was further reduced by splitting the main aerosol stream into four paths integrated within a custom-designed conducting 3D airway tree model that approximately mimics mid-bronchial generations in an average adult human lung (Ménache et al., 2008; **Figure 1c** and **Supplementary Figure S1**).

Using the 3D airway connecting model enables to simultaneously perform $n = 4$ *airway-on-chip* experiments, directly integrated within an anatomically inspired conducting airway tree. The overall flow rate selected was 0.2 l/min, as measured using a flow meter (TSI, 4100) at the aerosol generator outlet; the ensuing flow rate at the entrance of each (four) device was 0.05 l/min, i.e., corresponding to physiological airflow conditions representative of flow phenomena in small bronchial airways. Specifically, we replicate quiet breathing conditions (Pedley, 2003; Sznitman, 2013), such that the characteristic Reynolds numbers (Re) range between approximately 22 and 10 across the three generations of the *airway-on-chip*, where $Re = ud/\nu$ and represents the relative magnitude of the inertial forces to viscous forces (i.e., ν is the kinematic viscosity of air, u is the characteristic mean airflow velocity in each generation of diameter d).

In each experiment, four *airway-on-chip* devices are positioned in a horizontal orientation relative to gravity and directly tight-fitted to the four outlets of the 3D airway tree connector along the streamwise flow direction (see **Figure 1c** and **Supplementary Figure S1**). Unlike cell seeding via the top of the device (**Figures 1a,b**), this design ensures anatomical continuity and thereby adequate respiratory airflows during aerosol exposure assays. Note that the influence of gravity, and thus particle deposition, can be modified with the present design by changing the device position relative to the connector's outlet (**Supplementary Figure S3**). Each exposure assay was conducted for 30 min in an effort to yield representative ensemble depositions of aerosols and in parallel compare these with numerical simulation (see the section "Results"); in the case of cell viability assays a continuous exposure was conducted for 5 min. Note that here, constant steady-state inhalation flow conditions are mimicked, giving rise to fully developed laminar flow conditions; the range of Re across the 3D airway connector ranges approximately between Re ~ 50–22, in line with physiological respiratory conditions (Pedley, 2003; Sznitman, 2013).

To quantify ensuing aerosol deposition patterns, the models were subsequently imaged under microscopy using an inverted fluorescent microscope (Nikon eclipse Ti) at 20× magnification. A resulting single, high-resolution image of the complete *airway-on-chips* was obtained by tiling multiple images where the location of each deposited fluorescent particle was identified by locating local intensity maxima (ImageJ).

Numerical Simulations
Computational Fluid Dynamics Simulations
In an effort to interpret the underlying physical aerosol transport determinants governing deposition outcomes and further compare the experimentally obtained particle deposition patterns, *in silico* flow simulations were carried out using a commercial software (Fluent 18.2, ANSYS Inc.) that solves the mass and momentum (i.e., Navier–Stokes) equations

numerically. An airway model identical to the *airway-on-chip* design was first discretized with tetrahedral cell elements using the original CAD model and subsequently refined and converted into a polyhedral mesh (Inthavong et al., 2019). Flow convergence tests were conducted on three different mesh sizes, ranging between 240,000 and 660,000 polyhedral cells in size. A final mesh consisting of approximately 540,000 polyhedral cells was selected for flow simulations. To accurately mimic experimental conditions, a steady-state, fully developed velocity profile was imposed at the model inlet. A no-slip boundary condition was implemented at the walls, and any particles impacting the walls were assumed to be deposited. All four outlets were set to identical, zero-pressure outlet conditions. Given the relatively low-Reynolds-number regime (Re $<<$ 100), a laminar solver was chosen to simulate airflows. A SIMPLE pressure–velocity coupling scheme with least squares cell-based gradient discretization, second-order for pressure and second-order upwind scheme for momentum was implemented.

Particle Deposition Simulations

We simulated $\sim$6,400 monodisperse 2 μm diameter PS particles (ρ_p = 1.05 g/cm^3), tracked using a Lagrangian one-way coupled, steady-state discrete phase model. As particle mass flow through a cross-section may be assumed proportional to flow rate, particles were seeded at the inlet with a quasi-parabolic initial distribution using a truncated normal probability density function. For such particle size, the main forces governing transport are viscous drag (i.e., low-Re Stokes drag) and gravitational sedimentation; that is Brownian motion, electrostatic charge, or other forces are neglected (Koullapis et al., 2016). Locations of the deposited particles on the bottom wall (analogous to the apical side of the PET membrane) were extracted and identified according to airway branch generation.

Cell Culture

Cell Culture Maintenance

In the footsteps of recent small *airway-on-chip* models led by Benam et al. (2015), Normal Human Bronchial Epithelial (NHBE) cells (Lonza, CC-2540S) were cultured under immersed conditions with B-ALI growth medium (Lonza, 00193516) and 50% of supplemented BEGM SingleQuots (Lonza, CC-4175) in a tissue culture T75-flask (TPP, 90025). The medium was changed every second or third day until cells reached $\sim$90% confluency. A Trypsin–EDTA solution (Lonza, CC-5034) was then used to detach cells from culture dishes. Thereafter, cells were used for experiments as described in detail below. Cells were incubated at 37°C in a humidified atmosphere containing 5% CO$_2$. Cells were cultured up to passage (Rayner et al., 2019) four; mycoplasma controls were performed routinely using MycoAlert mycoplasma detection kit (Lonza, BELT07-218) without exhibiting infection.

Air–Liquid Interface (ALI)

For *airway-on-chip* cultures, 1.8 $\times$ 10^5 NHBE cells (in 135 μl medium) were seeded on top of the apical side of a 0.03 mg/ml collagen type I coated (Corning, 354236) PET membrane inside the devices, and 1 ml of medium was added to the basal compartment. For Transwell inserts culture (Corning, CLS3470), 5 $\times$ 10^4 NHBE cells (in 200 μl medium) were seeded on a collagen type I-coated PET membrane inside inserts, and 500 μl of medium was added to the basal compartment. Both cell cultures on chip and on inserts were first conducted under immersed conditions with B-ALI growth complete medium and 1% Antibiotic Antimycotic Solution (Sigma-Aldrich, A5955). By day 4 the NHBE culture was exposed to air (i.e., ALI) by removing the medium from the apical side of the *airway-on-chip* devices and the inserts, respectively. B-ALI differentiation medium (StemCell, 05001) was introduced in the basal chamber of the devices and inserts, respectively. Differentiated NHBE cell cultures were imaged under microscopy starting from day 21 after exposure to ALI.

Imaging

Scanning Electron Microscopy

Samples were washed three times with PBS and fixed in primary fixative buffer [1% para formaldehyde (PFA) and 2% GA in 0.1 M NaP pH 7.4 and 3% sucrose] for 60 min at RT. Following three washes with 0.1 M cacodylate buffer (pH 7.4) samples were fixed with 1% Osmium tetroxide in 0.1 M cacodylate buffer for 15 min at RT. Next, samples were dehydrated through a graded ethanol series and further processed by critical point drying and sputter coating with chromium (5 nm). Images were acquired with a Zeiss ULTRA plus field emission scanning electron microscope (SEM).

Mucus Visualization

Following perfusion of PBS, NHBE cells were fixed within the devices and inserts using 4% PFA (Sigma–Aldrich, 47608) for 20 min at RT and were washed again three times with PBS. For detection of glycoproteins typically present in mucus (Leonard et al., 2010; Lechanteur et al., 2018), samples were treated with 10 mg/ml alcian Blue 8G$\times$ (Sigma–Aldrich, A5268) in 3% acetic acid (1% w/v) for 15 min at RT and were washed three times with PBS. Images were then acquired with a light inverted microscope (Nikon Eclipse TS100) at 10$\times$.

Immunofluorescence Microscopy

Directly after cell fixation using 4% PFA, cells were treated with 0.05% Triton X-100 (Sigma–Aldrich, T8787) for 3 min at RT to increase membrane permeability and were blocked for non-specific binding using 2% BSA for 1 h at RT. For F-actin staining, NHBE cells were incubated with Alexa Fluor 568 Phalloidin (ThermoFisher Scientific, A12380) diluted with PBS (ratio of 1:200) for 40 min at RT. For DAPI nucleic acid staining cells were incubated with DAPI solution (ThermoFisher Scientific, D1306), diluted with PBS (ratio of 1:400) for 5 min at RT. For tight junction proteins, Zonula occludens-1 (ZO1), cells were incubated with the primary antibodies rabbit anti-ZO1 (ThermoFisher Scientific, 617300) diluted with PBS (ratio of 1:200) overnight at 4°C, followed by incubation with secondary antibody Alexa Fluor 488 anti-rabbit (Jackson ImmunoResearch, 111-545-144), diluted with PBS (ratio of 1:400) for 1 h at RT. After each step, cells were washed three times with PBS. Finally, confocal microscopy imaging of fluorescent immunostaining was performed (Nikon Eclipse Ti with spinning disk, Yokogawa, Japan).

Apoptosis Quantification

Following 5–8 days under immersed conditions, NHBE cells in the devices were exposed for 5 min to the PS-αVR1 particles and then incubated for 48 h. To ensure that apoptosis resulted solely from the exposure assay, the response of two control groups was monitored: (i) NHBE cells treated with airflow and (ii) cells exposed to PS-BSA particles (without the αVR1 antibody). To quantify apoptosis, following 48 h of incubation, cells were fully harvested using a Trypsin–EDTA solution, collected and then incubated with Alexa Fluor 488 conjugated Annexin V (Abcam, ab14085) in the dark for 5 min at RT. The cells were then imaged using an imaging flow cytometer (Amnis, ImageStreamX Mark II) at 40×. As a positive control, the NHBE cells' apoptotic response was measured over time following exposure to αVR1 antibody. Briefly, 5×10^4 NHBE cells per well were seeded in a 96-well plate (Nunc, 167008). Two days after seeding, medium containing 0.66 μM αVR1 antibody was added, followed by incubation of 24 and 48 h. Next, apoptotic cells were stained using Annexin V (see details above), and imaging of fluorescent immunostaining was performed. In parallel, as an additional positive control, we checked the toxicity effects of PS-VR1 particles using NHBE cells which were seeded on top of an insert for 7 days under immersed conditions, followed by incubation of 48 h with PS-BSA and PS-VR1 in a particle:cell ratio of 1:50. Finally, confocal imaging of fluorescent immunostaining was performed.

Particles Toxicity Assays

To ensure that apoptosis was due to the exposure assay using αVR1 antibody, a toxicity test was first performed. Briefly, 5×10^4 NHBE cells per well were seeded in a 96-well plate; 2 days following seeding, medium containing 2 μm PS-BSA particles with particle:cell ratios of 5:1, 2.5:1, 1:1, 1:2.5, 1:5, 1:10, 1:100, and 1:200 were added, respectively. NHBE cells were returned for 48 h incubation. Next, a cell viability reagent (almarBlue; Bio-Rad, BUF012A) with 10% volume in culture medium was added to each well followed by 4 h incubation. Finally, absorbance measurements were performed using a plate reader (Varioskan LUX, ThermoFisher Scientific) at 570 and 600 nm wavelengths, respectively. Each test was repeated independently three times. As a positive control, medium containing 2 μm PS-VR1 particles with a particle:cell ratio of 1:100 was added in the same experiment and a viability assay using almarBlue was performed.

Statistical Analysis

A student's t-test (two-tailed) was used to determine the level of significance among different experiments device. Error bars are presented as the standard error and asterisks indicating significance in the figures correspond to $p < 0.05$, 0.005, and 0.001 shown as *, **, and ***, respectively.

RESULTS AND DISCUSSION

To emulate a small conducting airway environment in view of cytotoxicity exposure evaluations, we designed a tree-like device featuring two planar, symmetric branching airway channels, broadly resembling the anatomy of small bronchial airways of an average adult lung (**Figures 1a,b**). The device consists of three layers (see the section "Materials and Methods"), including the apical side of the PDMS airway tree, in which the two small punches (1 mm in diameter) first allow to seed the pulmonary cells on top of the PET membrane (10 μm thick with 0.4 μm pores size). The PET membrane is bonded to the bottom PDMS compartment and sealed above by the airway channels. This permeable membrane allows nutrient supply from the medium in the reservoir and prevents cell leakage to the basal side. Notably, our custom design allows to culture the seeded pulmonary cells at ALI conditions; a necessary condition for adequate differentiation (Grainger et al., 2006; Lin et al., 2007). Our design mimics the *in vivo* environment by combining a 3D true scale pulmonary tree geometry with realistic airflow conditions and recapitulating *in situ*-like aerosol inhalation exposure to the deep TB regions of the lungs.

Aerosol Inhalation Exposure Assay

We first explore deposition patterns of inhaled aerosols during the inhalation maneuver and present ensemble deposition patterns for 2 μm particles on the bottom surface of the *airway-on-chips* (i.e., PET membrane). Such results follow a steady (i.e., constant flow rate) inhalation aerosol exposure assay across the anatomically realistic 3D airway connector (**Supplementary Figure S1**). Devices were exposed for 30 min to a steady stream of aerosols at a controlled flow rate matching physiological airflow conditions representative of small bronchial (with an entrance flow rate of $Q = 0.05$ l/min). We recall that our inhalation assays omit the oscillatory nature of respiratory flows and instead focus on inhalation phenomena. We recently explored in *in silico* simulations particle deposition occurring during inhalation and exhalation phases across extensive deep lung models (Koullapis P.G. et al., 2018) and assessed the contribution of each phase, respectively. Here, rather, the focus of the present proof-of-concept lies in recapitulating for the first time real mechanistic deposition determinants of inhaled aerosols within *lung-on-chip* platforms.

To mimic the hydrophilic environment of the bronchial lumen surrounded by mucus, we used collagen-coated devices (0.03 mg/ml collagen type I); we recall that in view of quantifying solely mechanistic aerosol transport characteristics devices are first void of epithelium. **Figure 2A** presents ensemble results of particle deposition patterns inside the *airway-on-chips* under physiological airflow conditions; the color-coded heat map quantifies particle concentration, defined as the number of neighboring particles within a 0.5 mm radius (results are normalized by the highest concentration in the tree). We begin by observing a heterogeneous deposition pattern with high particle concentrations along the centerline of each generation compared to the peripheral areas (i.e., nearer the airway side walls), in line with Poiseuille velocity profiles characteristics at such Re. When examining the average particle density (defined as the average number of deposited particles in each branch, normalized by the branch's surface area) as shown in **Figure 2B**, a consistent monotonic decrease in particle density is apparent with each deeper generation as

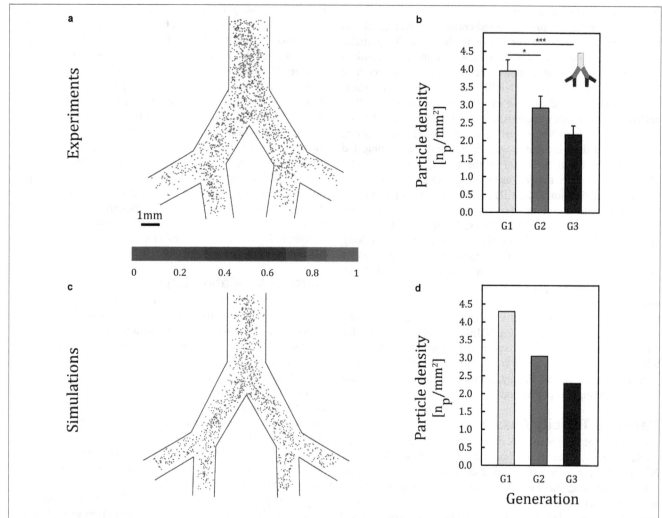

FIGURE 2 | Particle deposition patterns following exposure. Two micrometers of PS particles were aerosolized into the *airway-on-chips* in a horizontal position with respect to gravity at physiological airflow conditions corresponding to quiet breathing. **(a)** Ensemble deposition patterns imaged under fluorescence microscopy (*n* = 8 models). The color-coded heat map quantifies particle concentration, defined as the number of neighboring particles within an 0.5 mm radius (results are normalized by the highest concentration in the tree). **(b)** Histogram of particle deposition density quantifying the average particle number in each generation normalized by airway area (mm^2). Error bars represent the standard error. Asterisks indicate significance corresponding to p < 0.05, 0.001 shown as * and ***, respectively. Corresponding **(c)** aerosol deposition patterns and **(d)** histograms of deposition density obtained from *in silico* CFD simulations.

anticipated in the deep TB lung regions (Zhang et al., 2009). Namely, average particle density is observed to decrease by nearly half between the first and third generation, with a mean of 3.9 particles/mm^2 in generation 1 (G1) compared to 2.2 particles/mm^2 in generation 3 (G3). With our current design and exposure assay, we were able to reproduce spatial particle deposition density gradients across the airway trees and mimic anticipated *in situ* situations. Demonstrating this ability in a proof-of-concept holds ramifications for future cytotoxicity as well as drug screening assays (e.g., inhalation therapy), where local deposition patterns and thereby concentrations hotspots (Imai et al., 2012; Hofemeier and Sznitman, 2015; Islam et al., 2017), can lead to various differences in local inflammatory responses and disease onset. Such feature lies beyond reach using traditional assays (e.g., Transwell) or conversely straight channels.

To date, direct *in vivo* exposure studies of aerosol deposition have focused mainly on olfactory and upper trachea–bronchial regions in both animals (Gerde et al., 1991; Petitot et al., 2013) and humans (Cheng et al., 1996), with little explorations in the small bronchi and bronchioles. In addition, since *in vivo* data are conducted mostly with 2D gamma scintigraphy, the resolution of current imaging modalities remains inadequate to quantify deposition at small scales (Koullapis P. et al., 2018). Such limitations have driven the appeal of *in vitro–in silico* based strategies to deliver insight into deposition determinants. To date, however, efforts have been focused mainly on upper airways (Byron et al., 2010; Carrigy et al., 2014) with few studies exploring deposition endpoints in the mid- to small-bronchi. For example, Fishler et al. (2015) characterized the deposition of PS particles (i.e., 0.2–1 μm in diameter) in an *acinus-on-chip* platform and correlated findings *in silico*. In the footsteps of such endeavors, computational fluid dynamics (CFD) simulations were presently sought to gain quantitative insight into the deposition mechanisms at play. Results exhibit strong consistency when compared with the experimentally obtained deposition patterns (**Figures 2C,D**), with a maximum difference of 8% between experimental and numerical results. Notably, the deposition of 2 μm particles in small bronchi is principally governed by sedimentation, in line with the general understanding of inhalation aerosol deposition theory (Zhang et al., 2009). Dimensional analysis (see **Supplementary Material**) supports that deposition patterns under a horizontal orientation with respect to gravity are the result of the coupling between convective flow (i.e., viscous drag) along the streamwise airway direction and gravitational sedimentation in the normal direction, thereby giving rise to gradients in deposition density along each generation.

In addition, our *in vitro* exposure platform allows to examine the effect of gravity on ensuing deposition patterns by changing the orientation of the *airway-on-chips* (see **Supplementary Material**). Briefly, models were attached at a 45° tilt with respect to gravity and were exposed for 30 min to aerosolized 2 μm particles under physiological inhalation airflows. A decrease in the total number of deposited particles on the bottom PET membrane was observed as well as higher particle density in branches oriented lower with respect to gravity (see **Supplementary Figure S3**). Note that due to the imaged plane of the device (i.e., PET membrane), only deposited particles are identified (compared with those deposited on the PDMS side walls). Altogether, our *in vitro* exposure assays capture realistic aerosol transport determinants that still remain widely absent in more traditional PM instillations or direct spraying techniques (Blank et al., 2006; Lenz et al., 2014; Röhm et al., 2017) on plates and inserts. Furthermore, our *airway-on-chips* highlight for the first time that exposure assays can be configured to explore localized deposition effects, capturing for example deposition outcomes pertinent to regional lung lobes (e.g., upper versus lower lobes) that span broad orientation angles across the chest cavity (Sauret et al., 2002).

Reconstituting a Bronchial Epithelium on Chip

To reconstitute an epithelial cell population lining the conducting airways (e.g., ciliated and secretory cells), primary NHBE cells originating from healthy human bronchi (biopsy) were seeded on the apical side of the ALI device (**Figure 3a**). Although the use of primary cells is limited by difficulties in sample isolation, the small number of cells that can be produced and the large variation between different donors (Skardal et al., 2016), such strategy represents a well-acknowledged *in vitro* approach in mimicking generic airway models (Rayner et al., 2019) that capture the *in vivo* environment; a point advocated in recent *airway-on-chip* designs (Benam et al., 2015). By using NHBE cells, we have thus followed a similar approach, including the recent work of Bovard et al. (2018) who developed a *lung/liver-on-a-chip* platform with NHBE cells to study the toxicity of inhaled aerosols. Moreover, many studies have used such cells as an airway model to study

cell exposure to ambient air pollution (Becker et al., 2005), using traditional assays with Transwell inserts. Among other, Wu et al. (2001) studied the expression of IL-8 through the activation of the EGF receptor signaling after NHBE cells were exposed to environmental PM.

To evaluate differentiation, following 21 days at ALI conditions, we visualized mucus secretion from the differentiated cells using SEM as shown in **Figure 3b**, where mucus microstructure is similar to that observed in previous lungs mucus studies (Schuster et al., 2013). Since washing off the mucus layer from the epithelial culture could potentially damage the differentiated NHBE cells (i.e., ciliated and secretory cells), we have reverted to SEM imaging of the epithelium layer that was seeded on top of an insert and cultured at an ALI for 21 days (**Supplementary Figure S4a**), in parallel to those within the devices and under the same growth conditions. As a control, the undifferentiated NHBE cells were also investigated using SEM imaging (**Supplementary Figures S4c,d**) to emphasize the fundamental changes in morphology. In addition, we visualized specific glycoproteins, present in mucus (**Figure 3c**; see **Supplementary Figure S4f** for staining control). A confluent cell monolayer was observed by staining the whole device for F-actin, as shown in **Figure 3d**, and cell nuclei (**Figure 3e** represents an inset of the white square in **Figure 3d**). Finally, to assess the barrier formation in the chip, expression of one of the tight junction proteins (i.e., ZO1) was examined (**Figure 3f**). In parallel, for control, each of the cells passages was seeded on an insert under the same growth conditions (see for example **Supplementary Figure S4**).

Cell Viability Assay Following PM-Like Aerosol Exposure

Next, we explored the influence of PM-like particles on the NHBE cells cultured inside the device for cytotoxicity evaluation. To mimic the toxic characteristics of a PM group [e.g., oil fly ash (Agopyan et al., 2004), soils dust (Veranth et al., 2006), and coal fly ash (Deering-Rice et al., 2016) among others], we chose to simulate a well-known ligand that activates the Vanilloid receptor by preparing PM-like particles consisting of a PS-core conjugated to αVR1 antibodies (see the section "Particle Preparation"). We note that this activation can induce diverse biological cascades, including the release of pro-inflammatory cytokines such as IL-6, IL-8, and TNFα (Veronesi et al., 1999). Here, in a proof-of-concept, we specifically chose to demonstrate one well-known apoptosis pathway in the footsteps of previous studies (Agopyan et al., 2003, 2004).

The conjugation of the αVR1 antibody to the PS particles (i.e., PS-VR1) was confirmed by incubating the PS-VR1 with a secondary antibody (**Supplementary Figure S2**). As previously shown *in vitro*, the binding of the αVR1 antibody to the VR1 receptor, which is expressed on the epithelial surface, induces an apoptosis pathway (Agopyan et al., 2003, 2004). Thus, a qualitative measurement of the apoptotic response as a function of time of the NHBE cells after a αVR1 antibody stimulation was first performed using an Annexin V staining which stains for cells that enter the

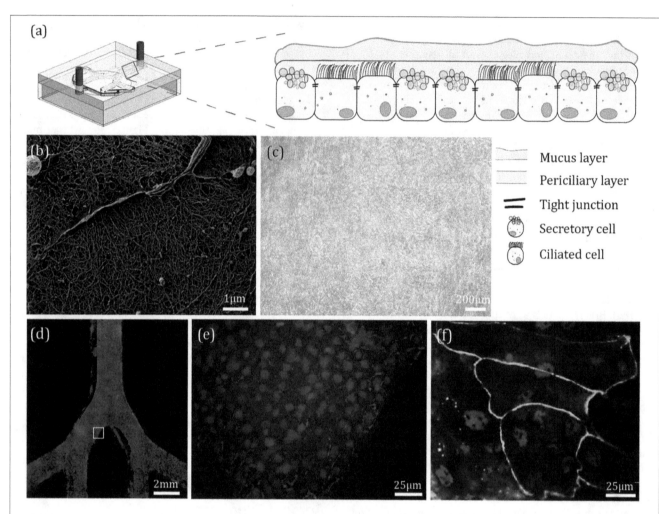

FIGURE 3 | Epithelial barrier reconstitution inside *airway-on-chips*. **(a)** Schematic illustration of the bronchial epithelium environment and the general differentiated cellular make-up. **(b)** Following device fabrication, NHBE cells were seeded on the apical side of the PET membrane under immersed conditions for 4 days, then cultured at ALI conditions for 21 days. Shown here is a scanning electron microscope (SEM) image of the mucus layer covering NHBE cells. **(c)** After 21 days at ALI conditions, NHBE cells were stained for glycoproteins typically present in mucus. **(d)** NHBE cells were cultured for 7 days under immersed conditions, then stained for F-actin. **(e,f)** After 21 days at ALI conditions, NHBE cells were stained for F-actin (red), ZO1 (green), and cell nuclei (blue).

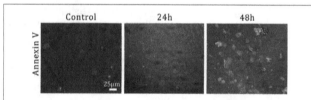

FIGURE 4 | Examination of αVR1 antibody effect on NHBE cells over time. The apoptotic response over time for αVR1 antibody on NHBE cells was investigated as a positive control. 5×10^4 NHBE cells per well are seeded in a 96-well plate. Two days after seeding, medium containing 0.66 μM αVR1 antibody was added, followed by incubation of 24 and 48 h. Next, apoptotic cells were stained using Annexin V (see the section "Apoptosis Quantification"), and imaging of fluorescent immunostaining was performed.

apoptotic pathway. Following an incubation period of 48 h, an increase in the apoptotic cell population was observed (**Figure 4**). As a positive control, to demonstrate the influence of our PM-like particles on the NHBE cells, cells were incubated with PS-BSA and PS-VR1, in a particle:cell ratio of 1:50, for an incubation period of 48 h. A qualitative measurement of the apoptotic cells was performed using Annexin V staining (**Supplementary Figure S5**) showing an increase in apoptotic cells which were incubated with the PS-VR1 particles, compared to control (incubation with PS-BSA particles). In addition, the PS toxicity level was assessed by titration of the PS-BSA particles which were incubated for 48 h with NHBE cells in a range of particles:cells ratios (**Supplementary Figure S6a**). A decrease in cell viability was detected starting from a particles:cells ratio of 5:1 (the selected ratio is ~1:500). The PS-VR1 toxicity effect was evaluated via viability assay following an incubation period of 48 h with NHBE cells in a particles:cells ratio of 1:100, resulting in a decrease in viability (**Supplementary Figure S6b**). This comprehensive examination allows us to refer to the manufactured PS-VR1 as PM-like particles, in line with seminal

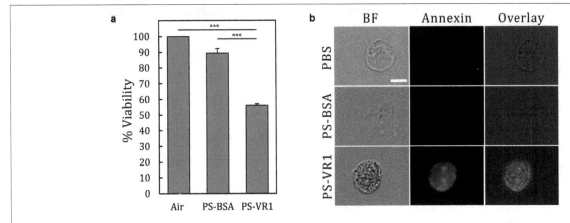

FIGURE 5 | Viability and apoptosis assay following NHBE cell exposure to PM-like particles. **(a)** Following inhalation exposure assays, *airway-on-chip* devices were returned to the incubator for 48 h prior to conducting a viability assay. The presented results are normalized to the air exposure, representing 100% viability ($n = 4$ for each treatment). **(b)** Single cell imaging using Annexin V staining which stained apoptotic cells with green (BF corresponds to bright field). Error bar represent the standard error and asterisks indicate significance ($p < 0.001$ shown as ***).

in vitro studies using traditional macroscopic assays on plate (Agopyan et al., 2003, 2004).

Our developed *in situ*-like airway exposure platform is suitable for diverse applications in the field of human inhalation toxicity *in vitro*. As a proof-of-concept, our *airway-on-chips* were exposed to harmful PM-like particles and their effect on the human bronchial epithelium was monitored. Following previous studies (Agopyan et al., 2003, 2004), cells were grown under immersed conditions and only exposed to air during the specific exposure assay. Prior to the exposure assay, cells were grown inside the *airway-on-chips* until confluency was reached (5–8 days following seeding). The models were then taken out of the incubator and connected to the larger conducting 3D airway model (**Figure 1c**) where a 5 min inhalation exposure was performed inside the biological hood (at RT). Next, the devices were placed back at the incubator for 48 h incubation (see the section "Materials and Methods"). Experiments were carried out for three independent exposure protocols: air, PS-BSA, and PS-VR1, respectively, using four replicates. Viability measurements were then performed 48 h post exposure, as shown in **Figure 5A**. The final percentage viability was normalized to the averaged value of the measurements for the air exposed group (defined as 100% viability). Our results indicate that the PS-BSA treatment was not toxic to the cells with around 90% viability. In contrast to the PS-BSA particles, the exposure to PS-VR1 particles led to a stark reduction in cell viability down to around 50% with standard error of 1.04%, demonstrating the high potency of PS-VR1 as an apoptosis inducer.

As the viability assay measures the level of the cellular metabolite and is not directly correlated with the level of apoptotic cells, a complementary assay was furthermore performed using Annexin V staining. The complete monolayer of cultured NHBE cells was trypsinized and harvested from the model, and was then incubated with Annexin V staining, followed by single cell imaging (see the section "Apoptosis Quantification") for each group. Here we present in **Figure 5B** a characteristic image for each treatment illustrating the ensuing

apoptotic levels; in the bright field (BF) column, single cells exhibiting a circular shape under each treatment show a typical morphology. When staining the cell membrane with Annexin V, only the cells under the PM-like treatment (i.e., PS-VR1) are stained compared with the controls (i.e., air and PS-BSA). This latter procedure further underlines one of the advantages of the present *airway-on-chip* platform; namely the ability to harvest cultured cells post exposure and conduct advanced single cell analyses. Together, these findings reinforce our setup as the first *in situ*-like platform suitable for aerosol exposure assays that combine realistic aerosol transport pathways in the lungs (i.e., from mouth to lumen) with biological toxicity that corroborates biological endpoints discussed in previous studies (Agopyan et al., 2003, 2004).

CONCLUSION

While past efforts with *lung-on-chips* have been widely restricted to simple isolated airway channels, in the present work we have established an advanced *in vitro* platform to recapitulate *in situ*-like aerosol exposure to PM under ALI conditions. Multigenerational *airway-on-chip* devices, mimicking bifurcating airway structures at true scale, were exposed to inhaled aerosols under physiological airflows within an integrated anatomically inspired bronchial airway tree model. Using *in vitro–in silico* strategies, our experimental efforts underscore the importance of the small airway tree anatomy and its orientation to gravity in determining mechanistically driven lung deposition outcomes; an important step toward *in vitro* pathways to explore deposition outcomes for various real lung-like deposition scenarios. Such efforts are anticipated to help shed light on inhaled particle deposition in deep airways and mimic more realistically representative *in vivo* deposition outcomes in human lungs with heterogeneous patterns.

Furthermore, we demonstrated the aptitude to culture human primary cells under ALI conditions for 21 days, guaranteeing them to differentiate to ciliated and secretory cells and thereby deliver a functional *in vivo*-like barrier. Such design allows additionally to incorporate in future studies the presence for example of immune cells as well as other co-/multi-cell cultures for specific endpoints. As a proof-of-concept, we manufactured monodisperse particles that mimic PM-induced apoptosis through the activation of the Vanilloid receptor and used two complementary techniques to demonstrate the effect of such harmful PM-like particles on the human bronchial epithelium (i.e., a viability assay and imaging ensuing apoptotic levels). At this stage, our aim was foremost to demonstrate how PS-VR1-conjugated particles deposited under physiological airflow conditions lead to loss of viability of the epithelium via an apoptotic cascade. In future studies, our devices can lend use for example toward physiological-based particle size screens. Future directions include also quantifying the effects of occupational environments on the epithelium barrier as our platform can be leveraged for more general *in vitro* exposure with the potential to expand our current knowledge on the mechanisms in which the PM injure the bronchial epithelium.

AUTHOR CONTRIBUTIONS

SE-K conceived the project and devised the experiments, designed the device, performed the experiments, analyzed the data, and wrote the manuscript. AA-S designed the experiments, performed the experiments, and wrote the manuscript. PD and MH-A performed the numerical simulations. NK assisted with manuscript drafting. JS conceived the project, supervised the analyses, and wrote the manuscript.

ACKNOWLEDGMENTS

The authors thank Simon Dorfman for technical assistance and Dr. Rami Fishler, Hikaia Zidan, Nofar Azulay, Eyal Habif, Mendel Kiperman, Moran Levi, and Mark Epshtein for helpful discussions and experimental support. They also thank Dr. Shaulov from the Biomedical Core Facilities (Technion) for technical support with the electron microscopy and Dr. Barak from Life Sciences and Engineering Infrastructure Center, Lorry I. Lokey Interdisciplinary Center (Technion) for technical support with the ImageStream.

REFERENCES

Abaci, H. E., Gledhill, K., Guo, Z., Christiano, A. M., and Shuler, M. L. (2015). Pumpless microfluidic platform for drug testing on human skin equivalents. *Lab Chip* 15, 882–888. doi: 10.1039/c4lc00999a

Agopyan, N., Bhatti, T., Yu, S., and Simon, S. (2003). Vanilloid receptor activation by 2- and 10-μm particles induces responses leading to apoptosis in human airway epithelial cells. *Toxicol. Appl. Pharmacol.* 192, 21–35. doi: 10.1016/S0041-008X(03)00259-X

Agopyan, N., Head, J., Yu, S., and Simon, S. A. (2004). TRPV1 receptors mediate particulate matter-induced apoptosis. *Am. J. Physiol. Lung. Cell Mol Physiol.* 286, L563–L572.

Anderson, J. O., Thundiyil, J. G., and Stolbach, A. (2012). Clearing the air: a review of the effects of particulate matter air pollution on human health. *J. Med. Toxicol.* 8, 166–175. doi: 10.1007/s13181-011-0203-1

Artzy-schnirman, A., Hobi, N., Schneider-daum, N., and Guenat, O. T. (2019a). European journal of pharmaceutics and biopharmaceutics advanced in vitro lung-on-chip platforms for inhalation assays: from prospect to pipeline. *Eur. J. Pharm. Biopharm.* 144, 11–17. doi: 10.1016/j.ejpb.2019.09.006

Artzy-Schnirman, A., Zidan, H., Elias-Kirma, S., Ben-Porat, L., Tenenbaum-Katan, J., Carius, P., et al. (2019b). Capturing the onset of bacterial pulmonary infection in acini-on-chips. *Adv. Biosyst.* 3:1900026. doi: 10.1002/adbi.20190 0026

Bair, W. J. (1989). Human respiratory tract model for radiological protection: a revision of the icrp dosimetric model for the respiratory system. *Health Phys.* 57, 249–253. doi: 10.1097/00004032-198907001-00032

Baker, C., Rodrigues, T., de Almeida, B. P., Barbosa-Morais, N. L., and Bernardes, G. J. L. (2019). Natural product–drug conjugates for modulation of TRPV1-expressing tumors. *Bioorg. Med. Chem.* 27, 2531–2536. doi: 10.1016/j.bmc.2019.03.025

Bals, R., and Hiemstra, P. S. (2004). Innate immunity in the lung: how epithelial cells fight against respiratory pathogens. *Eur. Respir. J.* 23, 327–333. doi: 10.1183/09031936.03.00098803

Barnes, P. J., Shapiro, S. D., and Pauwels, R. A. (2003). Chronic obstructive pulmonary disease: molecular and cellularmechanisms. *Eur. Respir. J.* 22, 672–688. doi: 10.1183/09031936.03.00040703

Becker, S., Mundandhara, S., Devlin, R. B., and Madden, M. (2005). Regulation of cytokine production in human alveolar macrophages and airway epithelial cells in response to ambient air pollution particles: further mechanistic studies. *Toxicol. Appl. Pharmacol.* 207, 269–275. doi: 10.1016/j.taap.2005.01.023

Becker, S., Soukup, J. M., Gilmour, M. I., and Devlin, R. B. (1996). Stimulation of human and rat alveolar macrophages by urban air particulates: effects on oxidant radical generation and cytokine production. *Toxicol. Appl. Pharmacol.* 141, 637–648. doi: 10.1006/TAAP.1996.0330

Benam, K. H., Villenave, R., Lucchesi, C., Varone, A., Hubeau, C., Lee, H.-H., et al. (2015). Small airway-on-a-chip enables analysis of human lung inflammation and drug responses in vitro. *Nat. Methods* 13, 151–157. doi: 10.1038/nmeth.3697

Benam, K. H., Novak, R., Nawroth, J., Hirano-Kobayashi, M., Ferrante, T. C., Choe, Y., et al. (2016). Matched-comparative modeling of normal and diseased human airway responses using a microengineered breathing lung chip. *Cell Syst.* 456.e4–466.e4. doi: 10.1016/j.cels.2016.10.003

Blank, F., Rothen-Rutishauser, B. M., Schurch, S., and Gehr, P. (2006). An Optimized In Vitro Model Of The Respiratory Tract Wall To Study Particle Cell Interactions. *J. AEROSOL Med.* 19, 392–405. doi: 10.1089/jam.2006.19.392

Bovard, D., Sandoz, A., Luettich, K., Frentzel, S., Iskandar, A., Marescotti, D., et al. (2018). Lab on a Chip A lung/liver-on-a-chip platform for acute and chronic toxicity studies †. *Lab Chip* 18, 3814–3829. doi: 10.1039/c8lc01029c

Brulle, R. J., and Pellow, D. N. (2006). Human health and environmental inequalities. *Annu. Rev. Public Heal.* 27, 103–127. doi: 10.1146/annurev.publhealth.27.021405.102124

Bueters, T., Ploeger, B. A., and Visser, S. A. G. (2013). The virtue of translational PKPD modeling in drug discovery: selecting the right clinical candidate while sparing animal lives. *Drug Discov. Today* 18, 853–862. doi: 10.1016/J.DRUDIS.2013.05.001

Button, B., Cai, L.-H., Ehre, C., Kesimer, M., Hill, D. B., Sheehan, J. K., et al. (2012). A periciliary brush promotes the lung health by separating the mucus layer from airway epithelia. *Science* 337, 937–941. doi: 10.1126/science.1223012

Byron, P. R., Hindle, M., Lange, C. F., Longest, P. W., McRobbie, D., Oldham, M. J., et al. (2010). *In vivo-in vitro* correlations: predicting pulmonary drug deposition from pharmaceutical aerosols. *J. Aerosol Med. Pulm. Drug Deliv.* 23, S59–S69.

doi: 10.1089/jamp.2010.0846

Carrigy, N. B., Ruzycki, C. A., Golshahi, L., and Finlay, W. H. (2014). Pediatric *in vitro* and *in silico* models of deposition via oral and nasal inhalation. *J. Aerosol Med. Pulm. Drug Deliv.* 27, 149–169. doi: 10.1089/jamp.2013.1075

Cheng, K.-H., Cheng, Y.-S., Yeh, H.-C., Guilmette, R. A., Simpson, S. Q., Yang, Y.-H., et al. (1996). *In vivo* measurements of nasal airway dimensions and ultrafine aerosol deposition in the human nasal and oral airways. *J. Aerosol Sci.* 27, 785–801. doi: 10.1016/0021-8502(96)00029-8

Conibear, L., Butt, E. W., Knote, C., Arnold, S. R., and Spracklen, D. V. (2018). Residential energy use emissions dominate health impacts from exposure to ambient particulate matter in India. *Nat. Commun.* 9:617. doi: 10.1038/s41467-018-02986-7

Daniels, C. B., and Orgeig, S. (2003). Pulmonary surfactant: the key to the evolution of air breathing. *Physiology* 18, 151–157. doi: 10.1152/nips.01438.2003

Deering-Rice, C. E., Stockmann, C., Romero, E. G., Lu, Z., Shapiro, D., Stone, B. L., et al. (2016). Characterization of transient receptor potential vanilloid-1 (TRPV1) variant activation by coal fly ash particles and associations with altered transient receptor potential ankyrin-1 (TRPA1) expression and asthma . *J. Biol. Chem.* 291, 24866–24879. doi: 10.1074/jbc.M116.746156

Douville, N. J., Zamankhan, P., Tung, Y.-C., Li, R., Vaughan, B. L., Tai, C.-F., et al. (2011). Combination of fl uid and solid mechanical stresses contribute to cell death and detachment in a microfl uidic alveolar model Combination of fluid and solid mechanical stresses contribute to cell death and detachment in a microfluidic alveolar model. *Lab Chip* 11, 557–760. doi: 10.1039/c0lc00251h

Drasler, B., Sayre, P., Steinhäuser, K. G., Petri-Fink, A., and Rothen-Rutishauser, B. (2017). In vitro approaches to assess the hazard of nanomaterials. *NanoImpact* 8, 99–116. doi: 10.1016/j.impact.2017.08.002

Fahy, J. V., and Dickey, B. F. (2010). Airway mucus function and dysfunction. *N. Engl. J. Med.* 363, 2233–2247. doi: 10.1056/NEJMra0910061

Fishler, R., Hofemeier, P., Etzion, Y., Dubowski, Y., and Sznitman, J. (2015). Particle dynamics and deposition in true-scale pulmonary acinar models OPEN. *Sci. Rep.* 5:14071. doi: 10.1038/srep14071

Gerde, P., Cheng, Y. S., and Medinsky, M. A. (1991). *In vivo* deposition of ultrafine aerosols in the nasal airway of the rat. *Toxicol. Sci.* 16, 330–336. doi: 10.1093/toxsci/16.2.330

Grainger, C. I., Greenwell, L. L., Lockley, D. J., Martin, G. P., and Forbes, B. (2006). Culture of calu-3 cells at the air interface provides a representative model of the airway epithelial barrier. *Pharm. Res.* 23, 1482–1490. doi: 10.1007/s11095-006-0255-0

Grotberg, J. B. (2011). Respiratory fluid mechanics. *Phys. Fluids* 23:021301. doi: 10.1063/1.3517737

Hassell, B. A., Goyal, G., Lee, E., Sontheimer-Phelps, A., Levy, O., Chen, C. S., et al. (2017). Human organ chip models recapitulate orthotopic lung cancer growth. Therapeutic Responses, and Tumor Dormancy In Vitro. *Cell Rep.* 21, 508–516. doi: 10.1016/j.celrep.2017.09.043

Hinds, W. C. (1999). *Aerosol Technology: Properties, Behavior, and Measurement of Airborne Particles.* Hoboken, NJ: John Wiley & Sons.

Hittinger, M., Schneider-Daum, N., and Lehr, C.-M. (2017). Cell and tissue-based in vitro models for improving the development of oral inhalation drug products. *Eur. J. Pharm. Biopharm.* 118, 73–78. doi: 10.1016/j.ejpb.2017.02.019

Hofemeier, P., and Sznitman, J. (2015). Revisiting pulmonary acinar particle transport: convection, sedimentation, diffusion, and their interplay. *J. Appl. Physiol.* 118, 1375–1385. doi: 10.1152/japplphysiol.01117.2014

Holian, A., Hamilton, R. F., Morandi, M. T., Brown, S. D., and Li, L. (1998). *Urban Particle-induced Apoptosis and Phenotype Shifts in Human Alveolar Macrophages.* Available at: https://www.ncbi.nlm.nih.gov/pmc/articles/PMC1533042/pdf/envhper00526-0053.pdf (accessed January 15, 2019).

Horsfield, K., Dart, G., Olson, D. E., Filley, G. F., Cumming, G., and Olson, E. (1971). Models of the human bronchial tree. *J. Appl. Physiol. Pri. U.S.A* 31, 207–217. doi: 10.1152/jappl.1971.31.2.207

Huh, D., Leslie, D. C., Matthews, B. D., Fraser, J. P., Jurek, S., Hamilton, G. A., et al. (2012). A human disease model of drug toxicity–induced pulmonary edema in a lung-on-a-chip microdevice. *Sci. Transl. Med.* 4:159ra147. doi: 10.1126/SCITRANSLMED.3004249

Huh, D., Matthews, B. D., Mammoto, A., Montoya-Zavala, M., Hsin, H. Y., and Ingber, D. E. (2010). Reconstituting organ-level lung functions on a chip.

Science 328, 1662–1668. doi: 10.1126/science.1188302

Humayun, M., Chow, C.-W., and Young, E. W. K. (2018). Microfluidic lung airway-on-a-chip with arrayable suspended gels for studying epithelial and smooth muscle cell interactions. *Lab Chip* 18, 1298–1309. doi: 10.1039/c7lc01357d

Imai, Y., Miki, T., Ishikawa, T., Aoki, T., and Yamaguchi, T. (2012). Deposition of micrometer particles in pulmonary airways during inhalation and breath holding. *J. Biomech.* 45, 1809–1815. doi: 10.1016/j.jbiomech.2012.04.017

Inoue, K., Takano, H., Sakurai, M., Oda, T., Tamura, H., Yanagisawa, R., et al. (2006). Pulmonary exposure to diesel exhaust particles enhances coagulation disturbance with endothelial damage and systemic inflammation related to lung inflammation. *Exp. Biol. Med.* 231, 1626–1632. doi: 10.1177/153537020623101007

Inthavong, K., Ma, J., Shang, Y., Dong, J., Chetty, A. S. R., Tu, J., et al. (2019). Geometry and airflow dynamics analysis in the nasal cavity during inhalation. *Clin. Biomech.* 66, 97–106. doi: 10.1016/j.clinbiomech.2017.10.006

Islam, M. S., Saha, S. C., Sauret, E., Gemci, T., and Gu, Y. T. (2017). Pulmonary aerosol transport and deposition analysis in upper 17 generations of the human respiratory tract. *J. Aerosol Sci.* 108, 29–43. doi: 10.1016/j.jaerosci.2017.03.004

Janssen, W. J., Stefanski, A. L., Bochner, B. S., and Evans, C. M. (2016). Control of lung defence by mucins and macrophages: ancient defence mechanisms with modern functions. *Eur. Respir. J.* 48, 1201–1214. doi: 10.1183/13993003.00120-2015

Kim, K.-H., Kabir, E., and Kabir, S. (2015). A review on the human health impact of airborne particulate matter. *Environ. Int.* 74, 136–143. doi: 10.1016/J.ENVINT.2014.10.005

Kleinstreuer, C., and Zhang, Z. (2010). Airflow and particle transport in the human respiratory system. *Annu. Rev. Fluid Mech* 42, 301–334. doi: 10.1146/annurev-fluid-121108-145453

Koullapis, P. G., Hofemeier, P., Sznitman, J., and Kassinos, S. C. (2018). An efficient computational fluid-particle dynamics method to predict deposition in a simplified approximation of the deep lung. *Eur. J. Pharm. Sci.* 113, 132–144. doi: 10.1016/j.ejps.2017.09.016

Koullapis, P., Kassinos, S. C., Muela, J., Perez-Segarra, C., Rigola, J., Lehmkuhl, O., et al. (2018). Regional aerosol deposition in the human airways: the SimInhale benchmark case and a critical assessment of in silico methods. *Eur. J. Pharm. Sci.* 113, 77–94. doi: 10.1016/j.ejps.2017.09.003

Koullapis, P. G., Kassinos, S. C., Bivolarova, M. P., and Melikov, A. K. (2016). Particle deposition in a realistic geometry of the human conducting airways: effects of inlet velocity profile, inhalation flowrate and electrostatic charge. *J. Biomech.* 49, 2201–2212. doi: 10.1016/j.jbiomech.2015.11.029

Lai, S. K., Wang, Y.-Y., and Hanes, J. (2008). Mucus-penetrating nanoparticles for drug and gene delivery to mucosal tissues ☆. *Adv. Drug Deliv. Rev.* 61, 158–171. doi: 10.1016/j.addr.2008.11.002

Lechanteur, A., das Neves, J., and Sarmento, B. (2018). The role of mucus in cell-based models used to screen mucosal drug delivery. *Adv. Drug Deli. Re* 124, 50–63. doi: 10.1016/j.addr.2017.07.019

Leggat, P. A., Kedjarune, U., and Smith, D. R. (2007). Occupational health problems in modern dentistry: a review. *Ind. Health* 45, 611–621. doi: 10.2486/indhealth.45.611

Lenz, A.-G., Stoeger, T., Cei, D., Schmidmeir, M., Semren, N., Burgstaller, G., et al. (2014). Efficient bioactive delivery of aerosolized drugs to human pulmonary epithelial cells cultured in air-liquid interface conditions. *Am. J. Respir. Cell Mol. Biol.* 51, 526–535. doi: 10.1165/rcmb.2013-0479OC

Leonard, F., Collnot, E.-M., and Lehr, C.-M. (2010). A three-dimensional coculture of enterocytes, monocytes and dendritic cells to model inflamed intestinal mucosa in vitro. *Mol. Pharm.* 7, 2103–2119. doi: 10.1021/mp1000795

Li, E., Xu, Z., Zhao, H., Sun, Z., Wang, L., Guo, Z., et al. (2015). Macrophages promote benzopyrene-induced tumor transformation of human bronchial epithelial cells by activation of NF-κB and STAT3 signaling in a bionic airway chip culture and in animal models. *Oncotarget* 6, 8900–8913. doi: 10.18632/oncotarget.3561

Lin, H., Li, H., Cho, H.-J., Bian, S., Roh, H.-J., Lee, M.-K., et al. (2007). Air-Liquid Interface (ALI) culture of human bronchial epithelial cell monolayers as an in vitro model for airway drug transport studies. *J. Pharm. Sci.* 96, 341–350. doi: 10.1002/JPS.20803

Ménache, M. G., Hofmann, W., Ashgarian, B., and Miller, F. J. (2008). Airway geometry models of children's lungs for use in dosimetry modeling. *Inhal. Toxicol.* 20, 101–126. doi: 10.1080/08958370701821433

Merck (2015). *Microsphere Coupling – Two-step EDC / Sulfo NHS Covalent Coupling Procedure for Estapor ® Carboxyl-modified Dyed Microspheres.* Kenilworth, NJ: Merck.

Mustafiz, M., Vaughan, A., Stevanovic, S., Morrison, L. E., Mohammad Pourkhesalian, A., Rahman, M., et al. (2015). Removal of organic content from diesel exhaust particles alters cellular responses of primary human bronchial epithelial cells cultured at an air-liquid interface. *J. Environ. Anal. Toxicol.* 5, 100316–100317. doi: 10.4172/2161-0525.1000316

Nemmar, A., Al-Salam, S., Dhanasekaran, S., Sudhadevi, M., and Ali, B. H. (2009). Pulmonary exposure to diesel exhaust particles promotes cerebral microvessel thrombosis: protective effect of a cysteine prodrug l-2-oxothiazolidine-4-carboxylic acid. *Toxicology* 263, 84–92. doi: 10.1016/J.TOX.2009.06.017

Nemmar, A., Al-Salam, S., Zia, S., Marzouqi, F., Al-Dhaheri, A., Subramaniyan, D., et al. (2011). Contrasting actions of diesel exhaust particles on the pulmonary and cardiovascular systems and the effects of thymoquinone. *Br. J. Pharmacol.* 164, 1871–1882. doi: 10.1111/j.1476-5381.2011.01442.x

Nemmar, A., Holme, J. A., Rosas, I., Schwarze, P. E., and Alfaro-Moreno, E. (2013). Recent advances in particulate matter and nanoparticle toxicology: a review of the in vivo and in vitro studies. *Biomed Res. Int.* 2013, 279371. doi: 10.1155/2013/279371

Nesmith, A. P., Agarwal, A., McCain, M. L., and Parker, K. K. (2014). Human airway musculature on a chip: an in vitro model of allergic asthmatic bronchoconstriction and bronchodilation. *Lab Chip* 14, 3925–3936. doi: 10.1039/C4LC00688G

Paur, H. R., Cassee, F. R., Teeguarden, J., Fissan, H., Diabate, S., Aufderheide, M., et al. (2011). In-vitro cell exposure studies for the assessment of nanoparticle toxicity in the lung-A dialog between aerosol science and biology. *J. Aerosol Sci.* 42, 668–692. doi: 10.1016/j.jaerosci.2011.06.005

Pedley, T. J. (2003). Pulmonary fluid dynamics. *Annu. Rev. Fluid Mech.* 9, 229–274. doi: 10.1146/annurev.fl.09.010177.001305

Petitot, F., Lestaevel, P., Tourlonias, E., Mazzucco, C., Jacquinot, S., Dhieux, B., et al. (2013). Inhalation of uranium nanoparticles: respiratory tract deposition and translocation to secondary target organs in rats. *Toxicol. Lett.* 217, 217–225. doi: 10.1016/j.toxlet.2012.12.022

Punde, T. H., Wu, W. H., Lien, P. C., Chang, Y. L., Kuo, P. H., Chang, M. D. T., et al. (2015). A biologically inspired lung-on-a-chip device for the study of protein-induced lung inflammation. *Integr. Biol* 7, 162–169. doi: 10.1039/c4ib00239c

Rayner, R. E., Makena, P., Prasad, G. L., and Cormet-Boyaka, E. (2019). Optimization of normal human bronchial epithelial (NHBE) cell 3D cultures for in vitro lung model studies. *Sci. Rep.* 9:500. doi: 10.1038/s41598-018-36735-z

Röhm, M., Carle, S., Maigler, F., Flamm, J., Kramer, V., Mavoungou, C., et al. (2017). A comprehensive screening platform for aerosolizable protein formulations for intranasal and pulmonary drug delivery. *Int. J. Pharm.* 532, 537–546. doi: 10.1016/j.ijpharm.2017.09.027

Ronaldson-Bouchard, K., and Vunjak-Novakovic, G. (2018). Organs-on-a-chip: a fast track for engineered human tissues in drug development. *Cell Stem Cell* 22, 310–324. doi: 10.1016/j.stem.2018.02.011

Sauret, V., Halson, P. M., Brown, I. W., Fleming, J. S., and Bailey, A. G. (2002). Study of the three-dimensional geometry of the central conducting airways in man using computed tomographic (CT) images. *J. Anat.* 200, 123–134. doi: 10.1046/j.0021-8782.2001.00018.x

Schuster, B. S., Suk, J. S., Woodworth, G. F., and Hanes, J. (2013). Nanoparticle diffusion in respiratory mucus from humans without lung disease. *Biomaterials* 34, 3439–3446. doi: 10.1016/j.biomaterials.2013.01.064

Shirure, V. S., Bi, Y., Curtis, M. B., Lezia, A., Goedegebuure, M. M., Goedegebuure, S. P., et al. (2018). Tumor-on-a-chip platform to investigate progression and drug sensitivity in cell lines and patient-derived organoids. *Lab Chip* 18, 3687–3702. doi: 10.1039/C8LC00596F

Skardal, A., Shupe, T., and Atala, A. (2016). Organoid-on-a-chip and body-on-a-chip systems for drug screening and disease modeling. *Drug Discov. Today* 21, 1399–1411. doi: 10.1016/j.drudis.2016.07.003

Stahlhofen, W., Rudolf, G., and James, A. C. (1989). Intercomparison of Experimental Regional Aerosol Deposition Data. *J. Aerosol Med.* 2, 285–308. doi: 10.1089/jam.1989.2.285

Stannard, W., and O'Callaghan, C. (2006). Ciliary function and the role of cilia in clearance. *J. AEROSOL Med* 19, 110–115. doi: 10.1089/jam.2006.19.110

Stucki, A. O., Stucki, J. D., Hall, S. R. R., Felder, M., Mermoud, Y., Schmid, R. A., et al. (2014). From chip-in-a-lab to lab-on-a-chip: towards a single handheld electronic system for multiple application-specific lab-on-a-chip (ASLOC). *Lab Chip* 15, 1302–1310. doi: 10.1039/c4lc01252f

Sznitman, J. (2013). Respiratory microflows in the pulmonary acinus. *J. Biomech.* 46, 284–298. doi: 10.1016/j.jbiomech.2012.10.028

Tenenbaum-Katan, J., Artzy-Schnirman, A., Fishler, R., Korin, N., and Sznitman, J. (2018). Biomimetics of the pulmonary environment in vitro: a microfluidics perspective. *Biomicrofluidics* 12:042209. doi: 10.1063/1.5023034

Veranth, J. M., Moss, T. A., Chow, J. C., Labban, R., Nichols, W. K., Walton, J. C., et al. (2006). Correlation of in vitro cytokine responses with the chemical composition of soil-derived particulate matter. *Environ. Health Perspect.* 114, 341–349. doi: 10.1289/ehp.8360

Veronesi, B., Oortgiesen, M., Carter, J. D., and Devlin, R. B. (1999). Particulate matter initiates inflammatory cytokine release by activation of capsaicin and acid receptors in a human bronchial epithelial cell line. *Toxicol. Appl. Pharmacol.* 154, 106–115. doi: 10.1006/taap.1998.8567

Weibel, E. R., Cournand, A. F., and Richards, D. W. (1963). *Morphometry of the Human Lung.* Berlin: Springer.

Whitsett, J. A. (2018). Airway epithelial differentiation and mucociliary clearance. *Ann. Am. Thorac. Soc.* 15, S143–S148. doi: 10.1513/AnnalsATS.201802-128AW

Wu, W., Jin, Y., and Carlsten, C. (2018). Inflammatory health effects of indoor and outdoor particulate matter. *J. Allergy Clin. Immunol.* 141, 833–844. doi: 10.1016/J.JACI.2017.12.981

Wu, W., Samet, J. M., Ghio, A. J., and Devlin, R. B. (2001). Activation of the EGF receptor signaling pathway in airway epithelial cells exposed to Utah Valley PM. *Am. J. Physiol. - Lung Cell. Mol. Physiol.* 281, 483–489. doi: 10.1152/ajplung.2001.281.2.l483

Zhang, Z., Kleinstreuer, C., and Kim, C. S. (2009). Comparison of analytical and CFD models with regard to micron particle deposition in a human 16-generation tracheobronchial airway model. *J. Aerosol Sci.* 40, 16–28. doi: 10.1016/j.jaerosci.2008.08.003

5

Humidified and Heated Cascade Impactor for Aerosol Sizing

Caroline Majoral[1,2], Allan L. Coates[3], Alain Le Pape[1,2] and Laurent Vecellio[1,2]*

[1] INSERM, Research Center for Respiratory Diseases, Tours, France, [2] Université de Tours, Tours, France, [3] Hospital for Sick Children, Toronto, ON, Canada

Aerosol sizing is generally measured at ambient air but human airways have different temperature (37°C) and relative humidity (100%) which can affect particle size in airways and consequently deposition prediction. This work aimed to develop and evaluate a new method using cascade impactor to measure particle size at human physiological temperature and humidity (HPTH) taking into account ambient air conditions. A heated and humidified trachea was built and a cascade impactor was heated to 37°C and humidified inside. Four medical aerosols [jet nebulizer, mesh nebulizer, Presurized Metered Dose Inhaler (pMDI), and Dry Powder Inhaler (DPI)] under ambient conditions and at HPTH were tested. MMAD was lower at HPTH for the two nebulizers; it was similar at ambient conditions and HPTH for pMDI, and the mass of particles smaller than 5 μm decreased for DPI at HPTH (51.9 vs. 82.8 μg/puff). In conclusion, we developed a new method to measure particle size at HPTH affecting deposition prediction with relevance. *In vivo* studies are required to evaluate the interest of this new model to improve the precision of deposition prediction.

Keywords: aerosol, cascade impactor, particle, inhalation, size, temperature, humidity

INTRODUCTION

Correspondence:
Laurent Vecellio
vecellio@med.univ-tours.fr

Aerosol particle size is a key parameter for predicting aerosol deposition in the airways of the lungs. Several methods of particle sizing can be used, cascade impactors and lasers being the most common. Cascade impactors offer the major advantage of measuring the aerodynamic diameter of the drug studied.

They are used in different regulatories (ISO 27427, 2012) and pharmacopeias (USP 28-Nf 23, 2005) with a continuous and constant air flow. However, this experimental set up does not take into account the effect of ventilation parameters from the patient which can modify the particle size. Sangwan et al. (2003) has used a low flow cascade impactor (1 L/min) with a breathing machine to mimic patient inhalation. They used clinically relevant breathing patterns to simulate aerosol delivery on the bench recognizing that, during a drug treatment the patient would be breathing a mixture of air at a certain tidal volume and frequency as well as air from the nebulizer and that this degree of ambient air mixing might influence the final inhaled distribution. Finally in a series of human studies demonstrated the relationship between predicting deposition via bench studies and effects on actual deposition measure particle size at different ventilation conditions. The low flow cascade impactor has the advantage to reduce the impact of air sampling on ventilation parameters and to reduce the particle evaporation effect in standing cloud set up (Solomita and Smaldone, 2009) but it has the unconvenient to collect a small fraction of aerosol which can be different to the aerosol cloud (Vecellio None et al., 2001).

In vitro measurements of aerosol particle size with a cascade impactor are usually made at ambient conditions of temperature and relative humidity (RH).

It has been shown that the temperature of a jet nebulizer outlet can decrease by more than 10°C, leading to evaporation of the droplets when entering the cascade impactor placed at ambient temperature. Previous studies have investigated the effect of temperature on aerosol sizing by cooling the impactor in order to limit droplet evaporation (Stapleton and Finlay, 1998; Kwong et al., 2000; Zhou et al., 2005a; Rao et al., 2010). Several studies have also investigated the effect of ambient air humidity on particle size distribution by sizing the aerosols at several different values of relative humidity (Prokop et al., 1995; Finlay et al., 1997; Nerbrink et al., 2003; Zhou et al., 2005b). However, the human respiratory tract is at 37°C and almost 100%RH (Ferron, 1977; Ferron et al., 1985; O'Doherty and Miller, 1993), which can alter particle size either through evaporation or condensation (i.e., hygroscopic growth) and can therefore affect the relevance of the prediction of deposition in the respiratory tract.

Studies have focused on mathematically modeling heat and water transport in the human respiratory tract (Daviskas et al., 1990; Eisner, 1992; Finlay and Stapleton, 1995; Zhang et al., 2006), or on establishing equations to predict the change in size of hygroscopic inhaled particles (Ferron, 1977; Ferron et al., 1988; Gradon and Podgórski, 1996; Broday and Georgopoulos, 2001; Longest and Hindle, 2012; Boudin et al., 2020). Particle growing in airways has been recently considered as a potential interest to reduce upper airways deposition and increase lung penetration, and deposition when using submicronic aerosols (Longest and Hindle, 2012; Spence et al., 2019). Martin et al. (1988) developed a model for particle sizing composed of a trachea and a cascade impactor at 37°C and either 30%RH or 97.5%RH. However, their model did not duplicate what happens *in vivo*. Instead of humidifying the aerosol after its generation, they humidified and heated the ambient air to 37°C before it entered the model. In fact, when a patient inhales an aerosol, the air he/she breathes comes from the atmosphere and is at ambient conditions of temperature, and humidity. In another study, Bell and Ho (1981) developed an experimental system which mixed a dry monodisperse aerosol with water-saturated air at 37°C at the top of a growth tube. They sized aerosol particles at the exit of this tube using an optical particle counter, thus measuring the geometric diameter, but neither the aerodynamic diameter nor the drug mass contained in the particles.

Consequently, temperature and humidity affect particle size. Particle size modification in airways depends on device and formulation. Different mathematical models have been developed to predict this size modification but they are complex to use. Different experimental measurement methods have been developed to measure *in vitro* aerosol size at 37°C and 100% but they have not measured the size of aerosol drug in realistic ambiant air mixing conditions, i.e., with ambiant temperature and humidity crossing the device and followed by a heating and humidifying just after aerosol delivery.

The purpose of the present study was (1) to develop an *in vitro* cascade impactor measurement method approaching human temperature and humidity with the respect of the ambient air before penetration in the trachea/induction port model, (2) to compare aerosol particle size measured at ambient conditions and at HPTH to evaluate the relevance of our method.

MATERIALS AND METHODS

Materials
Experimental Set Up at Ambient Air
The aerosol were sized using an 8-stage Andersen Cascade Impactor (ACI) (Mark II, Ecomesure, France) operating at 28.3 L/min for nebulizers and pMDI, and operating at 60 L/min for DPI. An artificial trachea for the ACI was created using a coarse screen wrapped with cotton with a heating coil running inside the walls which were then covered with aluminum foil and plastic (**Figure 1**). Absorbent glass fiber filters (Type A/E Glass, Pall Corporation, United States) were used on each plate of the impactor. The trachea was kept dry and not heated, and the cascade impactor was used with dry filters and at ambient temperature (22 ± 3°C; 50 ± 10%RH) (**Figure 2A**).

Experimental Set Up at 37°C and Ambient RH
Same cascade impactor and trachea as described above were used. The trachea was dry and heated to 37°C and the impactor was warmed in a water bath at 37°C. A potentiometer was used to regulate the temperature of the heating coil to 37°C and a temperature sensor was used to measure the temperature of the trachea and of the water bath. The filters on cascade impactor stages were dry so that humidity inside the impactor was the same as that of the ambient air, as the impactor was perfectly watertight (**Figure 2B**).

Experimental Set Up at 37°C and 100% RH
Same cascade impactor and trachea as described above were used. In this experimental set up, the trachea was humidified inside with water and heated to 37°C, and the cascade impactor filters were moistened with 3 mL of water and placed in a water bath at 37°C (**Figure 2C**).

Inhalation Drug Delivery Devices
Different inhalation drug were tested: Jet nebulizer (PariLC Star® with Turbo Boy N® compressor, Pari, Germany) filled with 2 mL of terbutaline (Bricanyl® 5 mg/2 mL, Astra Zeneca, France) or with 2 mL of 1%w/v NaF solution, a vibrating

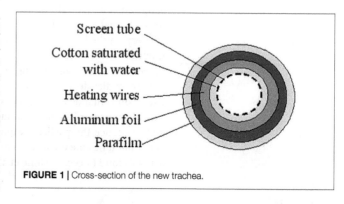

FIGURE 1 | Cross-section of the new trachea.

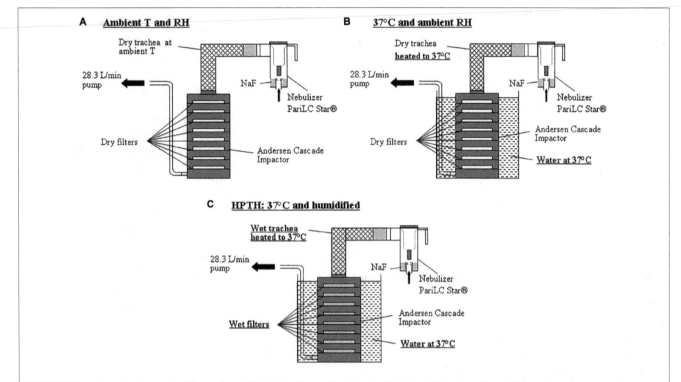

FIGURE 2 | Experimental set-ups using ACI sampling at 28.3 L/min with stage's substrates (filters) for 3 different conditions: **(A)** Aerosol measurement using cascade impactor at ambient temperature and ambient relative humidity. **(B)** Aerosol measurement using cascade impactor in a bath of water at 37°C and ambient relative humidity. **(C)** Aerosol measurement using cascade impactor in a bath of water at 37°C and humidified air inside the trachea model and the cascade impactor using the new trachea and wetted stage's substrates (HPTH: human physiological temperature and humidity).

mesh nebulizer (Aeroneb Go®, Ireland, United States) filled with 2 mL of terbutaline (Bricanyl® 5 mg /2 mL, Astra Zeneca, France), a salbutamol Presurized Metered Dose Inhaler (PMDI) (Ventoline® 100 µg/puff, GlaxoSmithKline, France), and a terbutaline Dry Powder Inhaler (DPI) (Bricanyl® Turbuhaler® 500 µg/puff, Astra Zeneca, France). Only the Pari LC Star® nebulizer with NaF was measured at 37°C-ambient humidity. Others inhalation drug delivery device were sized at ambient conditions (**Figure 2A**) and at HPTH (**Figure 2C**).

Methods
Experimental Setup Validation
Three milliliter of water were poured onto dry absorbent filters (Type A/E Glass, Pall Corporation, United States) laid on each impactor plate and they were each immediately weighed. The experimental set-up at HPTH described in **Figure 2C** was then carried out, substituting the nebulizer by an absolute filter to limit the risk of air particle contamination on wet filters. The impactor pump, operating at 28.3 L/min, was turned on for 5 min. The impactor was then dismantled and the filters were weighed again. The difference between the weights of the filters before and after the 5 min of sampling corresponded to the quantity of water evaporated inside the impactor during the 5 min. The experiment was performed three times. The relative humidity inside the trachea was measured after its humidification by a humidity measuring stick (Testo, France). Each experiment was carried out in triplicate.

Aerosol Sizing
For the two nebulizers, nebulization was stopped when no more aerosol was produced. After Naf nebulization, each filter and impactor stage were placed in 10 mL of 25% TISAB solution (TISAB IV, Riedel-de Haën, Germany) and was assayed with a fluoride electrode.

After terbutaline nebulization, each filter was placed in a centrifuge tube and each impactor stage was placed in 20 mL of sodium hydroxide 0.1M. The amount of drug was assayed by UV-spectrophotometry (Spectronic Unicam, Helios, United Kingdom). Residual drug mass in nebulizers was measured by drug assay method.

For pMDI, a total of 30 puffs of the were delivered for each experiment. The UV spectrophotometer was calibrated to measure salbutamol, and the filters were processed as described above for the nebulizers.

Terbutaline Turbuhaler® DPI required a 60 L/min pump instead of a 28.3 L/min pump. As the ACI was calibrated at 28.3 L/min, the usual values given for the cut-off diameters were only valid for the impactor operating at 28.3 L/min. The cut-off diameters were determined for a 60 L/min flow rate according to the following formula (Van Oort et al., 1996; Marple et al., 2003):

$$D_{60L/min} = D_{28.3L/min}\sqrt{\frac{28.3}{60}}$$

where $D_{60L/min}$ and $D_{28.3L/min}$ correspond to the cut-off diameters for the ACI operating at 60 and 28.3 L/min respectively.

The values of the cut-off diameters for a flow rate of 28.3 L/min were 9, 5.8, 4.7, 3.3, 2.1, 1.1, 0.7, and 0.4 μm for stages 0–7, respectively. The values of the cut-off diameters for a flow rate of 60 L/min were 6.2, 4.0, 3.2, 2.3, 1.4, 0.8, 0.5, and 0.3 μm for stages 0–7, respectively.

A total of 20 puffs of terbutaline Turbuhaler® DPI were generated for each experiment. The filters were processed as described above for the nebulizers.

Analysis of the Results

NaF aerosol particle size distributions were represented as mass deposited per stages in the cascade impactor. The percentage of recovery from the impactor and the trachea was expressed from the nebulizer load for the nebulizers, the difference from 100% corresponding to the residual volume. The deposition in the trachea was calculated by subtracting (total deposition on the impactor stages + residual volume) from the initial charge for nebulizers, and (total deposition on the impactor stages) from the emitted dose for the PMDI and DPI.

The results were also expressed in terms of Mass Median Aerodynamic Diameter (MMAD), total deposited mass on the stages of the impactor, % recovery from the impactor and the trachea of the nebulizer load for the nebulizers and of the emitted dose for the PMDI and DPI, and mass of particles smaller than 5 μm, also called the respirable mass or fine particle dose and predicting deposited mass in the lungs (Coates et al., 1998; ISO 27427, 2012).

RESULTS

Validation of the Method

A volume of 0.41 ± 0.07 mL of water was evaporated from each filter during the 5 min of sampling. There was no difference between each stage in term of evaporated volume water. These results validated the humidification of the air inside the impactor. The relative humidity inside the trachea after its humidification was superior to 95%, which corresponds to the relative humidity inside the respiratory tract.

Aerosol Sizing at Different Air Temperature and Humidity Conditions

MMAD, total deposited mass on the stages of the ACI and % recovery from the impactor and the trachea of the nebulizer load of 1%w/v NaF aerosol nebulized with PariLC Star® for the three experimental set-ups are summarized in **Table 1**. MMAD equaled 2.6 ± 0.2, 1.3 ± 0.1, and 1.8 ± 0.1 μm for ambient T and RH, 37°C and ambient RH, and HPTH respectively. Total deposited mass on the stages of the impactor was similar for the three experimental set-ups (10.0 ± 0.7, 9.2 ± 0.3, and 9.3 ± 0.7 mg).

Figure 3 shows the deposited mass on impactor stages with NaF aerosol nebulized by PariLC Star® for the three experimental set-ups.

MMAD, total deposited mass on the stages of the ACI, % recovery from the impactor and the trachea of the nebulizer load for the nebulizers and of the emitted dose for the PMDI and DPI,

and mass of particles smaller than 5 μm of terbutaline nebulized with PariLC Star® and Aeroneb Go® nebulizers, salbutamol PMDI and terbutaline Turbuhaler® DPI for both ambient conditions and HPTH are summarized in **Table 2**. MMAD values at ambient conditions and HPTH were, respectively, 2.1 ± 0.3 and 1.6 ± 0.1 μm for PariLC Star®, 3.3 ± 0.1 and 2.0 ± 0.2 μm for Aeroneb Go®, 3.1 ± 0.0 and 3.1 ± 0.1 μm for salbutamol PMDI, 3.7 ± 0.0 and 3.2 ± 0.1 μm for terbutaline Turbuhaler® DPI. Total deposited mass on the stages of the impactor was similar at ambient conditions and HPTH for all the devices except for terbutaline Turbuhaler® DPI: it was, respectively, 2.3 ± 0.2 and 2.5 ± 0.3 mg for PariLC Star®, 3.9 ± 0.3 and 3.9 ± 0.3 mg for Aeroneb Go®, 0.6 ± 0.0 and 0.6 ± 0.0 mg for salbutamol PMDI, 2.6 ± 0.2 and 1.5 ± 0.2 mg for terbutaline Turbuhaler® DPI. The mass of particles smaller than 5 μm was also similar at ambient conditions and HPTH for all the devices except for terbutaline Turbuhaler® DPI: it was, respectively, 2.0 ± 0.2 and 2.2 ± 0.2 mg for PariLC Star®, 2.9 ± 0.1 and 2.9 ± 0.2 mg for Aeroneb Go®, 15.8 ± 0.5 and 15.8 ± 1.3 μg/puff for salbutamol PMDI, 82.8 ± 8.7 μg/puff and 51.9 ± 3.3 μg/puff for terbutaline Turbuhaler® DPI. **Figure 4** shows the deposited mass on impactor stages with the differents devices at HPTH and ambient air conditions.

DISCUSSION

This study developed an operational method of aerosol sizing at human humidity and temperature conditions and taken into account inhaled air at ambient temperature and humidity. This study has not the objective to be an alternative of regulatories/standard methods but to provide scientific information regarding the effect of temperature and humidity in inhaled condition on particle size and consequently deposition. Standard methods measure particle sizes emitted by the device. Our method has the objective to measure the particle size in the airways.

The first step of the study, consisting in sizing 1%w/v NaF aerosol nebulized with PariLC Star® nebulizer for three intermediate experimental set-ups, highlighted the effect of temperature and humidity on particle size. It demonstrated that MMAD decreased significantly when heating to 37°C as the particles evaporated (2.6 vs. 1.3 μm); it then increased when RH was brought to saturation due to condensation, i.e., hygroscopic growth (1.3 vs. 1.8 μm). The second set-up may have been subjected to a decrease in relative humidity below ambient conditions, and thus conditions in the trachea and cascade impactor for this experimental set-up may have been drier than ambient conditions. The decrease of MMAD when comparing it at ambient temperature and RH and at HPTH (2.6 vs. 1.8 μm) leads to the conclusion that evaporation has more impact than condensation. This may be due to the functioning of the PariLC Star® nebulizer: the air circulates through the interior of the PariLC Star® and becomes saturated with humidity drawn from the large reservoir of solution (Nerbrink et al., 2003), so the air carrying the aerosol is already saturated when it comes out of the nebulizer. Prediction of lung deposition was

TABLE 1 | MMAD, total deposited mass on the stages of the ACI and % recovery from the impactor and the trachea of the nebulizer load of 1%w/v NaF aerosol nebulized with PariLC Star® for the three experimental set-ups [Ambient T and RH; 37°C and ambient RH; 37°C and humidified (HPTH: human physiological temperature and humidity)], expressed as mean ± standard deviation.

	MMAD (μm)	Total deposited mass on the stages of the ACI (mg) (% of the nebulizer load)	% recovery from the trachea of the nebulizer load
(1) Ambient T and RH	2.6 ± 0.2	10.0 ± 0.7 (47 ± 3%)	4 ± 4%
(2) 37°C and ambient RH	1.3 ± 0.1	9.2 ± 0.3 (46 ± 2%)	1 ± 2%
(3) HPTH	1.8 ± 0.1	9.3 ± 0.7 (43 ± 3%)	3 ± 3%

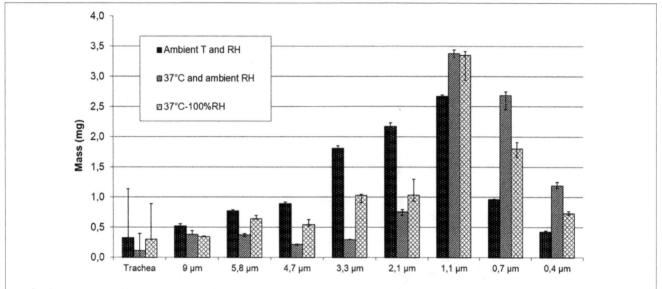

FIGURE 3 | Deposited mass on impactor stages using 1%w/v NaF aerosol nebulized with PariLC Star® for the three conditions of temperature (T) and relative humidity (RH): ambient T and ambient RH; 37°C and ambient RH; 37°C and 100% RH inside the trachea model and the cascade impactor.

TABLE 2 | MMAD, total deposited mass on the stages of the ACI, % recovery from the impactor and the trachea of the nebulizer load for the nebulizers and of the emitted dose for the pMDI and DPI, and mass of particles smaller than 5 μm of terbutaline (5 mg/2 mL) nebulized with PariLC Star and Aeroneb Go® nebulizers, salbutamol pMDI (100 μg/puff) and terbutaline Turbuhaler® DPI (500 μg/puff) for both ambient conditions and 37°C-humidified (HPTH: human physiological temperature and humidity), expressed as mean ± standard deviation.

		MMAD (μm)	Total deposited mass on the stages of the ACI (mg) (% of the nebulizer load or emitted dose)	% recovery from the trachea of the nebulizer load or emitted dose	Mass of particles < 5 μm
PariLC Star (1) + terbutaline	Ambient T and RH	2.1 ± 0.3	2.3 ± 0.2 (43 ± 3%)	6 ± 3%	2.0 ± 0.2 (mg)
	HPTH	1.6 ± 0.1	2.5 ± 0.3 (47 ± 4%)	6 ± 3%	2.2 ± 0.2 (mg)
Aeroneb Go® (2) + terbutaline	Ambient T and RH	3.3 ± 0.1	3.9 ± 0.3 (76 ± 1%)	6 ± 1%	2.9 ± 0.1 (mg)
	HPTH	2.0 ± 0.2	3.9 ± 0.3 (74 ± 5%)	10 ± 5%	2.9 ± 0.2 (mg)
Salbutamol pMDI (3)	Ambient T and RH	3.1 ± 0.0	0.6 ± 0.0 (26 ± 1%)	74 ± 1%	15.8 ± 0.5 (μg/puff)
	HPTH	3.1 ± 0.1	0.6 ± 0.0 (28 ± 2%)	72 ± 2%	15.8 ± 1.3 (μg/puff)
Terbutaline DPI (4)	Ambient T and RH	3.7 ± 0.1	2.6 ± 0.2 (41 ± 3%)	59 ± 3%	82.8 ± 8.7 (μg/puff)
	HPTH	3.2 ± 0.1	1.5 ± 0.2 (25 ± 3%)	75 ± 3%	51.9 ± 3.3 (μg/puff)

(1) jet nebulizer, (2) vibrating mesh nebulizer, (3) presurized metered-dose inhaler (pMDI), (4) dry powder inhaler (DPI).

consequently higher in the peripheral region at HPTH than at ambient conditions (MMAD smaller at HPTH than at ambiant condition), but both conditions (HPTH and ambient) predicted a significant deposition in the pulmonary region (mass of particles < 5 μm). These results could explain why Sangwan et al. (2003) have correlated cascade impaction data with deposition studies

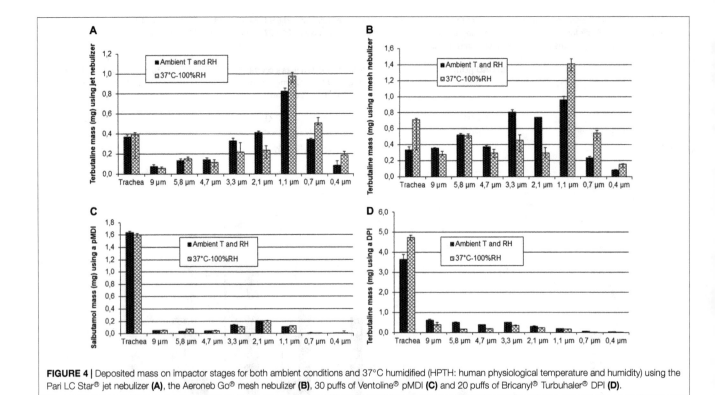

FIGURE 4 | Deposited mass on impactor stages for both ambient conditions and 37°C humidified (HPTH: human physiological temperature and humidity) using the Pari LC Star® jet nebulizer **(A)**, the Aeroneb Go® mesh nebulizer **(B)**, 30 puffs of Ventoline® pMDI **(C)** and 20 puffs of Bricanyl® Turbuhaler® DPI **(D)**.

and found that a more meaningful cut off is 2.5 μm instead of 5 μm. Our work also tested the three main types of device: two nebulizers (a jet nebulizer and a vibrating mesh nebulizer), a PMDI and a DPI. This enabled the behavior of each kind of device to be studied for the two conditions of temperature and humidity (ambient and HPTH), and to determine their respective sensitivity to high temperature and humidity. The comparison of particle size distributions sized at ambient conditions and at HPTH showed that MMAD at HPTH was smaller than at ambient conditions for the two nebulizers (PariLC Star® and Aeroneb Go®) with terbutaline, which is consistent with the results described above for NaF solution aerosolized with PariLC Star®. This indicates that particle evaporation was greater than hygroscopic growth.

An explanation of this low effect of condensation, even with the Aeroneb Go® nebulizer, could be the same as that given by Finlay and Smaldone (1998), who emphasized that much of the understanding of hygroscopic aerosols is based on considering the fate of single droplets which may behave quite differently from the clouds of droplets produced by nebulizers, as it is possible for such clouds to behave in a non-hygroscopic way. Aerosols with large numbers of droplets per unit volume, such as can occur with nebulized aerosols, can actually self-humidify the air around them and thereby prematurely stop hygroscopic size changes. This phenomenon, known as the "two-way coupled effect," occurs when each droplet shrinks only slightly, but the number of droplets is so great that the vapor evaporating off the droplets into the surrounding air causes the air to reach water vapor equilibrium (Finlay, 1998). Thus, the "two-way coupled effect" may stabilize some hygroscopic aerosols against

size alteration in the respiratory tract. While the airflow rate of our model was fixed, changing the airflow rate may change the dilution of the aerosol in the air, which could give different results.

This result is consistent with the study of Martin et al. (2005) who observed no significant difference in the evaporation rate of PMDI between dry and humid conditions at 37°C, i.e., PMDI particles did not evaporate more slowly in the presence of high levels of humidity. In their study, the droplets placed at 37°C evaporated under both humid and dry conditions, showing that evaporation was greater than condensation. Another study performed by Martin and Finlay (2005) led to the hypothesis that in humid conditions, PMDI particles initially undergo a rapid evaporation of propellant from residual drug particles which quickly reduces aerosol diameters, then a transient growth of propellant-cooled particles due to condensation of water, followed by a water re-evaporation at a steady, warmer temperature. Thus, given sufficient time, quasi-steady state evaporation of water from PMDI particles may largely negate the initial condensation.

For the nebulizers and the salbutamol PMDI, there was no difference in total drug deposition on the ACI stages between ambient conditions and HPTH, indicating that particles did not grow at the entrance of the trachea (before being impacted on the impactor stages) at HPTH. However, the results obtained for terbutaline Turbuhaler® DPI showed many fewer particles were deposited in the cascade impactor at HPTH than at ambient conditions, indicating that more particles were deposited in the trachea at HPTH. This would mean that at HPTH, particles grew very rapidly at the entrance of the trachea due to condensation, and impacted on the walls of the trachea and the cylinder. As a result, the mass of particles smaller than 5 μm at HPTH was nearly half that under ambient conditions. Terbutaline Turbuhaler® DPI was the only device tested whose particles grew, i.e., underwent more condensation than evaporation. This phenomenon may be explained by the fact that terbutaline Turbuhaler® DPI is a powder, and thus much more subject to hygroscopic growth than a solution. Moisture is well known to affect powder cohesion through capillary force at high relative humidity (Telko and Hickey, 2005; Chan, 2006).

There are clearly some limitations to this study. The flow chosen were constant and did not follow a pattern of breathing. The flow of 28.3 L/min was that recommended for the ACI and has stood the test of time with regard to accuracy. It is also a reasonable approximation of the mean inspiratory flow of an adult (tidal volume 750 mL and inspiratory time of 1.5 s). However, it would be too low to fully activate the DPI device so the flow of 60 L/min was chosen with a mathematical recalculation of the cut points which could have introduced some inaccuracies. This flow would be in the same order of magnitude as that expected from a patient inhaling forcefully from the device. These studies are in contrast to those of where Sangwan et al. (2003); Solomita and Smaldone (2009), Sagalla and Smaldone (2014), and Samuel and Smaldone (2020) used a low flow impactor to sample the aerosol rather than directing the entire output of the device into the impactor. This set up has the advantage to use a pattern of breathing but eliminated the "throat" where, in the present setup, it is expected that most of the changes in particle size occurred. NGI cascade impactor with a lower flow rate at 15 L/min is recommended for nebulizers particle size measurement (ISO 27427, 2012). Our method could be adapted with the NGI cascade impactor. A further issue is that they used either normal saline (Solomita and Smaldone, 2009; Sagalla and Smaldone, 2014) or γ interferon (Sangwan et al., 2003; Samuel and Smaldone, 2020) whereas the focus in the present study was asthma medication and the results suggest that changes in particle size due to exposure to HPTH conditions are specific for individual formulations. Finally, this was an *in vitro* study designed to evaluate temperature and humidity on various asthma medication and their delivery systems and does not have the power of *in vivo* deposition studies (Sangwan et al., 2003; Sagalla and Smaldone, 2014; Samuel and Smaldone, 2020) to predict pulmonary deposition in the face of significant disease.

The overall comparison of the four devices tested predicted a major deposition in the central and peripheral regions of the lung for the nebulizers (PariLC Star® and Aeroneb Go®), and in upper airways for the salbutamol PMDI and the terbutaline Turbuhaler® DPI. Thus PariLC Star® and Aeroneb Go® may allow the desired site of action to be targeted, i.e., the lung, whereas most of the drug delivered by salbutamol PMDI and terbutaline Turbuhaler® DPI may be lost in the upper airways. The high injection speed for the salbutamol PMDI and the 60 L/min sampling flow rate for the terbutaline Turbuhaler® DPI are mainly responsible for this large deposition in the trachea (Newman et al., 1996; Newman, 2003).

In this study, the nebulizers were associated with terbutaline solution. It is essential to consider the "nebulizer + solution to nebulize" couple and not the nebulizer alone, as one nebulizer can produce a different aerosol with different solutions. Results may have been different if another drug had been used. Formulation affects the particle growing/evaporation and consequently deposition prediction.

The potential change in cut-off diameters of the cascade impactor stages at 37°C was taken into account. Particle collection at the impactor stage is governed by the Stokes number. The cut-off diameter of the corresponding stage can be calculated from the Stokes number and depends on air viscosity. Air viscosity is defined by Willeke and Baron (1993), Baron and Willeke (2001):

$$\mu = \frac{\mu(\text{ref}) * (T(\text{ref}) + S)}{T + S} * \left(\frac{T}{T(\text{ref})}\right)^{3/2}$$

where $\mu(\text{ref})$ is the reference air viscosity (183.25 micropoise), $T(\text{ref})$ is the reference temperature (293.15 Kelvin), S is the Sutherland constant (110.4 Kelvin).

When comparing air viscosity at 20°C (ambient temperature) and 37°C, a deviation of 4% was observed. This deviation is not significant compared to the bias between the experiments.

The Stokes number can be defined by Hinds (1999), Willeke and Baron (1993), Baron and Willeke (2001):

$$St = \frac{\rho_p * d_p^2 * Q * C_p}{9 * \mu * W}$$

where ρ_p is the particle density (1,000 kg/m³), d_p is the particle diameter, Q is the jet velocity, C_p is the slip correction factor, μ is the air viscosity, W is the jet diameter.

For $d_p = 3$ μm and W = 0.0025 m, a deviation of 2% was observed when comparing air viscosity at 20°C (ambient temperature) and 37°C.

Mathematical models, which can be used to predict aerosol deposition in the respiratory tract, require knowledge of many parameters, including the characteristics of the drug, the aerosol generator and the aerosol itself. As the aerosol particle size has to be known, it seems more relevant to perform the sizing directly at HPTH to predict drug deposition. This is a considerable advantage of the method proposed in this study which allows study of the effect of temperature and humidity on the aerosol generated by the device and not on the device itself, a distinction which is not always clearly made. Moreover, our model is close to human physiological conditions where the air carrying the aerosol came from the ambient atmosphere, which is similar to the clinical setting. The continuous airflow may approximate the deep inhalation for PMDI and DPI, but did not simulate patient breathing for nebulizers. However, this study was an initial step in exploring the potential for hygroscopic growth and other changes to the aerosol that could take place while particle sizing with the ACI. The results obtained in this study for the nebulizers are consistent with the study of Fleming et al. (2006) which showed that alveolar deposition (i.e., small particles) was greater for *in vivo* experiments than for the LUDEP deposition modeling program. Our results could explain this difference. Finally, terbutaline Turbuhaler® DPI was the only device subject to hygroscopic growth, since its mass of particles smaller than 5 μm decreased at HPTH, whereas it did not change for the nebulizers and the salbutamol pMDI.

CONCLUSION

An aerosol sizing at controlled temperature and humidity with the respect of ambient air before aerosol delivery has been developed using a cascade impactor. Using physiological temperature (37°C) and humidity (100%RH) conditions vs. ambient air condition, we observed a decrease of particle size for liquid aerosol produced by nebulizers; no particle size change for PMDI, and a decrease of mass of particle smaller than 5 μm suggesting a rapid particle growing for powder aerosol produced

by a DPI. Scintigraphic measurement obtained by Sangwan et al. (2003) support our results obtained with nebulization. *In vivo* deposition studies have to be conducted to evaluate the relevance of this method for aerosol deposition prediction.

AUTHOR CONTRIBUTIONS

CM, AC, and LV conducted experiments and analyzed results. AC, AL, and LV provided scientific input and contributed to experiment design. CM and LV analyzed experiments and drafted the manuscript. AC, AL, and LV designed and coordinated the overall project. All authors contributed to the article and approved the submitted version.

REFERENCES

Baron, P. A., and Willeke, K. (2001). *Aerosol Measurement: Principles, Techniques, and Applications*, 2nd Edn. New York,NY: J Wiley and Sons.

Bell, K. A., and Ho, A. T. (1981). Growth rate measurements of hygroscopic aerosols under conditions simulating the respiratory tract. *J. Aerosol Sci.* 12, 247–254.

Boudin, L., Grandmont, C., Grec, B., Martin, S., Mecherbet, A., and Noël, F. (2020). Fluid-kinetic modelling for respiratory aerosols with variable size and temperature. *ESAIM: Proc. Surv.* 67, 100–119. doi: 10.1051/proc/20206 7007

Broday, D. M., and Georgopoulos, P. G. (2001). Growth and deposition of hygroscopic particulate matter in the human lungs. *Aerosol Sci. Technol.* 34, 144–159.

Chan, H. K. (2006). Dry powder aerosol delivery systems: current and future research directions. *J. Aerosol Med.* 19, 21–27.

Coates, A. L., MacNeish, C. F., Lands, L. C., Meisner, D., Kelemen, S., and Vadas, E. B. (1998). A comparison of the availability of Tobramycin for inhalation from vented vs unvented nebulizers. *Chest* 113, 951–956.

Daviskas, E., Gonda, I., and Anderson, S. (1990). Mathematical modeling of heat and water transport in human respiratory tract. *J. Appl. Physiol.* 69, 362–372.

Eisner, A. D. (1992). On the coupled mass and energy transport phenomena during breathing of high volume aqueous aerosols. *J. Aerosol Med.* 5, 241–250.

Ferron, G. A. (1977). The size of soluble aerosol particles as a function of the humidity of the air. Application to the human respiratory tract. *J. Aerosol Sci.* 8, 251–267.

Ferron, G. A., Haider, B., and Kreyling, W. G. (1985). A method for the approximation of the relative humidity in the upper human airways. *Bull. Math. Biol.* 47, 565–589.

Ferron, G. A., Kreyling, W. G., and Haider, B. (1988). Inhalation of salt aerosol particles - II. Growth and deposition in the human respiratory tract. *J. Aerosol Sci.* 19, 611–631.

Finlay, W. H. (1998). Estimating the type of hygroscopic behavior exhibited by aqueous droplets. *J. Aerosol Med.* 11, 221–229.

Finlay, W. H., and Smaldone, G. C. (1998). Hygroscopic behaviour of nebulized aerosols: not as important as we thought? *J. Aerosol Med.* 11, 193–195.

Finlay, W. H., and Stapleton, K. W. (1995). The effect on regional lung deposition of coupled heat and mass transfer between hygroscopic droplets and their surrounding phase. *J. Aerosol Sci.* 26, 655–670.

Finlay, W. H., Stapleton, K. W., and Zuberbuhler, P. (1997). Errors in regional lung deposition predictions of nebulized salbutamol sulphate due to neglect or partial inclusion of hygroscopic effects. *Int. J. Pharm.* 149, 63–72.

Fleming, J. S., Epps, B. P., Conway, J. H., and Martonen, T. B. (2006). Comparison of SPECT aerosol deposition data with a human respiratory tract model. *J. Aerosol Med.* 19, 268–278.

Gradon, L., and Podgórski, A. (1996). Deposition of Inhaled Particles: Discussion of Present Modeling Techniques. *J. Aerosol Med.* 9, 343–355.

Hinds, W. C. (1999). *Aerosol Technology.*, *2nd edition.* New York,NY: J Wiley and Sons.

Hindle, M., and Longest, P. W., (2012). Condensational growth of combination drug-excipient submicrometer particles for targeted high efficiency pulmonary delivery: evaluation of formulation and delivery device. *J. Pharm. Pharmacol.* 64, 1254–1263. doi: 10.1111/j.2042-7158.2012.01476.x

ISO 27427. (2012). *Anaesthetic and respiratory equipment — Nebulizing systems and components.* Geneva: ISO.

Kwong, W. T. J., Ho, S. L., and Coates, A. L., (2000). Comparison of nebulized particle size distribution with Malvern laser diffraction analyzer versus Andersen cascade impactor and low-flow Marple personal cascade impactor. *J. Aerosol Med.* 13, 303–314. doi: 10.1089/jam.2000.13.303

Longest, P. W., and Hindle, M. (2012). Condensational growth of combination drug-excipient submicrometer particles: Comparison of CFD predictions with experimental results. *Pharm. Res.* 29, 707–721.

Marple, V. A., Olson, B. A., Santhanakrishnan, K., Mitchell, J. P., Murray, S. C., and Hudson-Curtis, B. L. (2003). Next Generation Pharmaceutical Impactor (A New Impactor for Pharmaceutical Inhaler Testing). Part II: Archival Calibration. *J. Aerosol Med.* 16, 301–324.

Martin, A. R., and Finlay, W. H. (2005). The effect of humidity on the size of particles delivered from metered-dose inhalers. *Aerosol Sci. Technol.* 39, 283–289.

Martin, A. R., Kwok, D. Y., and Finlay, W. H. (2005). Investigating the evaporation of metered-dose inhaler formulations in humid air: single droplet experiments. *J. Aerosol Med.* 18, 218–224.

Martin, G. P., Bell, A. E., and Marriott, C. (1988). An in vitro method for assessing particle deposition from metered pressurized aerosols and dry powder inhalers. *Int. J. Pharm.* 44, 57–63.

Nerbrink, O. L., Pagels, J., Pieron, C. A., and Dennis, J. H. (2003). Effect of humidity on constant output and breath enhanced nebulizer designs when tested in the EN13544-1 EC Standard. *Aerosol Sci. Technol.* 37, 282–292.

Newman, S. P. (2003). Drug delivery to the lungs from dry powder inhalers. *Curr. Opin. Pulm. Med.* 9, S17–S20.

Newman, S. P., Steed, K. P., Reader, S. J., Hooper, G., and Zierenberg, B. (1996). Efficient delivery to the lungs of flunisolide aerosol from a new portable hand-held multidose nebulizer. *J. Pharm. Sci.* 85, 960–964.

O'Doherty, I. J., and Miller, R. F. (1993). Aerosols for therapy and diagnosis. *Eur. J. Nucl. Med.* 20, 1201–1213.

Prokop, R. M., Finlay, W. H., Stapleton, K. W., and Zuberbuhler, P. (1995). The effect of ambient relative humidity on regional dosages delivered by a jet nebulizer. *J. Aerosol Med.* 8, 363–372.

Rao, N., Kadrichu, N., and Ament, B. (2010). Application of a droplet evaporation model to aerodynamic size measurement of drug aerosols generated by a vibrating mesh nebulizer. *J. Aerosol Med. Pulm. Drug Deliv.* 23, 295–302.

Sagalla, R. B., and Smaldone, G. C. (2014). Capturing the efficiency of vibrating mesh nebulizers: minimizing upper airway deposition. *J. Aerosol Med. Pulm. Drug Deliv.* 27, 341–348.

Samuel, J., and Smaldone, G. C. (2020). Maximizing Deep Lung Deposition in

Healthy and Fibrotic Subjects During Jet Nebulization. *J. Aerosol Med. Pulm. Drug Deliv.* 33, 108–115.

Sangwan, S., Condos, R., and Smaldone, G. C. (2003). Lung deposition and respirable mass during wet nebulization. *J. Aerosol Med.* 16, 379–386.

Solomita, M., and Smaldone, G. C. (2009). Reconciliation of Cascade Impaction during Wet Nebulization. *J. Aerosol Med. Pulm. Drug Deliv.* 22, 11–18.

Spence, B. M., Longest, W., Wei, X., Dhapare, S., and Hindle, M. (2019). Development of a High Flow Nasal Cannula and Pharmaceutical Aerosol Combination Device. *J. Aerosol Med. Pulm. Drug Deliv.* 32, 224–241.

Stapleton, K. W., and Finlay, W. H. (1998). Errors in characterizing particle size distributions with cascade impactors. *J. Aerosol Med.* 11, S80–S83.

Telko, M. J., and Hickey, A. J. (2005). Dry powder inhaler formulation. *Respir. Care.* 50, 1209–1227.

USP 28-Nf 23. (2005). *Chapter 601 - Physical tests and determinations: Aerosols*.Rockville, MD: United States Pharmacopeia. 2359–2377.

Van Oort, M., Downey, B., and Roberts, W. (1996). Verification of operating the Andersen Cascade Impactor at different flow rates. *Pharmacopeia Forum* 22, 2211–2215.

Vecellio None, L., Grimbert, D., Becquemin, M. H., Boissinot, E., Le Pape, A., Lemarié, E., et al. (2001). Validation of laser diffraction method as a substitute for cascade impaction in the European Project for a Nebulizer Standard. *J. Aerosol Med.* 14, 107–114.

Willeke, K., and Baron, P. A. (1993). *Aerosol Measurement: Principles, Techniques, and Applications*. New York: Van Nostrand Reinhold.

Zhang, Z., Kleinstreuer, C., and Kim, C. S. (2006). Water vapor transport and its effects on the deposition of hygroscopic droplets in a human upper airway model. *Aerosol Sci. Technol.* 40, 1–16.

Zhou, Y., Ahuja, A., Irvin, C. M., Kracko, D. A., McDonald, J. D., and Cheng, Y. S. (2005a). Medical nebulizer performance: effects of cascade impactor temperature. *Respir. Care.* 50, 1077–1082.

Zhou, Y., Ahuja, A., Irvin, C. M., Kracko, D., McDonald, J. D., and Cheng, Y. S. (2005b). Evaluation of nebulizer performance under various humidity conditions. *J. Aerosol Med.* 18, 283–293.

6

PerfuPul—A Versatile Perfusable Platform to Assess Permeability and Barrier Function of Air Exposed Pulmonary Epithelia

Patrick Carius[1,2], Aurélie Dubois[1], Morvarid Ajdarirad[1,2], Arbel Artzy-Schnirman[3], Josué Sznitman[3], Nicole Schneider-Daum[1] and Claus-Michael Lehr[1,2]*

[1]Department of Drug Delivery (DDEL), Helmholtz-Institute for Pharmaceutical Research Saarland (HIPS), Helmholtz Centre for Infection Research (HZI), Saarbrücken, Germany, [2]Department of Pharmacy, Biopharmaceutics and Pharmaceutical Technology, Saarland University, Saarbrücken, Germany, [3]Department of Biomedical Engineering, Technion—Israel Institute of Technology, Haifa, Israel

*Correspondence:
Claus-Michael Lehr
Claus-Michael.Lehr@helmholtz-hips.de

Complex *in vitro* models, especially those based on human cells and tissues, may successfully reduce or even replace animal models within pre-clinical development of orally inhaled drug products. Microfluidic lung-on-chips are regarded as especially promising models since they allow the culture of lung specific cell types under physiological stimuli including perfusion and air-liquid interface (ALI) conditions within a precisely controlled *in vitro* environment. Currently, though, such models are not available to a broad user community given their need for sophisticated microfabrication techniques. They further require systematic comparison to well-based filter supports, in analogy to traditional Transwells®. We here present a versatile perfusable platform that combines the advantages of well-based filter supports with the benefits of perfusion, to assess barrier permeability of and aerosol deposition on ALI cultured pulmonary epithelial cells. The platform as well as the required technical accessories can be reproduced *via* a detailed step-by-step protocol and implemented in typical bio-/pharmaceutical laboratories without specific expertise in microfabrication methods nor the need to buy costly specialized equipment. Calu-3 cells cultured under liquid covered conditions (LCC) inside the platform showed similar development of transepithelial electrical resistance (TEER) over a period of 14 days as cells cultured on a traditional Transwell®. By using a customized deposition chamber, fluorescein sodium was nebulized *via* a clinically relevant Aerogen® Solo nebulizer onto Calu-3 cells cultured under ALI conditions within the platform. This not only allowed to analyze the transport of fluorescein sodium after ALI deposition under perfusion, but also to compare it to transport under traditional static conditions.

Keywords: air-liquid interface (ALI), permeability, perfusion, transepithelial electrical resistance (TEER), aerosol deposition, drug testing, pulmonary epithelia

INTRODUCTION

Animal models have undoubtedly been essential for the development of oral inhalation drug products, especially for demonstrating safety as well as, at least for some diseases, also efficacy in preclinical research. But it must be realized that, already in healthy state, animal models hardly reflect the human respiratory tract with regard to the administration and deposition of aerosolized medicines. While forced inhalation or tracheobronchial instillation may still allow to draw some conclusion about pulmonary toxicity, the problem becomes more challenging for efficacy studies. This is especially true for inhalable anti-infective drugs, where the available animal models fail to adequately replicate how such diseases affect the human respiratory tract (Lorenz et al., 2016). This can be attributed to evident species-species variations between humans and model organisms (e.g., in lung anatomy, airway histology, cellular composition of epithelial and sub epithelial compartments) that amongst other reasons eventually slow down the development of orally inhaled drug products (Barnes et al., 2015; Artzy-Schnirman et al., 2019a; Jimenez-Valdes et al., 2020).

In contrast to animal models, complex *in vitro* models, especially when human based, allow to focus on key elements of underlying (patho-) physiological conditions as observed in the clinic and to model such conditions within a controlled *in vitro* environment (Carius et al., 2021). Because at present no such predictive *in vitro* models are available yet, their technological development and subsequent validation represent important and demanding scientific tasks (European Commission Joint Research Centre, 2021). Pulmonary *in vitro* models thereby profited from utilizing well-based permeable growth supports (e.g., Transwell®) as a cell culture environment, because these substrates most importantly enable the establishment of air-liquid interface (ALI) conditions as well as polarized differentiation of pulmonary epithelial cells (Lacroix et al., 2018). The easy accessibility to the apical as well as to the basolateral compartment further supports aerosol deposition and/or permeability studies, along with the biophysical measurement of barrier properties *via* transepithelial electrical resistance (TEER). Various simple pulmonary *in vitro* models, usually consisting of bronchial or alveolar epithelial cell monocultures, but also complex models comprising pulmonary epi- and/or endothelial cells in co-culture with other cell types like immune cells (e.g., dendritic cells, macrophages or neutrophils) or fibroblasts have been extensively reviewed (Gordon et al., 2015; Hittinger et al., 2015; Hittinger et al., 2017; Ehrmann et al., 2020).

In moving beyond simple Transwell® cultures that are mainly limited by static culture conditions, organ-on-chip systems have advanced miniaturized biomimetic devices that allow the *in vitro* culture of human cells under physiological conditions similar to *in vivo*, including continuous perfusion and mechanical deflection (Tenenbaum-Katan et al., 2018). Lung-on-chip devices may moreover replicate the characteristics of specific regions of the lung (e.g., cell composition, exposure to air (flow), or breathing dynamics) and comprise tissue relevant cell types.

Among the earliest efforts, Nalayanda et al. (2009) described the ALI culture of the ATII-like carcinoma cell line A549 under low flow conditions (0.35 µl/min) in a PDMS-based lung-on-chip for up to 3 weeks. Following the pioneering work of Huh et al. (2010), that introduced an alveolar-capillary model able to co-culture pulmonary epithelial cells under ALI and flow conditions together with endothelial cells, both stretched by cyclic mechanical strain, the field rapidly advanced. Punde et al. (2015) followed the concept of a dynamic Transwell®-like device, thereby showing that the implementation of dynamic flow created a concentration gradient that effectively guided the transmigration of fibrocytes in an inflammation lung model. An anatomically inspired true-scale acini-on-chip allowed the investigation of the immune response of alveolar epithelial cells in co-culture with differentiated THP-1 macrophage-like cells to nebulized lipopolysaccharide (LPS) as a surrogate for bacterial infections (Artzy-Schnirman et al., 2019a). Recently, the same group used a branching airway-on-chip platform to realistically mimic the transport and deposition of aerosolized particulate matter and study its cytotoxic effect on normal human bronchial epithelial (NHBE) cells (Elias-Kirma et al., 2020). Other devices worth mentioning enable the displacement of a flexible membrane in a diaphragm-like motion (Stucki et al., 2015) in combination with perfusion (Cei et al., 2020) as well as the membrane-free culture of airway smooth muscle cells in co-culture with epithelial cells embedded within a hydrogel (Humayun et al., 2018) or the culture of human alveolar epithelial cells in a gelatin methacryloyl hydrogel resembling alveoli-like hemispheres in a breathing lung-on-chip (Huang et al., 2021).

Despite such advances, the lung-on-chip models described above are technically cumbersome to manufacture and unfortunately need either sophisticated microfabrication techniques, stemming from academic labs with a high level of bioengineering expertise and equipment, or are too costly to be introduced in a standard bio-/pharmaceutical laboratory. Inspired by these devices, we here provide the blueprint as well as a technical proof of principal study of a novel versatile perfusable platform to assess permeability and barrier function of air exposed pulmonary epithelia (PerfuPul), using the bronchial carcinoma cell line Calu-3. Furthermore, to mimic chronic infections of epithelial cells and to enable repetitive treatment of these cultures *in vitro* with aerosolized drug products, survival times should be spanning multiple days, ideally even weeks. Hence, we hypothesized that constant perfusion of cell culture medium could not only prolong the survival time of such complex infected co-culture models, by removal of bacterial toxins and virulence factors, but also accelerate and enhance cellular differentiation, as supported by others (Chandorkar et al., 2017). To this end, we identified ALI conditions, aerosol deposition, TEER measurements and especially perfusion as a physiological relevant clearance mechanism as needed prerequisites for the intended infection studies. Our platform fulfills the technical requirements for the intended infection models and can easily be reproduced in any bio-/pharmaceutical laboratory with a moderate time as well as financial investment.

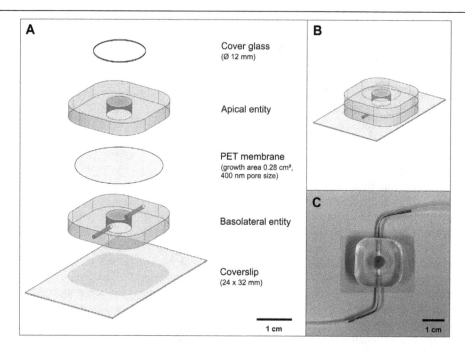

FIGURE 1 | Overview of the perfusable platform "PerfuPul". **(A)** Exploded computer-aided drawing (CAD) view of the perfusable platform made from PDMS. (B+C) The assembled platform **(B)** can be closed with a cover glass during cell culture **(C)**.

MATERIALS AND METHODS

Design and Fabrication of the Perfusable Platform

The perfusable platform consists of two well-based entities (apical and basolateral) separated *via* a permeable membrane and mounted on a glass coverslip (**Figure 1A**). The apical entity (chamber volume: 85 µl) can be closed with a removable cover glass (cover glass round 12 mm; Carl Roth GmbH, P231.1). Channels embedded in the basolateral entity (chamber volume: 85 µl) allow access to the basolateral chamber, to connect flexible 22ga polyethylene tubing (Instech, BTPE-50) or to insert a pair of electrodes for TEER measurements (**Figures 1B,C, 3A,B**).

The production of the perfusable platform is based on an adapted version of the protocol described by Artzy-Schnirman et al. (2019b), where the main steps of the production process are shown in **Figure 2**. Detailed engineering drawings and all steps that are needed to reproduce the platform are depicted in the Supplementary information (**Supplementary Figures S3–S25; Supplementary Table S1**). Engineering drawings and technical figures were created using Fusion360™ (Autodesk®; version 2.0.7402) under an education license. In short, two separate molds serve as a negative for the castings. The castings yield 6 apical or 6 basolateral entities respectively (**Supplementary Figure S5**). They were machined at the workshop of Saarland University (Saarbrücken, Germany) from polytetrafluoroethylene (PTFE). In case of the basolateral mold, the negatives for the channels were formed by insertion of 6 needles (Sterican size 12; B. Braun, 4657624). Polydimethylsiloxane (PDMS) (Sylgard 184 Elastomer Kit; Dow Corning, 1673921) was mixed with curing agent [10:1 (v/v)

ratio; base/curing agent] and degassed using a desiccator. After pouring degassed PDMS onto the molds, the molds were degassed additionally and baked for 60 min at 100°C. The cured castings were peeled off from the molds, the entities were excised out of the castings and centrally punched using a biopsy punch (6 mm; Kai medical, BP-60F) to generate the wells. Apical entities were attached to polyethylenterephthalat (PET) membranes (0.4 µm pore size; Corning, 3450) and basolateral entities to a 24 × 32 mm coverslip (coverslip 24 × 32 mm; Carl Roth GmbH, H 877) *via* a "stamping" method (Chueh et al., 2007). In brief, degassed liquid PDMS [10:1 (v/v) ratio] is poured on a microscopy slide (microscope slide 76 × 52 × 1 mm; Paul Marienfeld GmbH & Co. KG, 1,100,420) that was previously cleaned, first with water followed by 100% isopropanol and then dried. After that, PDMS was spin-coated (3,000 rpm; acceleration 100 rpm/s for 60 s), resulting in a thin layer. Entities were carefully applied on to the thin layer of PDMS and subsequently attached, either to PET membranes (apical entities) or to microscopy slides (basolateral entities). After degassing, the processed entities were baked for 15 min at 100°C. Basolateral entities were combined with the apical entities repeating this process, resulting in the final perfusable platform (**Figure 2**, step 5-6).

Cell Culture
General Cell Culture
Calu-3 cells (HTB-55™; ATCC) passages 35 to 55 were cultured in a T75-flask supplemented with 13 ml fresh minimum essential medium (MEM) containing Earle's salts and L-glutamine (11095080), 1% non-essential amino acids (NEAA, 40035), 1 mM sodium pyruvate (11360070), 100 U/ml penicillin,

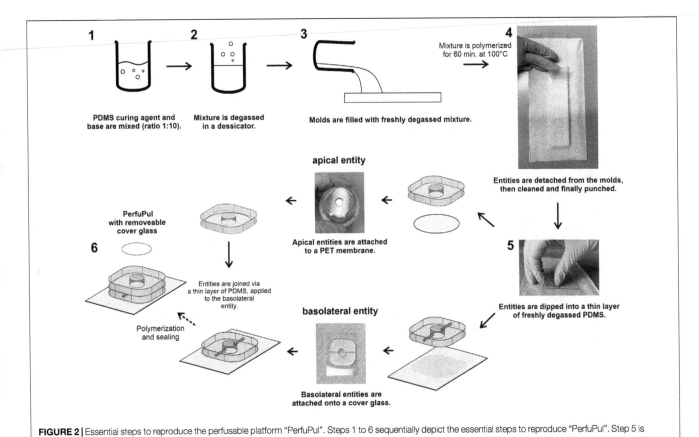

FIGURE 2 | Essential steps to reproduce the perfusable platform "PerfuPul". Steps 1 to 6 sequentially depict the essential steps to reproduce "PerfuPul". Step 5 is performed equally for two distinct manufacturing steps, one for the apical entity and a separate one for the basolateral entity. The apical and the basolateral entity are finally combined in the last step (6). A detailed step-by-step protocol is provided in the Supplementary information.

100 μg/ml streptomycin (15140122) and 10% fetal calf serum (FCS) (all Gibco™, Thermo Fisher Scientific Inc.) every two to 3 days. Cells were maintained at 37°C in a humidified atmosphere containing 5% CO_2. When reaching 80–90% confluency, cells were detached with Trypsin-EDTA 0.05% (Gibco™, Thermo Fisher Scientific Inc.) and then seeded into a new T75-flask (2 × 10^6 cells per flask) and/or used for the experiments detailed in the following paragraphs. All solutions were pre-warmed to 37°C before use.

Transwell® Experiments

$0.33 × 10^5$ Calu-3 cells were seeded in 200 μl MEM including all supplements per apical compartment of a Transwell® insert (0.33 cm²; 400 nm pore size; Corning, 3,470) (1 × 10^5 cells/cm²). The basolateral compartment was supplemented with 800 μl MEM including all supplements. Every two to 3 days used medium was aspirated from the basolateral compartment first and then from the apical compartment. Fresh MEM including all supplements was supplemented first in the apical compartment (200 μl) followed by the basolateral compartment (800 μl).

Perfusable Platform

Before cell culture, all platforms including tubing (**Supplementary Figure S24**) were transferred to one Petri dish (Petri dish 145 × 20 mm; Greiner Bio-One, 6052085) per

platform and decontaminated for 30 min on each side (apical side facing up first, then basolateral side facing up) *via* UV light (254 nm) within a safety cabinet. Filling of the perfusable platform was achieved by manually flushing 800 μl of MEM including all supplements carefully through the basolateral compartment using a bubble-free 1 ml syringe (Injekt®-F SOLO; B. Braun, TZ-2180), leaving 200 μl of medium in the syringe. $0.28 × 10^5$ Calu-3 cells were seeded apically in a volume of 85 μl MEM including all supplements (1 × 10^5 cells/cm²) and the perfusable platform was closed with an autoclaved cover glass. Every two to 3 days medium exchange was performed by carefully removing the cover glass with a sterile forceps, then aspirating the used medium from the apical compartment. After that the basolateral compartment was flushed with 800 μl from a bubble-free 1 ml syringe filled with MEM including all supplements leaving 200 μl medium in the syringe. The outlet of the basolateral compartment was closed with an autoclaved tubing clamp (Th.Geyer, 6200838). In a final step, 85 μl of MEM including all supplements was added to the apical compartment to restore LCC and the perfusable platform was closed apically with an autoclaved cover glass. The same procedure was performed for ALI conditions, with the exception, that when cells were confluent on day 7 or 8 of culture all medium in the apical compartment was aspirated. Additionally, the apical compartment of perfusable platforms containing Calu-3 cells grown under ALI conditions were washed with 85 μl pre-warmed PBS on days of medium exchange. If not stated otherwise, the perfusable platforms were always closed with an autoclaved cover glass and placed in a 145 mm diameter Petri dish at 37°C in a humidified atmosphere containing 5% CO_2.

Confocal Laser Scanning Microscopy
Immunofluorescence Staining

For the representative immunofluorescence staining only inserts with TEER values > 500 Ω^*cm^2 were selected. After washing the apical and basolateral entity with pre-warmed PBS (apical: 85 μl, basolateral: 800 μl) all liquid was flushed out the basolateral compartment by a bolus injection of air. Cells were fixated with 85 μl of 4% paraformaldehyde (in PBS) for 10 min at room temperature (RT) from apical only. Permeabilization and blocking of unspecific epitopes was performed with blocking buffer [1% BSA (Bovine Serum Albumin heat shock fraction; Sigma-Aldrich, A9647-50G), 0.05% Saponin (Saponin Quillaja sp.; Sigma-Aldrich, S4521-10G) in PBS (w/w/v)] for 1 h at RT. Primary antibodies against tight junction proteins Occludin (monoclonal antibody, Thermo Fisher Scientific, Cat# 33-1500, RRID:AB_2533101) and ZO-1 (monoclonal antibody, BD Biosciences, Cat# 610966, RRID:AB_398279) were both diluted [1:200 (v/v)] in blocking buffer and incubated for 12 h at 4°C. The secondary antibody [1:2000 (v/v) in blocking buffer] was incubated for 1 h at RT. Nuclei were stained with DAPI [1 μg/ml in PBS (v/v)] for 30 min at RT. All steps were performed with a volume of 85 μl and the perfusable platforms were washed in between steps with PBS at RT three times. After staining, the apical compartment including the membrane was carefully detached from the basolateral entity using a forceps, by slowly inserting a scalpel underneath the membrane but not touching the growth area. Briefly, the growth area of the membrane was cut from the basolateral side of the membrane as a squared shape, roughly 1 × 1 cm in size, using a scalpel, mounted on a microscope slide (Superfrost; Menzel, AAAA000080##32E) and embedded with fluorescence mounting medium (DAKO, S3023). Samples were always kept moist by careful addition of PBS during the cutting and mounting procedure.

Image Acquisition and Processing

Z-stacks were acquired with an inverted confocal laser scanning microscope (TCS SP8, Leica) equipped with a ×25 water objective, using a zoom of 1, a resolution of 1,024 × 1,024, and a scan speed of 200 Hz. Maximum projections were equally created for all images with FIJI/Image J (Schindelin et al., 2012) and further processed using the BIOP Channel tools plugin (https://c4science.ch/w/bioimaging_and_optics_platform_biop/image-processing/imagej_tools/ijab-biop_channel_tools/).

TEER Measurements
Transwell Insert

In case of Calu-3 cultured in Transwell® inserts under LCC, TEER was measured with a chopstick electrode connected to a Volt-Ohm-meter (STX2 and EVOM 2; World Precision instruments) according to the manufacturer's instructions. During the time of the measurement the Transwell® plate was placed on a heating plate (37°C). Ohmic resistance values were corrected for the area of the Transwell® insert (0.33 cm²) as well as the related value of a blank and reported as Ω^*cm^2. If not described differently, all cultures were fed after TEER measurement.

Perfusable Platform
Custom Electrode Fabrication

Two Ag/AgCl electrodes were created by following the procedure described by Rootare and Powers (1977), with the exception that the silver disk from the method described was replaced by a silver wire with an outer diameter of 0.5 mm (silver wire 0.5 mm diameter; neoLab, 2-3309) for each electrode. Pre-coated electrodes are also commercially available. The two Ag/AgCl electrodes (V1 and V2) and two additional pieces of silver wire (I1 and I2) were cut to a length of 15 mm, soldered to the stranded wires of a RJ14 (6P4C) telephone cable as described in **Supplementary Figure S3** and insulated with a shrinkage tube per strand. The custom-made electrode was equilibrated in 100 mM KCl overnight connected to a switched off EVOM 2 in "Ohm" mode before its first use, in order to stabilize its electrical potential. After this, the electrode was stored and handled in the same way as the STX2 electrode according to the manufacturer's instructions. To validate the custom-made electrode against the STX2 electrode, the TEER of the same Transwell® with Calu-3 cells (day 16–day 19) grown under LCC was first measured with the STX2 electrode and then with the custom-made electrode. For measuring TEER in the Transwell® with the custom-made electrode the electrode pair I2/V1 was placed in the basolateral compartment and I1/V2 in the apical compartment.

TEER Measurements in the Perfusable Platform

The custom-made electrode was first soaked in 70% isopropanol [in sterile MilliQ water (v/v)] for 5 min and then dried before each measurement. Briefly, TEER measurements of Calu-3 cells grown under LCC were performed as described for the Transwell®, by placing the electrode pair I2/V1 in the basolateral compartment and the electrode pair I1/V2 in the apical compartment (**Figure 3A**). In the case of Calu-3 cells grown under ALI conditions, LCC were reestablished by following the procedure described for medium exchange. After an incubation time of 1 h TEER measurements were performed as described for LCC. The TEER value for each platform measured on day 3 was used as a blank for the LCC cultures. In order to not disturb the development of an ALI, for all experiments under ALI conditions the blank was set to 178 Ω^*cm^2 for these experiments. This was the upper deviation from the mean of all blanks measured for the LCC cultures at day 3 (155 Ω^*cm^2 ± 23 Ω^*cm^2; n = 6). Ohmic resistance values were corrected for the area of the perfusable platform (0.28 cm²) as well as for the related value of a blank and reported as Ω^*cm^2.

Aerosol Deposition
Deposition Chamber Design and Fabrication

The custom-made deposition chamber was machined at the workshop of Saarland University (Saarbrücken, Germany) from a polyoxymethylene (POM) rod (**Supplementary Figure**

S4). The design was modified based on the device published by Horstmann et al. (2021) in order to fit the perfusable platform. The chamber was designed in such a way that the wider inlet of the cylindrical device fits tightly against an Aeroneb® Lab nebulizer (Aerogen®, Galway, Ireland) and the narrow outlet seals against the apical compartment of the perfusable platform (**Figure 5A**). In the upper to middle part of the deposition chamber, the inner diameter of the chamber matches the inner diameter of the nebulizer and then conically tapers towards the outlet, where a nozzle protrudes 2 mm from the main body of the deposition chamber. The nozzle is inserted into the apical entity of the perfusable platform and leaves a distance of 1 mm towards the apical surface area, ensuring that it will not interfere with any cells. The distance between the vibrating mesh of the nebulizer and the cell layer is ~50 mm and was chosen due to handling reasons. It can be extended by lenghthening the upper to middle part of the custom-made deposition chamber as needed. Aerosol loss is avoided by insertion of a sealing ring (22 mm inner diameter; 2 mm cord size) in the nebulizer-fitting cavity of the deposition chamber and a tight fit of the nozzle inside the perfusable platform.

Deposition Protocol

The Aeroneb® Lab nebulizer as well as the deposition chamber were disinfected with 70% isopropanol and allowed to dry before the experiments. Before each use, the Aeroneb® Lab nebulizer (standard VMAD, 2.5–4.0 μm droplet diameter) connected to an Aerogen® USB controller (both Aerogen®, Galway, Ireland) was tested for a constant liquid output rate which was not allowed to differ more than 10% from 0.5 ml/min. Therefore 200 μl of sterile PBS was nebulized and the time needed to nebulize all liquid was taken. For aerosol deposition experiments the Aeroneb® Lab nebulizer was connected to the custom-made deposition chamber and inserted into the open apical cavity of the perfusable platform. If not stated otherwise, 20 μl of a fluorescein sodium solution (1 mg/ml in PBS) were allowed to nebulize completely and the generated aerosol settled for 1 min before the nebulizer and the deposition chamber were removed from the perfusable platform. After aerosol deposition the perfusable platform was immediately closed with a sterile cover glass.

For the determination of the deposited dose (**Figure 5B**), single apical entities of the perfusable platform were directly attached to a 24 × 32 mm microscopy slide using the "stamping" method described for the fabrication of the perfusable platform. 20 μl of a fluorescein sodium solution (1 mg/ml in PBS) were nebulized into 30 μl of PBS which were previously pipetted into each apical entity and served as a surrogate for the cell layer. Fluorescence intensity of nebulized fluorescein sodium was measured in 96-well plates at 485 nm excitation and 530 nm emission wavelength with a plate reader (Infinite M200 Pro; Tecan Trading AG) and the deposited dose was calculated from a standard curve. This was done for 5 separate entities. The deposition efficiency was reported as the percentage of the measured dose from the invested dose before nebulization.

Transport Studies

Before each transport experiment, TEER values of Calu-3 cells cultured between day 17 and day 19 were measured while cells remained under LCC to ensure barrier integrity (before). Samples were only used for transport experiments when TEER values reached >300 Ω^*cm^2 before the transport study in accordance with Ehrhardt et al. (2002).

Transwell® System

Calu-3 cells were washed once with pre-warmed Hanks' Balanced Salt Solution (HBSS) with $CaCl_2$ as well as $MgCl_2$ (HBSS (1x); Gibco™, Thermo Fisher Scientific Inc., 14025050) and then equilibrated in HBSS (200 μl apical; 800 μl basolateral) for 1 h (1 h after switch). After measuring TEER, HBSS was aspirated from both, the apical and basolateral compartment. 200 μl fluorescein sodium solution (2.5 μg/ml in HBSS) were added apically (donor) and 800 μl HBSS were added to the basolateral compartment (acceptor). From the same solutions 200 μl each were transferred into a 96-well plate to determine the starting concentrations for each compartment. All steps were performed on a heating plate at 37°C. Afterwards, the Transwell® plates were placed on a MTS orbital shaker (150 rpm; IKA, Germany) in the incubator and 200 μl samples were taken every 1 h for a total of 7 h, from the basolateral compartment only. 200 μl sampled at time points were immediately replenished with 200 μl pre-warmed HBSS. TEER was measured 30 min after the last sample was taken (after 8 h), 200 μl from the apical as well as the basolateral compartment were sampled to determine the end concentrations and all samples were measured with a plate reader in a 96-well plate at 485 nm excitation and 530 nm emission wavelength. The concentration of fluorescein sodium in each sample was calculated using a calibration curve of defined concentrations of fluorescein sodium in HBSS.

Perfusable Platform

Calu-3 cells were washed once with pre-warmed HBSS, by repeating the procedures described for medium exchange. After 1 h of equilibration TEER was measured again (1 h after switch). After connecting a fresh set of tubing including a new syringe filled with pre-warmed HBSS, the basolateral compartment was filled bubble free, while the HBSS from the equilibration step remained in the apical compartment. Immediately after the basolateral compartment was filled and closed with a tubing clamp (receiver), the HBSS in the apical compartment was aspirated and 85 μl fluorescein sodium solution (2.5 μg/ml in HBSS) was added apically (donor). Shortly after, the syringe that was connected to the basolateral compartment was placed into a syringe pump (Harvard industries, PHD Ultra) and 80 μl samples were taken every 1 h for a total of 7 h, while the perfusable platform was placed on an orbital shaker (150 rpm). The flow rate of the syringe pump was set to 1 ml/min in order to sample 80 μl in a short period of time from the basolateral compartment while additionally preventing the sampling maneuver from exerting too much pressure on the cell layer. TEER was measured 30 min after the last sample was taken (after 8 h) and 80 μl from the apical as well as the basolateral compartment were sampled to determine end concentrations.

Transport studies under ALI conditions in the perfusable platform followed the same procedure as transport studies under LCC with only a few exceptions. Calu-3 cells were set to ALI conditions between day 7 or 8 of culture and cultured until day 16–18. The first TEER measurement (1 h after switch) was performed 1 h after LCC was restored by the addition of HBSS to both compartments. After the first TEER measurement ALI conditions were restored again and Calu-3 cells were allowed to equilibrate for 30 min. Then 20 µl of a sterile fluorescein sodium solution (1 mg/ml in PBS) were nebulized onto the apical compartment. The apical compartment was closed with an autoclaved cover glass immediately after the aerosol settled for 1 min. The perfusable platform was placed on an orbital shaker (150 rpm) and 80 µl samples (ALI discontinuous sampling) were taken every 1 h for a total of 5 h, while shortly perfused (1 ml/min) with a syringe pump during the time of sample collection. For transport studies of ALI cultures under perfusion, a peristaltic pump (flow rate: 80 µl/min; Gilson, minipuls 3) equipped with a PharMed® BPT tubing (internal diameter: 0.38 mm; Saint Gobain Performance Plastics™, 070539-04) was connected to the basolateral compartment and 80 µl samples (ALI continuous sampling) were taken every 1 h for a total of 5 h. Although the same dose of fluorescein sodium was used for the transport studies under ALI conditions and LCC, we reduced the duration of the transport studies under ALI conditions to 5 h due to an increased concentration gradient.

All samples were analyzed in the same way as described for the Transwell® samples. The area under the curve (AUC; a. u.), C_{max} (ng/ml) and t_{max} (min) were determined from the cumulative concentration-time curve using GraphPad Prism® 9 (GraphPad software).

Calculation of the Apparent Permeability Coefficient (Papp)

From the linear portion of a cumulative concentration-time curve (LCC: 240–360 min), where drug concentration in the receiver compartment did not exceed 10% of the drug concentration originally added to the donor compartment (**Supplementary Figure S2**) and at which no lag time was observed, the slope was calculated and divided by the area (A; cm^2) of the growth support to get the flux of fluorescein sodium (J; ng/cm^2*s). To obtain the Papp ($cm*s-1$) the following equation was applied, where c_0 (ng/cm^3) is the initial concentration in the donor compartment at the beginning of the experiment:

$$Papp = \frac{J}{c_0}$$

The measured concentrations were converted into absolute masses of compound by multiplication with the acceptor volume of the perfusable platform which was 120 µl (= 85 µl for the chamber +35 µl for the connected tubing).

Statistical Analysis

If not stated otherwise, numerical data were reported as individual values or mean values ± standard deviation (SD).

2-way ANOVA was performed not assuming sphericity and with a Šídák´s multiple comparisons test. Unpaired t-test was performed with Welch`s Correction. p values were defined as: ns: $p > 0.5$; *: $p < 0.05$; **: $p < 0.005$; ***: $p < 0.0005$. Calculations were made using GraphPad Prism® 9.

RESULTS

Concept of the Perfusable Platform

The perfusable platform has been designed in such a way, that it is both easy to produce and operable by non-experts. It encompasses an apical compartment, which is open to the top, and a basolateral compartment, which can be perfused *via* two lateral channels (**Figure 1A**). This design allows to keep experimental conditions similar to the established static Transwell® systems or analogues thereof, and to generate analogous readouts. The open design of the apical entity enables aerosol deposition as well as easy access to the apical cell layer, and the lateral orientation of the in- and outlet enables the insertion of a custom-made electrode for measuring TEER. In addition, the apical entity can be closed with a sterile cover glass to protect the cell layer during cell culture. The two entities are separated *via* a PET membrane that is cut from a Transwell®, which ensures that composition and quality of the growth support are essentially the same, requiring minimal adaptations of the protocol. By keeping the height of the assembled perfusable platform to a minimum, cell growth can be monitored microscopically under sterile conditions, while the assembled perfusable platform (**Figures 1B,C**) remains in a Petri dish. This was demonstrated in a model experiment for the growth of Calu-3 cells, which were seeded on the apical side of the membrane within the apical entity of the perfusable platform under LCC (**Supplementary Figure S1**). After seeding, Calu-3 cells reached confluency within 7–8 days of cell culture, indicating that neither the setup nor the handling of the platform impaired reproducible cell growth.

Analyzing Barrier Integrity Inside the Perfusable Platform

TEER measurements prove to be a non-destructive, reliable and functional tool for the assessment of barrier integrity. The increase in ohmic resistance of an *in vitro* culture grown on a permeable support thereby serves as a convenient readout to monitor the development of functional tight junctions and other cell-to-cell connections. To measure TEER in case of the Transwell®, the shorter leg of an Ag/AgCl chopstick electrode is inserted into the apical compartment, while the longer leg is simultaneously placed into the basolateral compartment. The electrode is then connected to an epithelial Volt-Ohm-Meter, which calculates the ohmic resistance.

The design of the perfusable platform, however, required another type of Ag/AgCl electrode to measure TEER values, since the narrow channels are incompatible with the commercial chopstick electrodes provided with a standard epithelial Volt-Ohm-Meter (EVOM 2) instrument. We decided

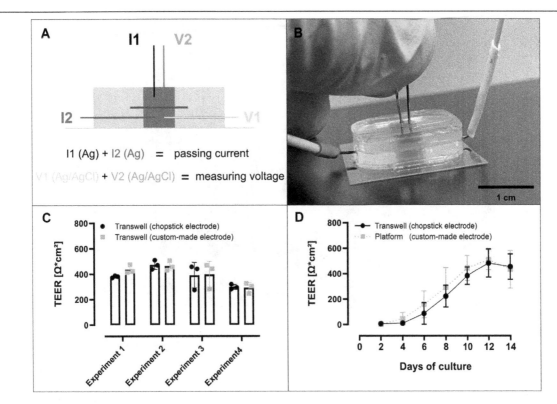

FIGURE 3 | TEER measurement inside the perfusable platform. (A + B) Working principle of the custom-made electrode **(A)** for TEER measurement inside the perfusable platform **(B)**. **(C)** The custom-made electrode was validated against the commercial chopstick electrode (STX-2), by measuring Transwells from 4 separate experiments each containing 14 day old Calu-3 cells grown at LCC. Transwells were first measured with the chopstick followed by the custom-made electrode. **(D)** No difference was observed between the TEER measurements from Calu-3 cells grown under LCC in the perfusable platform or on Transwell, over the course of 14 days n = 9 (d14 Platform n = 8) out of 3 independent experiments. Data represent mean ± S.D.

for a custom-made electrode connected to the four cords of a RJ14 (6P4C) telephone cable as described in the methods section. This is the same type of cable used to connect the chopstick electrode to a regular EVOM 2. As depicted in **Figure 3A**, two cords of the electrode are passing current [I1 (Ag) + I2 (Ag)] and voltage is measured *via* the other two cords [V1 (Ag/AgCl) + V2 (Ag/ AgCl)]. In order to measure TEER, I1/V2 need to be inserted into the apical compartment of the perfusable platform and I2/V1 need to be inserted into the basolateral compartment, while connected to an epithelial Volt-Ohm-Meter (**Figures 3A,B**).

The chopstick electrode, however, comprises a combination of Ag as well as Ag/AgCl electrodes per leg, one Ag pellet on the side of each leg that faces away from the Transwell® insert (passing current) and an Ag/AgCl pellet per leg that faces the Transwell® insert (measuring voltage). In order to show that the design of the custom-made electrode, which is based on individual silver wires and not on silver pellets attached to each leg, does not impair TEER measurements, the functionality of the custom-made electrode was compared to the chopstick electrode. Both measurements were conducted in the same Transwell® (**Figure 3C**). For this, TEER values from 12 Transwells® out of four experiments (3 Transwells® per experiment) carrying Calu-3 cells grown for 14 days under LCC were measured. After 14 days TEER values were measured first with the chopstick electrode and then with the custom-made electrode. The mean of all TEER

values determined with the custom-made electrode showed a deviation of +3% from the mean of all TEER values determined with the chopstick electrode (custom-made electrode: 398 ± 54 Ω*cm^2; chopstick electrode 386 ± 41 Ω*cm^2). These differences between the two electrodes were in an acceptable error range covering not more than 15 Ω*cm^2, which suffices for the determination of TEER values during *in vitro* culture of pulmonary epithelial cells.

The development of TEER values of Calu-3 cells inside the perfusable platform was compared side-by-side with Calu-3 cells grown on Transwells®, under LCC over the course of 14 days (**Figure 3D**). As displayed in **Figure 3D**, TEER values developed equally in the perfusable platform as well as in the Transwell® during 14 days of culture, reaching a maximum (perfusable platform: 510 ± 81 Ω*cm^2; Transwell®: 484 ± 112 Ω*cm^2) after 12 days of culture. These results indicated that the combination of the custom-made electrode and the perfusable platform could be used to reliably determine the development of TEER values in the same quality as the traditional combination of the chopstick electrode and the Transwell®.

Another common technique to demonstrate the integrity of a pulmonary epithelial barrier *in vitro* is the visualization of proteins that form functional tight junctions *via* fluorescent immunocytochemistry staining. **Figure 4** exemplifies how such methods can be conducted within the perfusable platform in the

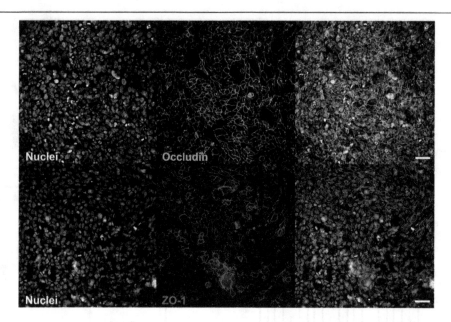

FIGURE 4 | Confocal microscopy possible with the perfusable platform. Micrograph showing Calu-3 cells cultured until d16 (top) or d18 (bottom) under LCC. Calu-3 cells were fixated with 4% paraformaldehyde and stained for tight junctions Occludin (top) or ZO-1 (bottom) as well as nuclei (DAPI) to show the versatility of the perfusable platform to apply immune staining methods (scale bar: 50 µm).

same manner as they are applied for the Transwell®. As described in the methods section, Calu-3 cells were fixated and treated with the respective antibodies to visualize the tight junction forming proteins Occludin (d16) and ZO-1 (d18). Both micrographs show the development of a densely connected network representative of functional tight junctions together with a homogenously distributed cell layer indicated *via* staining of cell nuclei with DAPI.

The combination of non-destructive TEER measurements to assess barrier integrity together with the ability to perform immunocytochemistry staining after cells have been fixated demonstrates that the perfusable platform can be used for the quantitative and mechansistic characterisation of barrier function during *in vitro* culture of pulmonary epithelial cells.

Pre-Metered Aerosol Deposition on the Perfusable Platform

The *in vitro* culture of pulmonary epithelial cells under ALI conditions exposes the epithelial cell layer apically to air, which creates a physiologically relevant interface to mimic the *in vivo* situation more closely. Other than LCC, which for good reasons are standard for intestinal epithelial or blood vessel forming endothelial cells, ALI conditions also allow the controlled deposition of aerosols to the apical surface of the cell layer. Since the apical compartment of the perfusable platform can be opened, by removing the cover glass whenever needed, switching to ALI conditions and the deposition of aerosols are easily possible. In this context, we adapted the design of a recently published custom-made deposition chamber (Horstmann et al., 2021) which fits to an Aeroneb® Lab vibrating mesh nebulizer (**Figure 5A**). The functional unit, consisting of an Aeroneb® Lab

nebulizer connected to an Aerogen® USB controller as well as to the deposition chamber, is placed on the apical compartment of the perfusable platform. The nebulizer generates an aerosol from an aqueous drug solution through a vibrating mesh, which is released into the deposition chamber and finally settles as a mist onto the apical compartment of the perfusable platform. Reproducible deposition of pre-metered doses of an aqueous drug solution, can be achieved by controlling the concentration and/or the volume of the solution before nebulization. While increasing the settling time beyond 30-s was found to not further affect the deposited dose, a settling time of 1 min was choosen as routine to facilitate the experimental procedure (Horstmann et al., 2021).

This was demonstrated by nebulizing 20 µl of fluorescein sodium solution (1 mg/ml in PBS) onto five perfusable platforms, which comprised only the apical compartment attached to a glass slide. By keeping the settling time of the mist to 1 min after each nebulization, a delivered dose of 212 ± 12 ng could be reproducibly deposited (**Figure 5B**).

Comparison of Fluorescein Sodium Transport Between the Transwell® and the Perfusable Platform

To carry out comparative transport experiments on Calu-3 cells grown under LCC on Transwell® versus cells grown under LCC in the perfusable platform, fluorescein sodium was used as a well-defined low-permeability marker.

Before, during and after each transport experiment, TEER values were measured to ensure that barrier integrity was not compromised by the transport buffer or over the duration of the experiment. In case of the cells grown under ALI conditions, the

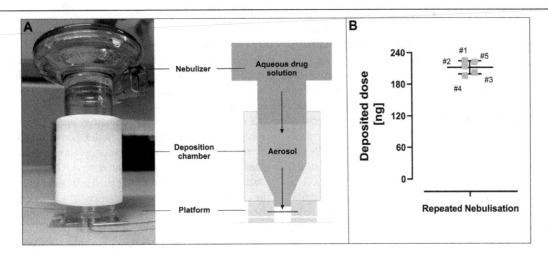

FIGURE 5 | Aerosol deposition on the perfusable platform. **(A)** By attaching an Aerogen Lab nebulizer to a custom made deposition chamber, aerosols can be deposited on the perfusable platform. **(B)** Repeated nebulisation (#1–#5) of 20 μl fluorescein sodium (1 mg/ml in PBS; cloud settling time 1 min) in five different devices led to a reproducible deposited dose (mean: 212 ± 12 ng). Data represent mean ± S.D.

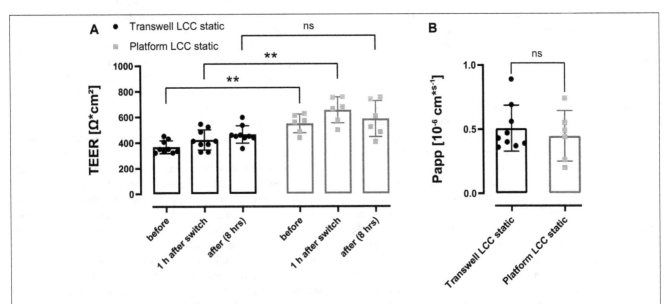

FIGURE 6 | Comparison of fluorescein sodium transport between Transwell and the perfusable platform under LCC. **(A)** Transport studies were performed on Calu-3 cells (LCC: d17-d19). TEER values were measured before the experiment (before), 1 h after the incubation in transport buffer (1 h after switch), as well as after the transport study (after) and indicated a stable barrier during the transport. **(B)** Apparent permeability (Papp) of fluorescein sodium (2.5 μg/ml (dose: 500 ng on Transwell; 212 ng on platform)) applied as a solution. Papp was determined after the transport study (7 h). Data represent mean ± S.D. **(A)** 2-way ANOVA was performed not assuming sphericity and with a Šídák's multiple comparisons test, ns: $p > 0.5$; *: $p < 0.05$; **: $p < 0.005$; **(B)** Unpaired t-test was performed with Welch's Correction; Transwell LCC: n = 9, Platform LCC: n = 6 out of 3 independent experiments.

first TEER measurements were performed 1 h after LCC conditions were re-established. Before the transport experiments, Calu-3 cells grown under LCC in the Transwell® presented a significantly lower TEER (before, 367 ± 49 Ω*cm^2) than Calu-3 cells grown in the perfusable platform under the same conditions (before, 548 ± 73 Ω*cm^2) (**Figure 6A**). After the switch to HBSS as a transport buffer (1 h after switch) TEER values slightly increased in both the Transwell® cultures (423 ±

78 Ω*cm^2) as well as in the cultures grown in the perfusable platform (to 653 ± 100 Ω*cm^2). After 7 h of transport experiments (Transwell®: 464 ± 67 Ω*cm^2; perfusable platform: 584 ± 140 Ω*cm^2), TEER values did not decline when compared to the condition before the transport experiments for either system, indicating that barrier properties remained intact during the course of the experiment. Without reaching statistical significance, however, it was observed that in the

perfusable platform TEER values after the transport slightly decreased ($-69 \pm 4 \, \Omega{*}cm^2$) compared to 1 h after the switch to transport buffer, whereas the TEER values of the cells cultured on Transwells® showed a slight inscrease ($41 \pm 3 \, \Omega{*}cm^2$).

The Papp values further supported the assumption of the formation of a functional diffusional barrier to fluorescein sodium within Calu-3 cell layers, which TEER value measurements already indicated (**Figure 6B**). The transport of fluorescein sodium over Calu-3 cell layers grown under LCC within Transwell® inserts showed no significant differences indicated by the respective Papp values when compared to cell layers grown in the perfusable platform (Transwell®: 0.51 ± 0.18 10–6 cm*s-1; perfusable platform: 0.45 ± 0.20 10–6 cm*s-1). In addition, permeability of fluorescein sodium in a perfusable platform without any cells grown inside was increased 20-fold (**Supplementary Figure S2**).

This set of experiments showed that the perfusable platform performs as good as the Transwell® under the experimental requirements of a transport study, in terms of reproducibility and consistency of results.

Transport Studies Under Perfusion

The essential advantage of the perfusable platform in comparison to the Transwell® system is the option to perfuse the basolateral compartment. In order to demonstrate one of the various possibilities enabled by perfusing the acceptor compartment, we compared the transport of fluorescein sodium after nebulization under static conditions and under the influence of perfusion (**Figure 7A**). For the static conditions, the experimental setup for sampling was the same as for the transport studies under LCC described earlier (**Figure 6**), where the basolateral compartment was only subjected to a short perfusion (80 µl, ALI discontinuous sampling) from a syringe pump during sample timepoints, while the platform remained on a shaker during the transport experiment. In the case of the samples that were taken from perfusion, samples were collected as fractions (80 µl, ALI continuous sampling) from perfusion (80 µl/h) generated by a peristaltic pump. During transport experiments TEER seemed not to be affected from perfusion when compared to static conditions (**Figure 7B**), demonstrating that perfusion did not disturb barrier properties during a 5 h transport experiments. Neither the comparison of the different concentration time curves nor the comparison of the area under the concentration time curve (AUC) (**Figure 7C**), yielded a significant difference between the two conditions (ALI continuous sampling: $22{,}525 \pm 6{,}248$ a. u.; ALI discontinuous sampling: $20{,}850 \pm 6{,}900$ a. u.), indicating that similar mass transport occurred under both conditions. When comparing the mean of C_{max} (ALI continuous sampling: 135 ± 47 ng/ml; ALI discontinuous sampling: 115 ± 41 ng/ml) as well as t_{max} (ALI continuous sampling: 140 ± 31 min; ALI discontinuous sampling: 165 ± 30 min) of the individual platforms, there seems to be - without being statistically significant - at least some trend towards higher C_{max} as well as shorter t_{max} for the transport studies under perfusion (**Figure 7D**), but this would need further investigation.

DISCUSSION

In spite of their physiological advantages, perfusable transport chambers have only rarely found their way into *in vitro* models of epithelial cell culture, in particular for the lungs (Artzy-Schnirman et al., 2020). Complex designs, mostly encompassing micron-sized rectangular channels, as well as the underlying problems of impaired aerosol deposition and/or complexity of handling by non-experts, might restrict the exploitation of the full potential of lung-on-chip devices as preclinical research tools (Junaid et al., 2017; Ehrmann et al., 2020). Perfusable systems offer particular advantages for studying infectious diseases, as concentration of e.g., bacterial virulence factors can be kept at lower levels by continuous supply and dilution with fresh media. Before this can be studied in more detail, however, it is necessary to ensure to what extent data generated on novel perfusabel setups can be compared to those obtained on established Transwells® under static conditions (Ainslie et al., 2019). We therefore here first describe the development as well as the characterization of a simple perfusable platform for pulmonary epithelial cell cultures at ALI conditions. This platform maintains the advantages of traditional Transwell®-based systems, but adds the possibility to implement perfusion as a prerequisite to develop longer-lasting *in vitro* models of chronic pulmonary diseases in the future. In addition, we want to share the protocol needed to produce the platform with a broad scientific community, in order to make this technology available to end-users that might not yet be familiar with microfabrication techniques.

Apart from standardized readouts to assess cell viability or cytotoxicity *in vitro*, such as the MTT or lactate dehydrogenase (LDH) assay respectively, information from TEER measurements or permeability studies appear extremely helpful for the preclinical evaluation of orally inhaled drug products (Wilson 2000; Hittinger et al., 2017). For such purposes, these models must allow ALI conditions together with the subsequent deposition of aerosols. Although pulmonary epithelial cells grown on Transwell® inserts meet all of these technical specifications, they are limited to static culture conditions. Recent studies, however, demonstrated that normal human bronchial epithelial (NHBE) cells cultured under ALI conditions and simultaneous perfusion of cell culture medium showed improved barrier properties in comparison to static conditions (Chandorkar et al., 2017; Bovard et al., 2018). Perfusion is, amongst other physiological important mechanical stimuli, also recognized as a central element to be implemented in organ-on-chip systems in general to improve cellular development (Thompson et al., 2020).

The new platform thus was designed to comply with the familiar technical standards and features of Transwell® inserts, but at the same time also enabling perfusion as a physiological relevant clearance mechanism not present in Transwell®-based culture plates. Major specifcations are: 1) a comparable surface area (24-well based Transwell®: 0.33 cm^2; perfusable platform: 0.28 cm^2), 2) the possibility to routinely inspect cell layers under a microscope while maintaining sterile culture conditions, 3) the option to measure TEER, and 4.) the implementation of ALI

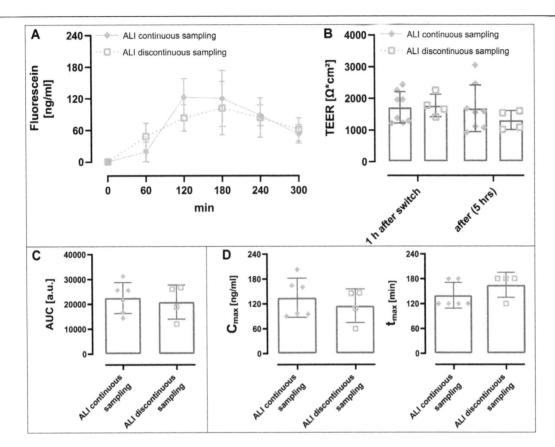

FIGURE 7 | Transport studies under perfusion after ALI deposition. **(A)** Concentration time curve of nebulized fluorescein sodium (dose: 212 ng in PBS). Samples were collected every hour either sampled continuously from perfusion (80 µl/h) generated by a peristaltic pump or discontinuously (80 µl) *via* a short perfusion with a syringe pump. During the transport study, samples termed "ALI continuous sampling" were thus constantly perfused, while samples termed "ALI discontinuous sampling" were shaken at 150 rpm and only shortly perfused with a syringe pump during sample collection. 80 µl sample volume was collected for both conditions every hour. **(B)** TEER values 1 h after switching from ALI to LCC in order to determine the TEER before the transport study (1 h after switch) and at the end of the 5 h transport experiment [after (5 h)] was unchanged, indicating that epithelial barrier function was not affected by perfusion. **(C)** The area under the concentration time curve (AUC) was comparable between the two conditions. **(D)** The maximal concentrations (Cmax; left) as well as the time to reach the highest concentration (tmax, right) did not significantly differ and were rather comparable for both conditions. Data represent mean ± S.D.; ALI continuous sampling n = 6 out of 3 independent experiments, ALI discontinuous sampling n = 4 out of 4 independent experiments.

conditions as well as subsequent aerosol deposition (**Figures 1, 3, 5; Supplementary Figure S1**). The access to the basolateral compartment *via* a combination of a channel-based inlet connected to a flexible tubing enables the culturing of cells under static culture conditions, but also adds the possibility to perform experiments under perfusion (**Figure 7**).

In a side-by-side comparison using Calu-3 cells grown on regular Transwell® inserts or within the perfusable platform we could show that both, the resistance readings from the two electrodes (chopstick vs. custom-made electrode) within the same Transwell® insert as well as the measurements performed in the perfusable platform and on Transwell® inserts under equal experimental conditions agree by good approximation (**Figure 3C, D**). Notably, this was irrespective of the fact that in the case of the custom electrode, when compared with the chopstick electrode within the same Transwell®, four separate cables needed to be arranged in each well. The custom-made Ag/AgCl electrode used by us can be connected to existing instrumentation (e.g., EVOM 2) with only little technical effort

needed to solder the different silver wires to a 4-cord cable (**Figure 3A**), as already described for organ-on-chip systems in similar ways (Douville et al., 2010; Ferrell et al., 2010; Huh et al., 2010; Kim et al., 2012; Griep et al., 2013). Most of these studies reported significantly higher TEER values in case of the organ-on-chip systems when compared to results obtained for the same cell models cultured on Transwell® inserts. However, these higher TEER values could be related to the geometry of the rectangular micron-sized channels within these organ-on-chips, that generate a non-uniformly distributed electrical current, rather than showing a biological effect (Odijk et al., 2015). The perfusable platform reported in the present paper, however, is based on a design encompassing two equally sized wells separated by a circular membrane that has a cell culture area identical to that of a 24-well Transwell® insert (**Figure 1A**). Limiting the use of micron-sized channels only to the in- and outlet that enable access to the basolateral well, further generates similarity to the Transwell®.

Especially during permeability studies within the same lab, TEER value measurements using an EVOM 2 or similar direct current based Voltohmmeters are widely accepted as a valuable non-invasive readout to routinely assess barrier integrity. This holds still true while some more advanced bioelectrical methods (e.g., impedance spectroscopy) might be more precise in determining information about actual barrier integrity (Günzel et al., 2012; Odijk et al., 2015; Srinivasan et al., 2015; Henry et al., 2017).

As already indicated by the stable TEER values during the course of the 7 h transport experiments, the apparent permeability of fluorescein sodium transported under LCC also did not reveal any significant differences between the perfusable platform and the Transwell® (**Figure 6B**). Further were the obtained Papp values in this study, in relation to the respective TEER values, consistent with reported Papp values in the literature performed under similar study conditions on Transwell® inserts using Calu-3 cells (Ehrhardt et al., 2002; Fiegel et al., 2003; Grainger et al., 2006; Haghi et al., 2010). To our knowledge, these historical data from Transwells® inserts have not been confirmed using any perfusable, microfluidic or lung-on-chip system so far.

To assess barrier integrity by staining for relevant cellular markers, techniques to perform immunofluorescence staining and subsequent confocal laser scanning microscopy or other imaging methods can be used with the perfusable platform in the same way as for Transwell® inserts. This was demonstrated by the example of the visualization of the proteins Occludin and ZO-1 that are involved in the formation of functional tight junctions (**Figure 4**). For that purpose, the apical as well as basolateral entity can be separated from the membrane, independently from each other. This procedure allows to flexibly conduct staining and cell fixation methods.

One of the unique features of the perfusable platform as presented here is the possibility to reproducibly deposit pre-metered aerosols from aqueous drug solutions on pulmonary epithelial cells grown at an ALI using a clinically relevant vibrating mesh nebulizer (Aeroneb® Lab). The removable cover glass, that allows to easily open and close the top of the apical compartment, thereby enables the establishment of ALI conditions after cells have been grown to confluency under LCC. The flexibility to open and close the top of the apical compartment is what creates the possibility to connect a vibrating mesh nebulizer to the perfusable platform by using the custom-made deposition chamber. The custom-made deposition chamber presented here was modified to fit the opening of the apical compartment of the perfusable platform, but mostly retains the design as well as dimensions of the device described by Horstmann et al. (2021) to be used with a single 12-well (12 mm) Transwell® insert or a single 24-well. Since we extensively discussed the obtained results and characterized the deposition chamber in the work mentioned above, we limited the characterization for its use with the perfusable platform to the experiments described in **Figure 5**, to ensure that reproducibility of results is consistent with our previous findings. While reproducibility could be maintained in good approximation (5.6% relative standard deviation (deposition on perfusable

platform) vs. 4.8% relative standard deviation [12-well Transwell®)], the deposition efficiency showed a 4-fold reduction [1.06 ± 0.06% (perfusable platform) vs. ~4% (12-well Transwell®)]. When all parameters, such as the used nebulizer, the volume to be nebulized in the same concentration and the settling time are kept constant, the deposition efficiency in these chambers is mainly limited by the inner diameter of the outlet (Horstmann et al., 2021). The inner diameter amounts to ~5 mm in the version for the perfusable platform and ~11 mm for the 12-well Transwell® version. A substantial amount of the aerosol mist generated by the vibrating mesh nebulizer thus deposits on the walls of the deposition chamber and therefore is not channeled through the outlet. A similar concept, also including a vibrating mesh nebulizer and a connected chamber, was recently introduced by Cei et al. (2020) in a dynamic *in vitro* stretch lung model. The outlet of the aerosol chamber in their model was about 20 mm in inner diameter and resulted in an impressive deposition efficiency of about 52% after nebulization.

Although we acknowledge the fact that a deposition efficiency of 1% from the invested dose seems relatively low, the dose delivered per surface area provides better comparability in this case. Based on an equally invested dose of 20 μg (20 μl from a 1 mg/ml solution) which would be nebulized, the delivered dose per surface area would result to ~0.7 μg/cm^2 (perfusable platform, 0.28 cm^2; deposition efficiency: 1%), ~0.8 μg/cm^2 (12-well Transwell®, 1.12 cm^2; deposition efficiency: 4.8%) or ~2.2 μg/cm^2 [(Cei et al., 2020), 4.67 cm^2; deposition efficiency: 52%]. Ultimately, between different devices the dose delivered per surface area should be used for comparison instead of the isolated deposition efficiency. This considerably mitigates the major differences observed when focusing on the isolated deposition efficiency while enhancing comparability, despite the fact that the delivered dose per surface area is still about three times higher in the device of Cei et al. (2020) when compared to the perfusable platform, since less compound is deposited on the walls of the deposition chamber. The foregoing notwithstanding, although the main share of compound is deposited on the walls of the deposition chamber and not reaching the cellular layer, the quantity of compound invested to obtain meaningful *in vitro* results with the devices mentioned before is still substantially lower than that normally required for conducting *in vivo* inhalation studies (Phalen and Mendez 2009).

As demonstrated by the data of **Figure 7**, transport studies under static as well as perfused conditions were successfully conducted after the reproducible deposition of a pre-metered aerosol from an aqueous fluorescein sodium solution. Interestingly enough, under perfusion we only observed a negligible decrease in TEER values (−2%) after 5 h of transport after ALI deposition of fluorescein sodium under perfusion (**Figure 7B**) while the difference after 5 h of transport under static conditions amounted to (−26%) when comparing only the mean values. Although this difference was not statistically supported, it could suggest a positive effect of perfusion on barrier properties during the course of the transport experiment in comparison to static conditions, but would need more thorough investigation. The ability to implement perfusion into the perfusable platform, further allowed the comparison of transport of nebulized fluorescein sodium as a model compound under static conditions to transport under perfusion. Although we also could only observe a slight trend towards higher C_{max} and lower t_{max} in case of the fluorescein sodium transported under continuous perfusion, we think that if such experiments would be performed under different parameters (shorter sampling intervals, drugs with different permeation, different flow rates etc.) meaningful insights into the transport of experimental drugs intended for inhalation under physiological relevant conditions could be provided.

We are well aware that the features that make up the perfusable platform are built upon the work of other researchers active in the lung-on-chip field. A similar concept comprising a PDMS-based chip which possessed an open apical compartment, thereby allowing the establishment of ALI conditions, which was also able to provide perfusion and TEER measurements was already introduced by Nalayanda et al., in 2009. Although the authors compared their findings systematically to Transwell® inserts at an ALI using the alveolar type 2-like cell line A549, they did not show the deposition of aerosols. The importance of flow in lung-on-chip systems initially demonstrated by Punde et al. (2015), was used by others to follow the concept of a flowable Transwell® (Blume et al., 2015; Blume et al., 2017; Chandorkar et al., 2017; Bovard et al., 2018; Schimek et al., 2020). The problem with such systems is that the Transwell® inserts where the cells are cultured during perfusion need to be taken out of the sophisticated culture devices that provide the perfusion, and are then transferred to separate culture wells or devices before TEER measurements can be performed or aerosols could be deposited. Especially for substances that are rapidly absorbed after aerosol deposition, such delays could aggravate subsequent analysis. Sophisticated aerosol deposition on cells grown at an ALI was described by Artzy-Schnirman et al. (2019a) for a morphologically inspired acinus-on-chip and also recently for a bronchial bifurcation mimic by Elias-Kirma et al. (2020). Unfortunately, these devices were not characterized in terms of TEER measurements nor in the application of perfusion. In addition, the former device needs sophisticated microfabrication during production and the latter device requires a complex set of devices for the generation of aerosols as well as the related physiologically relevant airflows. Researchers that consider implementing lung-on-chip devices for their research or just want to try out if the physiological features provided by these devices, such as perfusion, could benefit their work, are thus facing considerable difficulties, if they do not have the needed technical expertise in micro-fabrication or the financial resources to invest in commercial platforms. Although companies like Alveolix, CN bio, Emulate, Kirkstall or TissUse introduced innovative lung-on-chip devices or perfusable Transwells®, the material costs of the chips and the related infrastructure needed to operate them could add up to sums which are difficult to finance for academic labs (Kirkstall Ltd 2020; AlveoliX 2021; Chips - TissUse GmbH 2021; CN Bio Innovations 2021; Emulate 2021).

The perfusable platform presented here holds some limitations. The platform is based on a PET membrane, which is cut from Transwell® inserts and known to be rather rigid and bio-inert in comparison to the extracellular matrix found in vivo (Humayun et al., 2018). The used PDMS is also known to absorb small, hydrophobic molecules (Toepke and Beebe 2006). This technical characteristic can be corrected though, by pre-equilibrating the devices or adjusting for the loss of substance (Jimenez-Valdes et al., 2020). Depending on the skill of the operator but also on the used peristaltic pump, results obtained from the perfusable platform are in the low- to mid-throughput range depending on the extent of the intended studies.

CONCLUSION

The minimalistic design of the presented perfusable platform "PerfuPul" allows its production by non-experts in most lab environments without the need for specialized equipment. Furthermore, the platform combines TEER measurements, aerosol deposition as well as the implementation of perfusion as a physiological relevant clearance mechanism in a single device that matches the design as well as the quality of results known from Transwell® inserts. The open apical entity not only allows the establishment of ALI conditions but could be also utilized for working with cutting-edge techniques such as 3D bio printing. Moreover, the easy access to the basolateral compartment would permit co-culture studies, for instance, by also growing endothelial cells on the basal side of the membrane. Taking all of these factors in consideration, we are convinced that this perfusable platform will enable the development of novel pulmonary in vitro models especially to study long-term diseases, such as e.g., bacterial lung infections and their treatment by aerosolized drugs and nanoscale carriers therof.

AUTHOR CONTRIBUTIONS

PC had the idea for the perfusable platform, designed, planned as well as performed the experiments and wrote the manuscript. AD helped in the creation of the custom-made electrode and helped in improving the molds. MA helped in the creation of the Supplementary Information. JS, AA-S helped in planning the concept as well as the experiments for the perfusable platform. They further helped to write and enhance the manuscript. NS-D helped in revising the manuscript. C-ML shares the idea for the perfusable platform and helped in planning the experiments. He also helped writing and enhancing the manuscript.

ACKNOWLEDGMENTS

We would like to express our sincere thanks to Rudolf Richter (Workshop, Department of Physical Chemistry and Didactics of Chemistry, Saarland University) for his help in the technical realization and construction of the deposition device. In addition we would like to cordially thank Petra König and Jana Westhues for their help in routine cell culture.

REFERENCES

Ainslie, G. R., Davis, M., Ewart, L., Lieberman, L. A., Rowlands, D. J., Thorley, A. J., et al. (2019). Microphysiological Lung Models to Evaluate the Safety of New Pharmaceutical Modalities: a Biopharmaceutical Perspective. *Lab. Chip* 19, 3152–3161. doi:10.1039/c9lc00492k

AlveoliX (2021). *Information | the Latest News about Our Projects and Our Team - AlveoliX*. Available at: https://www.alveolix.com/information/ (Accessed March 30, 2021).

Artzy-Schnirman, A., Hobi, N., Schneider-Daum, N., Guenat, O. T., Lehr, C.-M., and Sznitman, J. (2019a). Advanced *In Vitro* Lung-On-Chip Platforms for Inhalation Assays: From prospect to Pipeline. *Eur. J. Pharm. Biopharm.* 144, 11–17. doi:10.1016/j.ejpb.2019.09.006

Artzy-Schnirman, A., Zidan, H., Elias-Kirma, S., Ben-Porat, L., Tenenbaum-Katan, J., Carius, P., et al. (2019b). Capturing the Onset of Bacterial Pulmonary Infection in Acini-On-Chips. *Adv. Biosys.* 3, 1900026. doi:10.1002/adbi.201900026

Artzy-Schnirman, A., Lehr, C.-M., and Sznitman, J. (2020). Advancing Human *In Vitro* Pulmonary Disease Models in Preclinical Research: Opportunities for Lung-On-Chips. *Expert Opin. Drug Deliv.* 17, 621–625. doi:10.1080/17425247.2020.1738380

Barnes, P. J., Bonini, S., Seeger, W., Belvisi, M. G., Ward, B., and Holmes, A. (2015). Barriers to New Drug Development in Respiratory Disease. *Eur. Respir. J.* 45, 1197–1207. doi:10.1183/09031936.00007915

Blume, C., Reale, R., Held, M., Millar, T. M., Collins, J. E., Davies, D. E., et al. (2015). Temporal Monitoring of Differentiated Human Airway Epithelial Cells Using Microfluidics. *PLoS One* 10, e0139872. doi:10.1371/journal.pone.0139872

Blume, C., Reale, R., Held, M., Loxham, M., Millar, T. M., Collins, J. E., et al. (2017). Cellular Crosstalk between Airway Epithelial and Endothelial Cells Regulates Barrier Functions during Exposure to Double-Stranded RNA. *Immun. Inflamm. Dis.* 5, 45–56. doi:10.1002/iid3.139

Bovard, D., Sandoz, A., Luettich, K., Frentzel, S., Iskandar, A., Marescotti, D., et al. (2018). A Lung/liver-On-A-Chip Platform for Acute and Chronic Toxicity Studies. *Lab. Chip* 18, 3814–3829. doi:10.1039/c8lc01029c

Carius, P., Horstmann, J. C., Souza Carvalho-Wodarz, C. de., and Lehr, C.-M. (2021). "Disease Models: Lung Models for Testing Drugs against Inflammation and Infection,," in *Organotypic Models in Drug Development*. Editors M. Schäfer-Korting, S. Stuchi Maria-Engler, and R. Landsiedel (Cham: Springer International Publishing), 157–186.

Cei, D., Doryab, A., Lenz, A. G., Schröppel, A., Mayer, P., Burgstaller, G., et al. (2020). Development of a Dynamic *In Vitro* Stretch Model of the Alveolar Interface with Aerosol Delivery. *Biotechnol. Bioeng.* 118, 690–702. doi:10.1002/bit.27600

Chandorkar, P., Posch, W., Zaderer, V., Blatzer, M., Steger, M., Ammann, C. G., et al. (2017). Fast-track Development of an *In Vitro* 3D Lung/immune Cell Model to Study Aspergillus Infections. *Sci. Rep.* 7, 11644. doi:10.1038/s41598-017-11271-4

Chips - TissUse GmbH (2021). HUMIMIC Chips – Superpowers for Superb Insights. Berlin, Germany: TissUse GmbH. Available at: https://www.tissuse.com/en/humimic/chips/ (Accessed March 29, 2021).

Chueh, B.-h., Huh, D., Kyrtsos, C. R., Houssin, T., Futai, N., and Takayama, S. (2007). Leakage-free Bonding of Porous Membranes into Layered Microfluidic Array Systems. *Anal. Chem.* 79, 3504–3508. doi:10.1021/ac062118p

CN Bio Innovations (2021). Barrier Models. Available at: https://cn-bio.com/barrier-models/ (Accessed March 29, 2021).

Douville, N. J., Tung, Y.-C., Li, R., Wang, J. D., El-Sayed, M. E. H., and Takayama, S. (2010). Fabrication of Two-Layered Channel System with Embedded Electrodes to Measure Resistance across Epithelial and Endothelial Barriers. *Anal. Chem.* 82, 2505–2511. doi:10.1021/ac9029345

Ehrhardt, C., Fiegel, J., Fuchs, S., Abu-Dahab, R., Schaefer, U. F., Hanes, J., et al. (2002). Drug Absorption by the Respiratory Mucosa: Cell Culture Models and Particulate Drug Carriers. *J. Aerosol Med.* 15, 131–139. doi:10.1089/089426802320282257

Ehrmann, S., Schmid, O., Darquenne, C., Rothen-Rutishauser, B., Sznitman, J., Yang, L., et al. (2020). Innovative Preclinical Models for Pulmonary Drug Delivery Research. *Expert Opin. Drug Deliv.* 17, 463–478. doi:10.1080/17425247.2020.1730807

Elias-Kirma, S., Artzy-Schnirman, A., Das, P., Heller-Algazi, M., Korin, N., and Sznitman, J. (2020). In Situ-Like Aerosol Inhalation Exposure for Cytotoxicity Assessment Using Airway-On-Chips Platforms. *Front. Bioeng. Biotechnol.* 8, 91. doi:10.3389/fbioe.2020.00091

Emulate (2021). Lung-Chip — Emulate. Available at: https://www.emulatebio.com/lung-chip (Accessed March 29, 2021).

European Commission Joint Research Centre (2021). *Establishing the Scientific Validity of Complex* in Vitro *Models: Results of a EURL ECVAM Survey*. Available at: https://publications.jrc.ec.europa.eu/repository/handle/JRC122394 (Accessed May 18, 2021).

Ferrell, N., Desai, R. R., Fleischman, A. J., Roy, S., Humes, H. D., and Fissell, W. H. (2010). A Microfluidic Bioreactor with Integrated Transepithelial Electrical Resistance (TEER) Measurement Electrodes for Evaluation of Renal Epithelial Cells. *Biotechnol. Bioeng.* 107, 707–716. doi:10.1002/bit.22835

Fiegel, J., Ehrhardt, C., Schaefer, U. F., Lehr, C.-M., and Hanes, J. (2003). Large Porous Particle Impingement on Lung Epithelial Cell Monolayers-Ttoward Improved Particle Characterization in the Lung. *Pharm. Res.* 20, 788–796. doi:10.1023/a:1023441804464

Gordon, S., Daneshian, M., Bouwstra, J., Caloni, F., Constant, S., Davies, D. E., et al. (2015). Non-animal Models of Epithelial Barriers (Skin, Intestine and Lung) in Research, Industrial Applications and Regulatory Toxicology. *ALTEX* 32, 327–378. doi:10.14573/altex.1510051

Grainger, C. I., Greenwell, L. L., Lockley, D. J., Martin, G. P., and Forbes, B. (2006). Culture of Calu-3 Cells at the Air Interface Provides a Representative Model of the Airway Epithelial Barrier. *Pharm. Res.* 23, 1482–1490. doi:10.1007/s11095-006-0255-0

Griep, L. M., Wolbers, F., de Wagenaar, B., ter Braak, P. M., Weksler, B. B., Romero, I. A., et al. (2013). BBB on Chip: Microfluidic Platform to Mechanically and Biochemically Modulate Blood-Brain Barrier Function. *Biomed. Microdevices* 15, 145–150. doi:10.1007/s10544-012-9699-7

Günzel, D., Zakrzewski, S. S., Schmid, T., Pangalos, M., Wiedenhoeft, J., Blasse, C., et al. (2012). From TER to Trans- and Paracellular Resistance: Lessons from Impedance Spectroscopy. *Ann. N. Y Acad. Sci.* 1257, 142–151. doi:10.1111/j.1749-6632.2012.06540.x

Haghi, M., Young, P. M., Traini, D., Jaiswal, R., Gong, J., and Bebawy, M. (2010). Time- and Passage-dependent Characteristics of a Calu-3 Respiratory Epithelial Cell Model. *Drug Dev. Ind. Pharm.* 36, 1207–1214. doi:10.3109/03639041003695113

Henry, O. Y. F., Villenave, R., Cronce, M. J., Leineweber, W. D., Benz, M. A., and Ingber, D. E. (2017). Organs-on-chips with Integrated Electrodes for Transepithelial Electrical Resistance (TEER) Measurements of Human Epithelial Barrier Function. *Lab. Chip* 17, 2264–2271. doi:10.1039/c7lc00155j

Hittinger, M., Juntke, J., Kletting, S., Schneider-Daum, N., de Souza Carvalho, C., and Lehr, C.-M. (2015). Preclinical Safety and Efficacy Models for Pulmonary Drug Delivery of Antimicrobials with Focus on *In Vitro* Models. *Adv. Drug Deliv. Rev.* 85, 44–56. doi:10.1016/j.addr.2014.10.011

Hittinger, M., Schneider-Daum, N., and Lehr, C.-M. (2017). Cell and Tissue-Based *In Vitro* Models for Improving the Development of Oral Inhalation Drug Products. *Eur. J. Pharm. Biopharm.* 118, 73–78. doi:10.1016/j.ejpb.2017.02.019

Horstmann, J. C., Thorn, C. R., Carius, P., Graef, F., Murgia, X., de Souza Carvalho-Wodarz, C., et al. (2021). A Custom-Made Device for Reproducibly Depositing Pre-metered Doses of Nebulized Drugs on Pulmonary Cells *In Vitro*. *Front. Bioeng. Biotechnol.* 9, 643491. doi:10.3389/fbioe.2021.643491

Huang, D., Liu, T., Liao, J., Maharjan, S., Xie, X., Pérez, M., et al. (2021). Reversed-engineered Human Alveolar Lung-On-A-Chip Model. *Proc. Natl. Acad. Sci. USA* 118, e2016146118. doi:10.1073/pnas.2016146118

Huh, D., Matthews, B. D., Mammoto, A., Montoya-Zavala, M., Hsin, H. Y., and Ingber, D. E. (2010). Reconstituting Organ-Level Lung Functions on a Chip. *Science* 328, 1662–1668. doi:10.1126/science.1188302

Humayun, M., Chow, C.-W., and Young, E. W. K. (2018). Microfluidic Lung Airway-On-A-Chip with Arrayable Suspended Gels for Studying Epithelial and Smooth Muscle Cell Interactions. *Lab. Chip* 18, 1298–1309. doi:10.1039/c7lc01357d

Jimenez-Valdes, R. J., Can, U. I., Niemeyer, B. F., and Benam, K. H. (2020). Where

We Stand: Lung Organotypic Living Systems that Emulate Human-Relevant Host-Environment/Pathogen Interactions. *Front. Bioeng. Biotechnol.* 8, 989. doi:10.3389/fbioe.2020.00989

Junaid, A., Mashaghi, A., Hankemeier, T., and Vulto, P. (2017). An End-User Perspective on Organ-On-A-Chip: Assays and Usability Aspects. *Curr. Opin. Biomed. Eng.* 1, 15–22. doi:10.1016/j.cobme.2017.02.002

Kim, H. J., Huh, D., Hamilton, G., and Ingber, D. E. (2012). Human Gut-On-A-Chip Inhabited by Microbial flora that Experiences Intestinal Peristalsis-like Motions and Flow. *Lab. Chip* 12, 2165–2174. doi:10.1039/c2lc40074j

Kirkstall Ltd (2020). *Quasi Vivo® | Commercially Available Organ-On-A-Chip Technology.* York, United Kingdom: Kirkstall Ltd. Available at: https://www.kirkstall.com/ (Accessed March 30, 2021).

Lacroix, G., Koch, W., Ritter, D., Gutleb, A. C., Larsen, S. T., Loret, T., et al. (2018). Air-Liquid Interface In Vitro Models for Respiratory Toxicology Research: Consensus Workshop and Recommendations. *Appl. Vitro Toxicol.* 4, 91–106. doi:10.1089/aivt.2017.0034

Lorenz, A., Pawar, V., Häussler, S., and Weiss, S. (2016). Insights into Host-Pathogen Interactions from State-Of-The-Art Animal Models of respiratoryPseudomonas Aeruginosainfections. *FEBS Lett.* 590, 3941–3959. doi:10.1002/1873-3468.12454

Nalayanda, D. D., Puleo, C., Fulton, W. B., Sharpe, L. M., Wang, T.-H., and Abdullah, F. (2009). An Open-Access Microfluidic Model for Lung-specific Functional Studies at an Air-Liquid Interface. *Biomed. Microdevices* 11, 1081–1089. doi:10.1007/s10544-009-9325-5

Odijk, M., van der Meer, A. D., Levner, D., Kim, H. J., van der Helm, M. W., Segerink, L. I., et al. (2015). Measuring Direct Current Trans-epithelial Electrical Resistance in Organ-On-A-Chip Microsystems. *Lab. Chip* 15, 745–752. doi:10.1039/c4lc01219d

Phalen, R. F., and Mendez, L. B. (2009). Dosimetry Considerations for Animal Aerosol Inhalation Studies. *Biomarkers* 14 (Suppl. 1), 63–66. doi:10.1080/13547500902965468

Punde, T. H., Wu, W.-H., Lien, P.-C., Chang, Y.-L., Kuo, P.-H., Chang, M. D.-T., et al. (2015). A Biologically Inspired Lung-On-A-Chip Device for the Study of Protein-Induced Lung Inflammation. *Integr. Biol. (Camb)* 7, 162–169. doi:10.1039/c4ib00239c

Rootare, H. M., and Powers, J. M. (1977). Preparation of Ag/AgCl Electrodes. *J. Biomed. Mater. Res.* 11, 633–635. doi:10.1002/jbm.820110416

Schimek, K., Frentzel, S., Luettich, K., Bovard, D., Rütschle, I., Boden, L., et al. (2020). Human Multi-Organ Chip Co-culture of Bronchial Lung Culture and Liver Spheroids for Substance Exposure Studies. *Sci. Rep.* 10, 7865. doi:10.1038/s41598-020-64219-6

Schindelin, J., Arganda-Carreras, I., Frise, E., Kaynig, V., Longair, M., Pietzsch, T., et al. (2012). Fiji: an Open-Source Platform for Biological-Image Analysis. *Nat. Methods* 9, 676–682. doi:10.1038/nmeth.2019

Srinivasan, B., Kolli, A. R., Esch, M. B., Abaci, H. E., Shuler, M. L., and Hickman, J. J. (2015). TEER Measurement Techniques for *In Vitro* Barrier Model Systems. *J. Lab. Autom.* 20, 107–126. doi:10.1177/2211068214561025

Stucki, A. O., Stucki, J. D., Hall, S. R. R., Felder, M., Mermoud, Y., Schmid, R. A., et al. (2015). A Lung-On-A-Chip Array with an Integrated Bio-Inspired Respiration Mechanism. *Lab. Chip* 15, 1302–1310. doi:10.1039/c4lc01252f

Tenenbaum-Katan, J., Artzy-Schnirman, A., Fishler, R., Korin, N., and Sznitman, J. (2018). Biomimetics of the Pulmonary Environmentin Vitro: A Microfluidics Perspective. *Biomicrofluidics* 12, 042209. doi:10.1063/1.5023034

Thompson, C. L., Fu, S., Heywood, H. K., Knight, M. M., and Thorpe, S. D. (2020). Mechanical Stimulation: A Crucial Element of Organ-On-Chip Models. *Front. Bioeng. Biotechnol.* 8, 602646. doi:10.3389/fbioe.2020.602646

Toepke, M. W., and Beebe, D. J. (2006). PDMS Absorption of Small Molecules and Consequences in Microfluidic Applications. *Lab. Chip* 6, 1484–1486. doi:10.1039/B612140C

Wilson, A. P., and Richards, S. A. (2000). Consuming and Grouping: Recource-Mediated Animal Aggregation. *Ecol. Lett.* 3, 175–180. doi:10.1046/j.1461-0248.2000.00135.x

7

Rho-Kinase 1/2 Inhibition Prevents Transforming Growth Factor-β-Induced Effects on Pulmonary Remodeling and Repair

Xinhui Wu[1,2], Vicky Verschut[3], Manon E. Woest[1,2,3], John-Poul Ng-Blichfeldt[1,2], Ana Matias[1,2], Gino Villetti[4], Alessandro Accetta[4], Fabrizio Facchinetti[4], Reinoud Gosens[1,2] and Loes E. M. Kistemaker[1,2,3]*

[1]Department of Molecular Pharmacology, Faculty of Science and Engineering, University of Groningen, Groningen, Netherlands, [2]Groningen Research Institute for Asthma and COPD, University Medical Center Groningen, University of Groningen, Groningen, Netherlands, [3]AQUILO BV, Groningen, Netherlands, [4]Corporate Pre-Clinical R and D, Chiesi Farmaceutici S.p.A., Parma, Italy

*Correspondence:
Loes E. M. Kistemaker
l.e.m.kistemaker@quilo.nl

Transforming growth factor (TGF)-β-induced myofibroblast transformation and alterations in mesenchymal-epithelial interactions contribute to chronic lung diseases such as chronic obstructive pulmonary disease (COPD), asthma and pulmonary fibrosis. Rho-associated coiled-coil-forming protein kinase (ROCK) consists as two isoforms, ROCK1 and ROCK2, and both are playing critical roles in many cellular responses to injury. In this study, we aimed to elucidate the differential role of ROCK isoforms on TGF-β signaling in lung fibrosis and repair. For this purpose, we tested the effect of a non-selective ROCK 1 and 2 inhibitor (compound 31) and a selective ROCK2 inhibitor (compound A11) in inhibiting TGF-β-induced remodeling in lung fibroblasts and slices; and dysfunctional epithelial-progenitor interactions in lung organoids. Here, we demonstrated that the inhibition of ROCK1/2 with compound 31 represses TGF-β-driven actin remodeling as well as extracellular matrix deposition in lung fibroblasts and PCLS, whereas selective ROCK2 inhibition with compound A11 did not. Furthermore, the TGF-β induced inhibition of organoid formation was functionally restored in a concentration-dependent manner by both dual ROCK 1 and 2 inhibition and selective ROCK2 inhibition. We conclude that dual pharmacological inhibition of ROCK 1 and 2 counteracts TGF-β induced effects on remodeling and alveolar epithelial progenitor function, suggesting this to be a promising therapeutic approach for respiratory diseases associated with fibrosis and defective lung repair.

Keywords: pulmonary remodeling, lung repair, rock inhibition, lung organoid, TGFβ signaling

INTRODUCTION

Fibroblast to myofibroblast differentiation represents an essential event during wound closure and tissue repair. Transforming growth factor (TGF)-β plays a major role in promoting myofibroblast differentiation. However, excessive and persistent TGF-β-induced myofibroblast differentiation and extracellular matrix (ECM) deposition contribute to pathological tissue remodeling that occurs in a broad range of lung diseases, such as chronic obstructive pulmonary disease (COPD) (Grzela et al., 2016), asthma (Fehrenbach et al., 2017), and idiopathic pulmonary fibrosis (IPF) (King et al., 2011;

Hirota and Martin, 2013; Ohgiya et al., 2017). Myofibroblasts are contractile cells possessing morphologic and biochemical features that are intermediate between fibroblast and smooth muscle cells. These contractile fibroblasts secrete ECM proteins such as collagens, which are the most important load-bearing component of the parenchymal lung connective tissue, crucial for maintaining structural and mechanical organ functionality (El Agha et al., 2017). Moreover, the differentiated myofibroblasts are characterized by enhanced expression of α-smooth muscle actin (α-SMA) and other cytoskeletal proteins contributing to the contractile activity of these cells (Meng et al., 2016; Florian et al., 2019; Winters et al., 2019).

As such, the persistent presence of myofibroblasts in disease may actually contribute to defective repair by airway and alveolar epithelial cells. Mesenchymal-epithelial interactions normally contribute to epithelial regeneration after injury, yet myofibroblasts are less effective in supporting epithelial repair (Demayo et al., 2002; Horowitz and Thannickal, 2006; Meng et al., 2016). Previously, we reported that TGF-β-induced myofibroblast differentiation profoundly skews the canonical WNT/β-catenin signaling in human lung fibroblasts, and results in reduced secretion of factors that nurture epithelial repair such as FGF7, FGF10 and HGF (Ng-Blichfeldt et al., 2019). Furthermore, TGF-β increases the expression of WNT-5A and WNT-5B by myofibroblasts (Ng-Blichfeldt et al., 2019), and such mesenchymal WNT-5A/5B signaling represses alveolar epithelial repair by inhibition of canonical WNT signaling (Wu et al., 2019a). Currently, there are no pharmacological treatments available in the clinic that effectively prevent or reverse the aberrant TGF-β-induced changes in remodeling and lung repair.

Rho-associated coiled-coil containing kinases (ROCK) are part of the AGC (cAMP-dependent protein kinase/protein kinase G/protein kinase C) kinase family that play crucial roles in several vital cellular functions including gene transcription, proliferation, differentiation, and apoptosis (Klein et al., 2019; Majolée et al., 2019; Park et al., 2019; Wang et al., 2019). Two isoforms, ROCK1 and ROCK2, were described as being part of this family of RhoA-GTP interacting proteins. Several studies have revealed a diverse range of functions of ROCK1 and 2 in the context of lung diseases (Htwe et al., 2017) and ROCK inhibitors have potential therapeutic applicability in lung diseases such as asthma, COPD and pulmonary fibrosis (Hallgren et al., 2012; Vigil et al., 2012; Htwe et al., 2017; dos Santos et al., 2018; Knipe et al., 2018). A recent study also showed that the gene expression of both ROCK1 and ROCK2 were increased in the lungs of the patients who died from Covid-19 (Ackermann et al., 2020). Pharmacological inhibition of ROCK using ROCK inhibitors has been shown to prevent airway remodeling and lung fibrosis in animal models (Qi et al., 2015; Knipe et al., 2018). Fasudil, a classic non-selective ROCK inhibitor and vasodilator approved in Japan for the treatment of brain vessel vasospasm induced by subarachnoid haemorrhage, is reported playing protective roles in bleomycin-induced pulmonary fibrosis in animal models (Jiang et al., 2012); however, its clinical applications are limited by the modest ROCK inhibition efficacy and poor selectivity (Tumbarello and Turner, 2006;

Hallgren et al., 2012; Pireddu et al., 2012; Rath and Olson, 2012; Vigil et al., 2012; Xueyang et al., 2016; Huang et al., 2018).

The differential role of ROCK isoforms on TGFβ signaling in fibrosis and repair has not been thoroughly investigated, yet. To fill this gap, we have selected from existing patents two potent ROCK-inhibitors: compound 31, a dual ROCK1 and ROCK2 inhibitor, and compound A11, a ROCK2 selective inhibitor. We then evaluated their efficacies in three in vitro models to identify their potential in restoring TGF-β-induced changes in myofibroblast differentiation and impaired alveolar epithelial progenitor cell function. Our results show that dual ROCK1 and 2 inhibition prevents myofibroblast differentiation and ECM deposition induced by TGF-β in lung fibroblasts and PCLS, whereas ROCK2 selective inhibition did not. Furthermore, our results reveal that dual ROCK1/2 and ROCK2 inhibition restores the defective TGF-β-induced changes in mesenchymal-epithelial progenitor interactions during organoid formation, suggesting ROCK inhibition as a promising therapeutic target for pulmonary diseases characterized by defective lung repair.

MATERIALS AND METHODS

Synthesis of compound 31 and compound A11

3,4-dimethoxy-N-((R)-1- (3 - (((S) - 6 - (propylamino) - 4, 5, 6, 7 tetrahydrobenzo [d]thiazol-2-yl) carbamoyl) phenyl) ethyl) benzamide (example 31 from WO 2012/006202) and N-(3-(5-((4-chloro-1H-indazol-5-yl)amino)-1,3,4-thiadiazol-2-yl)phenyl)-1-methyl-1H-pyrazole-4-carboxamide (example A11 from WO 2016/138335) were prepared by adapting the general synthesis procedures reported in the patent references.

Inhibition of ROCK1 and ROCK2 Enzymatic Activity

ROCK enzymatic activity inhibition was measured as described previously (Cantoni et al., 2019). Glutathione S-transferase (GST)-tagged 1–535 human ROCK1 and GST-tagged 1–552 human ROCK2 (Fisher Scientific United Kingdom Ltd., Loughborough, Leicestershire, United Kingdom) were diluted into assay buffer containing 40 mM Tris pH7.5, 20 mM MgCl2 0.1 mg/ml BSA, 50 μM DTT and 2.5 μM peptide substrate (myelin basic protein). Compounds to be tested were dissolved in dimethyl sulphoxide (DMSO) to a final concentration of 1%. All reactions/incubations were performed at 25°C. The compounds and either ROCK1 or 2 were mixed and incubated for 30 min. Reactions were initiated by addition of ATP (10 μM). After a 1 h incubation, 10 μl of ADP-Glo Reagent (Promega United Kingdom Ltd., Southampton, United Kingdom) was added and after another 45 min incubation, 20 μl of kinase Detection Buffer were added and then the mixture was incubated for 30 min. The luminescent signal was measured on a luminometer. Compounds were tested in a dose-response format. To determine the IC50, data were fit to a plot of % inhibition vs. Log10 compound concentration with a sigmoidal fit

TABLE 1 | Investigational compounds and concentrations in the current study.

Compound	IC50 ROCK1	IC50 ROCK2	Concentration	Selectivity
Compound 31	2.9 ± 0.5 nM	4 ± 0.6 nM	0.01, 0.1 and 1 µM	ROCK1 and 2
Compound A11	341.1 ± 38 nM	6.1 ± 1.4 nM	0.1, 1 and 10 µM	ROCK2 selective

using activitybase software (v 8.05, ID Business Solutions Limited, Guildford, United Kingdom).

Animals

Animals were housed conventionally under a 12-h light-dark cycle and received food and water ad libitum. All experiments were performed in accordance with the national guidelines and approved by the University of Groningen Committee for Animal Experimentation.

Precision-Cut Lung Slices

PCLS were harvested from 8–12 week old female Balb/c mice as described previously (Oenema et al., 2013; Van Dijk et al., 2017; Wu et al., 2019b). Briefly, animals were euthanized by subcutaneous injection of ketamine (40 mg/kg, Alfasan, Woerden, The Netherlands) and dexdomitor (0.5 mg/kg, Orion Pharma, Mechelen, Belgium), and the trachea was exposed and cannulated. Lungs were filled with 1.5 ml of 1.5% low melting-point agarose solution (Gerbu Biotechnik GmbH, Wieblingen, Germany) in $CaCl_2$ (0.9 mM), $MgSO_4$ (0.4 mM), KCl (2.7 mM), NaCl (58.2 mM), NaH_2PO_4 (0.6 mM), glucose (8.4 mM), $NaHCO_3$ (13 mM), Hepes (12.6 mM), sodium pyruvate (0.5 mM), glutamine (1 mM), MEM-amino acids mixture (1:50), and MEM-vitamins mixture (1:100), pH = 7.2). Agarose was allowed to solidify at 4°C for 15 min and lungs were then harvested. Lobes were separated and sliced individually, at a thickness of 250 µm in medium composed of $CaCl_2$ (1.8 mM), $MgSO_4$ (0.8 mM), KCl (5.4 mM), NaCl (116.4 mM), NaH_2PO_4 (1.2 mM), glucose (16.7 mM), $NaHCO_3$ (26.1 mM) andHepes (25.2 mM), set at pH = 7.2, using a tissue slicer (Leica VT1000S, Vibratome line, Amsterdam, The Netherlands). Slices were transferred in cell culture dishes, at 37°C in a humidified atmosphere of 5% CO_2 and medium ($CaCl_2$ (1.8 mM), $MgSO_4$ (0.8 mM), KCl (5.4 mM), NaCl (116.4 mM), NaH_2PO_4 (1.2 mM), glucose (16.7 mM), $NaHCO_3$ (26.1 mM), Hepes (25.2 mM), sodium pyruvate (1 mM), glutamine (2 mM), MEM-amino acids mixture (1:50), MEM-vitamins mixture (1:100) penicillin (100 U/mL) and streptomycin (100 µg/ml), pH = 7.2.) was refreshed every 30 min for four times to remove any remaining agarose and cell debris.

Treatments on PCLS

PCLS were incubated in Dulbecco's Modification of Eagle's Medium (DMEM) supplemented with sodium pyruvate (1 mM), MEM non-essential amino acid mixture (1:100; Gibco® by Life Technologies), gentamycin (45 µg/ml; Gibco® by Life Technologies), penicillin (100 U/mL), streptomycin (100 µg/ml), and amphotericin B (1.5 µg/ml; Gibco® by Life Technologies) at 37°C-5% CO_2 in a 12-well plate (three slices per well). Slices were treated with vehicle, 2 ng/ml TGF-β_1 (2 ng/ml, R&D systems, Abingdon, United Kingdom) and/or investigational compounds (**Table 1**) for 48 h. The PCLS were then stored at −80°C until PCR analysis, Western Blot analysis.

Fibroblast Cell Culture and Treatments

Human lung fibroblasts MRC5 (CCL-171; ATCC, Wesel, Germany) were cultured in Ham's F12 medium (Life technologies, Carlsbad, United States) supplemented with 10% (v/v) fetal bovine serum (FBS, PAA Laboratories, Pasching, Austria), 2 mM L-glutamine (Life Technologies #35050–061), 100 U/mL penicillin/streptomycin, and 1% amphotericin B (1x, Gibco). CCL-206 mouse lung fibroblasts ([MLg2908, CCL206], ATCC, Wesel, Germany) were cultured in DMEM/F12 medium supplemented with 10% FBS, penicillin/streptomycin (100 U/mL), glutamine (1%) and Amphotericin B. Cells were incubated at 37°C, 5% CO_2 humidified environment. MRC5 or CCL206 fibroblasts were starved once grown to 80% confluence in the 6-well culture plates. The starvation medium contains the same components as culture medium described above, but with only 0.5% FBS. After 24 h starvation, cells were then incubated with either vehicle, TGF-β1 and/or investigational compounds (**Table 1**) in serum deprivation medium for 48 h. MRC5 fibroblasts were collected for gene expression analysis. CCL206 fibroblasts were washed three times with warm PBS and proliferation-inactivated by incubation in mitomycin C (10 µg/ml, Sigma #M4287) for 2 h, followed by three washes in warm PBS and trypsinization prior to mixing with epithelial cells, as described previously (Ng-Blichfeldt et al., 2018; Ng-Blichfeldt et al., 2019).

Mouse Epithelial Cell Isolation

Epithelial (EpCAM$^+$) cells were isolated from lungs of 8–12 week old male and female C57Bl6 mice with microbeads as described previously (Ng-Blichfeldt et al., 2018; Ng-Blichfeldt et al., 2019; Wu et al., 2019a). Lungs of mice were flushed through the heart with PBS, instilled with dispase (BD Biosciences, Oxford, United Kingdom, #354235) and low-melt agarose (Sigma Aldrich, Poole, United Kingdom #A9414), and incubated at room temperature (RT) for 45 min. Trachea and extrapulmonary airways were removed, and the remaining lobes were homogenized in DMEM medium with dnase1 (Applichem, Germany #A3778). The resulting suspension was passed through a cell strainer with the size of 100 µm, incubated with microbeads conjugated to antibodies for CD45 (Miltenyi Biotec, Teterow, Germany #130–052–301) and CD31 (Miltenyi, #130–097–418), and passed through LS columns (Miltenyi #130–091–051). The CD31$^-$/CD45$^-$ suspension was then enriched for epithelial cells by positive selection using EpCAM (CD326) microbeads (Miltenyi #130–105–958). EpCAM$^+$ cells were resuspended in DMEM with 10% FBS.

Organoid Culture

The organoid assay was established as described previously (Ng-Blichfeldt et al., 2018; Ng-Blichfeldt et al., 2019; Wu et al., 2019a). EpCAM$^+$ cells were combined with fibroblasts at a 1:1 ratio in DMEM/F12 (10% FBS) at a density of 2 * 10^5 cells/ml. The cell suspension was then diluted 1:1 (v/v) with Matrigel (Fisher Scientific, Landsmeer, The Netherlands) and were seeded into transwell inserts (Thermo Fischer Scientific, Waltham, United States #10421761) witin 24-well plates (100 µl/insert). Cultures were maintained in DMEM/F12 with 5% (v/v) FBS, 2 mM glutamine, antibiotics, insulin-transferrin-selenium (1x, Gibco #15290018), recombinant mouse EGF (0.025 µg/ml, Sigma #SRP3196), bovine pituitary extract (30 µg/ml, Sigma #P1476), and freshly added all-trans retinoic acid (0.01µM, Sigma #R2625) at 37°C with 5% CO2. Media was refreshed every 2–3 days. The total number of organoids per well was counted manually 14 days after seeding using a light microscope at ×20 magnification. Organoid diameter was measured at the same day using a light microscope connected to NIS-Elements software. Thereafter, organoid cultures were fixed for immunofluorescence.

Gene Expression Analysis

Total RNA was extracted from PCLS by automated purification using the Maxwell 16 instrument and the corresponding Maxwell 16 LEV simply RNA tissue kit (Promega, Madison, United States) according to the manufacturer's instructions. Total RNA was extracted form MRC5 fibroblasts using the TRIzol method. RNA concentrations were determined using a ND-1000 spectrophotometer and equal amounts of total mRNA were then reverse transcribed (Promega, Madison, United States 0). The cDNA was subjected to real-time qPCR (Westburg, Leusden, The Netherlands) using SYBR green as the DNA binding dye (Roche Applied Science, Mannheim, Germany) on an Illumina Eco Real-Time PCR system (Westburg, Leusden, the Netherlands), with denaturation at 94°C for 30 s, annealing at 59°C for 30 s and extension at 72°C for 30 s for 40 cycles followed by 10 min at 72°C. Real-time qPCR data were analyzed using LinRegPCR analysis software and the amount of target gene was normalized to the endogenous reference gene 18S ribosomal RNA for mouse PCLS and to SDHA for human fibroblasts. The specific forward and reverse primers used are listed in **Supplementary Table S1**.

Immunofluorescence

MRC5 fibroblasts were cultured on the coverslips within the culture plate to perform immunofluorescence experiments. Cells were washed twice with PBS and fixed with 4% paraformaldehyde (PFA) for 10 min at RT. Then cells were washed again twice with PBS and were incubated with Alxea Fluor™ 488 Phalloidin (ThermoFisher, A12379) 1:40 diluted in PBS for 20 min at RT. After washing three times with PBS, the coverslips were transferred onto glass slides and were mounted by mounting medium contains DAPI (Abcam #ab104139).

Organoid were fixed within ice-cold acetone/methanol (1:1) medium for 15 min at −20°C, then were blocked in PBS, supplemented with 5% BSA (Ng-Blichfeldt et al., 2018; Ng-

Blichfeldt et al., 2019; Wu et al., 2019a). Cultures were incubated with primary antibodies Rb anti-pro-surfactant protein C (pro-SPC, Millipore AB3786) and mouse anti-acetylated tubulin (ACT, Santa Cruz sc-23950) diluted 1:200 in PBS with 0.1% BSA and 0.1% Triton-X100 at 4°C overnight. Thereafter, cultures were washed 3 times in PBS (>1 h between washes) and incubated with secondary antibodies donkey anti-rabbit (Jackson Immunoresearch, 711–165–152) and donkey anti-mouse (Jackson Immunoresearch, 711–165–152) diluted 1: 200 at room temperature for 2.5 h. Cultures were excised from inserts and mounted on glass slides with mounting media containing DAPI (Abcam #ab104139) and glass coverslips.

Immunofluorescence was visualized using a Leica SP8 confocal microscope (Wetzlar, Germany), and images obtained with Leica LAS software.

Data Analysis

Statistical evaluation of differences was performed using one-way ANOVA followed by a Student-Newman Keuls post-hoc test. Differences were considered to be statistically significant when $p < 0.05$. GraphPad Prism eight software was used to perform statistical analysis.

RESULTS

Novel ROCK Inhibitors and Their Kinase Selectivity

Over the past decades, numerous ROCK inhibitors have been developed from a variety of distinct scaffolds, however, few examples of selective ROCK2 inhibitors have been described. We selected two potent ROCK inhibitors (ROCKi) spotted in public patents, one is a dual ROCK1 and 2 (ROCK1/2) inhibitor naming compound 31 (example 2 of WO 2012/006202); and the other is a ROCK2 selective inhibitor naming compound A11 (example A11 of WO 2016/138335). The enzymatic potency of these two compounds is shown in **Table 1**. Compound 31 and compound A11 were screened in a competitive assay against a large panel (>400) of human kinases (Kinome Scan®, Discoverx) at the concentration of 100 nM, >10-fold higher than the enzymatic IC$_{50}$ against ROCK2. The graphical view of kinome scan is reported in **Figure1** where only interactions under the threshold for residual activity of 35% are displayed and potentially indicating off-target interactions. Compound 31 shows three spots, two related to ROCKs (ROCK1: 0% CTRL and ROCK2: 0% CTRL) and only one off-target interaction at 9.3% related to VRK2. Compound A11 showed only interaction with ROCK2 at 0.35% vs CTRL.

Effects of Dual ROCK1/2 and ROCK2 Selective Inhibition on Transforming Growth Factor-β-Induced Myofibroblast Differentiation

To induce myofibroblast differentiation, MRC5 human lung fibroblasts were treated with TGF-β1 (2 ng/ml) for 48 h.

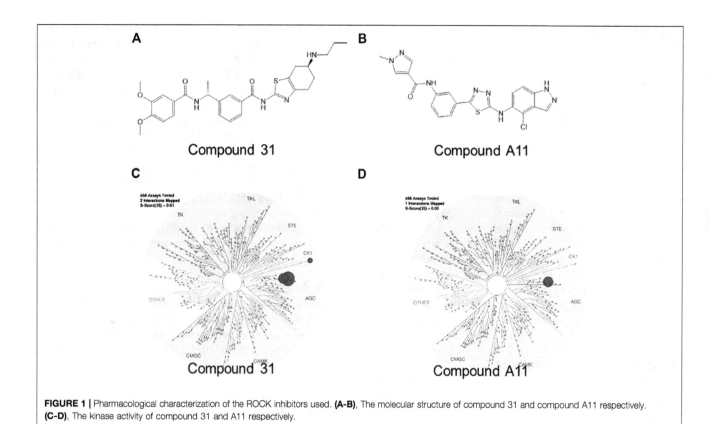

FIGURE 1 | Pharmacological characterization of the ROCK inhibitors used. **(A-B)**, The molecular structure of compound 31 and compound A11 respectively. **(C-D)**, The kinase activity of compound 31 and A11 respectively.

TGF-β1 increased the mRNA levels of α-smooth muscle actin (α-SMA), collagen 1α1 (Col1α1) and fibronectin (FN) significantly (**Figure 2**). To investigate the effect of ROCK inhibition on TGF-β driven airway remodeling, compound 31 (0.01-, 0.1-, and 1 μM) and compound A11 (0.1-, 1-, and 10 μM) were applied to the fibroblasts treated with TGF-β. Compound 31 had no effect on mRNA expression of FN in response to TGF-β, but significantly decreased the α-SMA gene expression level and tended to decrease the Col1α1 expression level in a concentration dependent manner (**Figures 2A–C**). In contrast, the ROCK2 selective compound A11 was not able to alter the expression of α-SMA, and if anything, tended to increase the expression of Col1α1 and FN in combination with TGF-β (**Figure 2D–F**). Neither compound 31 (1 μM) nor compound A11 (10 μM) had an effect on its own (i.e. in the absence of TGF-β). Next, we stained the MRC5 fibroblasts with phalloidin, which is able to bind and stabilize the filamentous actin (F-actin). As shown in **Figure 2G**, TGF-β treatment gave more F-actin stress fibers than the vehicle control, whereas treatment with compound 31 reduced stress fiber formation in combination with TGF-β (**Figure 2H**). Compound A11 on the other hand had no inhibitory effect and if anything, tended to enhance the formation of stress fibers (**Figure 2I**), similar to the previous findings on the gene expression of α-SMA.

In the murine PCLS, the mRNA levels of α-SMA, Col1α1 and FN were significantly increased by TGF-β treatment (**Figure 3**). In this model system, the increased mRNA expression of α-SMA, Col1α1 and FN were all significantly reduced by compound 31

in a concentration-dependent manner (**Figures 3A–C**). Interestingly, in line with the fibroblast data, compound A11 had no effect on the increased level of α-SMA, but significantly enhanced levels of Col1α1 and FN in the presence of TGF-β (**Figures 3D–F**). Taken together, these results indicate that dual ROCK 1/2 inhibition but not ROCK 2 selective inhibition is able to reduce the increased mRNA level of α-SMA, Col1α1 and FN in response to TGF-β. Unfortunately, the already high background expression of α-SMA, collagen 1 and fibronectin in the lung slice prevented us from being able to pick up strong enough effects of TGF-β at the protein level with semi-quantitative methods such as western blot and immunofluorescence microscopy (not shown), supporting the idea that the lung slice is suitable to pick up early changes, but not later stage changes associated with TGF-β induced fibrosis (Kasper et al., 2004).

Effects of Dual ROCK1/2 and ROCK2 Selective Inhibition on Transforming Growth Factor-β Induced Alterations in Alveolar Epithelial Organoid Formation

Previous studies from our group demonstrated that TGF-β activation impairs the fibroblast ability to support adult lung epithelial progenitor cells to form organoids (Ng-Blichfeldt et al., 2019). To investigate whether the novel ROCK inhibitors are able to restore the defective organoid formation, we designed the organoid assay as shown in **Figure 4A**. Murine CCL206 lung fibroblasts were

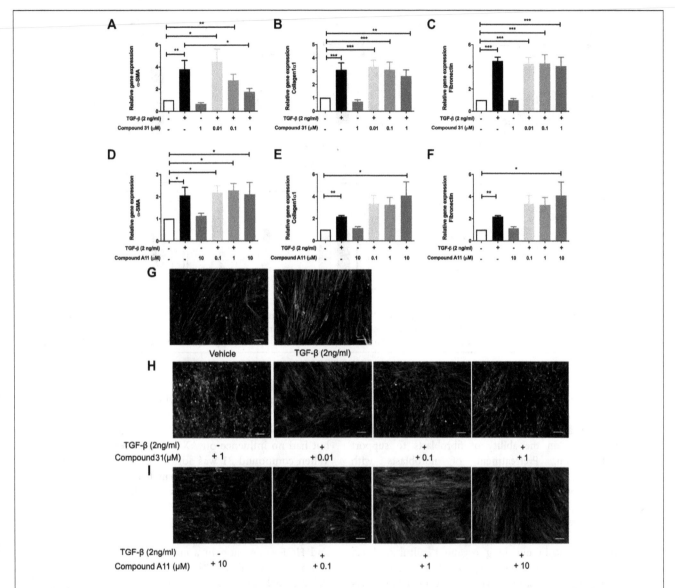

FIGURE 2 | Effects of dual ROCK1/2 vs ROCK2 selective inhibition on TGF-β induced myofibroblast differentiation of human lung fibroblasts. **(A–C)**, mRNA expression of α-sm-actin (α-SMA), collagen 1α1, and fibronectin (FN) in MRC5 cells treated with TGF-β (0-, 2 ng/mL) + compound 31 (0.01 μM, 0.1 μM and 1 μM). **(D–F)**, mRNA expression of α-sm-actin (α-SMA), collagen 1α1, and fibronectin (FN) in MRC5 cells treated with TGF-β (0-, 2 ng/mL) ± compound A11 (0.1 μM, 1 μM and 10 μM). **(G)**, Representative phalloidin staining of MRC5 cells treated with TGF-β (0-, 2 ng/mL). **(H)**, Representative phalloidin staining of MRC5 fibroblasts cells treated with TGF-β (0-, 2 ng/mL) + compound 31 (0-, 0.01-, 0.1-, 1- μM). **(I)**, Representative phalloidin staining of MRC5 cells treated with TGF-β (0-, 2 ng/mL) ± compound A11 (0-, 0.1-, 1-, 10- μM). Blue: dapi; green: F-actin. Scale bar = 100 μm.

differentiated into myofibroblasts by TGF-β (2 ng/ml) in the absence or presence of compound 31/compound A11 for 24 h. Afterward, the pretreated fibroblasts were extensively washed to remove the stimuli and co-cultured with freshly isolated mouse lung epithelial cells (CD31⁻/CD45⁻/EpCAM⁺ cells). Myofibroblast differentiation with TGF-β reduced the number of epithelial organoids formed at day 14, in line with our previous findings (12). Both compound 31 and compound A11 were able to restore the reduced numbers of organoids in a concentration-dependent manner to levels seen in the control cultures (**Figures 4C, D**). TGF-β induced myofibroblast differentiation had no impact on

the median diameter of the organoids formed (**Figures 4E, F**). In combination with compound A11, however, the median diameter was slightly decreased by 1 μM yet increased by 10 μM compound compared to TGF-β stimulation alone (**Figure 4F**). Myofibroblast differentiation with TGF-β significantly reduced the proportion of alveolar (proSPC⁺/ACT⁻) organoids yet increased the proportion of airway organoids (proSPC⁻/ACT⁺) quantified after immunofluorescence staining (**Figures 4G–I**). This was partially restored by dual ROCK1/2 inhibition with compound 31, whereas ROCK2 selective inhibition by compound A11 had no such effect (**Figures 4H, I**).

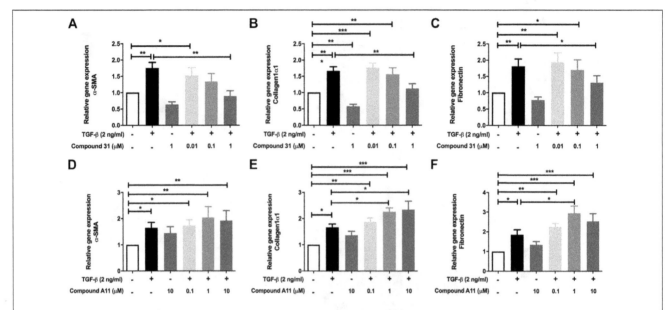

FIGURE 3 | Effects of dual ROCK1/2 vs ROCK2 selective inhibition on TGF-β induced myofibroblast differentiation in murine PCLS. **(A–C)**, mRNA expression of α-sm-actin (α-SMA), collagen 1α1, and fibronectin (FN) in murine PCLS treated with TGF-β (0-, 2 ng/mL) ± compound 31 (0.01 μM, 0.1 μM and 1 M). **(D–F)**, mRNA expression of α-smooth-actin (α-SMA), collagen 1α1, and fibronectin (FN) in murine PCLS treated with TGF-β (0-, 2 ng/mL) ± compound A11 (0.1 μM, 1 μM and 10 μM).

As the main effect of ROCK inhibition on the fibroblast was to reduce α-sm-actin expression and stress fiber formation (**Figure 2**), we also investigated the role of stress fiber formation in itself on the ability of fibroblasts to support organoid formation. Pretreatment of fibroblasts with jasplakinolide, a compound that restricts mobility by promoting actin polymerization, appeared sufficient to mimic the effect of TGF-β (**Figure 4J**). Interestingly, we spotted direct cell-cell contact between fibroblasts and developing epithelial organoids in the assay (**Figure 4K**). This is consistent with our observation that in our lung organoid cultures, direct contact of fibroblasts and alveolar epithelial cells is essential for organoid growth. Thus, organoids only form if fibroblasts and epithelial progenitors are in direct contact within the Matrigel. Organoids do not form if fibroblasts are cultured on the adjacent bottom chamber or if conditioned media of fibroblasts is used, confirming the essential role of fibroblasts in alveolar organoid formation (**Supplementary Figure S1**).

ROCK Inhibition Effects Secreted Factors From Fibroblasts That Support Organoid Formation

Fibroblasts secrete several growth factors that are essential to alveolar organoid formation, which is skewed by TGF-β treatment (Ng-Blichfeldt et al., 2019). Thus, we investigated whether ROCK inhibition may impact on the expression of these secreted factors. We focused these studies on compound 31 as this compound had the strongest impact on reversing the TGF-β effects throughout this study. We examined the mRNA expression level of several key components of WNT signaling

and FGF signaling pathways, which play an important role in tissue regeneration. Intriguingly, TGF-β increased the mRNA level of WNT-5A ($p < 0.05$) and WNT-2B in MRC5 fibroblasts but had no influence on AXIN2 (**Figures 5A–C**) expression. When compound 31 was added, the increased expression of those WNT ligands was normalized in a concentration-dependent manner (**Figures 5A–C**). Moreover, TGF-β stimulation increased FGF2 mRNA expression and decreased FGF-7 and HGF expression (**Figures 5D–F**). Compound 31 reduced FGF2 expression and restored FGF7 and HGF expression in a concentration-dependent manner (**Figure 5D–F**). Thus, TGF-β activation in fibroblasts distorts the mesenchymal-epithelial interactions via WNT signaling and FGF signaling pathways, which was reversed by dual ROCK 1/2 inhibition.

DISCUSSION

A better understanding of the mechanisms that regulate phenotype and function of lung (myo)fibroblasts may lead to the identification of therapeutic targets. TGF-β is a master regulator of myofibroblast differentiation in fibrosis, as evident from several *in vitro* and *in vivo* studies (Meng et al., 2016; Nagai et al., 2019; Ng-Blichfeldt et al., 2019; Noe et al., 2019; Saidi et al., 2019). In this study, we investigated the potential of two novel ROCK inhibitors with different selectivity against two ROCK isoforms in counteracting TGF-β induced effects on myofibroblast differentiation and alveolar epithelial progenitor organoid formation. Interactions between pulmonary fibroblasts and epithelial cells not only contributes to homeostasis but also to

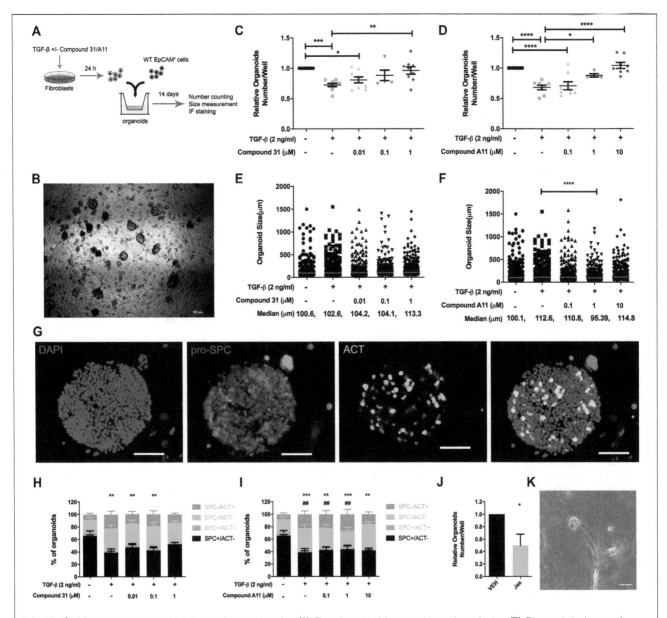

FIGURE 4 | ROCK inhibition restored the reduction of organoid number. **(A)**, The schematic of the organoid experimental setup. **(B)**, Representative images of epithelial organoids obtained, scale bar = 100 μm. **(C-D)**, Total organoid number at day 14 after co-culture of mouse CD31-/CD45-/EpCam+ cells with CCL206 lung fibroblasts pretreated with TGF-β (0-, 2 ng/mL) ± compound 31 (0.01 μM, 0.1 μM and 1 μM; panel C) or ompound A11 (0.1 μM, 1 μM and 10 μM; panel D), N = 4 - 6, mean ± SEM is shown, *$p < 0.05$, **$p < 0.01$. **(E-F)**, Organoid size measured at day 14 for the same experimental conditions as shown in C-D. **(G)**, Representative images of immunofluorescence staining of organoids, blue: dapi, red: pro-spc, green: acetylated tubulin (ACT), the scale bar = 100 μm. **(H-I)**, Quantification of organoid proportion expressing pro-proSPC+ or ACT+ at day 14. *$p < 0.05$, **$p < 0.01$, ***$p < 0.001$ compared to vehicle for proSPC+/ACT- alveolar organoids, #; $p < 0.05$, #$p < 0.01$ compared to vehicle for proSPC-/ACT+ airway organoids. **(J)**, Total organoid number at day14 of mouse CD31-/CD45-/EpCam+ cells with CCL206 lung fibroblasts pretreated with with jasplakinolide (100 nM). **(K)**, Image of a fibroblast cell touching an early formed organoid from day-3, scale bar = 100 μm.

lung repair in many pathological conditions (Demayo et al., 2002; Horowitz and Thannickal, 2006; Hirota and Martin, 2013; El Agha et al., 2017; Wu et al., 2019a; Ng-Blichfeldt et al., 2019; Noe et al., 2019; Zepp and Morrisey, 2019). We previously showed (Ng-Blichfeldt et al., 2019) that this interaction is disturbed if fibroblasts are transdifferentiated into myofibroblasts by TGF-β. A reduction in SPC+ alveolar organoids was observed after TGF-β treatment and an increase in the number of ACT+ airway

organoids. ROCK 1 and ROCK 2 inhibition was able to restore the reduced organoid formation in response to TGF-β in current study and dual inhibition partially restored the number of SPC+ alveolar organoids, whereas selective ROCK2 inhibition did not. We propose two mechanistic explanations for this TGF-β effect, being restriction of fibroblast motility and alterations in secreted factors, both of which are normalized by dual ROCK1/2 inhibition. Indeed, fibroblasts are needed in co-culture with

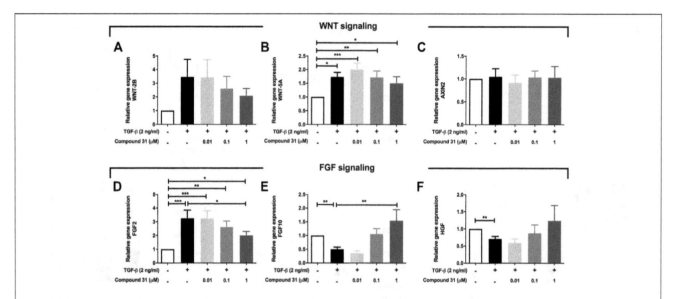

FIGURE 5 | Expression of WNT signaling and FGF signaling pathway genes in response to TGF-β and compound 31. **(A-F)**, The mRNA expression of WNT-2B, WNT-5A, AXIN2, FGF2, FGF10 and HGF in MRC5 cells treated with TGF-β (0-, 2 ng/mL) ± compound 31 (0.01 µM, 0.1 µM and 1 µM). *$p < 0.05$, **$p < 0.01$, ***$p < 0.001$.

epithelial cells in order to form organoids and organoids form only if fibroblasts are in direct cell-cell contact. We speculated that fibroblast motility is required for this effect. TGF-β restricts fibroblast motility by increasing α-sm-actin stress fibers. In support, we show that dual ROCK1/2 inhibition can inhibit both the stress fiber formation and the reduced organoid numbers in response to TGF-β. Furthermore, pretreatment of fibroblasts with jasplakinolide, which restricts fibroblast mobility by inducing α-sm-actin stress fiber formation, is sufficient to disturb the organoid formation to a similar extent as TGF-β (Ng-Blichfeldt et al., 2019).

In the past 2 decades, the development of pharmacological ROCK inhibitors has gained increasing interest; however, in the majority of published studies classic ROCK inhibitors, such as Y27632 and (hydroxy) fasudil, both of which target the ATP-dependent kinase domain of ROCK1 and ROCK2, are utilized. The two ROCK isoforms, ROCK1 and ROCK2, are structurally similar sharing ~60% overall amino acid identity, and within the N-terminal kinase domain, they are ~90% homologous. Accordingly, the design of isoform selective inhibitors has until now been very challenging. Unfortunately, both these first generation ROCK inhibitors have poor ROCK inhibition potency, and are additionally unselective against a range of other kinases, especially those in the AGC family (Tumbarello and Turner, 2006; Hallgren et al., 2012; Pireddu et al., 2012; Rath and Olson, 2012; Vigil et al., 2012; Xueyang et al., 2016; Huang et al., 2018; Cantoni et al., 2019). To fill this gap, we selected, as tool compounds, two ROCK inhibitors previously described in two distinct patents, a ROCK 1 and 2 inhibitor (compound 31), and a ROCK2 selective inhibitor (compound A11). Our results show that they elicit non-identical effects in TGF-β-induced remodeling. We show an increase of α-SMA expression in TGF-β activated human fibroblasts and the murine PCLS, and only

compound 31 was able to downregulate the contractile marker expression in both models, indicating that dual ROCK 1/2 inhibition is necessary for preventing contractile activity in pulmonary fibroblasts. A recent study (Knipe et al., 2018) using genetic ROCK inhibition showed that there is no significant decrease in α-SMA expression with individual ROCK1 or ROCK2 knockdown as compared with nontargeting siRNA in response to TGF-β, however, they showed a reduction of α-SMA expression when ROCK1 and ROCK2 were simultaneously knocked down. Together, this indicates that dual ROCK1 and ROCK2 inhibition profoundly attenuates the contractility of fibroblasts. Interestingly, we found dual ROCK1 and ROCK2 inhibition prevented the synthesis of collagen expression induced by TGF-β, however, ROCK2 inhibition tended to enhance it, suggesting the activity of each ROCK isoform may play counteractive roles in response to TGF-β signaling. Knipe R.S., et al., also observed a reduction in collagen expression with the knockdown of ROCK1 or with both isoforms in response to TGF-β (Knipe et al., 2018). Additionally, Yu Zhang, et al., showed that ROCK2-siRNA on TGF-β-stimulated ARE luciferase reporter expression was blocked by co-expression of ROCK2; and the inhibition of human ROCK2 overexpression in response to TGF-β was blocked in the presence of ROCK kinase inhibitor Y27632 in human liver cells, suggesting that ROCK2 acts as a negative regulator of the TGF-β signaling pathway (Zhang et al., 2009).

Rho kinases may regulate multiple signaling pathways via different substrates. In addition, ROCK inhibition is presumably playing a major role in regulating secreted factors. We examined several key components of the WNT signaling and FGF signaling pathway, which are known to contribute to epithelial development and regeneration (KathernMyrna et al., 2012;

Ornitz and Itoh, 2015; Dean and Lloyd, 2017; Kim et al., 2018; Prince, 2018; Puschhof and Clevers, 2018; Villar et al., 2019). Increasing evidence demonstrated aberrant WNT signaling results in fibrotic lung diseases (Baarsma and Königshoff, 2017; Cao et al., 2018; Martin-Medina et al., 2018). Vuga et al. (2009) showed enhanced WNT-5A signaling that contributes to ECM deposition, suggesting ROCK inhibition may repress the ECM deposition via WNT signaling (Vuga et al., 2009). Our results show that the non-canonical WNT ligand WNT-5A was significantly increased in response to TGF-β, whereas this was normalized by compound 31. This is consistent with our previous findings (Wu et al., 2019a) showing that the mesenchymal WNT-5A signaling represses alveolar epithelial progenitor growth, and suggests that pharmacological inhibition of ROCK1/2 in fibroblasts may help to promote canonical WNT signaling in lung repair.

Furthermore, functional alterations in the FGF signaling pathway were observed. Fibroblast growth factors (FGFs) are members of the heparin-binding growth factor family that are often involved in morphogenesis and wound repair and FGF signaling dysregulations is implicated in many disorders (Ornitz and Itoh, 2015; Fehrenbach et al., 2017; Ohgiya et al., 2017; Plikus et al., 2017; Shiraishi et al., 2019; Weiner et al., 2019). FGF2 has attracted increasing attention in lung biology recently and is reported as an important factor in airway remodeling by increasing the deposition of proteoglycans resulting in bronchial hyperresponsiveness in asthmatic airways (Kim et al., 2018). FGF10, a member of the FGF7-subfamily, is widely reported as a primary regulator for branching morphogenesis, cellular differentiation, and response to injury (Prince, 2018; Weiner et al., 2019; Zepp and Morrisey, 2019). We reported previously (Ng-Blichfeldt et al., 2018, 2019) that mesenchymal FGF7, HGF, and FGF10 support alveolar organoid growth, and exogenous FGF7 and HGF rescue TGF-β-induced reduction in organoid number when added to the organoid culture. Our transcriptional analysis also showed that TGF-β upregulated the expression of FGF2 but downregulated the expression of FGF10 and HGF in human fibroblasts and compound 31 counteracts TGF-β effects. Additionally, a recent publication showed that the gene expression of Col1α1, FN1, FGF2 and HGF were all increased in lungs of the patients who died from Covid-19 (Ackermann et al., 2020), genes that are all TGF-β responsive, yet inhibited by dual ROCK1/2 as we show in this study. Taken together, these results suggest that TGF-β elicits modifications of contractility and secreted factors in fibroblasts, and ROCK 1 and 2 inhibition is able to counteract such effects.

According to the human lung cell atlas (https://asthma. cellgeni.sanger.ac.uk/) (Schiller et al., 2019) and the IPF lung cell atlas (http://www.ipfcellatlas.com/) (Adams et al., 2019), the expression of ROCK1 is much higher than ROCK2 in both pulmonary epithelial cells and stromal cells (**Supplementary Figure S2**). Interestingly, ROCK1 increased in (myo)fibroblasts in response to IPF pathology, however, ROCK2 shows opposite alterations in fibroblasts and myofibroblasts (**Supplementary Figure S3**). These data suggest that the role of ROCK1 in IPF pathology (at least at transcriptomic level) might be more

profound as compared to that of ROCK2 and might explain why the protective effect of dual ROCK1/2 inhibition is more profound than ROCK2 selective inhibition in the current study. In further support of this contention, the level of ROCK1 has been demonstrated to function as a clinical progression marker for IPF (Park et al., 2014; Knipe et al., 2016). This is consistent with our functional studies showing that ROCK2 selective inhibition is less effective than ROCK1/2 inhibition. An earlier study (Hallgren et al., 2012) showed that fibroblasts isolated from the parenchyma of severe COPD patients that have more contractile phenotypes are associated with enhanced ROCK1 expression, and the ROCK inhibitor Y27632 blocked this contraction. Thus, it would be interesting to evaluate the effect of selective pharmacological inhibition of ROCK1 in future studies; unfortunately, ROCK1 selective inhibitors are currently not available. Giving the structural similarity between ROCK1 and ROCK2, there are no immediate structural features that can be exploited to design ROCK1 selective inhibitors, while in case of ROCK2, the optimization of van der Waals contacts between the more flexible glycine rich loop and the portion of the molecule underneath P-loop can favor selectivity. However, it is hard to use these observations to guide the design of a ROCK1 selective inhibitor. In addition, hypotensive effects of systemic ROCK inhibition appear to be associated mainly with ROCK1 and this may have driven for discovery of ROCK2 selective inhibitors as safer drugs. Since ROCK1 isoform-selective inhibitors are not currently available, additional studies using genetic approach to specifically delete ROCK1 or ROCK2 will be necessary to elucidate specific roles of these two isoforms in the development of pulmonary remodeling and repair. Such studies will be needed to determine whether an inhibitor for either ROCK1 or ROCK2 may be as effective as a nonselective inhibitor and may be better tolerated.

In conclusion, pharmacological inhibition of both ROCK 1 and 2 isoforms effectively prevents TGF-β-induced fibroblast myofibroblast differentiation and counteracts TGF-β induced growth inhibition of alveolar epithelial progenitors. Selective ROCK2 inhibition does not affect TGF-β effects on extracellular matrix and contractile proteins but does reverse the TGF-β induced inhibition of organoid growth. Our results indicate that mesenchymal ROCK1/2 inhibition may be a potential therapeutic target to promote lung repair.

ETHICS STATEMENT

The animal study was reviewed and approved by University of Groningen Committee for Animal Experimentation.

AUTHOR CONTRIBUTIONS

LEMK, and RG designed and supervised the project; XW, VV, MEW, J-P-N-B, and AM performed the experiments. LEMK, RG, XW, VV, MEW, analyzed data; LEMK, RG, XW, GV, AA and FF, interpreted results or experiments; XW, GV, AA, and

FF, prepared the figures; XW, LEMK, and FF, drafted manuscript; all authors edited and revised manuscript; LEMK, RG, XW, VV, MEW, J-P-N-B, GV, AA, FF, and AM, approved final version of manuscript.

REFERENCES

Ackermann, M., Verleden, S. E., Kuehnel, M., Haverich, A., Welte, T., Laenger, F., et al. (2020). Pulmonary vascular endothelialitis, thrombosis, and angiogenesis in covid-19. *N. Engl. J. Med.*, 383, 120–128. doi:10.1056/NEJMoa2015432

Adams, T. S., Schupp, J. C., Poli, S., Ayaub, E. A., Neumark, N., Ahangari, F., et al. (2019). Single Cell RNA-seq reveals ectopic and aberrant lung resident cell populations in idiopathic pulmonary fibrosis. bioRxiv. 10.1101/759902

Baarsma, H. A., and Königshoff, M. (2017). "WNT-er is coming": WNT signalling in chronic lung diseases. *Thorax.* 72 (8), 746–759. doi:10.1136/thoraxjnl-2016-209753

Cantoni, S., Cavalli, S., Pastore, F., Accetta, A., Pala, D., Vaccaro, F., et al. (2019). Pharmacological characterization of a highly selective Rho kinase (ROCK) inhibitor and its therapeutic effects in experimental pulmonary hypertension. *Eur. J. Pharmacol.* 850, 126–134. doi:10.1016/j.ejphar.2019.02.009

Cao, H., Wang, C., Chen, X., Hou, J., Xiang, Z., Shen, Y., et al. (2018). Inhibition of Wnt/β-catenin signaling suppresses myofibroblast differentiation of lung resident mesenchymal stem cells and pulmonary fibrosis. *Sci. Rep.* 8, 1–14. doi:10.1038/s41598-018-28968-9

Dean, C. H., and Lloyd, C. M. (2017). Lung alveolar repair: not all cells are equal. *Trends Mol. Med.* 23, 871–873. doi:10.1016/j.molmed.2017.08.009

Demayo, F., Minoo, P., Plopper, C. G., Schuger, L., Shannon, J., and Torday, J. S. (2002). Mesenchymal-epithelial interactions in lung development and repair: are modeling and remodeling the same process? *Am. J. Physiol. Lung Cell Mol. Physiol.* 283 (3), L510–L517. doi:10.1152/ajplung.00144.2002

dos Santos, T. M., Righetti, R. F., Camargo, L. d. N., Saraiva-Romanholo, B. M., Aristoteles, L. R. C. R. B., de Souza, F. C. R., et al. (2018). Effect of anti-IL17 antibody treatment alone and in combination with Rho-kinase inhibitor in a murine model of asthma. *Front. Physiol.* 9, 1–19. doi:10.3389/fphys.2018.01183

El Agha, E., Kramann, R., Schneider, R. K., Li, X., Seeger, W., Humphreys, B. D., et al. (2017). Mesenchymal stem cells in fibrotic disease. *Cell Stem Cell.* 21, 166–177. doi:10.1016/j.stem.2017.07.011

Fehrenbach, H., Wagner, C., and Wegmann, M. (2017). Airway remodeling in asthma: what really matters. *Cell Tissue Res.* 367, 551–569. doi:10.1007/s00441-016-2566-8

Florian, J., Watte, G., Teixeira, P. J. Z., Altmayer, S., Schio, S. M., Sanchez, L. B., et al. (2019). Pulmonary rehabilitation improves survival in patients with idiopathic pulmonary fibrosis undergoing lung transplantation. *Sci. Rep.* 9, 1–6. doi:10.1038/s41598-019-45828-2

Grzela, K., Litwiniuk, M., Zagorska, W., and Grzela, T. (2016). Airway remodeling in chronic obstructive pulmonary disease and asthma: the role of matrix metalloproteinase-9. *Arch. Immunol. Ther. Exp.* 64, 47–55. doi:10.1007/s00005-015-0345-y

Hallgren, O., Rolandsson, S., Andersson-Sjöland, A., Nihlberg, K., Wieslander, E., Kvist-Reimer, M., et al. (2012). Enhanced ROCK1 dependent contractility in fibroblast from chronic obstructive pulmonary disease patients. *J. Transl. Med.* 10, 1–11. doi:10.1186/1479-5876-10-171

Hirota, N., and Martin, J. G. (2013). Mechanisms of airway remodeling. *Chest.* 144, 1026–1032. doi:10.1378/chest.12-3073

Horowitz, J. C., and Thannickal, V. J. (2006). Epithelial-mesenchymal interactions in pulmonary fibrosis. *Semin. Respir. Crit. Care Med.* 27 (6), 600–612. doi:10.1055/s-2006-957332

Htwe, S. S., Cha, B. H., Yue, K., Khademhosseini, A., Knox, A. J., and Ghaemmaghami, A. M. (2017). Role of Rho-Associated coiled-coil forming kinase isoforms in regulation of stiffness-induced myofibroblast differentiation in lung fibrosis. *Am. J. Respir. Cell Mol. Biol.* 56, 772–783. doi:10.1165/rcmb.2016-0306OC

Huang, L., Dai, F., Tang, L., Bao, X., Liu, Z., Huang, C., et al. (2018). Distinct roles for ROCK1 and ROCK2 in the regulation of oxldl-mediated endothelial dysfunction. *Cell. Physiol. Biochem.* 49, 565–577. doi:10.1159/000492994

ACKNOWLEDGMENTS

The authors gratefully acknowledge the University Medical Center Groningen Imaging and Microscopy Center (UMIC), which is sponsored by NWO-grants 40–00506-98–9021 and 175–010–2009–023.

Jiang, C., Huang, H., Liu, J., Wang, Y., Lu, Z., and Xu, Z. (2012). Fasudil, a Rho-kinase inhibitor, attenuates bleomycin-induced pulmonary fibrosis in mice. *Int. J. Mol. Sci.* 13 (7), 8293–8307. doi:10.3390/ijms13078293

Kasper, M., Seidel, D., Knels, L., Morishima, N., Neisser, A., Bramke, S., et al. (2004). Early signs of lung fibrosis after *in vitro* treatment of rat lung slices with CdCl2 and TGF-β1. *Histochem. Cell Biol.* 121 (2), 131–140. doi:10.1007/s00418-003-0612-6

KathernMyrna, E. D. V. M., SimonPot, A. D. V. M., Christopher, J., and Murphy, D. V. M. (2012). Transformation in corneal wound healing and pathology. *Vet. Ophthalmol.* 12, 25–27. doi:10.1111/j.1463-5224.2009.00742.x.Meet

Kim, Y. S., Hong, G., Kim, D. H., Kim, Y. M., Kim, Y. K., Oh, Y. M., et al. (2018). The role of FGF-2 in smoke-induced emphysema and the therapeutic potential of recombinant FGF-2 in patients with COPD. *Exp. Mol. Med.* 50 1–10. doi:10.1038/s12276-018-0178-y

King, T. E., Pardo, A., and Selman, M. (2011). Idiopathic pulmonary fibrosis. *Lancet.* 378, 1949–1961. doi:10.1016/S0140-6736(11)60052-4

Klein, S., Frohn, F., Magdaleno, F., Reker-Smit, C., Schierwagen, R., Schierwagen, I., et al. (2019). Rho-kinase inhibitor coupled to peptide-modified albumin carrier reduces portal pressure and increases renal perfusion in cirrhotic rats. *Sci. Rep.* 9, 1–11. doi:10.1038/s41598-019-38678-5

Knipe, R., Probst, C., Ahluwalia, N., Shea, B., Franklin, A., Grasberger, P., et al. (2016). ROCK isoforms ROCK 1 and ROCK 2 are critical for the development of pulmonary fibrosis in several different cell specific mechanisms. *QJM An Int. J. Med.* 109, S2. doi:10.1093/qjmed/hcw118.005

Knipe, R. S., Probst, C. K., Lagares, D., Franklin, A., Spinney, J. J., Brazee, P. L., et al. (2018). The rho kinase isoforms ROCK1 and ROCK2 each contribute to the development of experimental pulmonary fibrosis. *Am. J. Respir. Cell Mol. Biol.* 58, 471–481. doi:10.1165/rcmb.2017-0075OC

Majolée, J., Pronk, M. C. A., Jim, K. K., van Bezu, J. S. M., van der Sar, A. M., Hordijk, P. L., et al. (2019). CSN5 inhibition triggers inflammatory signaling and Rho/ROCK-dependent loss of endothelial integrity. *Sci. Rep.* 9, 1–12. doi:10.1038/s41598-019-44595-4

Martin-Medina, A., Lehmann, M., Burgy, O., Hermann, S., Baarsma, H. A., Wagner, D. E., et al. (2018). Increased extracellular vesicles mediate WNT5A signaling in idiopathic pulmonary fibrosis. *Am. J. Respir. Crit. Care Med.* 198 (12), 1527–1538. doi:10.1164/rccm.201708-1580OC

Meng, X. M., Nikolic-Paterson, D. J., and Lan, H. Y. (2016). TGF-β: the master regulator of fibrosis. *Nat. Rev. Nephrol.* 12 (6), 325–338. doi:10.1038/nrneph.2016.48

Nagai, Y., Matoba, K., Kawanami, D., Takeda, Y., Akamine, T., Ishizawa, S., et al. (2019). ROCK2 regulates TGF-β-induced expression of CTGF and profibrotic genes via NF-κB and cytoskeleton dynamics in mesangial cells. *Am. J. Physiol. Ren. Physiol.* 317 (4), F839–F851. doi:10.1152/ajprenal.00596.2018

Ng-Blichfeldt, J. P., Schrik, A., Kortekaas, R. K., Noordhoek, J. A., Heijink, I. H., Hiemstra, P. S., et al. (2018). Retinoic acid signaling balances adult distal lung epithelial progenitor cell growth and differentiation. *EBioMedicine.* 36, 461–474. doi:10.1016/j.ebiom.2018.09.002

Ng-Blichfeldt, J. P., de Jong, T., Kortekaas, R. K., Wu, X., Lindner, M., Guryev, V., et al. (2019). Tgf-β activation impairs fibroblast ability to support adult lung epithelial progenitor cell organoid formation. *Am. J. Physiol. Lung Cell Mol. Physiol.* 317 (1), L14–L28. doi:10.1152/ajplung.00400.2018

Noe, N., Shim, A., Millette, K., Luo, Y., Azhar, M., Shi, W., et al. (2019). Mesenchyme-specific deletion of Tgf-β1 in the embryonic lung disrupts branching morphogenesis and induces lung hypoplasia. *Lab. Invest.* 99, 1363–1375. doi:10.1038/s41374-019-0256-3

Oenema, T. A., Maarsingh, H., Smit, M., Groothuis, G. M. M., Meurs, H., and Gosens, R. (2013). Bronchoconstriction induces TGF-β release and airway remodelling in Guinea pig lung slices. *PLoS One.* 8 (6), e65580. doi:10.1371/journal.pone.0065580

Ohgiya, M., Matsui, H., Tamura, A., Kato, T., Akagawa, S., and Ohta, K. (2017). The evaluation of interstitial abnormalities in group B of the 2011 global initiative for chronic obstructive lung disease (GOLD) classification of chronic obstructive pulmonary disease (COPD). *Intern. Med.* 56, 2711–2717. doi:10.2169/internalmedicine.8406-16

Ornitz, D. M., and Itoh, N. (2015). The fibroblast growth factor signaling pathway. *Wiley Interdiscip. Rev. Dev. Biol.* 4, 215–266. doi:10.1002/wdev.176

Park, J. S., Park, H. J., Park, Y. S., Lee, S. M., Yim, J. J., Yoo, C. G., et al. (2014). Clinical significance of mTOR, ZEB1, ROCK1 expression in lung tissues of pulmonary fibrosis patients. *BMC Pulm. Med.* 14 (1), 168. doi:10.1186/1471-2466-14-168

Park, J. S., Kim, D. H., Shah, S. R., Kim, H. N., Kshitiz, Kim, P., et al. (2019). Switch-like enhancement of epithelial-mesenchymal transition by YAP through feedback regulation of WT1 and Rho-family GTPases. *Nat. Commun.* 10, 1–15. doi:10.1038/s41467-019-10729-5

Pireddu, R., Forinash, K. D., Sun, N. N., Martin, M. P., Sung, S. S., Alexander, B., et al. (2012). Pyridylthiazole-based ureas as inhibitors of Rho associated protein kinases (ROCK1 and 2). *Medchemcomm.* 3, 699–709. doi:10.1039/c2md00320a

Plikus, M. V., Guerrero-Juarez, C. F., Ito, M., Li, Y. R., Dedhia, P. H., Zheng, Y., et al. (2017). Regeneration of fat cells from myofibroblasts during wound healing. *Science 84.* 355, 748–752. doi:10.1126/science.aai8792

Prince, L. S. (2018). FGF10 and human lung disease across the Life spectrum. *Front. Genet.* 9, 1–6. doi:10.3389/fgene.2018.00517

Puschhof, J., and Clevers, H. (2018). The myofibroblasts' war on drugs. *Dev. Cell.* 46, 669–670. doi:10.1016/j.devcel.2018.09.008

Qi, X. J., Ning, W., Xu, F., Dang, H. X., Fang, F., and Li, J. (2015). Fasudil, an inhibitor of Rho-associated coiled-coil kinase, attenuates hyperoxia-induced pulmonary fibrosis in neonatal rats. *Int. J. Clin. Exp. Pathol.* 8, 12140–12150

Rath, N., and Olson, M. F. (2012). Rho-associated kinases in tumorigenesis: Re-considering ROCK inhibition for cancer therapy. *EMBO Rep.* 13, 900–908. doi:10.1038/embor.2012.127

Saidi, A., Kasabova, M., Vanderlynden, L., Wartenberg, M., Kara-Ali, G. H., Marc, D., et al. (2019). Curcumin inhibits the TGF-β1-dependent differentiation of lung fibroblasts via PPARγ-driven upregulation of cathepsins B and L. *Sci. Rep.* 9, 491. doi:10.1038/s41598-018-36858-3

Schiller, H. B., Montoro, D. T., Simon, L. M., Rawlins, E. L., Meyer, K. B., Strunz, M., et al. (2019). The human lung cell atlas: a high-resolution reference map of the human lung in health and disease. *Am. J. Respir. Cell Mol. Biol.* 61 (1), 31–41. doi:10.1165/rcmb.2018-0416TR

Shiraishi, K., Shichino, S., Ueha, S., Nakajima, T., Hashimoto, S., Yamazaki, S., et al. (2019). Mesenchymal-epithelial interactome analysis reveals essential factors required for fibroblast-free alveolosphere formation. *iScience.* 11, 318–333. doi:10.1016/j.isci.2018.12.022

Tumbarello, D. A., and Turner, C. E. (2006). Hic-5 contributes to transformation through a RhoA/ROCK-dependent pathway. *J. Cell. Physiol.* 211 (3), 736–747. doi:10.1002/JCP.

Van Dijk, E. M., Culha, S., Menzen, M. H., Bidan, C. M., and Gosens, R. (2017). Elastase-induced parenchymal disruption and airway hyper responsiveness in mouse precision cut lung slices: toward an *ex vivo* COPD model. *Front. Physiol.* 7, 657. doi:10.3389/fphys.2016.00657

Vigil, D., Kim, T. Y., Plachco, A., Garton, A. J., Castaldo, L., Pachter, J. A., et al. (2012). ROCK1 and ROCK2 are required for non-small cell lung cancer anchorage-independent growth and invasion. *Cancer Res.* 72, 5338–5347. doi:10.1158/0008-5472.CAN-11-2373

Villar, J., Zhang, H., and Slutsky, A. S. (2019). Lung repair and regeneration in ARDS: role of PECAM1 and wnt signaling. *Chest.* [Epub ahead of print]. doi:10.1016/j.chest.2018.10.022

Vuga, L. J., Ben-Yehudah, A., Kovkarova-Naumovski, E., Oriss, T., Gibson, K. F., Feghali-Bostwick, C., et al. (2009). WNT5A is a regulator of fibroblast proliferation and resistance to apoptosis. *Am. J. Respir. Cell Mol. Biol.* 41 (5), 583–589. doi:10.1165/rcmb.2008-0201OC

Wang, Y. C., Chen, Q., Luo, J. M., Nie, J., Meng, Q. H., Shuai, W., et al. (2019). Notch1 promotes the pericyte-myofibroblast transition in idiopathic pulmonary fibrosis through the PDGFR/ROCK1 signal pathway. *Exp. Mol. Med.* 51, 1–11. doi:10.1038/s12276-019-0228-0

Weiner, A. I., Jackson, S. R., Zhao, G., Quansah, K. K., Farshchian, J. N., Neupauer, K. M., et al. (2019). Mesenchyme-free expansion and transplantation of adult alveolar progenitor cells: steps toward cell-based regenerative therapies. *Npj Regen. Med.* 4, 1–10. doi:10.1038/s41536-019-0080-9

Winters, N. I., Burman, A., Kropski, J. A., and Blackwell, T. S. (2019). Epithelial injury and dysfunction in the pathogenesis of idiopathic PulmonaryFibrosis. *Am. J. Med. Sci.* 357, 374–378. doi:10.1016/j.amjms.2019.01.010

Wu, X., van Dijk, E. M., Bos, I. S. T., Kistemaker, L. E. M., and Gosens, R. (2019a). Mesenchymal WNT-5A/5B signaling represses lung alveolar epithelial progenitors. *Cells.* 8 (10), 1147. doi:10.3390/cells8101147

Wu, X., van Dijk, E. M., Bos, I. S. T., Kistemaker, L. E. M., and Gosens, R. (2019b). Mouse lung tissue slice culture. *Methods Mol. Biol.,* 1940: 297–311. doi:10.1007/978-1-4939-9086-3_21

Xueyang, D., Zhanqiang, M., Chunhua, M., and Kun, H. (2016). Fasudil, an inhibitor of Rho-associated coiled-coil kinase, improves cognitive impairments induced by smoke exposure. *Oncotarget.* 7, 78764–78772. doi:10.18632/oncotarget.12853

Zepp, J. A., and Morrisey, E. E. (2019). Cellular crosstalk in the development and regeneration of the respiratory system. *Nat. Rev. Mol. Cell Biol.* 20, 551–566. doi:10.1038/s41580-019-0141-3

Zhang, Y., Li, X., Qi, J., Wang, J., Liu, X., Zhang, H., et al. (2009). Rock2 controls TGFβ signaling and inhibits mesoderm induction in zebrafish embryos. *J. Cell Sci.* 122, 2197–2207. doi:10.1242/jcs.040659

8

A High-Throughput System for Cyclic Stretching of Precision-Cut Lung Slices during Acute Cigarette Smoke Extract Exposure

Jarred R. Mondoñedo[1,2], Elizabeth Bartolák-Suki[1], Samer Bou Jawde[1], Kara Nelson[1], Kun Cao[1], Adam Sonnenberg[3], Walter Patrick Obrochta[1], Jasmin Imsirovic[1], Sumati Ram-Mohan[4], Ramaswamy Krishnan[4] and Béla Suki[1]*

[1] Department of Biomedical Engineering, College of Engineering, Boston University, Boston, MA, United States, [2] Boston University School of Medicine, Boston, MA, United States, [3] Department of Systems Engineering, College of Engineering, Boston University, Boston, MA, United States, [4] Department of Emergency Medicine, Beth Israel Deaconess Medical Center, Harvard Medical School, Boston, MA, United States

*Correspondence:
Béla Suki
bsuki@bu.edu

Rationale: Precision-cut lung slices (PCLSs) are a valuable tool in studying tissue responses to an acute exposure; however, cyclic stretching may be necessary to recapitulate physiologic, tidal breathing conditions.

Objectives: To develop a multi-well stretcher and characterize the PCLS response following acute exposure to cigarette smoke extract (CSE).

Methods: A 12-well stretching device was designed, built, and calibrated. PCLS were obtained from male Sprague-Dawley rats ($N = 10$) and assigned to one of three groups: 0% (unstretched), 5% peak-to-peak amplitude (low-stretch), and 5% peak-to-peak amplitude superimposed on 10% static stretch (high-stretch). Lung slices were cyclically stretched for 12 h with or without CSE in the media. Levels of Interleukin-1β (IL-1β), matrix metalloproteinase (MMP)-1 and its tissue inhibitor (TIMP1), and membrane type-MMP (MT1-MMP) were assessed via western blot from tissue homogenate.

Results: The stretcher system produced nearly identical normal Lagrangian strains (E_{xx} and E_{yy}, $p > 0.999$) with negligible shear strain ($E_{xy} < 0.0005$) and low intra-well variability $0.127 \pm 0.073\%$. CSE dose response curve was well characterized by a four-parameter logistic model ($R^2 = 0.893$), yielding an IC_{50} value of 0.018 cig/mL. Cyclic stretching for 12 h did not decrease PCLS viability. Two-way ANOVA detected a significant interaction between CSE and stretch pattern for IL-1β ($p = 0.017$), MMP-1, TIMP1, and MT1-MMP ($p < 0.001$).

Conclusion: This platform is capable of high-throughput testing of an acute exposure under tightly-regulated, cyclic stretching conditions. We conclude that the acute mechano-inflammatory response to CSE exhibits complex, stretch-dependence in the PCLS.

Keywords: stretcher, IL-1b, MMP-1, mechanotrasduction, emphysema

INTRODUCTION

Precision-cut lung slices (PCLSs) have emerged as a valuable tool in lung biology (Tepper et al., 2005; Henjakovic et al., 2008; Khan et al., 2010; Lavoie et al., 2012; Schlepütz et al., 2012; Rosner et al., 2014; Hiorns et al., 2016; Van Dijk et al., 2016). A key advantage of this preparation is that the PCLS can be acutely exposed to disease-modifying conditions, such as enzymatic parenchymal digestion in emphysema (Van Dijk et al., 2016), while recording corresponding structural and functional changes in both space and time (Hiorns et al., 2016; Lavoie et al., 2012). PCLSs also benefit by preserving the native extracellular environment (Sanderson, 2011) and retaining nearly all of the resident cell types in the lung. These technical advantages have thus promoted widespread adoption of the PCLS in models of exposure assessment (Langer et al., 2012; Lauenstein et al., 2014; Uhl et al., 2015; Hess et al., 2016; Watson et al., 2016; Neuhaus et al., 2017), pharmacologic therapy (Switalla et al., 2010; van Rijt et al., 2015; Donovan et al., 2016; Kistemaker et al., 2017), and disease modeling, including chronic obstructive pulmonary disease (COPD) (Chronic Obstructive Lung Disease [COLD], 2017).

The overwhelming majority of this prior work has examined the PCLS under static conditions. However, the lung is continuously and rhythmically stretched during tidal breathing *in vivo* and thus, a more accurate recapitulation of native lung responsiveness demands similar dynamic conditions be imposed *ex vivo* (Suki et al., 2013). For example, the absence of stretch has been shown to influence cellular and enzymatic maintenance of tissue properties (Yi et al., 2016; Jesudason et al., 2010) by impacting the biological phenomenon known as mechanotransduction (Ingber, 2006). One of the few models incorporating cyclic stretching of PCLS showed that stretch magnitude in ventilator induced lung injury (VILI) modulated the nuclear translocation of NF-κB and oxidative stress responses in lung slices (Song et al., 2016; Davidovich et al., 2013b). It has been suggested that analogous mechanisms could facilitate emphysema progression in the lung via stretch-dependent secretion of pro-inflammatory cytokines and enzymes accelerating matrix turnover (Suki et al., 2013). Yet, comparable and potentially transformative studies aimed at elucidating the possible role of mechanotransduction in COPD pathogenesis and progression are lacking.

Here, we report the design and implementation of a multi-well equibiaxial device to cyclically stretch PCLSs obtained from excised rat lungs. Its primary advantages include high-throughput, low variance, and the ability to deliver complex, user-defined stretch patterns to the entire slice. To demonstrate the feasibility of this system in studying the mechano-inflammatory response to an acute pharmacologic exposure, we use cigarette smoke extract (CSE) during cyclic stretching to mimic cigarette smoking *in vivo*. We hypothesize the corresponding physiological response is stretch-pattern dependent. To test this, we first confirm tissue viability in this system and then compare the effects of stretch and CSE exposure on biochemical changes in several molecular markers known to play a role in COPD.

MATERIALS AND METHODS

Device Design

The multi-well stretching system pictured in **Figure 1** was built and calibrated based on previous designs (Arold et al., 2009; Imsirovic et al., 2015). Briefly, one or two 6-well plates with deformable elastic membranes are secured in the upper stage of the stretcher. A linear actuating motor (A1 Series: Servo Cylinder, Ultra Motion, Cutchogue, NY, United States) is used to move the stage vertically. As the stage moves down, the elastic membrane in each well is stretched around a fixed, cylindrical indenter post. As the stage moves back up, the elastic membrane relaxes to its initial configuration. Cyclic stretching is achieved by repeating this process at a prescribed rate and displacement depth, which corresponds to the area strain translated to the elastic membrane. Ball bearings (McMaster-Carr, Elhmhurst, IL, United States) affixed to the top of the indenter posts reduce friction, heat generation, and hysteresis. Detailed designs available by request.

A custom software interface (Embarcadero C++ Developer, Austin, TX, United States) was developed to prescribe any simple or complex stretch pattern with parameters including

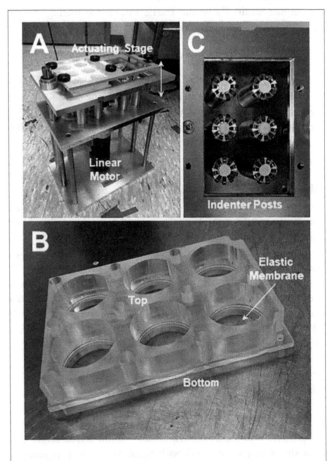

FIGURE 1 | (A) Multi-well device for cyclic stretching of precision-cut lung slices (PCLSs), see text for design details. **(B)** Reusable 6-well flexframe with interchangeable elastic membrane. **(C)** Ball bearings affixed to the indenter posts minimized friction during stretch.

88

waveform type, frequency, amplitude, and duration. The entire system was constructed from stainless steel and could be moved to a cell culture incubator for stretching under controlled, sterile conditions.

We also designed and fabricated a lightweight, reusable 6-well plate acrylic "flexframe" with an interchangeable elastic, silicone membrane (Specialty Manufacturing, Inc., Saginaw, MI, United States), which we validated by comparison with a commercially available alternative (BioFlex® Culture Plates, Flexcell International Corp., Burlington, NC, United States). The top and bottom components of the flexframe are separable, allowing for replacement of the elastic membrane between experiments.

Device Calibration

To calibrate the relationship between stage displacement and membrane surface area, colored acrylic markers (Pēbēo, Cedex, France) were adhered to the membrane in a circular arrangement and then tracked during quasi-static stretch to compute local radial area change. The corresponding area strain-displacement curve was used to calibrate the stretcher and prescribe area strains for cyclic stretching. Delaunay triangulation and radial displacement of individual beads were used to calculate the Lagrangian strain E_{ij} of the elastic membrane during stretch according to the following relation (Holzapfel, 2000):

$$ds^2 - ds_0^2 = 2E_{ij}da_i da_j$$

where ds and ds_0 are the segment lengths before and after deformation, respectively, of each triangle, while da_i and da_j are the changes in position of the bead vertices. To assess whether repeated stretch induced plastic deformation of the elastic membrane, this calibration procedure was repeated following 12 h of stretch.

Animal Protocol

Protocol #16-025 was reviewed and approved by the Boston University Institutional Animal Care and Use Committee. Male Sprague-Dawley rats ($N = 10$) with body weight 343.8 ± 60.2 g were sedated via intraperitoneal injection of xylazine (10 mg/kg) and ketamine (90 mg/kg). After ensuring appropriate depth of anesthesia and analgesia, animals were euthanized via abdominal aortic exsanguination. The lungs were excised and insufflated via tracheostomy with 10–12 mL of 1.5% low melt agarose (HyAgarose, ACTGene Inc., Piscataway, NJ, United States) in Hanks' buffered salt solution (HBSS, Sigma) at 37°C, according to previous techniques (Watson et al., 2016). Excised lungs were then placed on ice for 15 min to allow for solidification of the agarose.

Precision-Cut Lung Slices (PCLSs)

Lung lobes were separated, trimmed to fit the tissue stage, and then sliced in cooled HBSS with thickness ~500 μm using a vibratome (752M Vibroslice, Campden Instruments Ltd., United Kingdom). The vibratome tissue stage was modified to include an adjustable, cylindrical sleeve that was filled with agarose to help stabilize the lung lobe during slicing. PCLSs were then

"punched" using either a 6 or 10 mm coring tool (Acuderm Inc., Fort Lauderdale, FL, United States) to generate round, symmetric slices. Punching the tissues after slicing the entire lobe was found to yield a greater amount of material compared to coring the lung lobes prior to slicing. PCLSs were then moved to Dulbecco's Modified Eagle's Medium (DMEM, Gibco) supplemented with penicillin, streptomycin, and amphotericin B (Antimycotic-Antibiotic, Gibco). To facilitate removal of residual agarose and other cellular debris, media was changed every 30 min for 0–2 h after slicing, 1 h for 2–4 h, 2 h for 4–8 h, and 24 h thereafter, similar to previous methods (Davidovich et al., 2013a,b; Song et al., 2016). Lung slices were incubated under standard conditions (5% CO_2 at 37°C) and allowed to recover overnight.

MTS Assay

PCLS viability was assessed via MTS assay, which is a colorimetric measure of cell metabolic activity (Berridge et al., 2005). The formazan product yielded by this reaction is proportional to the number of metabolically healthy or active cells and is quantified by measuring the absorbance at 490 nm. The colorimetric MTS assay was used according to manufacturer's specifications. Lung slices (6 mm) were incubated in individual wells with 20 μL of MTS reagent in 200 μL of HBSS for 1.5 h at 37°C. The supernatant was then removed to a 96-well plate for measurement of optical density.

Preparation and Potency of Cigarette Smoke Extract (CSE)

Cigarette smoke extract solutions were prepared fresh by bubbling two cigarettes (Marlboro Red, Philip Morris USA, Richmond, VA, United States) with the filters removed, through 20 mL of DMEM at a rate of 1.0 L/min to yield a stock solution of 0.1 cig/mL. Next, the solutions were sterile filtered using a 0.22 μm pore size membrane vacuum filtration system (Steriflip, EMD Millipore) to remove large tobacco debris and other small particles. To determine the CSE dose response curve, the stock solution was diluted and 6 mm lung slices ($N = 93$) were incubated in 6-well plates for 12 h with CSE concentrations ranging from 0.001 to 0.050 cig/mL (~3 slices per 3 mL of solution in each well). Following incubation, individual slices were rinsed with warmed HBSS to remove any residual solution containing the CSE-media mix. PCLS were transferred to a 96-well plate for assessment of viability via MTS assay as described above.

Experimental Protocol

Individual lung slices were attached to the center of the elastic membranes in each well using four evenly spaced beads of cyanoacrylate glue along the tissue perimeter. Initial pilot studies confirmed appropriate local tissue stretch with this preparation (**Supplementary Figure S1**). PCLSs were covered with 3 mL of media with or without CSE (0.01 cig/mL) for the treated and control groups, respectively, then sinusoidally stretched for 12 h at 1 Hz under standard incubation conditions. To assess the effect of different stretch patterns, PCLS were randomly assigned to one of the following three stretch amplitude groups: unstretched (US); low-stretch (LS), 5% peak-to-peak amplitude with no static stretch; and high-stretch (HS), 5% peak-to-peak amplitude superimposed on 10% static stretch. These waveforms were arbitrarily selected to simulate regions of lung experiencing different stretch during tidal breathing; a schematic is shown in **Figure 2**. Following cyclic stretch, the PCLSs were collected from each well for biochemical analysis (N = 48). Protease inhibitors EDTA and Halt Protease Inhibitor cocktail (Thermo Scientific) were added to the homogenized tissue samples, then stored at −20°C until further use. PCLSs were also collected to assess tissue viability after stretching (N = 49). Lung slices were trimmed using a 6 mm coring tool to reduce edge effects from slicing and the attachment procedure, then evaluated via MTS as before.

Western Blot

Protein concentrations for the homogenized tissues were determined using the BCA colorimetric protein assay kit (Pierce, Thermo Scientific). The assay was used according to manufacturer's specifications. Equal amounts of protein (~3.7 μg) from each sample were separated via sodium dodecyl sulfate polyacrylamide gel electrophoresis (SDS-PAGE), transferred to a polyvinylidene difluoride (PVDF) membrane, and blocked using 5% bovine serum albumin in phosphate buffered saline containing 0.05% Tween 20 (PBS-T). All groups were run on the same membrane. After blocking for 2 h, the membrane was incubated for 1 h at room temperature with primary antibodies anti-IL-1β (1:250, Abcam), anti-MMP-1 (1:1000, Thermo Fisher Scientific), TIMP1 (1:1000, Abcam), MT1-MMP (1:5000, Abcam), and anti-GAPDH (loading control, 1 μg/ml, Abcam), washed in PBS-T 4 × 15 min, incubated with secondary antibody (anti-mouse, 1:7000, anti-rabbit, 1:10000, Vector Laboratories) for 1 h, and again washed in PBS-T 4 × 15 min. Quantitative densitometry was performed after chemiluminescence detection (SuperSignal West Pico Chemiluminescent Substrate, Pierce) with picomolar sensitivity

similar to that of ELISA, with corrections for background and loading control.

Statistical Analysis

Data analysis and fitting were performed using MATLAB (R2016a, MathWorks, Natick, MA, United States) and SigmaPlot (SigmaPlot v12.3, Systat Software, Inc., San Jose, CA, United States). CSE dose response data was fitted using a four-parameter logistic regression as follows:

$$y = a + \frac{b - a}{1 + \left(\frac{x}{c}\right)^d}$$

where y is normalized absorbance; x is CSE concentration a and b are the minimum and maximum values possible, respectively, c is the point of inflection; and d is a coefficient characterizing the slope of the curve. Two-Way analysis of variance (ANOVA) was used to evaluate the influence of stretch and CSE on PCLS viability as well as on IL-1β, MT1-MMP, MMP-1, and TIMP1. Holm-Sidak method was used for *post hoc* comparisons. For all, $p < 0.05$ was considered significant.

RESULTS

Figure 3 presents the calibration and validation of the multi-well stretcher and FlexFrame devices. Vertical displacement of the actuating stage yielded a non-linear relation between area strain and motor position (**Figure 3A**), which was used to prescribe waveforms for cyclic stretching. Note the minimal hysteresis between loading and unloading of the flexframe elastic membrane, 6.34%. Normal Lagrangian strains, E_{xx} and E_{yy}, were nearly identical, $\rho > 0.999$, with negligible shear strain, $E_{xy} < 0.0005$, demonstrating equibiaxial strain of the elastic membrane (**Figure 3B**). Compared to the commercially available BioFlex Culture Plates, our custom fabricated flexframe demonstrated lower intra-well variance for area strain, 0.473 ± 0.717% vs. 0.127 ± 0.073% (Variance Mean ± SD), particularly at larger prescribed strains (**Figure 3C**). Finally, there was no detectable plastic deformation of the membrane due to stretch as there was no difference in measured area strains before and after 12 h of cyclic stretching (slope: 0.998 with R^2 = 0.997; **Figure 3D**).

Figure 4 shows the effects of CSE and cyclic stretch on tissue viability. We first established a sub-toxic concentration mimicking acute cigarette smoke exposure *in vivo* (**Figure 4A**). As expected, PCLS viability decreased with CSE concentration. The corresponding dose response curve was well characterized by a four-parameter logistic model (R^2 = 0.893), yielding an IC_{50} value of 0.018 cig/mL corresponding to the CSE concentration at half-maximal viability. Based on this curve, the CSE concentration was selected to be 0.01 cig/mL for all subsequent experiments. We then confirmed tissue viability following 12 h of cyclic stretching ± CSE (**Figure 4B**). Two-way ANOVA detected no statistical difference in PCLS viability

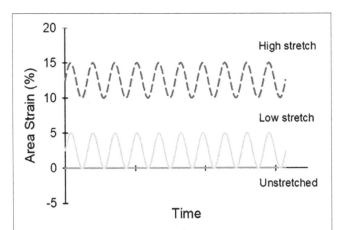

FIGURE 2 | Lung slices were randomly assigned to one of three stretch patterns: unstretched (0%), low stretch (0–5% area strain), or high stretch (10–15% area strain).

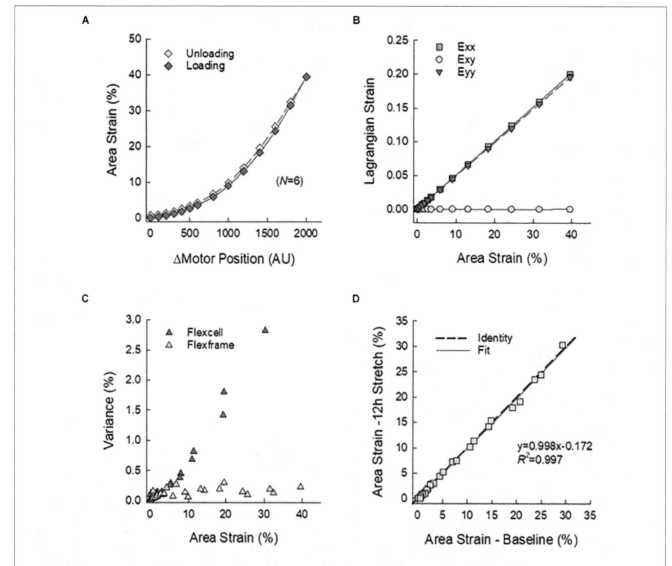

FIGURE 3 | (A) Calibration curve used to prescribe membrane area strain as a function of motor position. Symbols represent means of $N = 6$ wells with standard deviations smaller than symbol sizes. **(B)** Nearly identical normal strains, E_{xx} and E_{yy}, and negligible shear strain, E_{xy}, as estimated by Delaunay triangulation, confirmed equibiaxial strain of the elastic membrane. **(C)** The reusable flexframe exhibited lower variance of area strain in comparison to a commercially available disposable alternative. **(D)** There was no observable mechanical change in the elastic membrane after 12 h of cyclic stretching.

among different stretch patterns ($p = 0.070$), CSE exposure ($p = 0.594$), or their interaction ($p = 0.277$).

As shown in **Figure 5**, Two-Way ANOVA detected a significant interaction between stretch pattern and CSE exposure on the tissue content of all measured molecular markers (IL-1β, $p = 0.017$; MT1-MMP, MMP-1, TIMP1, $p < 0.001$). Each had a unique response to stretch and CSE. We found that IL-1β (**Figure 5A**) exhibited the greatest response to stretching ($p < 0.001$) among the group, and was statistically higher with CSE exposure ($p < 0.001$) for all stretch patterns. CSE also had a significant effect ($p < 0.001$) on MT1-MMP (**Figure 5C**), though regulation directionality depended on stretch pattern ($p < 0.001$). In contrast, stretch pattern had a significant effect on MMP-1 (**Figure 5B**) in the presence of CSE ($p < 0.001$), whereas it only had an effect on TIMP1 (**Figure 5D**) in the absence of

CSE ($p < 0.001$). The enzymes MT1-MMP and MMP-1 had the greatest tissue content for LS with CSE exposure, while the tissue content of the inhibitor TIMP1 was the greatest for the same stretch pattern when CSE was absent.

DISCUSSION

In this study, we present the design and implementation of a multi-well stretcher to investigate the mechano-inflammatory response in lung tissue following an acute pharmacologic insult. This is the first report to combine CSE exposure with cyclic PCLS stretching as an *ex vivo* model of the dynamic changes in lung volume that occur during cigarette smoke inhalation *in vivo*. First, we demonstrated this device delivered repeatable,

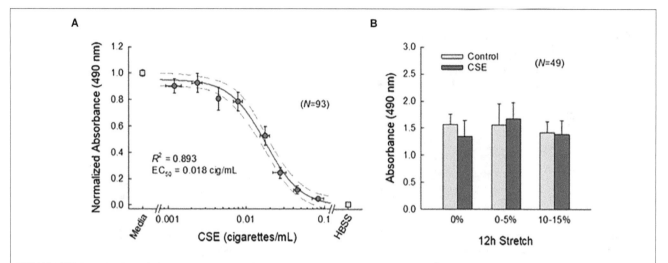

FIGURE 4 | (A) Lung slice (N = 93) viability decreased with CSE concentration and was well characterized (R^2 = 0.893) by a four-parameter logistic curve (solid line) shown with 95% confidence intervals (dashed lines). Binned data across multiple CSE concentrations are shown, vertical and horizontal error bars represent SE and SD, respectively. **(B)** The sub-toxic CSE concentration was selected to be 0.01 cig/mL. Two-way ANOVA detected no effects for stretch and CSE at this concentration, indicating tissue viability was not compromised with this system. Error bars represent SD.

low-variance, equibiaxial stretch. We then characterized the CSE dose response curve in PCLSs and confirmed that cyclic stretching did not compromise tissue viability. Finally, we found the interaction between stretch pattern and CSE exposure had a significant effect on all of the molecular markers, with each exhibiting a unique response pattern. Together, these findings demonstrate the feasibility of using this system to recapitulate tidal breathing-like conditions in PCLS, while identifying specific stretch-dependent molecular responses to acute CSE exposure.

Various approaches have been reported for stretching PCLS. Techniques range from suturing (Davidovich et al., 2013a,b) or clamping (Dassow et al., 2010) the PCLS to a deformable elastic membrane, to compressing it between a polyacrylamide gel and a hollow indenter (Lavoie et al., 2012). While such devices allow for real-time imaging, they can be time consuming, limited to a single lung slice, or constrained to a small area-of-stretch. In contrast, the multi-well device described here provides simultaneous, whole-slice stretching of up to 12 samples with minimal preparation time. A commercially available alternative capable of accommodating multiple lung slices operates by applying a negative pressure vacuum to deform an elastic membrane around a rigid post. However, we found that indenter posts with integrated ball bearings improved hysteresis, stretch homogeneity, and inter-cycle repeatability compared to other designs using grease to reduce friction, which can also cause heat-induced cell damage (Arold et al., 2009). Moreover, the flexframe design introduced here is considerably more economic, easy to build, reusable, and customizable with significantly lower intra-well variance. Although stretcher selection is generally dictated by application and familiarity, our device as described above is ideal for higher throughput testing of acute exposures, either pathologic or therapeutic, under tightly-regulated, physiologic stretching conditions.

This platform is uniquely appropriate for investigating mechano-inflammatory interactions, such as those underlying

COPD. Biomechanical forces are known to facilitate emphysema progression (Mishima et al., 1999; Kononov et al., 2001; Yi et al., 2016) along with inflammatory stimuli (*i.e.*, cigarette smoking) that weaken and predispose tissue to failure (Suki et al., 2003). Yet, there is a paucity of data describing their relationship. CSE has been used with *in vitro* (Nana-Sinkam et al., 2007; Stringer et al., 2007; Thaikoottathil et al., 2009; Farid et al., 2013; Ballweg et al., 2014; Chen et al., 2014) and small animal (Chen et al., 2009, 2010; Hanaoka et al., 2011; Lee et al., 2012; He et al., 2015; Chai et al., 2016) models of cigarette smoke exposure given its relatively short incubation time and similarity to pathophysiology *in vivo*. As a proof of concept, we used our system to characterize the PCLS response to acute CSE exposure under various stretch patterns, simulating cigarette smoke inhalation during tidal breathing-like conditions.

IL-1β and MMP-1 expression are often upregulated in patients with COPD (Imai et al., 2001; Ostridge et al., 2016), while MT1-MMP and TIMP1 imbalance can lead to improper lung tissue maintenance (Vandenbroucke et al., 2011; Woode et al., 2015). We observed that the interaction between stretch pattern and CSE exposure had a significant effect on these markers. IL-1β increased with CSE and showed the most robust response to stretch, whereas the enzymes MT1-MMP and MMP-1 and the inhibitor TIMP1 could be either up- or down-regulated by CSE depending on the level of stretch. Interestingly, the low stretch group showed the greatest tissue content of MT1-MMP and MMP-1 when CSE was present, and conversely when it was absent for TIMP1, suggesting this stretch pattern may be most sensitive to an acute exposure. Additional silver staining revealed similar regulatory effects on protein species across a range of molecular weights (**Supplementary Figure S2** and **Supplementary Table S1**). While not a comprehensive model of COPD, the stretch-dependent response to acute CSE exposure observed here suggests a role for mechanotransduction in modulating regional inflammation and enzyme burden on

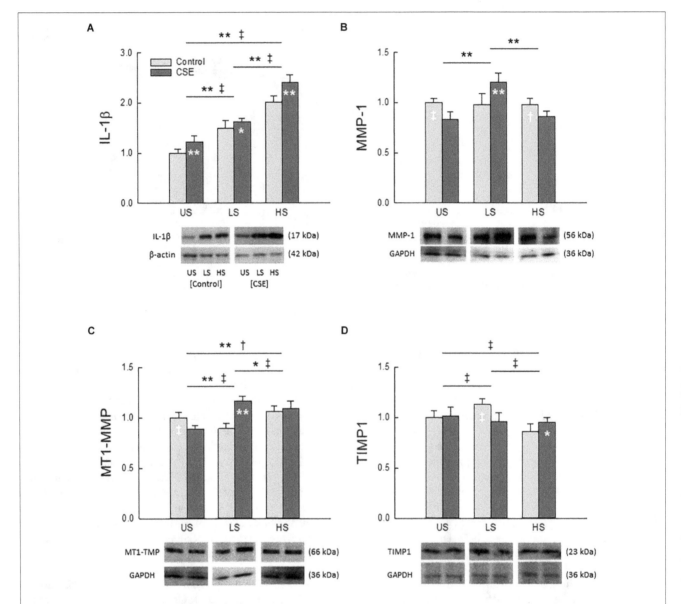

FIGURE 5 | Effects of stretch pattern, CSE, and their interaction on tissue content of IL-1β **(A)**, MMP-1 **(B)**, MT1-MMP **(C)**, and TIMP1 **(D)**. Representative bands with loading controls are also shown. Data ($N = 8$) are shown as normalized mean and SD ($*^†p < 0.05$ and $**^‡p < 0.001$ for CSE and Control groups, respectively). For presentation purposes the original images were cut to smaller ones including representative bands in the desired order and, according to standard publication guideless, white spaces were left between them.

the alveoli. One may speculate this could further exacerbate structural disease heterogeneity and emphysema progression, particularly in tissue experiencing abnormal stretch (Mishima et al., 1999; Suki et al., 2003; Bhatt et al., 2016, 2017; Bodduluri et al., 2017; Mondoñedo and Suki, 2017). In any case, these findings show a clear and definitive difference in PCLS response to an acute exposure between cyclically stretched and unstretched conditions, highlighting the need to provide a comparable dynamic environment as experienced by the lung during tidal breathing *in vivo*.

There are some limitations of this study. (1) Bathing the lung slices directly in media simultaneously exposes all cell types to CSE, whereas exposure to inhaled cigarette smoke initially occurs at the airway and alveolar wall interfaces primarily involving epithelial cells. This is an inherent limitation of the PCLS design. Similarly, the MTS analysis does not specify local tissue viability, but could be extended with immunohistochemistry to verify cell origin. (2) The low-melt agarose is likely incompletely removed despite frequent media changes after slicing as in previous studies (Tepper et al., 2005; Sanderson, 2011; Davidovich et al., 2013b), which could affect the apparent stiffness and residual area of the lung slice. Thus, excised lungs were carefully prepared in the same manner each time to minimize disparities between animals. (3) The lack of circulation in the PCLS limits the study of chemotactic factors, including neutrophil recruitment, which participate in the inflammatory response to cigarette smoking (van der Vaart et al., 2004). (4) While this platform does not facilitate real-time imaging, flexframes are easily removed to visualize lung slices immediately after stretching. (5) Although the deformation provided by the equibiaxial stretching is not 3-dimensional uniform expansion, cells experience physiologically appropriate stretch as the aspect ratio is approximately 1 to 16.

In summary, we demonstrated the feasibility of using this device to perform high-throughput testing of an acute exposure under tightly-regulated, cyclic stretching conditions. We showed that pro-inflammatory and enzyme expression-related effects of acute exposure to cigarette smoke extract are stretch-dependent. These findings identify a fundamental difference between static and tidal breathing-like conditions in precision-cut lung slices. Additional studies in PCLS are required to determine whether mechanotransduction could be a key mediator in COPD disease pathogenesis and progression.

ETHICS STATEMENT

This animal study was reviewed and approved by the IACUC of Boston University.

AUTHOR CONTRIBUTIONS

JM designed the stretcher and experiments, carried out studies, analyzed the data, and wrote the manuscript. EB-S carried out the biochemical assays and analyzed the data. SB analyzed the data. AS analyzed the data and designed the stretcher. KN, KC, AS, WO, and SR-M carried out the experiments. RK designed the experiments. JI designed the stretcher. BS designed the stretcher and experiments, analyzed the data, and wrote the manuscript.

ACKNOWLEDGMENTS

The authors thank Dr. Niccole Schaible and Ms. Ariana Harvey for their contributions in the early stages of this study.

REFERENCES

Arold, S. P., Bartolák-Suki, E., and Suki, B. (2009). Variable stretch pattern enhances surfactant secretion in alveolar type II cells in culture. Am. J. Physiol. Lung Cell. Mol. Physiol. 296, L574–L581. doi: 10.1152/ajplung.90454.2008

Ballweg, K., Mutze, K., Königshoff, M., Eickelberg, O., and Meiners, S. (2014). Cigarette smoke extract affects mitochondrial function in alveolar epithelial cells. Am. J. Physiol. Lung Cell. Mol. Physiol. 307, L895–L907. doi: 10.1152/ajplung.00180.2014

Berridge, M. V., Herst, P. M., and Tan, A. S. (2005). Tetrazolium dyes as tools in cell biology: new insights into their cellular reduction. Biotechnol. Annu. Rev. 11, 127–152. doi: 10.1016/s1387-2656(05)11004-7

Bhatt, S. P., Bodduluri, S., Hoffman, E. A., Newell, J. D. Jr., Sieren, J. C., Dransfield, M. T., et al. (2017). CT measure of lung at-risk and lung function decline in chronic obstructive pulmonary disease. Am. J. Respir. Crit. Care Med. 196, 569–576.

Bhatt, S. P., Bodduluri, S., Newell, J. D., Hoffman, E. A., Sieren, J. C., Han, M. K., et al. (2016). CT-derived biomechanical metrics improve agreement between spirometry and emphysema. Acad. Radiol. 23, 1255–1263. doi: 10.1016/j.acra.2016.02.002

Bodduluri, S., Bhatt, S. P., Hoffman, E. A., Newell, JD Jr, Martinez, C. H., Dransfield, M. T., et al. (2017). Biomechanical CT metrics are associated with patient outcomes in COPD. Thorax 72, 409–414. doi: 10.1136/thoraxjnl-2016-209544

Chai, X.-M., Li, Y.-L., Chen, H., Guo, S.-L., Shui, L.-L., and Chen, Y.-J. (2016). Cigarette smoke extract alters the cell cycle via the phospholipid transfer protein/transforming growth factor-β1/CyclinD1/CDK4 pathway. Eur. J. Pharmacol. 786, 85–93. doi: 10.1016/j.ejphar.2016.05.037

Chen, L., Ge, Q., Tjin, G., Alkhouri, H., Deng, L., Brandsma, C. A., et al. (2014). Effects of cigarette smoke extract on human airway smooth muscle cells in COPD. Eur. Respir. J. 44, 634–646. doi: 10.1183/09031936.00171313

Chen, Y., Hanaoka, M., Chen, P., Droma, Y., Voelkel, N. F., and Kubo, K. (2009). Protective effect of beraprost sodium, a stable prostacyclin analog, in the development of cigarette smoke extract-induced emphysema. Am. J. Physiol. Lung Cell. Mol. Physiol. 296, L648–L656. doi: 10.1152/ajplung.90270.2008

Chen, Y., Hanaoka, M., Droma, Y., Chen, P., Voelkel, N. F., and Kubo, K. (2010). Endothelin-1 receptor antagonists prevent the development of pulmonary emphysema in rats. Eur. Respir. J. 35, 904–912. doi: 10.1183/09031936.00003909

Chronic Obstructive Lung Disease [GOLD] (2017). From the Global Strategy for the Diagnosis, Management and Prevention of COPD, Global Initiative for Chronic Obstructive Lung Disease (GOLD) 2017. Available from: http://goldcopd.org (accessed 5 February, 2017).

Dassow, C., Wiechert, L., Martin, C., Schumann, S., Müller-Newen, G., Pack, O., et al. (2010). Biaxial distension of precision-cut lung slices. J. Appl. Physiol. 108, 713–721. doi: 10.1152/japplphysiol.00229.2009

Davidovich, N., Chhour, P., and Margulies, S. S. (2013a). Uses of remnant human lung tissue for mechanical stretch studies. Cell. Mol. Bioeng. 6, 175–182. doi: 10.1007/s12195-012-0263-6

Davidovich, N., Huang, J., and Margulies, S. S. (2013b). Reproducible uniform equibiaxial stretch of precision-cut lung slices. Am. J. Physiol. Lung Cell. Mol. Physiol. 304, L210–L220. doi: 10.1152/ajplung.00224.2012

Donovan, C., Seow, H. J., Bourke, J. E., and Vlahos, R. (2016). Influenza A virus infection and cigarette smoke impair bronchodilator responsiveness to β-adrenoceptor agonists in mouse lung. Clin. Sci. (Lond). 130, 829–837. doi: 10.1042/cs20160093

Farid, M., Kanaji, N., Nakanishi, M., Gunji, Y., Michalski, J., Iwasawa, S., et al. (2013). Smad3 mediates cigarette smoke extract (CSE) induction of VEGF release by human fetal lung fibroblasts. Toxicol. Lett. 220, 126–134. doi: 10.1016/j.toxlet.2013.04.011

Hanaoka, M., Droma, Y., Chen, Y., Agatsuma, T., Kitaguchi, Y., Voelkel, N. F., et al. (2011). Carbocisteine protects against emphysema induced by cigarette smoke extract in rats. Chest 139, 1101–1108. doi: 10.1378/chest.10-0920

He, Z. H., Chen, P., Chen, Y., He, S. D., Ye, J. R., Zhang, H. L., et al. (2015). Comparison between cigarette smoke-induced emphysema and cigarette smoke extract-induced emphysema. Tob. Induc. Dis. 13:6. doi: 10.1186/s12971-015-0033-z

Henjakovic, M., Martin, C., Hoymann, H. G., Sewald, K., Ressmeyer, A. R., Dassow, C., et al. (2008). Ex vivo lung function measurements in precision-cut lung slices (PCLS) from chemical allergen-sensitized mice represent a suitable alternative to in vivo studies. Toxicol. Sci. 106, 444–453. doi: 10.1093/toxsci/kfn178

Hess, A., Wang-Lauenstein, L., Braun, A., Kolle, S. N., Landsiedel, R., Liebsch, M., et al. (2016). Prevalidation of the ex-vivo model PCLS for prediction of respiratory toxicity. Toxicol. In Vitro 32, 347–361. doi: 10.1016/j.tiv.2016.01.006

Hiorns, J. E., Bidan, C. M., Jensen, O. E., Gosens, R., Kistemaker, L. E., Fredberg, J. J., et al. (2016). Airway and parenchymal strains during bronchoconstriction in the precision cut lung slice. Front. Physiol. 7:309.

Holzapfel, G. A. (2000). *Nonlinear Solid Mechanics: A Continuum Approach for Engineering, New Edition.* Chichester, NY: Wiley.

Imai, K., Dalal, S. S., Chen, E. S., Downey, R., Schulman, L. L., Ginsburg, M., et al. (2001). Human collagenase (matrix metalloproteinase-1) expression in the lungs of patients with emphysema. *Am. J. Respir. Crit. Care Med.* 163(Pt 1), 786–791. doi: 10.1164/ajrccm.163.3.2001073

Imsirovic, J., Wellman, T. J., Mondoñedo, J. R., Bartolák-Suki, E., and Suki, B. (2015). Design of a novel equi-biaxial stretcher for live cellular and subcellular imaging. *PLoS One* 10:e0140283. doi: 10.1371/journal.pone.014 0283

Ingber, D. E. (2006). Cellular mechanotransduction: putting all the pieces together again. *FASEB J.* 20, 811–827. doi: 10.1096/fj.05-5424rev

Jesudason, R., Sato, S., Parameswaran, H., Araujo, A. D., Majumdar, A., Allen, P. G., et al. (2010). Mechanical forces regulate elastase activity and binding site availability in lung elastin. *Biophys. J.* 99, 3076–3083. doi: 10.1016/j.bpj.2010.09.018

Khan, M. A., Ellis, R., Inman, M. D., Bates, J. H. T., Sanderson, M. J., and Janssen, L. J. (2010). Influence of airway wall stiffness and parenchymal tethering on the dynamics of bronchoconstriction. *Am. J. Physiol. Lung Cell. Mol. Physiol.* 299, L98–L108. doi: 10.1152/ajplung.00011.2010

Kistemaker, L. E. M., Oenema, T. A., Baarsma, H. A., Bos, I. S. T., Schmidt, M., Facchinetti, F., et al. (2017). The PDE4 inhibitor CHF-6001 and LAMAs inhibit bronchoconstriction-induced remodeling in lung slices. *Am. J. Physiol. Lung Cell. Mol. Physiol.* 313, L507–L515. doi: 10.1152/ajplung.00069.2017

Kononov, S., Brewer, K., Sakai, H., Cavalcante, F. S., Sabayanagam, C. R., Ingenito, E. P., et al. (2001). Roles of mechanical forces and collagen failure in the development of elastase-induced emphysema. *Am. J. Respir. Crit. Care Med.* 164(Pt 1), 1920–1926. doi: 10.1164/ajrccm.164.10.210 1083

Langer, M., Duggan, E. S., Booth, J. L., Patel, V. I., Zander, R. A., Silasi-Mansat, R., et al. (2012). Bacillus anthracis lethal toxin reduces human alveolar epithelial barrier function. *Infect. Immun.* 80, 4374–4387. doi: 10.1128/IAI.010 11-12

Lauenstein, L., Switalla, S., Prenzler, F., Seehase, S., Pfennig, O., Förster, C., et al. (2014). Assessment of immunotoxicity induced by chemicals in human precision-cut lung slices (PCLS). *Toxicol. In Vitro* 28, 588–599. doi: 10.1016/j.tiv.2013.12.016

Lavoie, T. L., Krishnan, R., Siegel, H. R., Maston, E. D., Fredberg, J. J., Solway, J., et al. (2012). Dilatation of the constricted human airway by tidal expansion of lung parenchyma. *Am. J. Respir. Crit. Care Med.* 186, 225–232. doi: 10.1164/rccm.201202-0368OC

Lee, J. H., Hanaoka, M., Kitaguchi, Y., Kraskauskas, D., Shapiro, L., Voelkel, N. F., et al. (2012). Imbalance of apoptosis and cell proliferation contributes to the development and persistence of emphysema. *Lung* 190, 69–82. doi: 10.1007/s00408-011-9326-z

Mishima, M., Hirai, T., Itoh, H., Nakano, Y., Sakai, H., Muro, S., et al. (1999). Complexity of terminal airspace geometry assessed by lung computed tomography in normal subjects and patients with chronic obstructive pulmonary disease. *Proc. Natl. Acad. Sci. U.S.A.* 96, 8829–8834. doi: 10.1073/pnas.96.16.8829

Mondoñedo, J. R., and Suki, B. (2017). Predicting structure-function relations and survival following surgical and bronchoscopic lung volume reduction treatment of emphysema. *PLoS Comput. Biol.* 13:e1005282. doi: 10.1371/journal.pcbi.1005282

Nana-Sinkam, S. P., Lee, J. D., Sotto-Santiago, S., Stearman, R. S., Keith, R. L., Choudhury, Q., et al. (2007). Prostacyclin prevents pulmonary endothelial cell apoptosis induced by cigarette smoke. *Am. J. Respir. Crit. Care Med.* 175, 676–685. doi: 10.1164/rccm.200605-724oc

Neuhaus, V., Schaudien, D., Golovina, T., Temann, U. A., Thompson, C., Lippmann, T., et al. (2017). Assessment of long-term cultivated human precision-cut lung slices as an ex vivo system for evaluation of chronic cytotoxicity and functionality. *J. Occup. Med. Toxicol.* 12:13. doi: 10.1186/s12995-017-0158-5

Ostridge, K., Williams, N., Kim, V., Bennett, M., Harden, S., Welch, L., et al. (2016). Relationship between pulmonary matrix metalloproteinases and quantitative CT markers of small airways disease and emphysema in COPD. *Thorax* 71, 126–132. doi: 10.1136/thoraxjnl-2015-207428

Rosner, S. R., Ram-Mohan, S., Paez-Cortez, J. R., Lavoie, T. L., Dowell, M. L., Yuan, L., et al. (2014). Airway contractility in the precision-cut lung slice after cryopreservation. *Am. J. Respir. Cell Mol. Biol.* 50, 876–881. doi: 10.1165/rcmb.2013-0166MA

Sanderson, M. J. (2011). Exploring lung physiology in health and disease with lung slices. *Pulm. Pharmacol. Ther.* 24, 452–465. doi: 10.1016/j.pupt.2011.05.001

Schlepütz, M., Rieg, A. D., Seehase, S., Spillner, J., Perez-Bouza, A., Braunschweig, T., et al. (2012). Neurally mediated airway constriction in human and other species: a comparative study using precision-cut lung slices (PCLS). *PLoS One* 7:e47344. doi: 10.1371/journal.pone.0047344

Song, M. J., Davidovich, N., Lawrence, G. G., and Margulies, S. S. (2016). Superoxide mediates tight junction complex dissociation in cyclically stretched lung slices. *J. Biomech.* 49, 1330–1335. doi: 10.1016/j.jbiomech.2015.10.032

Stringer, K. A., Tobias, M., O'Neill, H. C., and Franklin, C. C. (2007). Cigarette smoke extract-induced suppression of caspase-3-like activity impairs human neutrophil phagocytosis. *Am. J. Physiol. Lung Cell. Mol. Physiol.* 292, L1572–L1579.

Suki, B., Lutchen, K. R., and Ingenito, E. P. (2003). On the progressive nature of emphysema: roles of proteases, inflammation, and mechanical forces. *Am. J. Respir. Crit. Care Med.* 168, 516–521. doi: 10.1164/rccm.200208-908pp

Suki, B., Sato, S., Parameswaran, H., Szabari, M. V., Takahashi, A., and Bartolák-Suki, E. (2013). Emphysema and mechanical stress-induced lung remodeling. *Physiology (Bethesda)* 28, 404–413. doi: 10.1152/physiol.00041.2013

Switalla, S., Lauenstein, L., Prenzler, F., Knothe, S., Förster, C., Fieguth, H. G., et al. (2010). Natural innate cytokine response to immunomodulators and adjuvants in human precision-cut lung slices. *Toxicol. Appl. Pharmacol.* 246, 107–115. doi: 10.1016/j.taap.2010.04.010

Tepper, R. S., Ramchandani, R., Argay, E., Zhang, L., Xue, Z., Liu, Y., et al. (2005). Chronic strain alters the passive and contractile properties of rabbit airways. *J. Appl. Physiol.* 98, 1949–1954. doi: 10.1152/japplphysiol.00952.2004

Thaikoottathil, J. V., Martin, R. J., Zdunek, J., Weinberger, A., Rino, J. G., and Chu, H. W. (2009). Cigarette smoke extract reduces VEGF in primary human airway epithelial cells. *Eur. Respir. J.* 33, 835–843. doi: 10.1183/09031936.00080708

Uhl, F. E., Vierkotten, S., Wagner, D. E., Burgstaller, G., Costa, R., Koch, I., et al. (2015). Preclinical validation and imaging of Wnt-induced repair in human 3D lung tissue cultures. *Eur. Respir. J.* 46, 1150–1166. doi: 10.1183/09031936.00183214

van der Vaart, H., Postma, D. S., and Timens, W.. and ten Hacken, N. H. T., (2004). Acute effects of cigarette smoke on inflammation and oxidative stress: a review. *Thorax* 59, 713–721. doi: 10.1136/thx.2003.012468

Van Dijk, E. M., Culha, S., Menzen, M. H., Bidan, C. M., and Gosens, R. (2016). Elastase-induced parenchymal disruption and airway hyper responsiveness in mouse precision cut lung slices: toward an Ex vivo COPD model. *Front. Physiol.* 7:657.

van Rijt, S. H., Bölükbas, D. A., Argyo, C., Datz, S., Lindner, M., Eickelberg, O., et al. (2015). Protease-mediated release of chemotherapeutics from mesoporous silica nanoparticles to ex vivo human and mouse lung tumors. *ACS Nano* 9, 2377–2389. doi: 10.1021/nn5070343

Vandenbroucke, R. E., Dejonckheere, E., and Libert, C. (2011). A therapeutic role for matrix metalloproteinase inhibitors in lung diseases? *Eur. Respir. J.* 38, 1200–1214. doi: 10.1183/09031936.00027411

Watson, C. Y., Damiani, F., Ram-Mohan, S., Rodrigues, S., de Moura Queiroz P, Donaghey, T. C., et al. (2016). Screening for chemical toxicity using cryopreserved precision cut lung slices. *Toxicol. Sci.* 150, 225–233. doi: 10.1093/toxsci/kfv320

Woode, D., Shiomi, T., and D'Armiento, J. (2015). Collagenolytic matrix metalloproteinases in chronic obstructive lung disease and cancer. *Cancers (Basel)* 7, 329–341. doi: 10.3390/cancers70 10329

Yi, E., Sato, S., Takahashi, A., Parameswaran, H., Blute, T. A., Bartolák-Suki, E., et al. (2016). Mechanical forces accelerate collagen digestion by bacterial collagenase in lung tissue strips. *Front. Physiol.* 7:287. doi: 10.3389/fphys.2016.00287

9

A Novel Fibroblast Reporter Cell Line for *in vitro* Studies of Pulmonary Fibrosis

Julia Nemeth[1†], Annika Schundner[1†], Karsten Quast[2], Veronika E. Winkelmann[1] and Manfred Frick[1]*

[1] *Institute of General Physiology, Ulm University, Ulm, Germany,* [2] *Boehringer Ingelheim Pharma GmbH & Co. KG, Biberach, Germany*

*Correspondence:
Manfred Frick
manfred.frick@uni-ulm.de
orcid.org/0000-0002-4763-1104

[†] *These authors have contributed equally to this work*

Idiopathic pulmonary fibrosis (IPF) is a fatal disease of the lower respiratory tract with restricted therapeutic options. Repetitive injury of the bronchoalveolar epithelium leads to activation of pulmonary fibroblasts, differentiation into myofibroblasts and excessive extracellular matrix (ECM) deposition resulting in aberrant wound repair. However, detailed molecular and cellular mechanisms underlying initiation and progression of fibrotic changes are still elusive. Here, we report the generation of a representative fibroblast reporter cell line (10-4A^{BFP}) to study pathophysiological mechanisms of IPF in high throughput or high resolution *in vitro* live cell assays. To this end, we immortalized primary fibroblasts isolated from the distal lung of Sprague-Dawley rats. Molecular and transcriptomic characterization identified clone 10-4A as a matrix fibroblast subpopulation. Mechanical or chemical stimulation induced a reversible fibrotic state comparable to effects observed in primary isolated fibroblasts. Finally, we generated a reporter cell line (10-4A^{BFP}) to express nuclear blue fluorescent protein (BFP) under the promotor of the myofibroblast marker alpha smooth muscle actin (*Acta2*) using CRISPR/Cas9 technology. We evaluated the suitability of 10-4A^{BFP} as reporter tool in plate reader assays. In summary, the 10-4A^{BFP} cell line provides a novel tool to study fibrotic processes *in vitro* to gain new insights into the cellular and molecular processes involved in fibrosis formation and propagation.

Keywords: idiopathic pulmonary fibrosis, lung, myofibroblast, TGF-β, extracellular matrix, alpha smooth muscle actin

INTRODUCTION

Idiopathic pulmonary fibrosis (IPF) is a progressive, irreversible and usually fatal lung disease with poor prognosis. IPF is characterized by subpleural fibrosis, subepithelial fibroblast foci, and microscopic honeycombing (Raghu et al., 2011; Wuyts et al., 2013; Lederer and Martinez, 2018; Sgalla et al., 2018). Various risk factors, including air pollution and smoking, have been associated with the development of IPF (Selman and Pardo, 2001; Kage and Borok, 2012; Liang et al., 2016; Kasper and Barth, 2017; Richeldi et al., 2017). In recent years, it has become clear that IPF is also strongly associated with genetic aberrations (Armanios et al., 2007; Seibold et al., 2011; Ryu et al., 2014; Stuart et al., 2015; Evans et al., 2016). Hence, an approach in understanding IPF pathogenesis is to consider it as a three-stage process: predisposition, initiation, and progression.

The conceptual model for the pathogenesis of IPF postulates that recurrent micro-injuries to the bronchoalveolar epithelium, superimposed on accelerated epithelial aging, result in aberrant wound repair. The reduced renewal capacity of bronchoalveolar stem cells, including alveolar type II cells, leads to reduced alveolar-epithelial cell proliferation, and secretion of profibrotic mediators (Selman and Pardo, 2001; Plantier et al., 2011; Kage and Borok, 2012; Ryu et al., 2014; Chambers and Mercer, 2015; Liang et al., 2016; Xu et al., 2016; Kasper and Barth, 2017; Richeldi et al., 2017; Lederer and Martinez, 2018). The main and most studied profibrotic cytokine is transforming growth factor beta 1 (TGF-β1). Several other cytokines play a major role in immune and inflammation responses for fibrosis formation, including interleukins (IL) like IL-13 (Zhu et al., 1999; Kolodsick et al., 2004; O'Reilly, 2013), IL-33 (Yanaba et al., 2011; Luzina et al., 2012, 2013) and IL-4 (Huaux et al., 2003; Saito et al., 2003), tumor necrosis factor alpha (TNFα) (Sime et al., 1998; Oikonomou et al., 2006; Epstein Shochet et al., 2017) as well as thymic stromal lymphopoietin (TSLP) (Datta et al., 2013; Lee et al., 2017). Profibrotic cytokines promote fibroblast activation and proliferation (Sime et al., 1997; Hinz, 2009; Luzina et al., 2015).

Fibroblast activation results in altered and increased ECM production, deposition, and accumulation (Liu et al., 2010; Bagnato and Harari, 2015). This causes remodeling processes of the pulmonary interstitium, forming scar tissue and modifying its mechanical properties (Booth et al., 2012; Parker et al., 2014). Scarring is accompanied by a strong increase in the tissue stiffness and an overall thickening of the alveolar septae (Horowitz and Thannickal, 2006; Hinz, 2009; Richeldi et al., 2017). During this progression phase, the matrix stiffness can increase from ~ 0.5 to 15 kPa in healthy lung tissue to up to 100 kPa in fibrotic tissue depending on the measured lung compartment (Liu et al., 2010; Booth et al., 2012). The pathologically stiff matrix further propagates remodeling independent of epithelial cell dysfunction. In a feed-forward loop, increased matrix stiffness promotes additional differentiation of fibroblasts to myofibroblasts and matrix deposition (Hinz, 2009; Enomoto et al., 2013; Burgess et al., 2016; Tschumperlin et al., 2018). Overall, these processes result in the destruction of the overall alveolar architecture, leading to a strong impairment of lung function and eventually resulting in the death of the patient (Wuyts et al., 2013).

Studies regarding the onset and progress of IPF are mainly conducted in animal models by the application of fibrosis inducing agents like bleomycin (Gabazza et al., 2004; Xiao et al., 2006; Löfdahl et al., 2018). However, animal models of IPF do not fully recapitulate human pathophysiology (Lederer and Martinez, 2018). These models only partially mimic the events hallmarking IPF but it's challenging to gain a deep insight into cellular and molecular processes. Hence, studies investigating molecular alterations of affected cell populations in response to pro-fibrotic stimuli are essential to get a more in-depth understanding of

key processes responsible for development and progression of IPF. In this context, *in vitro* studies mimicking the *in vivo* situation hold great promise to elucidate molecular mechanisms underlying IPF initiation and progression. Sophisticated "lung on a chip" approaches recapitulating the alveolar microenvironment were developed and optimized by different groups (Huh, 2015; Stucki et al., 2018; Felder et al., 2019). These enable co-culture of differentiated alveolar epithelial and mesenchymal cells at air-liquid conditions whilst mimicking breathing motion and blood flow. However, the impact of these *in vitro* models depends on the use of cells representative of the *in vivo* situation.

In order to promote *in vitro* models for studying fibrotic processes, we generated an immortalized pulmonary fibroblast reporter cell line (10-4A^{BFP}) using CRISPR/Cas9 gene-editing. 10-4A^{BFP} cells express nuclear blue fluorescent protein (BFP) under the promotor of the myofibroblast marker alpha smooth muscle actin (*Acta2*). To this end, we isolated primary cells from the distal lung of Sprague-Dawley rats and immortalized them using a recently described technology (Kuehn et al., 2016). We characterized several clones and validated selected clones for suitability in fibrosis studies, directly comparing responsiveness to either mechanical or chemical stimuli to responses observed in primary isolated fibroblasts. We identified clone 10-4A as a matrix fibroblast subpopulation that can be (reversibly) induced to a fibrotic state comparable to primary isolated fibroblasts. The 10-4A clone was then used for generation of a reporter cell line (10-4A^{BFP}) expressing nuclear BFP under the promotor of the myofibroblast marker alpha smooth muscle actin (*Acta2*) using CRISPR/Cas9 technology. Finally, we evaluated the use of 10-4A^{BFP} cells as screening tool in plate reader assays. In summary, the 10-4A^{BFP} cell line provides a novel tool to study fibrotic processes in an *in vitro* co-culture system at high resolution and/or high throughput and thereby enables new insights into the cellular and molecular processes involved in fibrosis formation and propagation.

MATERIALS AND METHODS

Chemicals and Antibodies

Human TGF-β1 was obtained from Proteintech (cat. # HZ-1011, Manchester, United Kingdom), rat IL-13 (cat. # 1945-RL-025) and rat TNF-α (cat. # 510 RT) from R&D Systems (Minneapolis, MN, United States), rat IL-33 (cat. # ab200250) from Abcam (Cambridge, United Kingdom) and rat IL-1β (cat. # 80023-RNAE) from Sino Biological (Vienna, Austria). All other chemicals were obtained from Sigma-Aldrich GmbH (Steinheim, Germany) if not stated otherwise. The following primary and secondary antibodies were used for immunofluorescence staining: αSMA (1:200, cat. # ab5694; Abcam; RRID:AB_2223021), vimentin (1:500, cat. # ab73159; Abcam; RRID:AB_1271458), EpCAM (1:200, cat. # ab71916; Abcam, RRID:AB_1603782), ABCa3 (1:500, cat. # ab24751; Abcam, RRID:AB_448287), Aqp5 (1:200, cat. # ab92320; Abcam, RRID:AB_2049171), caveolin 1 (1:200, cat. # ab2910, Abcam, RRID:AB_303405), CD45 (1:500, cat. # 12-0461-80, Thermo Fisher Scientific, Bonn, Germany, RRID:AB_2572560).

Alexa Fluor® 488 goat anti-chicken (1:300, cat. # A11039; Thermo Fisher Scientific, RRID:AB_142924); Alexa Fluor® 568 goat anti-rabbit (1:300, cat. # A11011; Thermo Fisher Scientific, RRID:AB_143157) Alexa Fluor® 488 goat anti-mouse (1:300, cat. # A11029; Thermo Fisher Scientific, RRID:AB_138404).

Cell Isolation and Cultivation

All lung cells were isolated from 12 to 14-week-old male Sprague-Dawley rats.

Primary alveolar type II (ATII) cells were isolated according to a modified protocol described by Jansing et al. (2018) In short, rats were anesthetized with ketamine (10%) and xylazil (2%) and injected with heparin (400 IU/kg). Lungs were perfused, removed, washed with BSS-A supplemented with EGTA, BSS-A w/o EGTA and BSS-B solution. The tissue was incubated with 0.5 mg/ml elastase (Elastin Products Co., Owensville, MO, United States) for 20 min. Then, 2 mg/ml DNase were added and the tissue was minced with sharp scissors into bits of about 1 mm^3. The enzymatic reaction was stopped by adding FCS (GIBCO® life technologies, Carlsbad, CA, United States) (37°C, 2 min). The digested tissue was filtered through gauze and nylon meshes (mesh sizes: 100, 40, and 10 μm) and the cell filtrate was centrifuged for 8 min at 130 rcf. For further cell separation, density gradient centrifugation was applied by mixing the cells in OptiPrep™ Density Gradient medium (1.077 g/mL) diluted in BSS-B. The cells were centrifuged for 20 min at 200 rcf. The layer containing ATII cells was collected and supplemented with BSS-B to a total volume of 40 ml. Cells were centrifuged at 130 rcf for 8 min, resuspended in MucilAir™ cell culture medium and 1 × 10^6 cells/cm^2 were seeded apically on 0.4 μm transparent Transwell® filter inserts (Sarstedt, Nümbrecht, Germany). Purity of the ATII cells (>90%) was determined by staining with 0.4 μM Lyso Tracker Red DND 99 for 10 min (Thermo Fisher Scientific, Waltham, MA, United States) and more specifically with an ABCa3 staining. The amount of LTR positive cells was determined using a Countess II FL Automated Cell Counter (Thermo Fisher Scientific, Waltham, MA, United States).

Primary lung fibroblasts and distal lung cells were isolated according to the method of Dobbs et al. (1986) with minor modifications as previously described (Miklavc et al., 2010).

For primary isolated fibroblasts further modifications were applied:

Anesthesia, lung perfusion and removal followed the protocol described for isolation of AT2 cells. The tissue was then incubated with 0.5 mg/ml elastase (Elastin Products Co., Owensville, MO, United States) and 0.05 mg/ml trypsin at 37°C for 30 min. 2 mg/ml DNase were added, the enzymatic reaction was stopped by FCS and the digested tissue was filtered through gauze and nylon meshes (mesh sizes: 100, 70, and 40 μm). For purification of primary fibroblasts, cell suspensions were depleted of leukocytes using anti-CD45 MicroBeads (Miltenyi Biotec, Bergisch Gladbach, Germany) before fibroblasts were isolated using anti- CD90.1 MicroBeads (Miltenyi Biotec, Bergisch Gladbach, Germany) according to manufacturer's instructions. Cells were seeded on polydimethylsiloxane (PDMS) gels or plastic substrate in MucilAir™ culture medium containing 25.6 μg/ml Gentamicin ± 5 ng/mL TGF-β1 at a density of 1 to 5 × 10^5 cells/cm^2. Cells were cultured at 37°C, 5% CO$_2$ and 95% humidity for up to 14 days. Culture media were changed every 2 days, with TGF-β1 being added freshly to the medium in corresponding experiments.

Generation of Immortalized Cell Lines

Immortalization was performed by InSCREENeX (Braunschweig, Germany) as previously described (Lipps et al., 2018). In short: Immortalization genes were incorporated with third generation self-inactivating lentiviral vectors. Gene expression is controlled by an internal SV 40 promoter. Integration of the transgenes was verified by PCR and subsequent gel electrophoresis.

Overall, 15 immortalized cell clones were generated, all displaying characteristics of different cell populations of the distal lung. The incorporated genes used for the immortalization process for the cell line 10-4A are TAg, ID2, ID3, Rex, Nanog, and E7.

10-4A cells were maintained in the chemically defined, standardized, cell culture medium MucilAir™ (Epithelix, Genève, Switzerland) containing 25.6 μg/ml Gentamicin (Thermo Fisher Scientific) at 37°C, 5% CO$_2$ and 95% humidity. Cells were detached upon reaching 80% confluence using TrypLE (Thermo Fisher Scientific), centrifuged, resuspended in cell culture medium ± 5 ng/mL TGF-β1 and seeded on PDMS gels or plastic dishes at a density of 0.5 × 10^3 to 40 × 10^3 cells/cm^2. Culture media were changed every 2 days, with TGF-β1 being added freshly to the medium in corresponding experiments. Cells from passage 11 to 25 were used for all experiments.

PDMS Gel Preparation and Coating of Cell Culture Dishes

PDMS gels were prepared with the Sylgard 527 Silicon Dielectric Gel Kit (Dow Europe GmbH, Wiesbaden, Germany) as previously described (Palchesko et al., 2012) with minor modifications. In brief, component A and B were thoroughly mixed in a 1:1 ratio and added to 24 Well Culture Plates (Sarstedt, Nümbrecht, Germany) or ibiTreat μSlide 8 well (ibidi GmbH, Gräfelfing, Germany), respectively. Culture containers were kept under vacuum for 2 h to remove potential air inclusions and then incubated at room temperature for 48 h for polymerization. Fully polymerized PDMS gels were sterilized in a UV Crosslinker (GE Healthcare Europe GmbH, Freiburg im Breisgau, Germany) for 30 min and then coated with a 0.01% w/v polydopamine solution [50 mM Tris–HCl, pH = 8.5, 0.01% (w/v) Dopamine Hydrochloride] for 1 h and a 38 μg/ml rat tail collagen I solution (Advanced BioMatrix Inc., San Diego, CA, United States), diluted in Dulbecco PBS (Biochrom, Berlin, Germany; pH 7.4) over night at 37°C, respectively.

Identical coating conditions were used for culture plastic dishes w/o PDMS to ensure comparability.

RNA Isolation, cDNA Synthesis and qPCR

Total RNA was isolated using the my-Budget RNA Mini Kit (Bio-Budget Technologies GmbH, Krefeld, Germany) with an additional DNA removal step using the RNase free DNase Set (QIAGEN GmbH, Hilden, Germany). cDNA synthesis was performed using the SuperScript® VILO™ cDNA Synthesis Kit (Thermo Fisher Scientific) and cDNA was diluted in a 1:3 ratio with DEPC treated H_2O (Carl Roth, Karlsruhe, Germany) prior qPCR.

Amplification was performed on a StepOnePlus qPCR cycle (Applied Biosystems, Foster City, CA, United States) using EvaGreen QPCR Mix II (Bio-Budget Technologies). The following QuantiTect® Primer assays (QIAGEN GmbH, Hilden Germany) were used: Rn_Plin2_2_SG (QT01624329), Rn_Acta2_1_SG (QT01615901), Rn_Col1a1_1_SG (QT01081059), Rn_Sftpc_1_SG (QT00179368), Rn_ABCa3_1_SG (QT01587936), Rn_Vim_1_SG (QT00178724), Rn_HOPX_1_SG (QT00182693), Rn_Cav1_1_SG (QT00398181), and Rn_Hmbs_1_SG (QT00179123). The relative quantification of mRNA expression was performed according to the method of Pfaffl (2001).

Illumina Library Preparation and Sequencing

The Sequencing library preparation has been done using 200 ng of total RNA input with the TruSeq RNA Sample Prep Kit v2-Set B (RS-122–2002, Illumina Inc., San Diego, CA, United States) producing a 275 bp fragment including adapters in average size. In the final step before sequencing, eight individual libraries were normalized and pooled together using the adapter indices supplied by the manufacturer. Pooled libraries have then been clustered on the cBot Instrument from Illumina using the TruSeq SR Cluster Kit v3 – cBot – HS (GD-401–3001, Illumina Inc., San Diego, CA, United States) sequencing was then performed as 50 bp, single reads and 7 bases index read on an Illumina HiSeq2000 instrument using the TruSeq SBS Kit HS- v3 (50-cycle) (FC-401–3002, Illumina Inc., San Diego, CA, United States).

mRNA-Seq Bioinformatics Pipeline

RNA-Seq reads were aligned to the rat genome using the STAR Aligner v2.5.2a (Dobin et al., 2013) with the Ensembl 84 reference genome[1]. Sequenced read quality was checked with FastQC v0.11.2[2] and alignment quality metrics were calculated using the RNASeQC v1.18 (Deluca et al., 2012). Following read alignment, duplication rates of the RNA-Seq samples were computed with bamUtil v1.0.11 to mark duplicate reads and the dupRadar v1.4 Bioconductor R package for assessment (Sayols et al., 2016). The gene expression profiles were quantified using Cufflinks software version 2.2.1 (Trapnell et al., 2013) to get the Reads Per Kilobase of transcript per Million mapped reads (RPKM) as well as read counts from the feature counts software package (Liao et al., 2014). The matrix of read counts and the design file were imported to R, normalization factors calculated using trimmed mean of M-values (TMM) and subsequently voom normalized, before subjected to downstream descriptive statistics analysis.

Western Blot

Cells were washed twice with PBS, collected with RIPA Buffer (Sigma-Aldrich) and sonicated (Sonifier 250, Branson Ultrasonics Corporation, Danbury, CT, United States) prior loading on gels. The protein concentration was determined by Pierce BCA Protein Assay (Thermo Fisher Scientific). Protein Loading Buffer and NuPAGE reducing agent (Thermo Fisher Scientific) were added in a 1:5 and 1:10 ratio, respectively. Samples were incubated at 70°C for 10 min, separated by SDS-PAGE and blotted on a nitrocellulose membrane. Immunodetection of αSMA and HSP90 was performed using Anti-alpha smooth muscle actin (1:200, cat # ab5694; Abcam, RRID:AB_2223021) and HSP90 α/β antibodies (F-8) (1:500, cat. # sc-13119; Santa Cruz Biotechnology, Dallas, TX, United States, RRID:AB_675659) in combination with fluorescent labeled secondary antibodies [1:20,000; IRDye® 800CW Donkey anti-Rabbit (cat. # 926-32213, RRID:AB_621848), IRDye® 680RD Donkey anti-Mouse (cat. # 926-68072, RRID:AB_10953628)] diluted in Intercept® Blocking Buffer (cat. # 927-60001) (all from LI-COR Biosciences, Lincoln, NE, United States). Primary antibodies were incubated over night at 4°C, secondary antibodies for 1 h at RT, respectively. Membranes were analyzed with the Odyssey Fc Imaging System (LI-COR Biosciences).

Immunofluorescence

For immunofluorescence staining, cells were washed with DPBS (Biochrom, Berlin, Germany; pH 7.4) and fixed in a 4% paraformaldehyde solution (dissolved in DPBS) for 10 min followed by a 1 min incubation in ice-cold 99.8% MeOH. Cells were permeabilized in a 0.2% w/v saponin solution (dissolved in DPBS) containing 10% FBS (Thermo Fisher Scientific) and 50 mM HEPES. Subsequently, cells were stained for 1 h with primary antibodies, washed twice with DPBS and stained with secondary antibodies diluted in saponin solution for 1 h. Images were taken on an iMIC digital microscope (FEI Munich GmbH, Gräfelfing, Germany) with an Olympus UApo/340 40x/1.35 Oil Iris, Infinity/0.17 lens (Olympus Europa SE & Co. KG, Hamburg, Germany) and the corresponding software (Live Aquisition v2.6.0.14).

Generation of the *Acta2*-BFP Reporter Cell Line

CRISPR/Cas9 dependent gene editing of 10-4A cells was performed according to the method described in Ran et al. (2013).

A 20 bp single guide RNA (sgRNA) (AAACAGGAGT ATGACGAAGC), binding at the end of the coding region of the *Acta2* gene was designed by using the R&D Benchling software[3]. The sgRNA was cloned into SpCas9(BB)-2A-GFP (Addgene plasmid ID: 48138). A donor vector was designed to allow for in-frame fusion of a T2A-BFP-NLS (BFP from Evrogen, Heidelberg, Germany) cassette at the 3′ end of the *Acta2* gene. Primers used were listed in **Table 1**. DNA sequences flanking the sgRNA cutting site at the 5′and 3′ end were amplified from genomic DNA isolated from 10-4A cells (isolated with DNeasy Blood ans Tissue Kit, QIAGEN GmbH), and

---

[1]http://www.ensembl.org

[2]http://www.bioinformatics.babraham.ac.uk/projects/fastqc/

[3]https://www.benchling.com

TABLE 1 | Primers used for cloning of T2A-BFP-NLS and homology arms into donor vector pGFX-6P-1.

Primer Name	Sequence 5′ → 3′
pGEX-6P-1_fwd	tgtggaattgtgagcggataac
pGEX-6P-1_rev	cattatacgcgatgattaattg
T2A-BFP-NLS_fwd	tcggctcgtataatggagggcagaggaag tctgct
T2A-BFP-NLS_rev	gctcacaattccacattataccttctcttcttt tttgga
*Acta2*_right_homologous_right_arm_fwd	tcggctcgtataatgccctctgtgttgggcag
*Acta2*_right_homologous_right_arm_rev	acttcctctgccctcccacatctgctgga aggtaga
*Acta2*_left_homologous_right_arm_fwd	caggaaacagtattcgtcacgccccaccct
*Acta2*_left_homologous_right_arm_rev	aacttccagatccgatgtaaacacatgtata attgttttacttatccggtcac
pGEX-6P-1_T2A-BFP-NLS_right_arm_rev	cattatacgcgatgattaattgtcaacag
pGEX-6P-1_T2A-BFP-NLS_right_arm_fw	gagggcagaggaagtctgctaac
pGEX-6P-1_T2A-BFP-NLS_left_arm_fw	tcggatctggaagttctgttccagg
pGEX-6P-1_T2A-BFP-NLS_left_arm_rev	gaatactgtttcctgtgtgaaattgttatccg

subcloned into the targeting pGEX-6P-1 Vector (GE Healthcare, 28-9546-48) using the In-Fusion kit (Clontech, Mountain View, CA, United States). 10-4A cells were co-transfected with the sgRNA/SpCas9(BB)-2A-GFP plasmid and the pGEX-6P-1 donor plasmid in a ratio of 2:1 using Lipofectamine LTX (Ratio: LTX Reagent: PLUS^TM Reagent, 1:1) (Thermo Fisher Scientific). The efficiency of sgRNA/Cas9-mediated integration of the BFP was evaluated after addition of 5 ng/ml TGF-β1 via fluorescence microscopy. 72 h after transfection, isolation of clonal cells was achieved by fluorescent activated cell sorting (FACS). Cells were selected for GFP and BFP expression using the BD FACSAria^TM III (Becton Dickinson GmbH) with the corresponding BD FACSDiva^TM v6.1.3 software. Single cells were seeded in 96-well plates containing cell culture medium.

Functional Testing of BFP Integration

The DNA of the cell clones was extracted as described above. The region of interest was amplified by PCR and the respective products (WT: 1000 bp, with BFP insert: 1880 bp) were verified by Sanger Sequencing (Eurofins).

Additionally, in order to verify the functionality of the *Acta2* coupled BFP reporter system, cells were seeded in plastic or 5 kPa PDMS coated ibiTreat μSlide 8 well at a density of 25000/cm² in MucilAir ± 5 ng/ml TGF-β1. Pictures were taken with an iMIC Digital Microscope (FEI Munich GmbH). All images were obtained using an Olympus Objective UApo/340 40x/1.35 Oil ∞/0.17 and a 405 nm excitation filter for BFP.

Microplate Reader Assay

Cells were seeded in PDMS coated 96-well plates (Sarstedt, Nümbrecht, Germany). Respective growth factors were added 24 h post-seeding and the BFP signal was measured at indicated time points. For fluorescence measurements, cells were trypsinized, transferred to a collagen (Advanced BioMatrix Inc.) coated black 96-well plate (Sarstedt) and let adhere for 3 h.

Cells were stained with Calcein AM (Thermo Fisher Scientific) for 30 min in bath solution (in mM: 140 NaCl, 5 KCl, 1 MgCl2, 2 CaCl2, 5 glucose, and 10 HEPES; pH 7.4), washed twice with PBS w/o Ca²⁺/Mg²⁺ and maintained in 200 μl bath solution during analysis of BFP signal with the plate reader (Tecan, Salzburg, Austria). Excitation wavelength were 385 nm and 485 nm and BFP and Calcein emissions were collected at 445 nm and 535 nm, respectively. BFP and Calcein signals were background subtracted and the BFP signal was normalized to the Calcein signal to adjust for cell number.

Statistical Analysis

GraphPad Prims7 software (GraphPad, La Jolla, CA, United States) was used for statistical analysis, curve fitting and data representation. Respective tests are given within the figure legend. Data are represented as means ± SEM unless stated otherwise. Statistical significance was determined using the non-parametric Mann–Whitney-U test for comparison of two independent samples at the same time point. The number of experiments (N) indicates individual animals for primary fibroblasts and cells from varying passages for immortalized fibroblasts. Data was considered significant if the p value was < 0.05 and is indicated with an asterisk. Statistical significance is indicated in the graphs as follows: p-values < 0.05: *, p-values < 0.01: **, p-values < 0.001: ***.

RESULTS

10-4A Cells Resemble Matrix Fibroblasts but Not Myo-/Lipofibroblasts

Isolation and immortalization of primary cells from the distal lung yielded 15 individual cell clones (**Figure 1A**). Subsequently, cell clones were analyzed for phenotypic expression patterns resembling primary epithelial and mesenchymal cells. Expression of marker genes for alveolar type II (ATII) [*Abca3*, *Sftpc* (Beers et al., 2017)], alveolar type I (ATI) [*Hopx*, *Aqp5*, *Cav1* (McElroy and Kasper, 2004; Beers et al., 2017)], pan-epithelial [*Epcam* (Hasegawa et al., 2017)], leukocyte [*CD45* (Barletta et al., 2012)], and mesenchymal [*Vim* (Cheng et al., 2016)] cells was analyzed on the gene and protein level. Both, semi-quantitative RT-PCR and immunofluorescence data identified the presence of mesenchymal and absence of epithelial and leukocyte cell markers in several clones (**Figures 1B,C**). Taking into consideration that *Cav1* is also expressed in lung fibroblasts (Xiao et al., 2006) the data indicate a fibroblast phenotype of all investigated cell clones.

Based on gene expression analysis and protein localization, clone 10-4A was selected for further analysis. In-depth characterization was performed by transcriptomic analysis. Gene expression in 10-4A cells was also compared to expression in healthy primary distal lung fibroblasts and primary ATII cells. The 10-4A cell line exhibits high expression of matrix fibroblast marker genes, in particular *Col1a1* and *Vim*, and low expression of myofibroblast marker genes. Lipofibroblast marker gene expression was low in 10-4A cells when compared to primary fibroblasts (**Figure 2**). Expression of specific pan- and alveolar

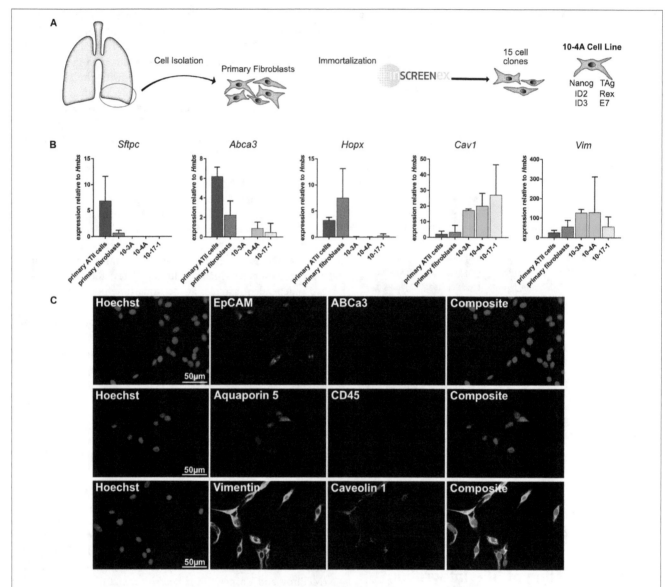

FIGURE 1 | Gene and protein expression pattern of the immortalized cell lines. **(A)** Schematic representation of the immortalization process. *Right:* Genes incorporated in 10-4A cells for immortalization **(B)** Semi-quantitative RT-PCR of ATII cell (*Sftpc*, *Abca3*), ATI cell (*Hopx*, *Cav1*), and mesenchymal cell (*Vim*) marker genes. $N = 5$ **(C)** Immunofluorescent staining of 10-4A cells for expression of epithelial cell (EpCAM), alveolar type II cell (ABCa3), alveolar type I cell (aquaporin 5, caveolin 1), leukocyte (CD45), and mesenchymal cell (vimentin) marker expression. 10-4A cells predominantly express mesenchymal marker vimentin and caveolin-1, that is also expressed in lung fibroblasts. Scale bar = 50 μm.

epithelial marker genes was very low. Together these data suggest that 10-4A cells exhibit a matrix fibroblast phenotype (Zepp et al., 2017; Xie et al., 2018).

Interestingly, 10-4A exhibited high expression of *Pdgfrα*, which is associated with the capability of myofibroblast differentiation (Li et al., 2018).

Increased Substrate Stiffness Exhibits of Myofibroblast Characteristics in 10-4A Cells

The high expression of *Pdgfrα* suggested that these cells may constitute a model to study activation/differentiation of fibroblast

cells observed in pulmonary fibrosis. To test whether 10-4A cells resemble a suitable surrogate cell model for *in vitro* fibrosis studies, we first investigated the responsiveness of 10-4A cells to mechanical stimuli (Hinz, 2009). We analyzed expression of myofibroblast marker genes in response to changes in substrate stiffness. Results in 10-4A cells were compared to effects on freshly isolated primary fibroblasts.

Expression of myofibroblast marker *Acta2* and ECM component *Col1a1* were unchanged over a 14 days period in 10-4A and primary fibroblasts when maintained on soft PDMS gels with physiological stiffness (Young's Modulus of 5 kPa) (Palchesko et al., 2012). In line, with maintenance of a quiescent phenotype, *Plin2*, a marker for lipofibroblasts, did not

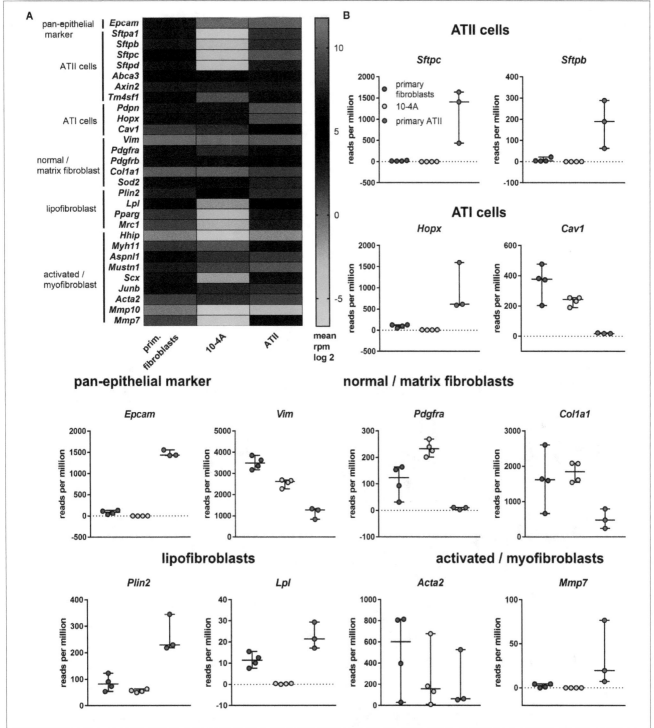

FIGURE 2 | Transcriptomic profile of 10-4A compared to freshly isolated rat fibroblasts and ATII cells. **(A)** Heat map of selected pan-epithelial, ATII, ATI and different fibroblast subtype marker genes. Values are given as log2-fold change of the mean reads per million base pairs. 10-4A and primary fibroblasts, $N = 4$, primary ATII cells, $N = 3$. **(B)** Detailed presentation of rpm values obtained for selected marker genes.

significantly change (**Figures 3A–C**). In some cases, a faint alpha smooth muscle actin (αSMA) signal (the product of *Acta2*) was detected in Western Blots at day 0 in 10-4A.

In contrast, culture on rigid plastic substrate resulted in significantly increased *Acta2* expression in 10-4A (day 4,

$p = 0.008$; day 7, $p = 0.03$; day 14, $p = 0.008$) and primary fibroblasts (day 4, $p = 0.007$; day 7, $p = 0.053$; day 14, $p = 0.03$) (**Figure 3A**). Consistently, αSMA stress fiber formation was detected from day 7 onward, in immunofluorescence experiments and was confirmed by Western Blot (**Figures 3D,E**).

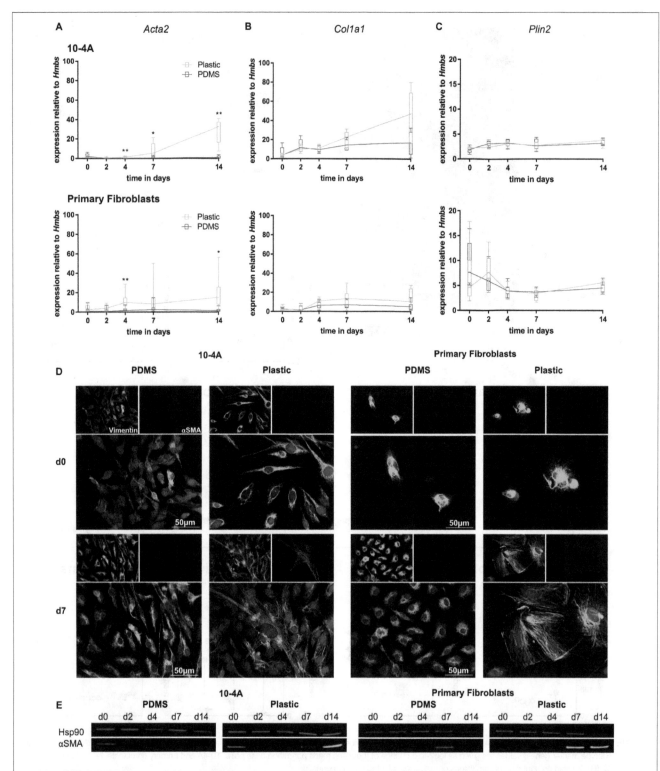

FIGURE 3 | Mechanical stimulation of 10-4A cells and primary fibroblasts. Semi-quantitative RT-PCR analysis of *Acta2* **(A)**, *Col1a1* **(B)**, and *Plin2* **(C)** expression in 10-4A cells **(top graph)** and primary fibroblasts **(bottom graph)** maintained on soft PDMS or stiff plastic substrate, respectively. Data are expressed as fold expression of the housekeeping gene hydroxymethylbilane synthase (*Hmbs*). Primary fibroblast data were obtained from seven different animals, 10-4A data from five different passages. Statistical significance for the respective time points was tested with the non-parametric Mann–Whitney-*U*-Test. Statistical significance is indicated as follows: *p*-values < 0.05: *, *p*-values < 0.01: **. Box plots show data as median values, the boxes represent percentiles, the whiskers indicate the minimum/maximum. **(D)** Immunofluorescence staining of 10-4A cells **(left)** or primary fibroblasts either seeded on PDMS or plastic directly after adherence (d0) or 7 days post-seeding. Cells were stained for the mesenchymal marker vimentin (green) and the pro-fibrotic protein αSMA (red). Scale bar = 50 μm. **(E)** Western Blot for αSMA in 10-4A cells and primary fibroblasts cultured over 14 days on soft (PDMS) and stiff (Plastic) matrices, respectively. HSP90 was used as loading control.

This likely originates from αSMA expressed during cell culture in plastic culture flasks that had not been degraded by the time samples were collected (approx. 6 h after seeding on PDMs substrate). Expression of *Col1a1* and *Plin2* were not affected by stiff substrate within the 14 days culture period, suggesting that the time course might not be sufficiently long enough for full differentiation and activation of fibroblasts. A weak αSMA signal was detected in Western blots for day 0 samples from 10-4A cells.

TGF-β1 Induces a Transient Myofibroblast Phenotype in 10-4A Cells

To further characterize the response of 10-4A cells to fibrotic stimuli, we stimulated the cells with the potent profibrotic cytokine TGF-β1.

Transforming growth factor beta 1 (5 ng/ml) treatment resulted in significantly increased *Acta2* gene expression after 2 days in 10-4A cells (day 2, $p = 0.008$; day 4, $p = 0.008$; day 7, $p = 0.057$; day 14, $p = 0.03$) and after 4 days in primary fibroblasts (day 4, $p = 0.003$; day 7, $p = 0.003$; day 14, $p = 0.003$) (**Figure 4A**). In line, αSMA stress fiber formation was more prominent from day 2 post-seeding onward in 10-4A cells as well as primary fibroblasts (**Figures 4D,E**). Interestingly, the TGF-β1-induced increase in *Acta2* expression followed a transient course in the 10-4A cells, peaking at day 2 after TGF-β1 addition and returning to baseline at day 4–5. A similar trend was noticeable in primary fibroblast post day 7. In contrast to mechanical stimulation, TGF-β1 administration also resulted in significantly increased *Col1a1* (day 2, $p = 0.008$, day 7, $p = 0.03$, day 14, $p = 0.03$) and a reduced *Plin2* (day 2, $p = 0.008$, day 4, $p = 0.02$) gene expression in 10-4A cells (**Figures 4B,C**) and primary fibroblasts (*Col1a1* day 4, $p = 0.003$, *Plin2*, day 4, $p = 0.003$). Together these data suggest that TGF-β1 administration triggers changes observed in fibrosis in 10-4A cells and primary fibroblasts, respectively. However, the effect was not sustained over a 14-day time course, despite constant exposure to TGF-β1.

Combination of Stiff Matrix and TGF-β1 Stimulation Leads to Strong and Persistent Expression of Myofibroblast Markers in 10-4A Cells

In pulmonary fibrosis mechanical and chemical cues act simultaneously. Therefore, we investigated the combination of mechanical and chemical stimulation seeding cells on plastic substrate and stimulated them with TGF-β1.

The combination of mechanical and chemical stimulation resulted in significantly increased *Acta2* gene expression in 10-4A cells from day 2 onward (day 2, $p = 0.008$, day 4, $p = 0.008$, day 7, $p = 0.008$, day 14, $p = 0.008$) and 4 days onward in primary fibroblasts (day 4, $p = 0.003$, day 7, $p = 0.003$, day 14, $p = 0.003$) (**Figure 5A**). This was also observed on the protein level (**Figures 5D,E**). Similar changes were observed for *Col1a1* (**Figure 5B**) (10-4A: day 2, $p = 0.008$, day 4, $p = 0.008$, day 7, $p = 0.008$, day 14, $p = 0.008$; primary fibroblasts: day 4, $p = 0.05$, day 7, $p = 0.003$, day 14, $p = 0.003$). In line, *Plin2* expression

(**Figure 5C**) was decreased in both cell types after 4 and 2 days, respectively (10-4A: day 2, $p = 0.008$, day 4, $p = 0.02$, day 14, $p = 0.03$; primary fibroblasts: day 4, $p = 0.005$, day 14, $p = 0.003$).

Overall, the combination of mechanical and chemical stimulation induced a robust and persistent expression of myofibroblast markers in 10-4A cells and primary fibroblasts. Interestingly the transient effect observed by TGF-β1 treatment alone was counteracted by increased substrate stiffness.

Generation of a 10-4A Reporter Cell Line to Monitor Fibroblast to Myofibroblast Differentiation in Live Cell *in vitro* Assays

In order to track fibroblast to myofibroblast differentiation within living cells, we designed a reporter system targeting the *Acta2* gene locus in 10-4A cells by generating a BFP-reporter of *Acta2* expression. We inserted a T2A-BFP-NLS sequence at the end of the *Acta2* CDS in 10-4A cells (10-4A^{BFP}). The correct integration of the BFP sequence was verified via PCR and Sanger sequencing. Induction of myofibroblast differentiation (TGF-β1) resulted in a nuclear BFP signal in 10-4A^{BFP} cells (**Figures 6A,B**).

To exclude changes in *Acta2* gene expression arising from genetic modifications, we compared the 10-4A^{BFP} cell line to wildtype 10-4A cells during quiescence (on PDMS, soft matrix) and after TGF-β1 stimulation, respectively. 10-4A^{BFP} cells showed similar responses to PDMS and TGF-β1 stimulation as 10-4A cells when analyzing *Acta2*, *Col1a1*, and *Plin2* gene expression (**Figures 6C–E**), indicating no adverse effects of T2A-BFP-NLS cassette integration.

Next, we tested on the protein level, whether the BFP signal correlated with αSMA expression. TGF-β1 treatment resulted in double-positive cells, whereas cells cultured on soft substrate without TGF-β1 were negative for BFP and αSMA (**Figure 6F**). Correlating the αSMA and BFP signal within individual cells, confirmed a linear correlation between BFP intensity and αSMA expression ($R^2 = 0.82$, $p < 0.0001$) (**Figure 6G**).

For a high throughput evaluation of fibrotic signals, a fluorescence-based 96-well assay was established. First, a linear correlation between BFP signal and cell count was verified under different culture conditions.

For a more thorough characterization and verification of the 10-4A^{BFP} cells, cytokines elevated during pulmonary fibrosis (TGF-β1, IL-33, IL-4, and TSLP) were screened to establish dose- and time-response curves (**Figure 7**). EC$_{50}$ values following a 2-day incubation post-seeding were 1.45 ng/ml for TGF-β1, 400 pg/ml for TSLP, 12 ng/ml for IL-4, and 22 pg/ml for IL-33. Time course analysis of BFP signal expression revealed that the BFP signal was transiently increasing following TGF-β1 and IL-33, respectively, similar to what was observed for wildtype 10-4A cells (**Figure 4**). In contrast, TSLP and IL-4 show an increase in BFP expression until day 2 and afterward a stable BFP expression up to day 7.

In summary, the 10-4A^{BFP} cell line resembles a valuable tool for high throughput analysis of factors driving fibroblast to myofibroblast differentiation in pulmonary fibrosis, enabling screening with limited sample preparation and processing.

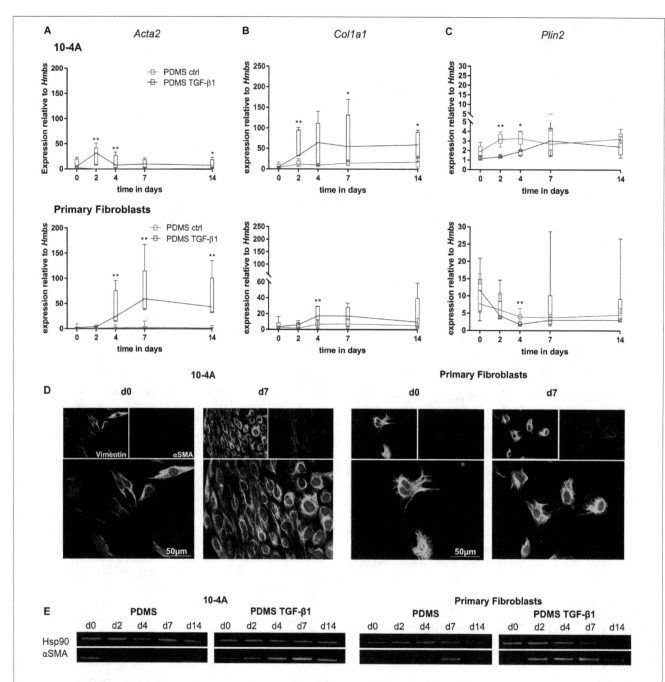

FIGURE 4 | Chemical stimulation of 10-4A cells and primary fibroblasts with TGF-β1 on a physiological substrate. Semi-quantitative RT-PCR of *Acta2* **(A)**, *Col1a1* **(B)**, and *Plin2* **(C)** expression in 10-4A cells **(top graph)** and primary fibroblasts **(bottom graph)** cultured in the presence or absence of 5 ng/ml TGF-β1 on a soft PDMS substrate, respectively. Data are expressed as fold expression of housekeeping gene *Hmbs*. Primary fibroblast data were obtained from 5 different animals, 10-4A data from five independent passages. The respective time points were tested with the non-parametric Mann–Whitney-*U*-Test. Statistical significance is indicated as follows: *p*-values < 0.05: *, *p*-values < 0.01: **. Box plots show data as median values, the boxes represent percentiles, the whiskers indicate the minimum/maximum. **(D)** Immunofluorescence staining of 10-4A cells **(left)** or primary fibroblasts seeded on PDMS with administration of 5 ng/ml TGF-β1 directly after adherence (d0) or 7 days post-seeding. Cells were stained for the mesenchymal marker vimentin (green) and the pro-fibrotic protein αSMA (red). Scale bar = 50 μm. **(E)** Western Blot for αSMA in 10-4A cells and primary fibroblasts cultured over 14 days on PDMS substrate in the presence or absence of TGF-β1, respectively. HSP90 was used as loading control.

DISCUSSION

Frequently, when studying molecular and cellular mechanisms in pulmonary fibrosis, primary fibroblasts are used for *in vitro*

experiments (Pierce et al., 2007; Huang et al., 2012; Pardo and Selman, 2016). However, use of primary cells is often limited by availability, restricted propagation, ethical hurdles, the cost and difficulty of repetitive cell isolations and often

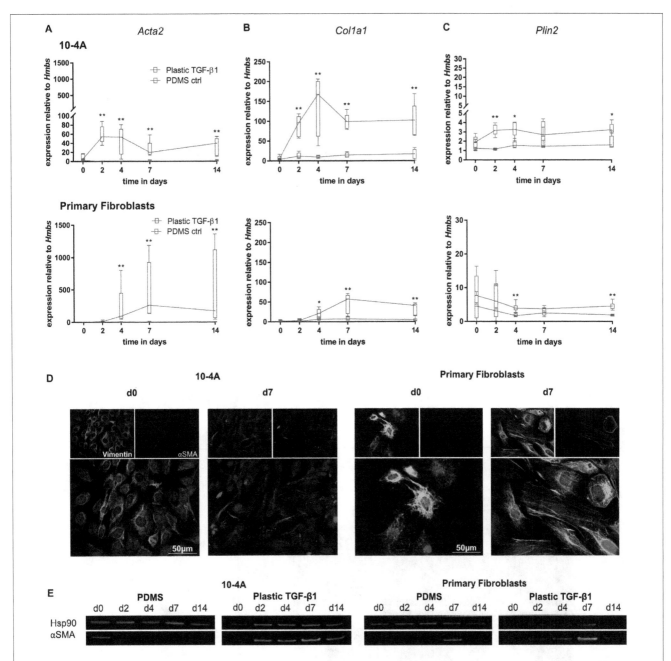

FIGURE 5 | Combination of chemical and mechanical stimulation of 10-4A cells and primary fibroblasts with TGF-β1 on a physiological substrate. Semi-quantitative RT-PCR of *Acta2* **(A)**, *Col1a1* **(B)**, and *Plin2* **(C)** expression in 10-4A cells (top graph) and primary fibroblasts (bottom graph) cultured on either soft substrate (PDMS) or in the presence of 5 ng/ml TGF-β1 stiff substrate (Plastic), respectively. Data are expressed as fold expression of housekeeping gene *Hmbs*. Primary fibroblast data were obtained from five different animals, 10-4A data from five independent cell culture experiments. The respective time points were tested with the non-parametric Mann–Whitney-*U*-Test. Statistical significance is indicated as follows: *p*-values < 0.05: *, *p*-values < 0.01: **. Box plots show data as median values, the boxes represent percentiles, the whiskers indicate the minimum/maximum. **(D)** Immunofluorescence staining of 10-4A cells (left) or primary fibroblasts seeded on PDMS with administration of 5 ng/ml TGF-β1 directly after adherence (d0) or 7 days post-seeding. Cells were stained for the mesenchymal marker Vimentin (green) and the pro-fibrotic protein αSMA (red). Scale bar = 50 μm. **(E)** Western Blot for αSMA in 10-4A cells and primary fibroblasts cultured over 14 days on PDMS substrate or on Plastic in the presence of TGF-β1, respectively. HSP90 was used as loading control.

a heterogeneity of isolated cells within or between isolations from different donors (Kaur and Dufour, 2012). Thus, well-characterized, representative cell lines provide a useful alternative for high-throughput, live-cell assays and can be used for *in vitro* disease modeling. Genetic modifications are easily

introduced to study specific signaling pathways. In addition, they offer the opportunity for long-term studies replicating diseases progression *in vitro*. The aim of our work was to generate a representative cell line to be used for *in vitro* fibrosis research. To this end, we immortalized primary rat lung cells, screened them

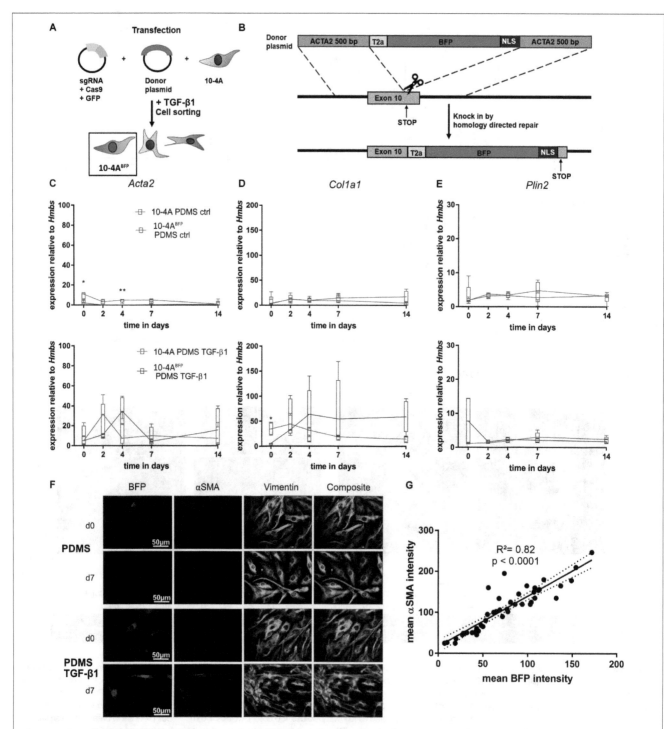

FIGURE 6 | Generation and verification of an *Acta2* coupled BFP reporter cell line. **(A,B)** Schematic representation of 10-4A cell transfection. Cells were transfected with a plasmid containing Cas9 and the sgRNA binding at the desired gene (exon 10) and a donor plasmid. The donor plasmid contained a BFP flanked by a self-cleaving T2A cassette, a nuclear localization sequence and two 500 bp homologous arms of the sgRNA cutting site. After cell transfection, *Acta2* gene expression was induced by addition of 5 ng/ml TGF- β1 and cells were FACS sorted for BFP. Semi-quantitative RT-PCR analysis of *Acta2* **(C)**, *Col1a1* **(D)**, and *Plin2* **(E)** expression in 10-4A and 10-4A^{BFP} cells with and without administration of 5 ng/ml TGF-β1 on a soft PDMS substrate, respectively. Values are means from five individual culture experiments. The respective time points were tested with the non-parametric Mann–Whitney-U-Test. Statistical significance is indicated as follows: p-values < 0.05: *, p-values < 0.01: **. Box plots show data as median values, the boxes represent percentiles, the whiskers indicate the minimum/maximum. **(F)** Immunofluorescence staining of 10-4A^{BFP} cells seeded on PDMS with and without administration of 5 ng/ml TGF-β1 directly after adherence (d0) or 7 days post-seeding. Cells were monitored for BFP and stained for the mesenchymal marker vimentin (green) and the pro-fibrotic protein αSMA (red). Scale bar = 50 μm. **(G)** Correlation of the BFP and αSMA signal intensity within individual cells 7 days post seeding. $N = 48$ cells. A linear regression line and the corresponding indicator R and p-value show the linear dependency of BFP and αSMA signal.

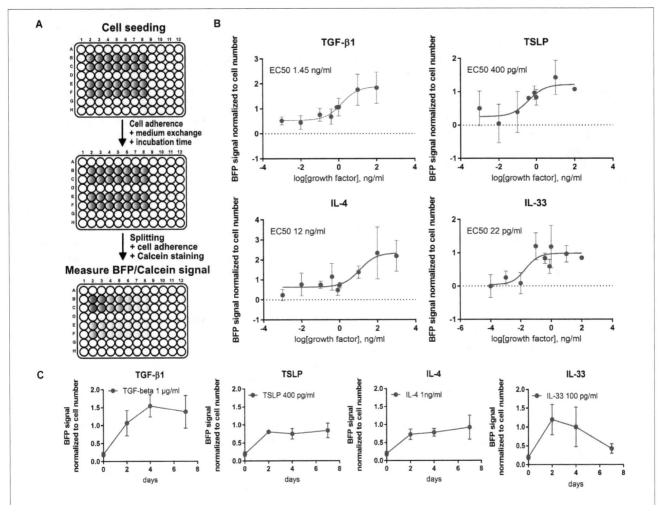

FIGURE 7 | High-throughput screening using the 10-4A^{BFP} cell line. **(A)** Schematic of plate reader assay to study the fibrotic response of 10-4A^{BFP} to cytokine treatment in live cell assays. For normalization to the cell number, cells were stained with Calcein AM. **(B)** Dose-response curves of BFP expression in 10-4A^{BFP} cells in response to 2 days exposure with increasing doses of TGF-β1, TSLP, IL-4, and IL-33. **(C)** Time-response curve of 10-4A^{BFP} cells to continuous exposure to TGF-β1, TSLP, IL-4, and IL-33.

for fibroblast characteristics and tested the induction of fibrosis after mechanical as well as chemical stimulation.

Within recent years, various cell and, in particular, fibroblast subpopulations were reported for the distal lung. Diverse roles in development, lung homeostasis, aging and injury repair were attributed to distinct populations, raising the complexity for modeling pulmonary fibrosis (Zepp et al., 2017; Xie et al., 2018). Interestingly, some myo-and lipofibroblast marker genes like *Mmp7*, *Mmp10* or *Plin2* (Adams et al., 2019; Reyfman et al., 2019; Strunz et al., 2019) were also expressed in ATII cells, emphasizing the importance to look in detail at a combination of distinct marker genes in order to assign cells to a cellular group. The presence of *Epcam* in the RNA sequencing data from primary fibroblasts likely indicates small impurities of epithelial cells, whereas the presence of *Vim* indicates minor impurities in the epithelial cell in the primary cell isolates. The presence of small fractions of other cell types after the isolation of primary lung cells is also described by other groups (Dobbs et al., 1986; Driscoll et al., 2012; Lee et al., 2018).

Regarding the fibroblast subpopulations stated by Xie et al. (2018), our 10-4A cell line neither exhibits a classical myofibroblast nor a lipofibroblast phenotype, but rather a matrix fibroblast phenotype with unexpected high expression of *Pdgfrα*. On a molecular level, the 10-4A cells could also be clearly differentiated from alveolar epithelial cells. The ATI-related genes *Cav1* as well as *Pdpn*, often used to discriminate ATI and ATII cells, are both also highly expressed in lung fibroblasts (Xiao et al., 2006; Quintanilla et al., 2019). Considering lineage-tracing and CRISPR/Cas9 *knock-in* experiments, *Pdgfrα* positive cells have been shown to give rise to either myofibroblasts or lipofibroblasts during development and to be able to differentiate into myofibroblasts in the adult lung (Ntokou et al., 2015; Zepp et al., 2017; Li et al., 2018). This directed differentiation of fibroblasts into myofibroblasts, as described for *Pdgfrα* positive cells, is one of the major requirements when studying pulmonary fibrosis. Thus, the gene and protein expression pattern of the 10-4A cell line indicates their suitability to study the mechanisms involved in the initiation and progression of pulmonary fibrosis.

Congruent with previous findings, we were also able to verify that myofibroblast differentiation can be induced mechanically (Wipff et al., 2007; Huang et al., 2012; Asano et al., 2017) and/or chemically (Chambers et al., 2003; Thannickal et al., 2003; Goffin et al., 2006; Blaauboer et al., 2011; Shi et al., 2013; El Agha et al., 2017) in 10-4A cells. Moreover, our data confirmed that fibroblasts grown on a substrate with physiological stiffness (Huang et al., 2012; Asano et al., 2017) and serum free medium (Baranyi et al., 2019) stay in a quiescent state over a time-course of 14 days. Since it is well established that fetal bovine serum exerts a heterogeneous influence on cellular behavior in cell culture due to batch-dependent variations and variable growth factor levels (Krämer et al., 2005; Mannello and Tonti, 2009; Baranyi et al., 2019), we decided to use a chemically defined, standardized, serum-free culture medium. Thereby, we were able to exclude potential variations in cellular responses due to heterogeneity of our culture conditions.

With regards to mechanical activation of the 10-4A cell line, the increase in gene and protein expression of αSMA was comparable to what has been described for primary fibroblasts as well as cell lines (Wipff et al., 2007; Huang et al., 2012; Asano et al., 2017). In line, a recent report from Tschumperlin et al., has shown that *Col1a1* mRNA levels were stable above a substrate stiffness of 0.1 kPa (Liu et al., 2010).

Transforming growth factor beta 1 in combination with a soft substrate resulted in an increase of *Acta2*, *Col1a1* and decrease of *Plin2* gene expression as well as an increase of αSMA on the protein level. These observations are in accordance to already published data in several studies of human (Chambers et al., 2003; Thannickal et al., 2003; Blaauboer et al., 2011; El Agha et al., 2017) and rodent lung fibroblasts (Goffin et al., 2006; Shi et al., 2013; El Agha et al., 2017). Interestingly, continuous stimulation with TGF-β1 induced an early but transient increase in profibrotic marker gene expression. *Acta2* expression was downregulated after 4 days in 10-4A cells continuously treated with TGF-β1. This effect was also observed in primary fibroblasts from two out of five animals after 7 days. In accordance, *Col1a1* and *Plin2* expression also adopt to control conditions for the primary fibroblasts. This indicates, that TGF-β1 stimulation alone, is not sufficient to maintain a myofibroblast phenotype and that changes in substrate stiffness are essential to induce a robust, persistent fibrotic response. The dependence of TGF-β1 on mechanical activation was already described by Shi et al. (2013). However, due to the lack of long-term studies examining the TGF-β1 effect beyond > 4 days, comparable data are not available. Likewise, it has been reported, that TGF-β1 requires mechanical induction to be able to regulate myofibroblast differentiation (Hinz, 2009). This is again in accordance with our data, that the combination of chemical and mechanical stimulation is necessary to fully resemble the aspects of myofibroblast differentiation. This is also more likely to reflect the *in vivo* situation where fibrosis might be triggered by chemical stimuli but shifts to a self-perpetuating state with increasing stiffening of the lung tissue (spreading from fibrotic foci). We limited the observation time to 14 days as cellular overgrowth under fibrotic conditions, due to increased proliferation rates, resulted in inconsistent findings at observation periods beyond 14 days.

In order to accelerate and facilitate the read-out of fibroblast differentiation in a live cell, high-throughput setting, we generated an *Acta2*-BFP coupled reporter system using CRISPR/Cas9 technology. This reporter system is intended for use in live-cell, long-term screening applications. CRISPR/Cas9 can lead to off-target mutations. Therefore, we have verified correct insertion of BFP-NLS by Sanger sequencing and that 10-4A[BFP] and 10-4A cells exhibit a similar behavior under physiological cell culture conditions and after fibrotic stimulation. Minor differences in expression of *Acta2* and *Col1a1* at day 0 might indicate a slightly delayed RNA turnover in 10-4A[BFP] during adjustment to non-fibrotic culture conditions after transfer from culture flasks (Kitsera et al., 2007). On the protein level, αSMA signal and the respective BFP signal correlated very well, confirming appropriate reporter characteristics. Similarly, the regulation of BFP expression under the αSMA promoter could be confirmed by the targeted induction of the BFP signal after TGF-β1 administration.

Finally, in order to confirm the proper functionality and the suitability to use 10-4A[BFP] cells in high throughput assays, we performed plate-reader based experiments to analyze the dose- and time-response of *Acta2* expression (i.e., myofibroblast induction) in response to exposure to distinct profibrotic cytokines. The effective concentrations were in agreement with previous reports for induction of fibrosis (Saito et al., 2003; Yanaba et al., 2011; Datta et al., 2013; Lee et al., 2017; Jones et al., 2019).

One potential limitation of the presented reporter cell line is its origin from rat rather than human. Several human pulmonary fibroblast cell lines are already available. However, in contrast to the cell line presented here, none of the currently available human cell lines has been characterized in detail with regards to the representation of a specific mesenchymal cell sub-population (Adams et al., 2019; Reyfman et al., 2019; Valenzi et al., 2019; Habermann et al., 2020; Liu et al., 2020; Travaglini et al., 2020). This might not only affect cellular responses to pro-fibrotic mechanical and chemical cues, but also affect epithelial-mesenchymal crosstalk and fibrotic remodeling when used in complex co-culture *in vitro* models (e.g., lung-on-a-chip). It is also accepted that *in vivo* animal models do not fully recapitulate all features of IPF pathogenesis (Moore et al., 2013). The reasons are not fully understood. The human lung contains structural and cellular differences to the rodent lung, however, the alveolus is one of the most conserved regions between rodents and human lungs and whether the mesenchymal and epithelial cells believed to be central to development of IPF are different is still a matter of debate. Even lipofibroblasts, a cell that's presence has been found in rodents but has long been controversial in the human lung (Tahedl et al., 2014), has recently been identified in human lung (Liu et al., 2020; Travaglini et al., 2020). Therefore, we believe that the cell line reported here provides a valuable tool for fibrosis research, offering the opportunity to investigate molecular and cellular responses of a representative mesenchymal cell to mechanical and/or chemical stimuli with high resolution and in high throughput formats.

In summary, our data clearly demonstrate that the 10-4A cell line can be used as a valuable, novel tool for studying the onset and progression of fibrotic changes observed in pulmonary fibrosis. Additionally, the deviated 10-4A^{BFP} reporter cell line is a useful tool for high-throughput live cell, *in vitro* assays to directly monitor fibrotic changes over time.

ETHICS STATEMENT

The animal study was reviewed and approved by the Regierungspräsidium Tübingen.

AUTHOR CONTRIBUTIONS

JN, AS, and MF conceived and designed the study, interpreted

results of the experiments, and edited and revised the manuscript. JN, AS, and VW performed the experiments. JN, KQ, and AS analyzed the data. JN and AS prepared the figures. JN, AS, KQ, and MF drafted the manuscript. All authors approved final version of manuscript.

ACKNOWLEDGMENTS

We thank Achim Riecker and Tatiana Felder for help with primary cell isolation, Susan Tavakoli and Kay Gottschalk for advice with PDMS gel preparation and handling, and Prof. Dr. C. Buske and the Core Facility Cytometry Ulm University for performance of cell sorting. We also want to thank Coralie Viollet, Head of the Genomics Lab at Boehringer Ingelheim, Biberach, for the Illumina library preparation.

REFERENCES

Adams, T., Schupp, J., Poli, S., Ayaub, E., Neumark, N., Ahangari, F., et al. (2019). Single Cell RNA-seq reveals ectopic and aberrant lung resident cell populations in idiopathic pulmonary fibrosis. *bioRxiv* [preprint]. doi: 10.1101/759902

Armanios, M. Y., Chen, J. J. L., Cogan, J. D., Alder, J. K., Ingersoll, R. G., Markin, C., et al. (2007). Telomerase mutations in families with idiopathic pulmonary fibrosis. *N. Engl. J. Med.* 356, 1317–1326. doi: 10.1056/NEJMoa066157

Asano, S., Ito, S., Takahashi, K., Furuya, K., Kondo, M., Sokabe, M., et al. (2017). Matrix stiffness regulates migration of human lung fibroblasts. *Physiol. Rep.* 5, 1–11. doi: 10.14814/phy2.13281

Bagnato, G., and Harari, S. (2015). Cellular interactions in the pathogenesis of interstitial lung diseases. *Eur. Respir. Rev.* 24, 102–114. doi: 10.1183/09059180.00003214

Baranyi, U., Winter, B., Gugerell, A., Hegedus, B., Brostjan, C., Laufer, G., et al. (2019). Primary human fibroblasts in culture switch to a myofibroblast-like phenotype independently of TGF Beta. *Cells* 8:721. doi: 10.3390/cells8070721

Barletta, K. E., Cagnina, R. E., Wallace, K. L., Ramos, S. I., Mehrad, B., and Linden, J. (2012). Leukocyte compartments in the mouse lung: distinguishing between marginated, interstitial, and alveolar cells in response to injury. *J. Immunol. Methods* 375, 100–110. doi: 10.1016/j.jim.2011.09.013

Beers, M. F., Moodley, Y., Stem, R., and Hall, E. J. S. (2017). When is an alveolar Type 2 cell an alveolar Type 2 Cell? A conundrum for lung stem cell biology and regenerative medicine. *Am. J. Respir. Cell Mol. Biol.* 57, 1–31. doi: 10.1165/rcmb.2016-0426PS

Blaauboer, M. E., Smit, T. H., Hanemaaijer, R., Stoop, R., and Everts, V. (2011). Cyclic mechanical stretch reduces myofibroblast differentiation of primary lung fibroblasts. *Biochem. Biophys. Res. Commun.* 404, 23–27. doi: 10.1016/j.bbrc.2010.11.033

Booth, A. J., Hadley, R., Cornett, A. M., Dreffs, A. A., Matthes, S. A., Tsui, J. L., et al. (2012). Acellular normal and fibrotic human lung matrices as a culture system for in vitro investigation. *Am. J. Respir. Crit. Care Med.* 186, 866–876. doi: 10.1164/rccm.201204-0754OC

Burgess, J. K., Mauad, T., Tjin, G., Karlsson, J. C., and Westergren-Thorsson, G. (2016). The extracellular matrix – the under-recognized element in lung disease? *J. Pathol.* 240, 397–409. doi: 10.1002/path.4808

Chambers, R. C., Leoni, P., Kaminski, N., Laurent, G. J., and Heller, R. A. (2003). Global expression profiling of fibroblast responses to transforming growth factor-β1 reveals the induction of inhibitor of differentiation-1 and provides evidence of smooth muscle cell phenotypic switching. *Am. J. Pathol.* 162, 533–546. doi: 10.1016/S0002-9440(10)63847-3

Chambers, R. C., and Mercer, P. F. (2015). Mechanisms of alveolar epithelial injury, repair, and fibrosis. *Ann. Am. Thoracic Soc.* 12, S16–S20. doi: 10.1513/AnnalsATS.201410-448MG

Cheng, F., Shen, Y., Mohanasundaram, P., Lindström, M., Ivaska, J., Ny, T., et al. (2016). Vimentin coordinates fibroblast proliferation and keratinocyte

differentiation in wound healing via TGF-β-Slug signaling. *Proc. Natl. Acad. Sci. U.S.A.* 113, E4320–E4327. doi: 10.1073/pnas.1519197113

Datta, A., Alexander, R., Sulikowski, M. G., Nicholson, A. G., Maher, T. M., Scotton, C. J., et al. (2013). Evidence for a functional thymic stromal lymphopoietin signaling axis in fibrotic lung disease. *J. Immunol.* 191, 4867–4879. doi: 10.4049/jimmunol.1300588

Deluca, D. S., Levin, J. Z., Sivachenko, A., Fennell, T., Nazaire, M. D., Williams, C., et al. (2012). RNA-SeQC: RNA-seq metrics for quality control and process optimization. *Bioinformatics* 28, 1530–1532. doi: 10.1093/bioinformatics/bts196

Dobbs, L. G., Gonzalez, R., and Williams, M. C. (1986). An improved method for isolating type II cells in high yield and purity. *Am. Rev. Respir. Dis.* 134, 141–145. doi: 10.1164/arrd.1986.134.1.141

Dobin, A., Davis, C. A., Schlesinger, F., Drenkow, J., Zaleski, C., Jha, S., et al. (2013). STAR: ultrafast universal RNA-seq aligner. *Bioinformatics* 29, 15–21. doi: 10.1093/bioinformatics/bts635

Driscoll, B., Kikuchi, A., Lau, A. N., Lee, J., Reddy, R., Jesudason, E., et al. (2012). Isolation and characterization of distal lung progenitor cells. *Methods Mol. Biol.* 879, 109–122. doi: 10.1007/978-1-61779-815-3_7

El Agha, E., Moiseenko, A., Kheirollahi, V., De Langhe, S., Crnkovic, S., Kwapiszewska, G., et al. (2017). Two-way conversion between lipogenic and myogenic fibroblastic phenotypes marks the progression and resolution of lung fibrosis. *Cell Stem Cell* 20, 261.e3–273.e3. doi: 10.1016/j.stem.2016.10.004

Enomoto, N., Suda, T., Kono, M., Kaida, Y., Hashimoto, D., Fujisawa, T., et al. (2013). Amount of elastic fibers predicts prognosis of idiopathic pulmonary fibrosis. *Respir. Med.* 107, 1608–1616. doi: 10.1016/j.rmed.2013.08.008

Epstein Shochet, G., Brook, E., Israeli-Shani, L., Edelstein, E., and Shitrit, D. (2017). Fibroblast paracrine TNF-α signaling elevates integrin A5 expression in idiopathic pulmonary fibrosis (IPF). *Respir. Res.* 18:122. doi: 10.1186/s12931-017-0606-x

Evans, C. M., Fingerlin, T. E., Schwarz, M. I., Lynch, D., Kurche, J., Warg, L., et al. (2016). Idiopathic pulmonary fibrosis: a genetic disease that involves mucociliary dysfunction of the peripheral airways. *Physiol. Rev.* 96, 1567–1591. doi: 10.1152/physrev.00004.2016

Felder, M., Trueeb, B., Stucki, A. O., Borcard, S., Stucki, J. D., Schnyder, B., et al. (2019). Impaired wound healing of alveolar lung epithelial cells in a breathing lung-on-a-chip. *Front. Bioeng. Biotechnol.* 7:3. doi: 10.3389/fbioe.2019.00003

Gabazza, E. C., Kasper, M., Ohta, K., Keane, M., D'Alessandro-Gabazza, C., Fujimoto, H., et al. (2004). Decreased expression of aquaporin-5 in bleomycin-induced lung fibrosis in the mouse. *Pathol. Int.* 54, 774–780. doi: 10.1111/j.1440-1827.2004.01754.x

Goffin, J. M., Pittet, P., Csucs, G., Lussi, J. W., Meister, J. J., and Hinz, B. (2006). Focal adhesion size controls tension-dependent recruitment of α-smooth muscle actin to stress fibers. *J. Cell Biol.* 172, 259–268. doi: 10.1083/jcb.200506179

Habermann, A. C., Gutierrez, A. J., Bui, L. T., Yahn, S. L., Winters, N. I., Carla, L., et al. (2020). Single-cell RNA-sequencing reveals profibrotic roles of distinct epithelial and mesenchymal lineages in pulmonary fibrosis. *Sci. Adv.* 6. doi: 10.1101/753806

Hasegawa, K., Sato, A., Tanimura, K., Uemasu, K., Hamakawa, Y., Fuseya, Y., et al. (2017). Fraction of MHCII and EpCAM expression characterizes distal lung epithelial cells for alveolar type 2 cell isolation. *Respir. Res.* 18, 1–13. doi: 10.1186/s12931-017-0635-5

Hinz, B. (2009). Tissue stiffness, latent TGF-β1 activation, and mechanical signal transduction: implications for the pathogenesis and treatment of fibrosis. *Curr. Rheumatol. Rep.* 11, 120–126. doi: 10.1007/s11926-009-0017-1

Horowitz, J. C., and Thannickal, V. J. (2006). Epithelial-mesenchymal interactions in pulmonary fibrosis. *Semin. Respir. Crit. Care Med.* 27, 600–612. doi: 10.1055/s-2006-957332

Huang, X., Yang, N., Fiore, V. F., Barker, T. H., Sun, Y., Morris, S. W., et al. (2012). Matrix stiffness-induced myofibroblast differentiation is mediated by intrinsic mechanotransduction. *Am. J. Respir. Cell Mol. Biol.* 47, 340–348. doi: 10.1165/rcmb.2012-0050OC

Huaux, F., Liu, T., McGarry, B., Ullenbruch, M., and Phan, S. H. (2003). Dual Roles of IL-4 in lung injury and fibrosis. *J. Immunol.* 170, 2083–2092. doi: 10.4049/jimmunol.170.4.2083

Huh, D. (2015). A human breathing lung-on-a-chip. *Ann. Am. Thoracic Soc.* 12, 42–44. doi: 10.1513/AnnalsATS.201410-442MG

Jansing, N. L., McClendon, J., Kage, H., Sunohara, M., Alvarez, J. R., Borok, Z., et al. (2018). Isolation of rat and mouse alveolar type II epithelial cells. *Methods Mol. Biol.* 1809, 69–82. doi: 10.1007/978-1-4939-8570-8_6

Jones, D. L., Haak, A. J., Caporarello, N., Choi, K. M., Ye, Z., Yan, H., et al. (2019). TGFβ-induced fibroblast activation requires persistent and targeted HDAC-mediated gene repression. *J. Cell Sci.* 132:jcs233486. doi: 10.1242/jcs.233486

Kage, H., and Borok, Z. (2012). EMT and interstitial lung disease: a mysterious relationship. *Curr. Opin. Pulm. Med.* 18, 517–523. doi: 10.1097/MCP.0b013e3283566721

Kasper, M., and Barth, K. (2017). Potential contribution of alveolar epithelial type I cells to pulmonary fibrosis. *Biosci. Rep.* 37:BSR20171301. doi: 10.1042/bsr20171301

Kaur, G., and Dufour, J. (2012). Cell lines: valuable tools or useless artifacts. *Spermatogenesis* 2, 1–5. doi: 10.4161/spmg.19885

Kitsera, N., Khobta, A., and Epe, B. (2007). Destabilized green fluorescent protein detects rapid removal of transcription blocks after genotoxic exposure. *BioTechniques* 43, 222–227. doi: 10.2144/000112479

Kolodsick, J. E., Toews, G. B., Jakubzick, C., Hogaboam, C., Moore, T. A., McKenzie, A., et al. (2004). Protection from fluorescein isothiocyanate-induced Fibrosis in IL-13-Deficient, but Not IL-4-Deficient, mice results from impaired collagen synthesis by fibroblasts. *J. Immunol.* 172, 4068–4076. doi: 10.4049/jimmunol.172.7.4068

Krämer, D. K., Bouzakri, K., Holmqvist, O., Al-Khalili, L., and Krook, A. (2005). Effect of serum replacement with Plysate on cell growth and metabolismin primary cultures of human skeletal muscle. *Cytotechnology* 48, 89–95. doi: 10.1007/s10616-005-4074-7

Kuehn, A., Kletting, S., De Souza Carvalho-Wodarz, C., Repnik, U., Griffiths, G., Fischer, U., et al. (2016). Human alveolar epithelial cells expressing tight junctions to model the air-blood barrier. *Altex* 33, 251–260. doi: 10.14573/altex.1511131

Lederer, D. J., and Martinez, F. J. (2018). Idiopathic pulmonary fibrosis. *N. Engl. J. Med.* 378, 1811–1823. doi: 10.1056/NEJMra1705751

Lee, D. F., Salguero, F. J., Grainger, D., Francis, R. J., MacLellan-Gibson, K., and Chambers, M. A. (2018). Isolation and characterisation of alveolar type II pneumocytes from adult bovine lung. *Sci. Rep.* 8:11927.

Lee, J. U., Chang, H. S., Lee, H. J., Jung, C. A., Bae, D. J., Song, H. J., et al. (2017). Upregulation of interleukin-33 and thymic stromal lymphopoietin levels in the lungs of idiopathic pulmonary fibrosis. *BMC Pulm. Med.* 17:39. doi: 10.1186/s12890-017-0380-z

Li, R., Bernau, K., Sandbo, N., Gu, J., Preissl, S., and Sun, X. (2018). Pdgfra marks a cellular lineage with distinct contributions to myofibroblasts in lung maturation and injury response. *eLife* 7, 1–20. doi: 10.7554/eLife.36865

Liang, J., Zhang, Y., Xie, T., Liu, N., Chen, H., Geng, Y., et al. (2016). Hyaluronan and TLR4 promote surfactant-protein-C-positive alveolar progenitor cell renewal and prevent severe pulmonary fibrosis in mice. *Na. Med.* 22, 1285–1293. doi: 10.1038/nm.4192

Liao, Y., Smyth, G. K., and Shi, W. (2014). FeatureCounts: an efficient general purpose program for assigning sequence reads to genomic features. *Bioinformatics* 30, 923–930. doi: 10.1093/bioinformatics/btt656

Lipps, C., Klein, F., Wahlicht, T., Seiffert, V., Butueva, M., Zauers, J., et al. (2018). Expansion of functional personalized cells with specific transgene combinations. *Nat. Commun.* 9:994. doi: 10.1038/s41467-018-03408-4

Liu, F., Mih, J. D., Shea, B. S., Kho, A. T., Sharif, A. S., Tager, A. M., et al. (2010). Feedback amplification of fibrosis through matrix stiffening and COX-2 suppression. *J. Cell Biol.* 190, 693–706. doi: 10.1083/jcb.201004082

Liu, X., Rowan, S. C., Liang, J., Yao, C., Huang, G., Deng, N., et al. (2020). Definition and signatures of lung fibroblast populations in development and fibrosis in mice and men. *bioRxiv* [preprint]. doi: 10.1101/2020.07.15.203141

Löfdahl, A., Rydell-Törmänen, K., Larsson-Callerfelt, A. K., Wenglén, C., and Westergren-Thorsson, G. (2018). Pulmonary fibrosis in vivo displays increased p21 expression reduced by 5-HT2B receptor antagonists in vitro - A potential pathway affecting proliferation. *Sci. Rep.* 8:1927. doi: 10.1038/s41598-018-20430-0

Luzina, I. G., Kopach, P., Lockatell, V., Kang, P. H., Nagarsekar, A., Burke, A. P., et al. (2013). Interleukin-33 potentiates Bleomycin-induced lung injury. *Am. J. Respir. Cell Mol. Biol.* 49, 999–1008. doi: 10.1165/rcmb.2013-0093OC

Luzina, I. G., Pickering, E. M., Kopach, P., Kang, P. H., Lockatell, V., Todd, N. W., et al. (2012). Full-Length IL-33 promotes inflammation but not Th2 response in vivo in an ST2-Independent fashion. *J. Immunol.* 189, 403–410. doi: 10.4049/jimmunol.1200259

Luzina, I. G., Todd, N. W., Sundararajan, S., and Atamas, S. P. (2015). The cytokines of pulmonary fibrosis: much learned, much more to learn. *Cytokine* 74, 88–100. doi: 10.1016/j.cyto.2014.11.008

Mannello, F., and Tonti, G. A. (2009). Concise review: no breakthroughs for human mesenchymal and embryonic stem cell culture: conditioned medium, feeder layer, or feeder-free; medium with fetal calf serum, human serum, or enriched plasma; serum-free, serum replacement nonconditioned medium, o. *Stem Cells* 25, 1603–1609. doi: 10.1634/stemcells.2007-0127

McElroy, M. C., and Kasper, M. (2004). The use of alveolar epithelial type I cell-selective markers to investigate lung injury and repair. *Eur. Respir. J.* 24, 664–673. doi: 10.1183/09031936.04.00096003

Miklavc, P., Frick, M., Wittekindt, O. H., Haller, T., and Dietl, P. (2010). Fusion-Activated Ca2+ entry: an "active zone" of elevated Ca2+ during the postfusion stage of lamellar body exocytosis in rat Type II Pneumocytes. *PLoS One* 5:e10982. doi: 10.1371/journal.pone.0010982

Moore, B. B., Lawson, W. E., Oury, T. D., Sisson, T. H., Raghavendran, K., and Hogaboam, C. M. (2013). Animal models of fibrotic lung disease. *Ame. J. Respir. Cell Mol. Biol.* 49, 167–179. doi: 10.1165/rcmb.2013-0094TR

Ntokou, A., Klein, F., Dontireddy, D., Becker, S., Bellusci, S., Richardson, W. D., et al. (2015). Characterization of the platelet-derived growth factor receptor-α-positive cell lineage during murine late lung development. *Am. J, Physiol. Lung Cell. Mol. Physiol.* 309, L942–L958. doi: 10.1152/ajplung.00272.2014

Oikonomou, N., Harokopos, V., Zalevsky, J., Valavanis, C., Kotaniduo, A., Szymkowski, D. E., et al. (2006). Soluble TNF mediates the transition from pulmonary inflammation to fibrosis. *PLoS One* 1:e108. doi: 10.1371/journal.pone.0000108

O'Reilly, S. (2013). Role of interleukin-13 in fibrosis, particularly systemic sclerosis. *BioFactors* 39, 593–596. doi: 10.1002/biof.1117

Palchesko, R. N., Zhang, L., Sun, Y., and Feinberg, A. W. (2012). Development of polydimethylsiloxane substrates with tunable elastic modulus to study cell mechanobiology in muscle and nerve. *PLoS One* 7:e0051499. doi: 10.1371/journal.pone.0051499

Pardo, A., and Selman, M. (2016). Lung fibroblasts, aging, and idiopathic pulmonary fibrosis. *Ann. Am. Thoracic Soc.* 13, S417–S421. doi: 10.1513/AnnalsATS.201605-341AW

Parker, M. W., Rossi, D., Peterson, M., Smith, K., Sikström, K., White, E. S., et al. (2014). Fibrotic extracellular matrix activates a profibrotic positive feedback loop. *J. Clin. Invest.* 124, 1622–1635. doi: 10.1172/JCI71386

Pfaffl, M. W. (2001). A new mathematical model for relative quantification in real-time RT-PCR. *Nucleic Acids Res.* 29:e45. doi: 10.1093/nar/29.9.e45

Pierce, E. M., Carpenter, K., Jakubzick, C., Kunkel, S. L., Evanoff, H., Flaherty, K. R., et al. (2007). Idiopathic pulmonary fibrosis fibroblasts migrate and proliferate to

CC chemokine ligand 21. *Eur. Respir. J.* 29, 1082–1093. doi: 10.1183/09031936.00122806

Plantier, L., Crestani, B., Wert, S. E., Dehoux, M., Zweytick, B., Guenther, A., et al. (2011). Ectopic respiratory epithelial cell differentiation in bronchiolised distal airspaces in idiopathic pulmonary fibrosis. *Thorax* 66, 651–657. doi: 10.1136/thx.2010.151555

Quintanilla, M., Montero, L. M., Renart, J., and Villar, E. M. (2019). Podoplanin in inflammation and cancer. *Int. J. Mol. Sci.* 20:707. doi: 10.3390/ijms20030707

Raghu, G., Collard, H. R., Egan, J. J., Martinez, F. J., Behr, J., Brown, K. K., et al. (2011). An Official ATS/ERS/JRS/ALAT statement: idiopathic pulmonary fibrosis: evidence-based guidelines for diagnosis and management. *Am. J. Respir. Crit. Care Med.* 183, 788–824. doi: 10.1164/rccm.2009-040GL

Ran, F. A., Hsu, P. D., Wright, J., Agarwala, V., Scott, D. A., and Zhang, F. (2013). Genome engineering using the CRISPR-Cas9 system. *Nat. Protoc.* 8, 2281–2308. doi: 10.1038/nprot.2013.143

Reyfman, P. A., Walter, J. M., Joshi, N., Anekalla, K. R., McQuattie-Pimentel, A. C., Chiu, S., et al. (2019). Single-cell transcriptomic analysis of human lung provides insights into the pathobiology of pulmonary fibrosis. *Am. J. Respir. Crit. Care Med.* 199, 1517–1536. doi: 10.1164/rccm.201712-2410OC

Richeldi, L., Collard, H. R., and Jones, M. G. (2017). Idiopathic pulmonary fibrosis. *Lancet* 389, 1941–1952. doi: 10.1016/S0140-6736(17)30866-8

Ryu, J. H., Moua, T., Daniels, C. E., Hartman, T. E., Yi, E. S., Utz, J. P., et al. (2014). Idiopathic pulmonary fibrosis: evolving concepts. *Mayo Clin. Proc.* 89, 1130–1142. doi: 10.1016/j.mayocp.2014.03.016

Saito, A., Okazaki, H., Sugawara, I., Yamamoto, K., and Takizawa, H. (2003). Potential action of IL-4 and IL-13 as fibrogenic factors on lung fibroblasts in vitro. *Int. Arch. Allergy Immunol.* 132, 168–176. doi: 10.1159/000073718

Sayols, S., Scherzinger, D., and Klein, H. (2016). dupRadar: a bioconductor package for the assessment of PCR artifacts in RNA-Seq data. *BMC Bioinformatics* 17:428. doi: 10.1186/s12859-016-1276-2

Seibold, M. A., Wise, A. L., Speer, M. C., Steele, M. P., Brown, K. K., Loyd, J. E., et al. (2011). A common MUC5B promoter polymorphism and pulmonary fibrosis. *N. Engl. J. Med.* 364, 1503–1512. doi: 10.1056/NEJMoa1013660

Selman, M., and Pardo, A. (2001). Idiopathic pulmonary fibrosis: an epithelial/fibroblastic cross-talk disorder. *Respir. Res.* 3, 1–8. doi: 10.1186/rr175

Sgalla, G., Iovene, B., Calvello, M., Ori, M., Varone, F., and Richeldi, L. (2018). Idiopathic pulmonary fibrosis: pathogenesis and management. *Respir. Res.* 19:32. doi: 10.1186/s12931-018-0730-2

Shi, Y., Dong, Y., Duan, Y., Jiang, X., Chen, C., and Deng, L. (2013). Substrate stiffness influences TGF-β1-induced differentiation of bronchial fibroblasts into myofibroblasts in airway remodeling. *Mol. Med. Rep.* 7, 419–424. doi: 10.3892/mmr.2012.1213

Sime, P. J., Marr, R. A., Gauldie, D., Xing, Z., Hewlett, B. R., Graham, F. L., et al. (1998). Transfer of tumor necrosis factor-α to rat lung induces severe pulmonary inflammation and patchy interstitial fibrogenesis with induction of transforming growth factor-β1 and myofibroblasts. *Am. J. Pathol.* 153, 825–832. doi: 10.1016/S0002-9440(10)65624-6

Sime, P. J., Xing, Z., Graham, F. L., Csaky, K. G., and Gauldie, J. (1997). Adenovector-mediated gene transfer of active transforming growth factor-β1 induces prolonged severe fibrosis in rat lung. *J. Clin. Invest.* 100, 768–776. doi: 10.1172/JCI119590

Strunz, M., Simon, L. M., Ansari, M., Mattner, L. F., Angelidis, I., Mayr, C. H., et al. (2019). Longitudinal single cell transcriptomics reveals Krt8+ alveolar epithelial progenitors in lung regeneration. *bioRxiv* [preprint]. doi: 10.1101/705244

Stuart, B. D., Choi, J., Zaidi, S., Xing, C., Holohan, B., Chen, R., et al. (2015). Exome sequencing links mutations in PARN and RTEL1 with familial pulmonary fibrosis and telomere shortening. *Nat. Genet.* 47, 512–517. doi: 10.1038/ng.3278

Stucki, J. D., Hobi, N., Galimov, A., Stucki, A. O., Schneider-Daum, N., Lehr, C. M., et al. (2018). Medium throughput breathing human primary cell alveolus-on-chip model. *Sci. Rep.* 8:14359. doi: 10.1038/s41598-018-32523-x

Tahedl, D., Wirkes, A., Tschanz, S. A., Ochs, M., and Mühlfeld, C. (2014). How common is the lipid body-containing interstitial cell in the mammalian lung? *Am. J. Physiol. Lung Cell. Mol. Physiol.* 307, L386–L394. doi: 10.1152/ajplung.00131.2014

Thannickal, V. J., Lee, D. Y., White, E. S., Cui, Z., Larios, J. M., Chacon, R., et al. (2003). Myofibroblast differentiation by transforming growth factor-β1 is dependent on cell adhesion and integrin signaling via focal adhesion kinase. *J. Biol. Chem.* 278, 12384–12389. doi: 10.1074/jbc.M208544200

Trapnell, C., Hendrickson, D. G., Sauvageau, M., Goff, L., Rinn, J. L., and Pachter, L. (2013). Differential analysis of gene regulation at transcript resolution with RNA-seq. *Nat. Biotechnol.* 31, 46–53. doi: 10.1038/nbt.2450

Travaglini, K. J., Nabhan, A. N., Penland, L., Sinha, R., Gillich, A., Sit, R. V., et al. (2020). A molecular cell atlas of the human lung from single cell RNA sequencing. *bioRxiv* [Preprint]. doi: 10.1101/742320

Tschumperlin, D. J., Ligresti, G., Hilscher, M. B., and Shah, V. H. (2018). Mechanosensing and fibrosis. *J. Clin. Invest.* 128, 74–84. doi: 10.1172/JCI93561

Valenzi, E., Bulik, M., Tabib, T., Morse, C., Sembrat, J., Trejo Bittar, H., et al. (2019). Single-cell analysis reveals fibroblast heterogeneity and myofibroblasts in systemic sclerosis-associated interstitial lung disease. *Ann. Rheumat. Dis.* 78, 1379–1387. doi: 10.1136/annrheumdis-2018-214865

Wipff, P. J., Rifkin, D. B., Meister, J. J., and Hinz, B. (2007). Myofibroblast contraction activates latent TGF-β1 from the extracellular matrix. *J. Cell Biol.* 179, 1311–1323. doi: 10.1083/jcb.200704042

Wuyts, W. A., Agostini, C., Antoniou, K. M., Bouros, D., Chambers, R. C., Cottin, V., et al. (2013). The pathogenesis of pulmonary fibrosis: a moving target. *Eur. Respir. J.* 41, 1207–1218. doi: 10.1183/09031936.00073012

Xiao, M. W., Zhang, Y., Hong, P. K., Zhou, Z., Feghali-Bostwick, C. A., Liu, F., et al. (2006). Caveolin-1: a critical regulator of lung fibrosis in idiopathic pulmonary fibrosis. *J. Exp. Med.* 203, 2895–2906. doi: 10.1084/jem.20061536

Xie, T., Wang, Y., Deng, N., Huang, G., Taghavifar, F., Geng, Y., et al. (2018). Single-cell deconvolution of fibroblast heterogeneity in mouse pulmonary fibrosis. *Cell Rep.* 22, 3625–3640. doi: 10.1016/j.celrep.2018.03.010

Xu, Y., Mizuno, T., Sridharan, A., Du, Y., Guo, M., Tang, J., et al. (2016). Single-cell RNA sequencing identifies diverse roles of epithelial cells in idiopathic pulmonary fibrosis. *JCI Insight* 1:e90558. doi: 10.1172/jci.insight.90558

Yanaba, K., Yoshizaki, A., Asano, Y., Kadono, T., and Sato, S. (2011). Serum IL-33 levels are raised in patients with systemic sclerosis: association with extent of skin sclerosis and severity of pulmonary fibrosis. *Clin. Rheumatol.* 30, 825–830. doi: 10.1007/s10067-011-1686-5

Zepp, J., Zacharias, W., and Frank, D. (2017). Distinct mesenchymal lineages and niches promote epithelial self-renewal and myofibrogenesis in the lung. *Cell* 170, 1134–1148. doi: 10.1016/j.cell.2017.07.034

Zhu, Z., Homer, R. J., Wang, Z., Chen, Q., Geba, G. P., Wang, J., et al. (1999). Pulmonary expression of interleukin-13 causes inflammation, mucus hypersecretion, subepithelial fibrosis, physiologic abnormalities, and eotaxin production. *J. Clin. Invest.* 103, 779–788. doi: 10.1172/JCI5909

10

A Bioinspired *in vitro* Lung Model to Study Particokinetics of Nano-/Microparticles under Cyclic Stretch and Air-Liquid Interface Conditions

Ali Doryab [1,2], *Mehmet Berat Taskin* [3], *Philipp Stahlhut* [3], *Andreas Schröppel* [1,2],
Sezer Orak [1,2], *Carola Voss* [1,2], *Arti Ahluwalia* [4,5], *Markus Rehberg* [1,2], *Anne Hilgendorff* [1,2,6],
Tobias Stöger [1,2], *Jürgen Groll* [3] and *Otmar Schmid* [1,2]*

[1] Comprehensive Pneumology Center Munich, Member of the German Center for Lung Research, Munich, Germany,
[2] Helmholtz Zentrum München—German Research Center for Environmental Health, Institute of Lung Biology and Disease,
Munich, Germany, [3] Department of Functional Materials in Medicine and Dentistry, Bavarian Polymer Institute, University of
Würzburg, Würzburg, Germany, [4] Research Center "E. Piaggio", University of Pisa, Pisa, Italy, [5] Department of Information
Engineering, University of Pisa, Pisa, Italy, [6] Center for Comprehensive Developmental Care (CDeC[LMU]), Dr. von Haunersches
Children's Hospital University, Hospital of the Ludwig-Maximilians University, Munich, Germany

Correspondence:
Otmar Schmid
otmar.schmid
@helmholtz-muenchen.de

Evolution has endowed the lung with exceptional design providing a large surface area for gas exchange area (ca. 100 m^2) in a relatively small tissue volume (ca. 6 L). This is possible due to a complex tissue architecture that has resulted in one of the most challenging organs to be recreated in the lab. The need for realistic and robust *in vitro* lung models becomes even more evident as causal therapies, especially for chronic respiratory diseases, are lacking. Here, we describe the **C**yclic **In VI**tro **C**ell-stretch (CIVIC) "breathing" lung bioreactor for pulmonary epithelial cells at the air-liquid interface (ALI) experiencing cyclic stretch while monitoring stretch-related parameters (amplitude, frequency, and membrane elastic modulus) under real-time conditions. The previously described biomimetic copolymeric BETA membrane (5 μm thick, bioactive, porous, and elastic) was attempted to be improved for even more biomimetic permeability, elasticity (elastic modulus and stretchability), and bioactivity by changing its chemical composition. This biphasic membrane supports both the initial formation of a tight monolayer of pulmonary epithelial cells (A549 and 16HBE14o$^-$) under submerged conditions and the subsequent cell-stretch experiments at the ALI without preconditioning of the membrane. The newly manufactured versions of the BETA membrane did not improve the characteristics of the previously determined optimum BETA membrane (9.35% PCL and 6.34% gelatin [w/v solvent]). Hence, the optimum BETA membrane was used to investigate quantitatively the role of physiologic cyclic mechanical stretch (10% linear stretch; 0.33 Hz: light exercise conditions) on size-dependent cellular uptake and transepithelial transport of nanoparticles (100 nm) and microparticles (1,000 nm) for alveolar epithelial cells (A549) under ALI conditions. Our results show that physiologic stretch enhances cellular uptake of 100 nm nanoparticles across the epithelial cell barrier, but the barrier becomes permeable for both nano- and micron-sized particles (100 and 1,000 nm). This suggests that currently used static *in vitro* assays may underestimate cellular uptake and transbarrier transport of nanoparticles in the lung.

Keywords: lung cell model, cyclic stretch, ALI culture, bioinspired membrane, particle study

INTRODUCTION

The lung is the largest organ of the human body built to accommodate the extraordinary size of required gas (oxygen-carbon dioxide) exchange surface area (ca. 100 m^2) corresponding to about half the size of a tennis court (Weibel, 1970, 2009) within a relatively small volume (ca. 6 l; <10% of body volume). Direct exposure to airborne particles, such as cigarette smoke particles, urban dust and particles from indoor sources (e.g., cooking and laser printer) jeopardizes the fragile architecture of this organ, causing pulmonary lung diseases, such as asthma and chronic obstructive pulmonary disease (Pope et al., 2009; Hänninen et al., 2010; Schaumann et al., 2014). Out of the wide size range of inhalable particles (up to 10 μm diameter), nanoparticles (NPs) with a diameter between 100 and 300 nm have been shown to undergo epithelial-endothelial translocation, i.e., they can cross the alveolar tissue barrier into the blood circulation and from there to other organs (Kreyling et al., 2013). Moreover, ultrafine NPs (<100 nm in diameter) have received increasing attention due to their enhanced surface area per mass of particles, which has been associated with both acute and chronic lung disease (Peters et al., 1997; Schmid and Stoeger, 2016).

Improvement of the predictive power of pre-clinical *in vitro* models as an alternative to animal experiments according to the 3R principles (replacement, refinement, and reduction) relies on enhancing their biomimetic features. Over the past decades *in vitro* cell culture models of the lung epithelial cells have evolved significantly from technologically simple, non-physiologic, submerged cell culture systems to an advanced level of *in vitro* cell culture models at the air-liquid interface (ALI) (Doryab et al., 2016). In these advanced lung models, epithelial lung cells are seeded on the apical (air) side of a porous/perforated membrane, which is in contact with the cell culture medium located on the basal side. This setup mimics *in vivo* conditions, initiating polarization of cells, and secretion of protective lining fluids (surfactant), which do not occur under submerged conditions where cells are completely covered with cell culture medium (Doryab et al., 2019). Hence, ALI cell cultures provide more physiologic conditions and potentially clinically more relevant results when testing drug/toxin effects on the lung as compared to submerged cultures (Paur et al., 2011).

Moreover, *in vitro* lung models have been developed to exert cyclic mechanical stretch to cells mimicking the breathing-induced cyclic stretch conditions in the alveolar lung tissue in order to include this important stimulus for cell physiology and

morphology in the cell culture models (Doryab et al., 2019). Hence, addition of this type of stimulus may prove useful for preclinical drug testing and assessment of toxin- and/or particle-induced toxicity. Most of the studies reported in the literature used commercially available cell-stretch technologies (e.g., Flexcell strain unit; Flexcell International Corp., USA) that are only suitable for submerged culture conditions (Edwards et al., 1999; Vlahakis et al., 1999; Hammerschmidt et al., 2004; Guenat and Berthiaume, 2018; Doryab et al., 2019).

Nevertheless, a variety of *in vitro* models has been developed to combine cyclic cell-stretch and ALI culture conditions for more biomimetic models of the alveolar air-blood barrier. Ideally, these advanced models enable (I) cyclic mechanical activation of the (multi-)cell cultures at the ALI, (II) basal perfusion of the culture medium, mimicking blood circulation, and (III) dose-controlled, aerosolized substance delivery. While the former two items have been implemented in various models, the latter is often missing (Doryab et al., 2019; Artzy-Schnirman et al., 2020). In 2010, the seminal work performed by Ingber et al. at the WYSS Institute of Harvard University introduced a microfluidic lung bioreactor often referred to as "lung-on-a-chip" (Huh et al., 2010). The concept of these systems is comparable to standard (multi-)cell culture models of the lung cultured at the ALI on an elastic, perforated membrane, which can be mechanically activated (stretched) combined with basal medium perfusion on a miniature-scale (shift from milli- to microfluidic system). Nowadays, these microfluidic systems have been evolved from a simple bi-channel structure (Huh et al., 2010; Stucki et al., 2015) to a complex airway network (acini-on-chips) (Artzy-Schnirman et al., 2019). However, wide-spread use of these systems is still hampered by the high degree of complexity associated with operating these systems (Ehrmann et al., 2020). These types of biomimetic alveolar barrier models not only have the potential to predict clinical outcome during early preclinical drug or toxin testing and accurate but also for mimicking drug/particle transport from the lung into the blood. In fact, the latter is part of the clinical testing (phase I of clinical trial) required for regulatory licensing of safety and efficacy of novel drugs.

All of these models and recent developments suffer from a lack of a suitable biomimetic membrane, acting as a cell-substrate. An appropriate membrane should emulate the main characteristics of the supporting extracellular matrix (ECM) of the cells, such as thickness, stiffness, permeability, and bioactivity. Commercially available polycarbonate (PC) and polyethylene terephthalate (PET) membranes are widely used in (static) ALI culture systems that do not mimic the stiffness (or rather "softness") of the ECM in the lung. Silicone-based materials, such as poly(dimethylsiloxane) (PDMS, Sylgard 184) are generally cast for cell-stretch applications due to their suitable mechanoelastic properties (Doryab et al., 2019). Nonetheless, adsorption of proteins/growth factors to and leaching of uncured oligomers from PDMS membranes has been recognized as potential cause of adverse effects on cell physiology (Regehr et al., 2009). Recently, synthetic/natural electrospun scaffolds with a thickness range of ≈20–200 μm have been fabricated with suitable properties for lung cells using co-polymers consisting of poly(ε-caprolactone) (PCL)/star-shaped polyethylene glycols (sPEG) functionalized with biomolecules (Nishiguchi et al., 2017), poly-L-lactic acid (PLLA)/decellularized pig lung ECM (PLECM) (Young et al., 2017), and PCL/gelatin (Higuita-Castro et al., 2017). The stretchability of these scaffolds/membranes has not been determined as they were employed only under static cell culture conditions.

We have recently introduced a novel porous and elastic membrane for *in vitro* cell-stretch models of the lung cultured under ALI conditions (Doryab et al., 2020). This innovative hybrid biphasic membrane, henceforth referred to as **B**iphasic **E**lastic **T**hin for **A**ir-liquid culture conditions (BETA) membrane, was developed to optimize membrane characteristics for the two phases of cell-stretch experiments under ALI conditions, namely the initial cell seeding, attachment and growth phase under submerged cell culture conditions (phase I) followed by an ALI acclimatization and cell-stretch phase at the ALI (phase II). As these phases require distinctly different membrane properties, the BETA membrane has been designed to be biphasic. As the pores are initially filled with a wettable, water-soluble and hence sacrificial material (gelatin), the BETA membrane provides initially a non-porous and wettable enough (WCA ≤ 70°) substrate for initial cell adhesion and growth into a confluent epithelial monolayer on the apical side of the membrane (closed pores avoid inadvertent transmembrane migration of cells) (phase I). Subsequently, dissolution of the sacrificial material results in sufficient porosity, permeability and stretchability for up to 25% reversible linear strain (without plastic deformation), granting suitable ALI cell culture conditions under cyclic mechanical stretch (phase II). In contrast to typically used stretchable poly(dimethylsiloxane) (PDMS) membranes, the BETA membrane is bioactive enough to support the proliferation and formation of a confluent layer of alveolar (A549) and bronchial (16HBE14o⁻) epithelial cells without pre-coating with ECM proteins (e.g., Matrigel) (Doryab et al., 2020).

Right now, the main limitations of the BETA membrane are the relatively larger thickness (ca. 5 μm) compared to the alveolar-capillary tissue barrier (ca. 1 μm) and higher stiffness [uniaxial Young's modulus: 1.8 ± 0.7 MPa (1D stretch); 0.78 ± 0.24 MPa (3D stretch)], which is similar to or better than other typically used porous membranes for lung cell-stretch cultures (e.g., PDMS), but still about 100-fold lager than the elastic modulus (3–6 kPa) reported for alveolar walls/tissue (Doryab et al., 2020). Moreover, the ideal membrane is as bioactive as possible to provide optimum growth conditions for (primary) cell cultures and perfectly permeable to minimize membrane effects on transbarrier transport measurements.

In the present study, we attempted to improve the previously described limitations of the "optimum" BETA membrane with respect to thickness, permeability, elasticity (elastic modulus and stretchability), and bioactivity by changing its chemical composition. This is supported by newly applied analytical parameters (e.g., 3D porosity and mapping of surface topology of the membrane). Moreover, we provide a detailed technical description of the recently introduced Cyclic *In VItro* Cell-stretch (CIVIC) bioreactor for cell-stretch experiments under ALI conditions (Doryab et al., 2020) with particular attention to refinements over its earlier version (MALI, **M**oving **A**ir-**L**iquid **I**nterface bioreactor) (Cei et al., 2020). Subsequently, the effect of cyclic stretch on the particokinetics of aerosol-delivered nano- (100 nm) and microparticles (1,000 nm) in an alveolar tissue barrier model (A549) cultured under ALI conditions was investigated quantitatively with respect to size-dependent cellular uptake and transepithelial transport of particles.

RESULTS

Advanced *in vitro* Cell-Stretch System (CIVIC)

The Cyclic *In VItro* Cell-stretch (CIVIC) system, which was employed for cell-stretch experiments with the BETA membrane, is a modified version of our previously described MALI system (Cei et al., 2020) mainly with respect to material stability, (BETA) membrane fixation, pressure sealing, and quality control including real-time monitoring of the amplitude and frequency of the cyclically stretched cell-covered membrane. The CIVIC system allows for culturing of lung epithelial cells under ALI, cyclic mechanical stretch, and medium (blood) perfusion conditions in combination with dose-controlled delivery of aerosolized substances to the cells. This *in vitro* scenario resembles closely aerosol deposition onto the air-blood barrier of the lung as encountered during inhalation therapy or breathing of ambient aerosol. The details of the technical aspects of the CIVIC system are presented in **Figures 1A,B** and the Methods and Materials section. A movie of the cyclically stretched membrane in the "breathing" CIVIC system can be found in the **Supplementary Video 1**.

Characterization and Optimization Bioinspired Stretchable Membrane (BETA)

As mentioned above, we recently described an optimized biphasic copolymeric membrane for cell growth inspired by the ECM in the alveolar region of the lung (Doryab et al., 2020). The initially non-porous membrane consists of two polymeric components namely poly(ε-caprolactone) (PCL) and gelatin, tailored to facilitate initial cell adhesion and growth under submerged condition (phase I) (**Figures 1C, 2A**). Upon contact with cell culture medium, the gelatin at the surface of the membrane turns into a hydrogel, which is conducive to cell growth (lowers water contact angle; provides favorable conditions for cell adhesion

A Bioinspired in vitro Lung Model to Study Particokinetics of Nano-/Microparticles under Cyclic Stretch...

115

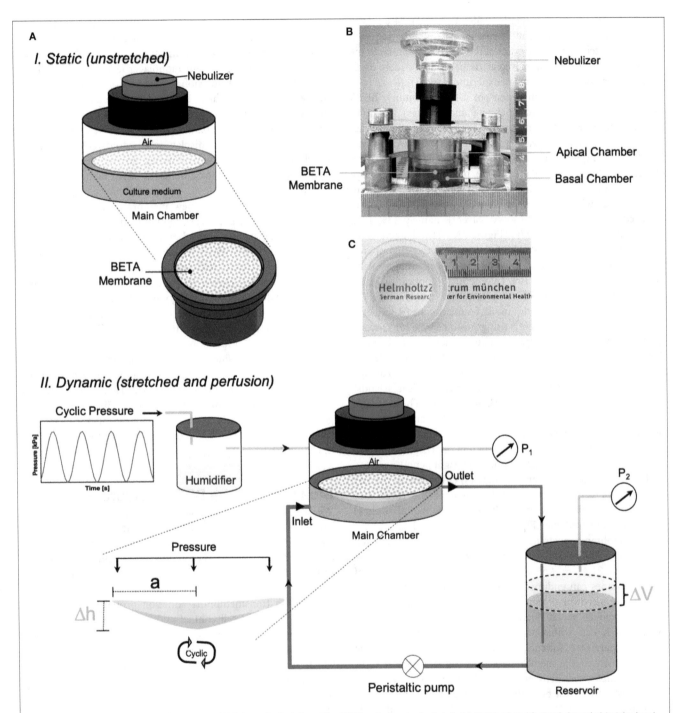

FIGURE 1 | The CIVIC system used in this study. **(A)** Schematic depiction of the CIVIC system under (top) static (unstretched) and (bottom) dynamic (stretched and perfusion) conditions with the pressure-based strain/elasticity monitoring system. A thin, permeable, and stretchable membrane (BETA) placed in the (PDMS-free) main chamber of the bioreactor separates the apical (air) and basal (medium) compartments. Lung cells are grown on the membrane at ALI and perfused with culture medium by circulating the medium in the basal compartment with a perfusion pump to mimic blood flow. Cyclic mechanical stretch is applied to the cells on the membrane by applying cyclic (positive) pressure (P_1) to the apical compartment. The cell/membrane stretch profile can be monitored via a pressure sensor in the air volume of the medium reservoir (P_2), which is connected to the main chamber. The apical compartment of the bioreactor can be connected to a nebulizer to deliver aerosolized particles/drugs to the cells. **(B)** Snapshot of the main chamber of the CIVIC bioreactor system. **(C)** Photograph of the BETA membrane in the PC holder of the CIVIC system, which is transparent, thus favorable for direct cell imaging applications.

and proliferation). Gelatin also serves as "sacrificial" material, i.e., it is gradually dissolved by the medium turning the initially non-porous, stiff membrane into a porous/permeable and more elastic membrane as required for nurturing ALI cell cultures via basolateral medium and during cell-stretch experiments (phase II) (**Figure 2B**). We previously determined the optimum concentrations of PCL and gelatin (9.35% PCL and 6.34% gelatin [w/v solvent]) for membrane fabrication by spin coating with respect to matching the properties of the BETA membrane to the basement membrane of the alveolar tissue using a widely used) optimization approach [design of experiment (DoE)].

Due to remaining limitations of the "optimum" BETA membrane with respect to thickness and stiffness (ca. 100-fold reduction needed to match alveolar basement membrane) (Polio et al., 2018; Doryab et al., 2019; Bou Jawde et al., 2020), we attempted to improve the performance characteristics of the membrane by expanding the previously tested range of PCL/gelatin mixing ratios. For this, new membranes were manufactured with PCL concentration larger than the previously explored upper limit of 10% [w/v solvent], namely 15% PCL mixed with 6, 8, and 10% [w/v] (**Figure 2A**). The characteristics of these three newly generated BETA membranes were compared with previously characterized membranes consisting of 10% PCL mixed with 6, 8, and 10% [w/v] and the optimum BETA membrane (9.35% PCL and 6.34% gelatin [w/v]).

Surface analysis of the optimum BETA membrane (9.35% PCL and 6.34% gelatin [w/v solvent]) using Atomic Force Microscopy (AFM) showed an average roughness height of 1.31 μm (**Figure 2C**). The cross-sectional structure of the membrane was studied using Focused Ion Beam-Scanning Electron Microscopy (FIB-SEM). The data show that gelatin forms spherical "islands" in the PCL membrane (**Figure 2D**, left panel). These gelatin islands also extend deep into the PCL membrane, leaving a favorable interconnected 3D network of pores after dissolution of the gelatin in phase II, as confirmed by Energy Dispersive X-ray Spectroscopy (EDS)-FIB-SEM (**Figure 2D**, right panel).

Analysis of the water contact angle (WCA)—one of the key properties of cell attachment and growth of the three new membranes reveals a range of 70–76° indicating that all of these membranes are wettable (**Figure 2E**). The uniaxial tensile test of the membranes prior to cell seeding (in phase I) revealed that Young's modulus (elastic modulus) varies between 5.33 ± 1.90 and 21.41 ± 4.65 MPa (**Figure 2F**). Moreover, all of the membranes can endure at least 8% linear reversible strain, which is required for physiologic cell stretch conditions in the lung (Doryab et al., 2019), except for PCL 10% gelatin 6% [w/v], which can withstand only 4% linear strain. Another important parameter for culturing of cells under ALI conditions is the porosity of the membrane at the end of phase II (ALI culture), which varies between 1.8 ± 2.5 and 49.7 ± 1.4%, where the highest and lowest porosity corresponds to the membrane consisting of PCL 10% gelatin 10% and PCL 15% gelatin 8% [w/v], respectively (**Figure 2G**). It is noteworthy, that there is excellent agreement between empirically determined porosity and theoretically derived (upper limit of) porosity (volume fraction of gelatin), if the composition-derived theoretical porosity exceeds 40% (here: PCL 10% gelatin 8% and PCL 10% gelatin 10%).

In addition, repeatedly performed WST1 assays showed that the metabolic activity (cell viability) of A549 cells increases with incubation time on the membranes (**Figure 2H**). This indicates that the relatively few initial seeded cells are proliferating and gradually covering the entire membrane as indicated by WST1

values near 100%, representing the WST1 signal obtained for standard Transwell PET inserts. After a 4–6 days growth period (depending on membrane composition), all of the membranes are covered with a confluent monolayer layer of epithelial cells (**Figure 3A**). As an additional measure of cytocompatibility, the release of intracellular lactate dehydrogenase (LDH) from the cytosol due to uncontrolled cell death was measured. The small release of LDH (<0.5% of totally available LDH) indicates that these membranes display low cytotoxicity (**Figure 2I**), which implies that the membranes do not release or leach significant amounts of toxic materials when incubated with the cell culture medium.

In summary, the three new membranes consisting of 15% [w/v] (with 6–10% [w/v] of gelatin) did not improve the key characteristics of a membrane for cell-stretch experiments at the ALI. While their wettability as quantified by WCA was not statistically different from that of the optimum BETA membrane (**Figure 2D**), the membrane with the lowest Young's modulus and hence highest elasticity (prior to removal of gelation) displayed an extremely low porosity of 2% as compared to the 15.32% of the optimum BETA membrane (**Figure 2F**). Such a low porosity value is a knock-out criterion for the membrane since it prevents efficient trans-membrane transport of nutrients (or drugs or nanoparticles) and hence nourishment of cells cultured at the ALI. Hence, the previously determined optimum BETA membrane (9.35% PCL and 6.34% gelatin [w/v solvent]) is superior to all of the 15% PCL membranes and therefore remains the composition of the optimum BETA membrane, which is used for cell experiments described below.

Bioactivity of the BETA Membrane

We also evaluated the bioactivity of the (optimum) BETA membrane using two lung epithelial cell lines namely human lung alveolar epithelial cells (A549) and human bronchial epithelial cells (16HBE14o$^-$). CLSM (confocal laser scanning microscopy) analysis showed that A549 cells grew on the membrane into a confluent cell monolayer resulted in the formation of E-cadherin—a transmembrane adhesion protein—which plays a pivotal role in cell-cell contact and polarization of cells at the ALI. Moreover, F-actin rich regions representing a network of polymeric microfilaments of the cytoskeleton were formed, which is essential for important cellular functions, such as cell motility, cell division, vesicle and organelle movement, cell signaling as well as the establishment and maintenance of cell-cell junctions and cell morphology (**Figure 3A**; images reflect day 6). From the DAPI-stained images (**Figure 3A**) the number of cells (nuclei) per surface area was determined (4.3×10^5 cells cm^{-2}). Since this value is 2.9-fold larger than the seeding density of the cells (1.5×10^5 cells cm^{-2}), this indicates that substantial cell proliferation has occurred during the 6 days of cell growth under submerged culture conditions. For reference, we also compared the bioactivity of the BETA membrane with that of a commercially available standard Transwell® insert (PET) membrane. It is evident that while initial cell growth/metabolic activity (WST1 signal) on the BETA membrane was slower/lower, this difference

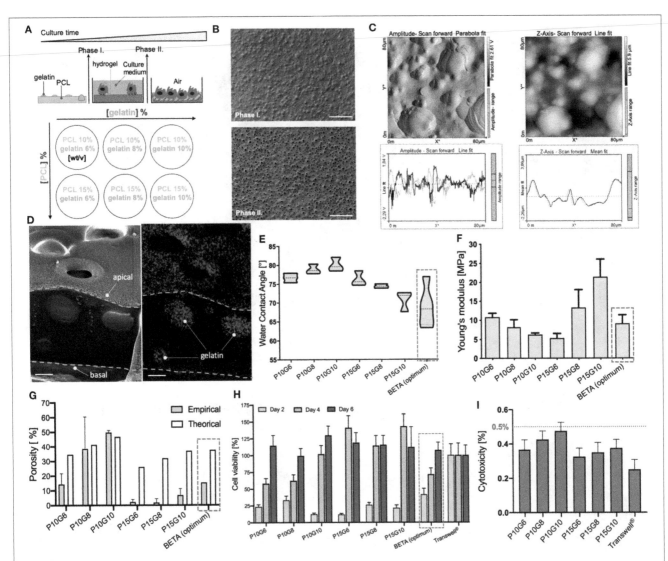

FIGURE 2 | Characterization of the biphasic (BETA) membrane used in this study. **(A)** Schematic depiction of the biphasic membrane concept. (Top) During phase I, gelatin forms a hydrogel due to contact with water (cell culture medium), which serves as adhesion point for epithelial cells of the lung and facilitates subsequent cell proliferation until a confluent epithelial cell layer is formed. After 4 days (phase II), the gelatin has been dissolved in water leaving behind a network of interconnected pores in the PCL membrane, which provides space for further cell spreading and at the same time enhances both membrane permeability and elastic modulus. (Bottom) Different membranes with various combinations of mixing ratio of PCL and gelatin—in the PCL/gelatin solution used for membrane manufacturing—expected to obtain a wide range of physicomechanical properties. **(B)** Top view of the ultrastructure of the "optimum" membrane (9.35% PCL and 6.34% gelatin [w/v of TFE], i.e., P/G = 9.35/6.34), which is also used for the analysis presented in **(C,D)**. The scale bar is 100 μm. **(C)** Surface topography of an 80 × 80 μm² section of the membrane analyzed by Atomic Force Microscopy (AFM; left) and its corresponding z-amplitude profile (right) showing an average roughness height of 1.31 μm. **(D)** Cross-sectional analysis of the membrane using Focused Ion Beam-Scanning Electron Microscopy (FIB-SEM, left panel) and Energy Dispersive X-ray Spectroscopy FIB-SEM (EDS-FIB-SEM, right panel), indicating that gelatin is distributed throughout the PCL membrane during the late stage of phase I. The thickness of the membrane thickness ca. 5 μm. The scale bar is 2 μm. The newly manufactured membranes (P15G6, P15G8, and P15G10) are analyzed (and compared to previously reported results (Doryab et al., 2020) with respect to **(E)** Water Contact Angle (WCA), **(F)** Young's modulus (uniaxial, phase I, under dry conditions), **(G)** porosity obtained empirically by the liquid displacement method—and theoretical (maximum) porosity (gelatin volume fraction), **(H)** cell viability analyzed by WST1 assay on days 2, 4, and 6 of culture relative to PET Transwell® cell culture insert **(H)**, and **(I)** cytotoxicity (LDH assay at day 6) of the three newly investigated membranes with different mixing ratios of PCL and gelatin. The LDH release for each membrane was normalized by the maximum possible LDH level (LDH contained in all cells). Typically, LDH < 10% is considered non-cytotoxic. There is no significant difference between the LDH release of Transwell® inserts and the different mixing ratios of BETA membranes. Optimum values for WCA, Young's modulus, empirical porosity, and theoretical (maximum) porosity were 69 ± 5 [°], 9.0 ± 1.9 [MPa], 15.32 [%] and 37.6 [%], respectively. Data are reported as the mean ± SD, $n = 3$.

had disappeared on day 4–6 (**Figure 2H**). The ultrastructural analysis exhibited a flattened cell morphology when cells grew on the BETA membrane (**Figure 3B**). Furthermore,

cells showed superior interaction and integration with the BETA membrane as compared to the Transwell® insert (**Figure 3B**).

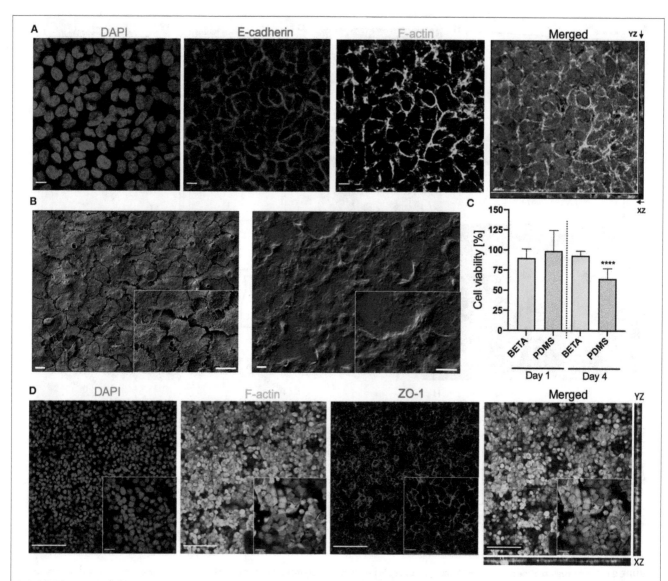

FIGURE 3 | Bioactivity of the BETA membrane (optimum: 9.35% PCL and 6.34% gelatin [w/v of TFE]). **(A)** Z-stack Confocal Laser Scanning Microscopy (CLSM) of human alveolar epithelial cells (A549) on the membrane (under static submerged culture conditions for 6 days) demonstrating the formation of a confluent uniform cell layer. The cell nuclei (DAPI, blue), expression of the cell-cell adhesion protein E-cadherin (red), and formation of F-actin filaments (green). The scale bar is 10 μm. **(B)** SEM image of A549 cells after proliferation on a (left) biphasic membrane and (right) a commercial Transwell® insert (6 days of submerged culture). The scale bar is 10 μm. **(C)** Effect of leaching from BETA and PDMS membrane on cell viability (WST1 assay; A549 cells). BETA and PDMS membranes were incubated for 2 days in cell culture medium and this medium was used to grow A549 cells for 1 and 4 days in a standard 12-well tissue culture well plate. The reduced cell viability for PDMS-conditioned medium after 4 days indicates that some substances (e.g., uncured oligomers) leaching from the PDMS have a cytotoxic effect. This effect is not seen for the BETA membrane. The viability data were normalized that of a standard 12- well cell culture plate with fresh medium. Data are reported as mean ± SD. *n* = 8; ****$P < 0.00001$ by one-way ANOVA with Dunnett test. **(D)** Z-stack and orthogonal CLSM view of (XY) with side views of YZ (right) and XZ (bottom) optical projection of the human bronchial epithelial cells (16HBE14o⁻) on the membrane visualizing a confluent cell monolayer and the formation of tight junctions (culture conditions: 6 days submerged and 24 h ALI culture); cell nucleus (DAPI, blue), F-actin filaments (green); ZO-1 tight junction (red). The scale bars are 100 μm (for the 20× projection view) and 20 μm (for the 63× projection view).

PDMS (Sylgard 184) membranes are commonly used in cell-stretch devices due to their mechano-elastic properties. However, it has been reported that uncured oligomers of PDMS are released into the culture medium during cell culture, which might be toxic for the cells (Regehr et al., 2009; Carter et al., 2020). Hence, we assessed the leaching of unwanted components of the PDMS membrane compared to the (optimum) BETA membrane (**Figure 3C**). Medium incubated for 48 h with PDMS and BETA membranes was used to culture A549 cells under submerged conditions. After 1 day, no significant difference was detected in cell viability for the two materials. However, after 4 days of incubation, a 36% reduction in cell viability was detected for the cells incubated with PDMS-leached medium, while only 6% of viability reduction was observed for the BETA membrane-leached medium as compared to cells cultured with pristine cell culture medium.

We also examined the bioactivity of the BETA membrane using the human bronchial epithelial cell line 16HBE14o⁻. Cells were grown on the (optimum) BETA membrane for 6 days under submerged and 1 day under ALI conditions. A confluent epithelial barrier with the formation of the F-actin was observed (**Figure 3D**). SEM analysis also confirmed the CLSM findings (**Supplementary Figure 2**). Excellent barrier integrity was also confirmed by a TEER value of $451 \pm 55 \, \Omega \, cm^2$, which is consistent with data reported for 16HBE14o⁻ cells in the literature (Ehrhardt et al., 2002) and higher than the TEER value for A549 epithelial confluent cell monolayer on the BETA ($136 \pm 23 \, \Omega \, cm^2$).

Nano- and Microparticle Kinetics Study

As an application of the *in vitro* cell-stretch lung model (CIVIC), we investigated the cellular uptake by and transepithelial transport of nano- and microparticles of A549 cells under physiologic cyclic mechanical stretch (10% linear, 0.33 Hz) applied for 2 h. The stability of the stretch parameters as well as the stiffness [Young's modulus: 0.78 ± 0.24 MPa (mean $\pm$ SD, $n = 5$)] of the membrane was monitored continuously during the entire experiment with the differential pressure monitoring system of the CIVIC system. The metabolic activity of the cells did not show any evidence of reduced viability due to aerosol exposure and 2 h of cyclic stretch (**Supplementary Figure 3**).

This study shows that 2 h of cyclic stretch affects cellular uptake and intracellular distribution, but not trans-cellular transport in a size-dependent way. The former is qualitatively evident from CLSM images revealing that cellular uptake of 100 and 1,000 nm particles under unstretched (static) ALI conditions was very limited and cell-associated particles were mostly located close to the air-facing, apical cell surface (**Figure 4B**). In contrast, 100 nm NPs were internalized more efficiently under stretch conditions and co-localized with the F-actin cytoskeleton deeper within the cell (**Figure 4B**). On the other hand, stretch did not enhance cellular uptake of 1,000 nm microparticles and particles were still localized close to the apical cell surface, but positioned preferably between adjacent cells rather than randomly as without stretch (**Figure 4B**). Quantitative fluorescence analysis of the CLSM images revealed a 2.4-fold increase of cellular uptake of 100 nm NPs under stretch, while there was no statistically significant effect of stretch on cellular uptake for 1,000 nm microparticles (**Figure 4C**).

In addition, spectrophotometric analysis of the basal medium revealed the transepithelial transport (translocation) of particles after 2 h under static and stretch-activated conditions of A549 cells on the BETA membrane or on 3 µm pore (static) PET membranes of 6-well Transwell® inserts (**Figure 4D**). For Transwell® inserts, the particles were delivered with a VITROCELL®Cloud 6 system to A549 cells (Lenz et al., 2014) and then cultured under (static) ALI conditions.

After 2 h of incubation time under static conditions, the transport fractions across A549 cells on both Transwell® inserts and BETA membranes for 100 and 1,000 nm particles were below the detection limit, except for the $1.8 \pm 0.4\%$ transport of 1,000 nm particles observed for Transwell® inserts (two-way ANOVA followed by *post-hoc* Tukey's multiple comparison test) (**Figure 4D** and **Table 1**).

For cell-stretch, the transepithelial transport of 100 and 1,000 nm particles across the A549 cell-covered BETA membrane was increased to 30.0 ± 1.7 and $21.0 \pm 11.3\%$, respectively, but no statistically significant dependence on size was observed (no stretch can be applied to Transwell® inserts). Hence, cell-stretch significantly increased the translocation of 100 and 1,000 nm particles across the alveolar epithelial barrier independent of particle diameter (see **Table 1** and **Figure 4D**).

DISCUSSION

In the quest for overcoming limitations of traditional *in vitro* models of the lung, the field of bioengineering has witnessed significant efforts toward developing advanced *in vitro* models striving to mimic more closely the human pulmonary environment (de Souza Carvalho et al., 2014). This has led the way from mono-cellular submerged cell lines to primary co-culture cell models at the ALI (air-blood barrier), from static cell culture media and cell layers to medium perfusion (pulmonary blood flow) and cyclic stretch (breathing-induced mechanical tissue strain), and from millifluidic ($\sim cm^2$ cell area, mL of media) into microfluidic systems often referred to as lung/acinar-on-a-chip technologies (Huh et al., 2012, 2013; de Souza Carvalho et al., 2014; Benam et al., 2015; Tenenbaum-Katan et al., 2018; Ainslie et al., 2019; Artzy-Schnirman et al., 2019). While lung-on-a-chip technologies are starting to become commercially available (e.g., Alveolix, Switzerland and Emulate, USA), also millifluidic lung bioreactors are expected to continue to play a role due to their ease-of-handling, a larger amount of cell samples suitable for many standard assay kits, and lower maintenance efforts.

At the core of any cell-stretch lung bioreactor/chip is a porous and elastic membrane on which the cell culture model is cultured. For lung/acinar-on-a-chip systems mainly 3.5–10 µm thick PDMS membranes are used for cell seeding and growth of an alveolar or bronchial tissue barrier (Huh et al., 2010; Stucki et al., 2015). PDMS membranes are widely used for their high mechano-elasticity, with Young's modulus of $\approx$1–3 MPa (Wang et al., 2014). While perforated PDMS membranes are suitable for small-sized lung-on-chip applications ($\sim mm^2$), they are too fragile for larger millifluidic ($\sim cm^2$) devices. Moreover, PDMS membranes have low wettability (WCA $\geq$ 115°) (**Supplementary Figure 1**) and therefore require pre-treatment and/or coating with ECM proteins to facilitate sufficient cell adhesion and proliferation (Wang et al., 2010). Another disadvantage is that uncured oligomers of PDMS can leach into the cell culture medium resulting in changes and cell physiology (Regehr et al., 2009; Carter et al., 2020). Our investigation of a PDMS film has confirmed reports from the literature that cells may experience reduced cell viability due to the leaching of toxins into the cultured in a medium (Regehr et al., 2009). Alternatively, commercial electrospun biocompatible

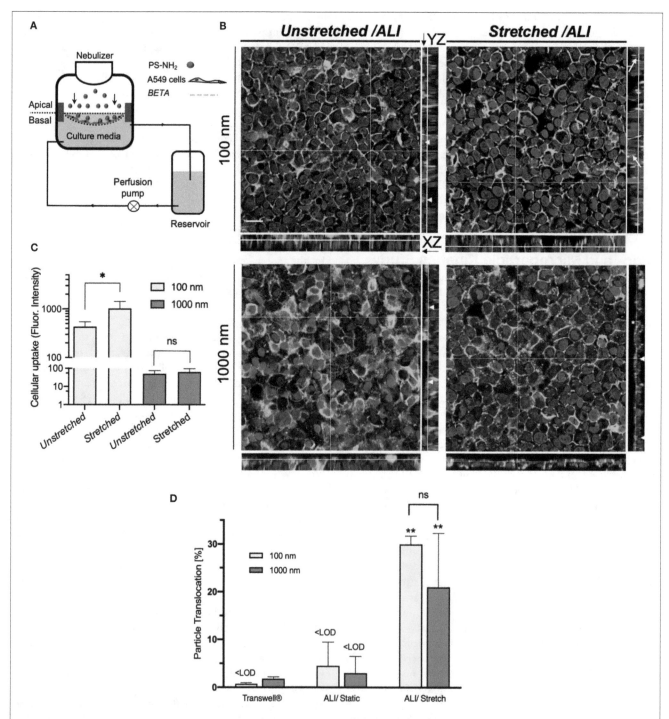

FIGURE 4 | Cellular uptake and membrane-association of aerosolized nano- and microparticles for alveolar epithelial (A549) cells and translocation across the epithelial barrier (2 h incubation). **(A)** Schematic of the CIVIC bioreactor system for particle study. A549 cells were seeded on the BETA membrane (cell density: 2 × 10⁵ cells cm⁻², 4 days LLC, and 1-day ALI culture). Amine-modified polystyrene (PS-NH₂) nano- and microparticles (100 and 1,000 nm diameter, respectively) are then nebulized onto the cells with the nebulizer of the bioreactor. After 2 h, the cells were fixed and prepared for CLSM analysis. **(B)** 3D reconstruction z-stack of CLSM images presented as orthogonal (XY) and side views (YZ, right) of monolayered, confluent cells on the membrane after nebulization of 100 and 1,000 nm fluorescently labeled, amine-modified polystyrene (PS-NH₂) particles under non-stretched and physiologically stretched (10% linear, 0.33 Hz for 2 h) under ALI conditions. Cell nucleus (DAPI, blue), particles (red) and F-actin filaments of the cytoskeleton (green). Arrows, arrowheads, and asterisk indicate internalized particles, cell-membrane associated (extracellular) particles (on the apical cell surface) and particles located between cells, respectively. (Scale bar: 20 μm). **(C)** Quantitative cellular uptake of particles measured by fluorescence intensity of z-stacks, showing that physiologic cyclic mechanical stretch enhances uptake of 100 nm NPs as compared to static conditions, while there is no effect on 1,000 nm microparticles [Representative images (z-stacks) were recorded at 5 independent fields of view for each sample (n = 4); region of interest: 134.95 × 134.95 μm]. Y-axis is presented fluorescence intensity data in a log scale. Data are reported as the mean ± SD;

(Continued)

FIGURE 4 | *P < 0.01 by two-way ANOVA and data were corrected by Sidac for multiple comparison tests. (D) Translocation of 100 and 1,000 nm particles across the cell layer grown on unstretched PET Transwell® inserts and on the BETA membrane (under unstretched and stretched conditions) (n = 3). ** Show the comparison between stretched with the corresponding experiment under unstretched conditions. Data are reported as the mean ± SD; **P < 0.001 by two-way ANOVA and data were corrected by Tukey for multiple comparison tests.

TABLE 1 | Transport of 100 and 1,000 nm particles across A549 cell-layer grown on BETA or PET Transwell® insert membrane (3 μm pores) at ALI within 2 h of particle exposure (mean ± SD; n = 3).

Run / Translocation [%]	100 nm	1,000 nm
Transwell®/Unstretched	<LOD*	1.8 ± 0.4
BETA/Unstretched	<LOD	<LOD
BETA/Stretched	30.0 ± 1.7	21.0 ± 11.3

* <LOD, below limit of detection.

poly(carbonate)urethane (PCU) membranes (Bionate® II 80A, The Electrospinning Company, UK) have been tested for cell growth in a millifluidic lung bioreactor. They proved inadequate due to their hydrophobic nature (in spite of pre-coating with ECM proteins) and associated poor cell proliferation, their relatively large thickness (ca. 75 μm), and their inability to prevent the formation of multilayered epithelial tissue deep within the membrane rather than at its apical side (Cei et al., 2020).

The BETA membrane, which overcomes some of these limitations (**Figure 5**), has a thickness of ≤5 μm, which is thinner than conventional PET or PC/PET membranes used in static Transwell® inserts (≈10 μm) and similar to the lower range of advanced PDMS membranes (≈3.5–10 μm) (Huh et al., 2010; Stucki et al., 2015). The two polymer components, i.e., gelatin and PCL were chosen for their wettability and mechanical properties, respectively. The presence of gelatin initial non-porous membrane (BETA in phase I) is conducive to cell adhesion/growth without requiring further surface modification and prevents apically seeded epithelial cells from unwanted migration through the membrane to the basal side, fostering the formation of a monolayer of epithelial cells on the apical side. The gradual dissolution of gelatin by cell culture medium induces sufficient porosity for culturing of cells at the ALI and even results in the secretion of innate ECM secreted by the cells. In contrast to PDMS, no adverse effect on cell viability due to leaching has been observed (**Figure 3C**).

As mentioned above, one of the main advantages of the PDMS membranes is their high mechano-elasticity with Young's modulus of ≈1–3 MPa (Wang et al., 2014), which is still ca. 100-fold larger than that of alveolar tissue with 3–6 kPa (Polio et al., 2018; Bou Jawde et al., 2020). Since the previously derived optimized BETA membrane (PCL/gelatin = 9.35%/6.34% [w/v solvent] or P/G = 9.35/6.34) (Doryab et al., 2020) has an initial Young's modulus of 9.0 ± 1.9 MPa (prior dissolution of gelatin), the present study tested the hypothesis that an increased PCL concentration of 15% (rather than 6–10% as tested previously) will result in a more elastic membrane. It became evident, that

while a ca. 2-fold lower (uniaxial) Young's modulus (5.3 ± 1.2 MPa for P15G6) could be obtained (**Figure 2F**), the porosity would be prohibitively low (2% for P15G6) for sufficient trans-membrane nutrient transport during ALI culture conditions. Hence, the previously determined optimum BETA membrane (P/G = 9.35/6.34) was used for the cell-stretch cell experiments.

It is important to note that albeit the (optimum) BETA membrane has an initial (uniaxial) Young's modulus of 9.0 ± 1.9 MPa prior to the dissolution of gelatin (prior to phase I), the (uniaxial) Young's modulus reduces to 1.84 ± 0.66 MPa after dissolving sacrificial gelatin (day 6 under submerged conditions; end of phase II) (Doryab et al., 2020). When measured under more realistic, triaxial stretch conditions in the CIVIC (pressure monitoring method), the elastic modulus of the BETA membrane decreased from 1.33 ± 0.14 MPa (day 1; partial gelatin dissolution) to 0.78 ± 0.24 MPa (day 6) (Doryab et al., 2020), which is ca. 2-fold lower than the corresponding uniaxial value (1.84 ± 0.66 MPa). Considering that the latter was measured under dry conditions these two values can be considered equal within expected experimental uncertainties, which indicates that the BETA membrane is quite isotropic.

In the present study, we recognized the limited value of 2D porosity (pore-area fraction at the surface of the membrane), did not correlate well with the gelatin volume fraction of the membrane, for membrane optimization with respect to 3D porosity (through pores) as only an interconnected 3D pore structure allows for sufficient contact between apically located cells and basal medium during ALI cell culturing. The measurement method for 3D porosity described here was in excellent agreement with the theoretically predicted porosity from gelatin volume fraction, if the latter was larger than 41% (**Figure 2G**). This indicates that for gelatin volume factions larger than 41% all of the available gelatin can eventually be reached and hence dissolved by culture medium, i.e., the gelatin-induced 3D pore structure is perfectly interconnected, which is optimum for ALI culture conditions. For gelatin factions below ca. 35%, the 3D porosity falls below 10% implying that increasing "islands" of gelatin are formed, which are completely engulfed by non-soluble PCL (Figure 2B of Doryab et al., 2020). Thus, future efforts for improved membrane composition should focus on gelatin volume fractions near or above 40% to provide sufficient 3D porosity.

In summary, the optimum BETA membrane is relatively thin (≤5 μm) with a suitable permeability (9.9 × 10^{-6} cm s^{-1} for FITC-dextran 4 kDa and 15.3% 3D porosity), which can provide sufficient contact between ALI cultured cells on the apical and medium on the basal side of the membrane (Weibel, 1970; Doryab et al., 2019). The BETA membrane is also stretchable up to 25% linear strain (during phase

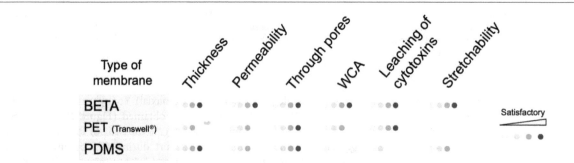

FIGURE 5 | Qualitative comparison between key properties of conventional porous membranes (PET and PDMS) used for static and dynamic (cell-stretch) *in vitro* lung models at the air-liquid interface and the BETA membrane presented here. The scores are based on biomimetic relevance as compared to the alveolar basement membrane. The permeability was measured as apparent permeability (Papp) for FITC-dextran (4 kDa). Stretchability and through pores refer to the elastic modulus and pores connecting the apical and basal sides of the membrane, respectively.

II), which includes the range of physiologic strain (up to 12% linear) and non-physiologic over-stretch conditions as discussed below. While the BETA membrane is more biomimetic than most other membranes currently available due to the low WCA (68°) and 3D interconnectivity of the pores, the BETA membrane still has a ca. 100-fold higher elastic modulus and thickness of the alveolar tissue and basement membrane, respectively (Polio et al., 2018; Doryab et al., 2019; Bou Jawde et al., 2020). The former is expected to alter cell physiology as compared to lung conditions and the latter may result in bias transbarrier transport studies. Future research on membrane technology mimicking the alveolar basement membrane should focus not only on matching the physicochemical properties of the basement membrane but also on its microstructural (network of ECM fibers) and molecular structure.

Thus, further research is needed to close this physiologic gap. Several alternative synthetic scaffolds have presented promising results for lung, such as biofunctionalized or synthetic-peptide-based synthetic scaffold (Nishiguchi et al., 2017). Despite the natural-based scaffold (e.g., collagen type I), synthetic scaffolds can be tailored to have selective tunable properties, mimicking the microenvironment of cells to facilitate cell adherence, proliferation, and differentiation. However, artificial scaffolds, i.e., natural, synthetic, and natural/synthetic introduced until now are unable to concurrently mimic all the physical, mechanical, and biological properties of the natural ECM or basement membrane of the pulmonary cells. The biomimetic biphasic scaffold reported here has excellent structural, mechanical, and biophysical characteristics and can be a suitable alternative for growing epithelial cells not only in the monoculture but also in co-culture and triple co-culture models (Lehmann et al., 2011; Heydarian et al., 2019).

Ultimately, sufficiently biomimetic *in vitro* models of the alveolar tissue should not only focus on the basement membrane but also include more advanced primary alveolar cell models, such as the commercially available primary-derived hAELVi cells (Kuehn et al., 2016) or EpiAlveolar cell model (MatTek, Inc.) (Barosova et al., 2020). The combination of both aspects should

lead to even more biomimetic and hence clinically predictive models of the alveolar barrier.

The millifluidic CIVIC bioreactor utilizes positive pressure to mechanically stretch a cell-covered elastic membrane activate stretchable and thus allows for ALI cell culture conditions with medium perfusion, cyclic stretch, and monitoring of the pressures in the apical and basal compartment of the bioreactor is leveraged for real-time monitoring of amplitude and frequency of cyclic stretch and of tri-axial Young's modulus of the cell-covered membrane. This allows for precise selection of stretch conditions and quality control of key experimental conditions during the course of the cell-stretch experiment. Moreover, an aerosol-cell delivery unit using a clinically relevant nebulizer enhances its applicability to drug testing suitable for inhalation therapy.

It is instructive to relate the characteristic stretch and perfusion parameters of the CIVIC equipped with the BETA membrane to clinical conditions. The BETA membrane can sustain linear stretch amplitudes of up to 25% (Doryab et al., 2020). Population-based averages for breathing frequency and tidal volume during heavy exercise are 26 breaths per minute (33 bpm for women) and 1.92 L (1.36 L), respectively (ICRP, 1994). For typical lung inflation of 3.3 L (2.7 L) at functional residual capacity (FRC, at end of exhalation), this tidal volume corresponds to a 58% (50%) increase in lung volume yielding a 17% (15%) linear and 36% (31%) area change (assuming the alveolar sacs are spherical). Analogous, the stretch conditions were chosen here for the particokinetics study (10% linear at 0.33 Hz = 20 bpm) correspond to a tidal volume of 1.09 L (female 0.89 L), which is similar to "light exercise" conditions (male: 1.25 L, 20 bpm; female: 0.99 L, 21 bpm) (ICRP, 1994). Consequently, linear strain larger than 17% (or 35% ΔSA), which may occur for instance during positive pressure ventilation, is considered over-distension or non-physiologic strain, possibly provoking apoptosis and necrosis, increase permeability and release of inflammatory mediators (such as Interleukin-8) in alveolar epithelial cells (Edwards et al., 1999; Vlahakis et al., 1999; Hammerschmidt et al., 2004).

The maximum positive differential pressure applied to the apical side of the cells during a cyclic stretch in the CIVIC

(2.5 kPa) is higher than exerted onto the lung tissue during normal exhalation (0.1–0.5 kPa), but similar to conditions during mechanical ventilation at the intensive care unit of a hospital (normal: 1.5–2.0 kPa, 2.5 kPa acceptable peak value; 3.0 kPa should not be exceeded for an extended period of time) (Hall, 2016). Finally, the medium perfusion rate of 400 μL min^{-1} has to be put into context with the area of gas exchange (membrane area: 5 cm^2) for comparison with the lung. The ratio of area and perfusion rate of the CIVIC is with 1.25 m^2/(L min^{-1})$^{-1}$ considerably lower than that of the lung [20 m^2/(L min^{-1})$^{-1}$ = 100 m^{-2}/(5 L min^{-1})], but the corresponding flow rate of 6.4 L min^{-1} in the CIVIC system technically not be difficult to establish since it would require tubing with much larger diameter enhancing the laboratory footprint unduly.

It is well known that the size of particles plays a key role in cellular uptake and internalization of the particles (Takenaka et al., 2012; Zhu et al., 2013). We found that both 100 and 1,000 nm amine-coated particles could not be internalized by alveolar epithelial cells (A549) under static/unstretched conditions (2 h after aerosolized particle delivery). Moreover, 1,000 nm microparticles were also not taken up by cells under stretched conditions, which can be explained by endocytic uptake (most relevant uptake mechanism for epithelial cells) being limited to ca. 500 nm particles (Winnik and Maysinger, 2013; Zhu et al., 2013; Annika Mareike Gramatke, 2014). In contrast, the relatively efficient cellular uptake of 100 nm NPs is consistent with previous observations that positively charged (amine-coated) NPs tend to interact with the negatively charged cell membrane, which enhances their uptake as compared to neutral or even negatively charged particles of the same size (Rothen-Rutishauser et al., 2006). The observed colocalization of NPs with the F-actin cytoskeleton in A549 cells is conducive for further intracellular trafficking and endocytosis of the NPs within cells (Foroozandeh and Aziz, 2018). For in vitro pharmacokinetic testing, ALI culture conditions have several advantages over submerged cell culture settings. In addition to more physiologic and tighter barrier function, burst-like pharmacokinetic profiles as typically seen in patients can only be observed for ALI conditions (Meindl et al., 2015; Schmid et al., 2017) since this resembles rapid depletion of the pulmonary drug reservoir due to drug transport into the blood. Moreover, the cell-delivered dose is often poorly known under submerged conditions due to variable particle-cell transport rates in cell culture medium (Teeguarden et al., 2007; Schmid and Cassee, 2017). In contrast, under ALI conditions, the aerosol dose is delivered immediately directly onto the epithelial barrier mimicking the conditions of inhaled particles in the lung. To date, in vitro particokinetic studies are mainly performed under submerged culture conditions, and to the best of our knowledge, no quantitative transbarrier particokinetic (translocation) studies under cell-stretch ALI conditions have been reported, yet.

For sub-100 nm NPs the translocated fraction of particles is inversely proportional to particle size in both static in vitro cell and in vivo animal models of the lung (Kreyling et al., 2014; Bachler et al., 2015). For A549 cells at ALI and rodent models after NP instillation, the first plateau of particle translocation is achieved within 2 h for 80 nm gold NPs, but it is considerably larger for (static) A549 cells (ca. 2% of the delivered dose) as compared to particle instillation in rats (ca. 0.2%) (Kreyling et al., 2014; Bachler et al., 2015). For A549 cells, receiving doses larger than 0.1 μg cm^{-2} for gold NPs has resulted in a decrease in the transport rate (Bachler et al., 2015).

The 2 h translocation fraction of 100 nm amine-modified polystyrene particles observed in this study was below the detection limit [ca. 1.0% (Transwell) and ca. 3% BETA], which is in general agreement well with the results from Bachler and colleagues (Bachler et al., 2015), if we consider that the larger than 0.1 μg cm^{-2} (here 2.1 μg cm^{-2}) cell-delivered dose may have lowered the transport fraction. On the other hand, the 1.8% of translocation fraction for 1,000 nm particles (Transwell inserts) appears relatively large considering that virtually no translocation of microparticles has been reported in in vivo biokinetics studies. The absence of 1,000 nm translocation for the BETA membrane (below detection limit of ca. 3%) is consistent with these in vivo results. While it may be expected that cyclic stretch affects the transepithelial mobility of particles by, e.g., additional convective particle transport, changes in paracellular barrier integrity, and effects on cellular uptake and transport mechanisms, the relatively large increase to 30 and 20% for 100 and 1,000 nm particles is unexpectedly high. Since these values even agree within experimental uncertainty it is unlikely that this is the result of an active cellular transport process especially since endo-/exocytosis as the most effective cellular uptake and transport mechanism for epithelial cells is limited to sizes below 500 nm. Moreover, substantially enhanced cellular uptake was only observed for 100 nm particles (**Figure 4B**). Therefore, we assume that this large increase in translocation fraction is due to a combination of passive mechanisms, such as rupture of the relatively weak tight junctions of A549 cells yielding intracellular gaps, which allows for enhanced convective transport of particles irrespective of particle size due to leakage of the medium in and out of the apical space where the particles are residing.

CONCLUSION

The "optimum" copolymeric BETA membrane (P/G = 9.35/6.34) applied here is biomimetic in the sense that it is thin ($\leq$5 μm), surface wettable, permeable with proper pore size for cell growth and interconnected 3D pore structure, elastic and bioactive, and somewhat comparable to the ECM in the alveolar region. However, it still is ca. 100-fold too thick and stiff as compared to the basement membrane of the alveolar region. These limitations could not be alleviated by enhancing the poly(ε-)caprolactone (PCL) concentration 15% (w/v). Using the "optimum" we showed that the CIVIC can be utilized for cellular uptake and transepithelial transport studies under physiologic stretch and ALI conditions including aerosolized substance delivery. While the results for static conditions are in general agreement with literature data, unexpectedly high translocation of both 100 and 1,000 nm particles under physiologic stretch (light exercise) was observed for an A549 alveolar lung barrier. This suggests that more appropriate cell (co-)culture models with more pronounced tight junctions and advanced primary cell culture models should be employed for cell-stretch experiments. Studies in the field of respiratory diseases are expected to benefit greatly from the development of more biomimetic and reliable *in vitro* models of the lung as currently available. We believe our system presents a valuable step toward improvement of the predictive value of advanced lung cell models.

MATERIALS AND METHODS
Cell Culture

Human alveolar type-II like epithelial cells (A549) were cultured and maintained in Dulbecco's Modified Eagle Medium: Nutrient Mixture F-12 (DMEM/F12, 1:1 v/v, Gibco) supplemented with 10% FCS (Gibco), 1% (v/v) Pen/Strep (100 U mL^{-1}, Gibco), 1% L-glutamine (2 mM, Gibco), and 2-phospho-L-ascorbic acid (0.1 mM, Sigma). Human bronchial epithelial cells (16HBE14o$^-$) were cultured in MEM/F12 medium (Gibco) supplemented with 10% FCS (Gibco), 1% (v/v) Pen/Strep (100 U mL^{-1}, Gibco) and 1% L-glutamine (2 mM, Gibco).

For longitudinal monitoring of cell viability (WST1), A549 cells were grown on the BETA membranes by seeding cells with a cell density of 1.5×10^5 cells cm^{-2} on a UV sterilized BETA membrane (effective growth area: 1.3 cm^2, depending on application). A PTFE holder was used for keeping the BETA membranes) and on Corning® Costar® Transwell® cell culture inserts (PET, 12-well, 1.1 cm^2; 3 μm pore) (control). Cells were then cultured for 6 days under submerged conditions (basal and apical medium volumes were 1.5 and 0.5 mL, respectively) followed by 24 h under ALI conditions. Similarly, 16HBE14o$^-$ cells were also grown on the BETA membrane (cell seeding density: 2×10^5 cells cm^{-2}; effective growth area: 1.3 cm^2) for 6 days under submerged and 24 h under ALI conditions.

Immediately prior to cell-stretch experiments the membrane was placed in the CIVIC and the media volume in the basal and reservoir chamber of the CIVIC were 4 and 12 mL (including 2 mL in the connecting tubing), respectively.

In vitro Cell-Stretch System (CIVIC)

We used the CIVIC system to apply cyclic stretch to cells grown on the BETA membrane under ALI culture conditions (**Figure 1**). The main chamber of the CIVIC bioreactor is separated by the BETA membrane into an apical (humidified air) and a basal (perfused cell culture medium) compartment mimicking the air-blood barrier of the lung including its breathing-related cyclic stretch induced by oscillation of the apical pressure (**Figures 1A,B** and **Supplementary Video 1**). The cell culture medium in the basal compartment is circulated using a peristaltic pump to mimic blood flow (400 μL min^{-1}). Cells grown on the membrane are subjected to a uniform cyclic triaxial strain by applying a cyclic (here: sinusoidal) positive pressure to the apical chamber by cyclic opening of a valve connected to pressurized cleaned house air and a valve connected to ambient air. The entire system is placed in an incubator (37°C) to maintain optimum cell culture conditions. The dry house air is entering the chamber for pressurization via a humidifier and the initially dry air in the apical compartment can be humidified by nebulization of small volume (2 μL) of saline using the nebulizer described

below (**Figures 1A,B**). Both amplitude and frequency of stretch can be set by an Arduino integrated development environment (or IDE) software (Arduino IDE 1.0.5 for Windows). For BETA membranes, the CIVIC bioreactor is able to apply physiologic linear strain: (0–17%) and non-physiologic (over-stretch; 17–25%) stretch conditions, as described below.

The CIVIC system is a modified version of the previously described MALI bioreactor system (Cei et al., 2020). The overall setup and geometry of the MALI system have not been changed. However, the following technical improvements were implemented. All of the components in contact with culture medium are now manufactured with PDMS-free material (namely polycarbonate, PC) to prevent potential artifacts due to leaching of toxicants from the PDMS into the cell culture medium. Moreover, an upgraded design of the PC holder more effectively prevents membrane slipping and leakage of culture medium during pressure oscillations required for inducing cyclic cell stretch as described below. The pressure sealing of the main chamber was improved and not only the pressure in the basal compartment (headspace of the medium reservoir, P_2), but also the pressure in the apical compartment was measured continuously (P_1) (**Figure 1A**) using two piezoresistive, monolithic silicon pressure transducers (MPX5050, Freescale Semiconductor, Munich, Germany).

A clinically used vibrating mesh nebulizer (Aeroneb Pro/Lab, Aerogen Inc., Galway, Ireland) is positioned at the top of the apical chamber for delivery of aerosolized substances to the cells on the BETA membrane. This type of nebulizer has liquid output rates and mass median droplet diameters ranging from 0.2 to 0.8 mL min^{-1} and 2.5 to 6 μm, respectively, depending on the specific type of nebulizer (Ding et al., 2020). Nebulization of 10 μL of liquid and subsequent spatially uniform deposition onto the cells cultured on the BETA membrane (5 cm^2) with a deposition efficiency of 52% occurs within 2 min due to cloud settling (Cei et al., 2020). These aerosol delivery parameters are, independent of nebulizer performance in terms of droplet diameter or liquid output rate (Lenz et al., 2014) since cloud settling depends on the fractional aerosol volume in the air only and hence on the nebulized aerosol volume (10 μL) and the volume of the apical compartment of the chamber. Vibrating mesh nebulizers contain a porous membrane for aerosol production, which may be affected by cyclic positive pressure. Since aerosolized substance delivery is short (2 min) relative to typical cell-stretch experiments (>2 h), aerosolized substance application is typically decoupled from cyclic cell stretch, i.e., cell-stretch is not applied during aerosolization. This patented aerosol-cell exposure unit has recently been made commercially available as VITROCELL®Cloud MAX (VITROCELL Systems, Waldkirch, Germany), albeit only for standard transwell inserts, which cannot be subjected to cyclic stretch. When positive pressure is applied apically to the membrane (P_1), the initially relaxed, flat, horizontally oriented membrane is stretched triaxially downwards expanding the volume of the apical compartment by a dome-shaped volume ΔV (**Figures 1A, 4A**). Due to the incompressible nature of water (culture medium), this change in apical volume reduces the air-filled headspace of the medium reservoir by ΔV and the corresponding increase in pressure (P_2) can be directly related to the linear/area amplitude of membrane stretch (**Figure 1A**).

This special feature of the CIVIC bioreactor enables real-time monitoring of the experimental stretch parameters (amplitude, frequency) and Young's modulus of the cell-covered membrane with thickness t during triaxial stretch under wet conditions (contact with culture medium) by continuously monitoring the apical and basal pressures (P_1 and P_2, respectively). While the stretch frequency can be directly derived from the time course of P_1 or P_2, the linear (1D) and area (2D) amplitude as well as Young's modulus (elastic modulus; E, kPa) of the membrane can be determined from the maximal values of P_1 and P_2 according to the Equations (1)–(3) (Flory et al., 2007).

$$\Delta V = \Delta P \left(\frac{V_0}{P_0} \right), \; where \; \Delta P = P_2 - P_0 \qquad (1)$$

$$\Delta V = \pi \Delta h \left(\frac{a^2}{2} + \frac{\Delta h^2}{6} \right) \qquad (2)$$

$$\Delta P' = (P_1 - P_2) = \frac{4E \left(\frac{\Delta h}{a} \right) t}{3a \left(\left(\frac{\Delta h}{a} \right)^2 + 1 \right)} \left(1 - \frac{1}{\left(1 + \left(\frac{\Delta h}{a} \right)^2 \right)^3} \right) \qquad (3)$$

Initially, the membrane is non-stretched and the pressure in both the apical and basal compartment is at ambient pressure P_0 (on average 98.0 kPa in Munich, Germany) (see **Figure 1A**). Under these conditions, the radius (area) of the membrane a is 1.26 cm (5 cm^2) and the headspace volume in the medium reservoir V_0 is 30 mL (40 mL vessel filled with 10 mL medium). The deflection of the membrane perpendicular to the membrane (Δh) can be obtained from the corresponding change in apical/basal air volume ΔV, which is determined from Equations (1), (2) and the measured pressures P_1 and P_2. Young's modulus (elastic modulus; E, kPa) of the membrane can then be obtained from Equation (3), where t is the thickness of the membrane (ca. 5 µm; calculated by cross-sectional SEM analysis). For dome-shaped geometry (spherical cap), one can find the relative linear and area strain according to Equation (4).

$$\frac{\Delta L}{L} = \frac{\Delta h}{a} \quad or \quad \frac{\Delta S}{S} = \left(\frac{\Delta h}{a} \right)^2 \qquad (4)$$

The amplitude of cell stretch can be calculated from Equation (4), where Δh is the membrane deflection ($0 \leq \Delta h \leq 0.11$ cm) (Equations 1–3) and ΔS is membrane change in surface area during the stretch. P_1 and P_2 are 100.5 and 99.5 kPa for physiologic stretch (10% linear strain or 21% ΔS), respectively.

For optimum BETA membrane, the CIVIC bioreactor is able to apply a linear mechanical strain of up to 17% (or 3, which covers both physiologic and non-physiologic (overstretch) conditions. For those conditions, the optimum BETA membrane is resilient to 48 h cyclic stretch with no deformation, rupture, and creep.

Membrane Fabrication

We recently introduced a novel ultra-thin co-polymeric membrane (BETA) transitioning from an initially stiff,

hydrophilic, non-porous membrane to an elastic, porous substrate, providing optimum cell culture conditions during the two phases of typical *in vitro* alveolar cell-stretch experiments at the ALI (Doryab et al., 2020). Briefly, we employed a two-component (hybrid) polymeric material consisting of poly(ε-caprolactone) (PCL: Sigma-Aldrich, Mn 80,000) and gelatin (Type A from porcine skin, Sigma) chosen for their mechano-elastic and bioactivity properties, respectively. Different mass ratios of PCL and gelatin were dissolved in TFE [(2,2,2-trifluoroethanol) with >99.8% purity, Carl Roth GmbH, Karlsruhe, Germany] and stirred until the blend became homogenous. The PCL/gelatin mixture was then added to a custom-made spin-coater (2,000 rpm) to produce a thin film which was left to dry under vacuum (**Figure 2A**). The initially non-porous membrane (phase I: initial cell adhesion and growth) becomes gradually permeable (phase II: ALI culture) upon contact with the cell culture medium. The underlying concept of a biphasic membrane for cell-stretch experiments under ALI conditions mimicking the conditions in the alveolar tissue has been described in the introduction. The optimum concentrations of PCL and gelatin was determined previously as 9.35% PCL and 6.34% gelatin [w/v solvent]; solvent: $\geq$99% TFE (2,2,2-trifluoroethanol) (Doryab et al., 2020). Here, three new membranes with 15% PCL and 6, 8, and 10% of gelatin were manufactured. The membranes were placed in a holder for placement in the CIVIC system during cell-stretch experiments as described below (**Figure 1C**). Membranes were sterilized before cell culture experiments with ethanol and ultraviolet (UV) light exposure. The membrane is optically transparent and hence suitable for modern cell microscopy technologies.

Membrane Characterization

The membranes were characterized in terms of thickness, ultrastructure, pore size, elemental and chemical composition, surface wettability, elastic modulus, 3D porosity, and cell proliferation (viability and cytotoxicity).

Physical, Elemental, and Chemical Characterization

Thickness, ultrastructure, and pore size of the membranes were analyzed by Scanning Electron Microscopy (SEM). The samples were fixed in 6% (v/v) glutaraldehyde (Sigma-Aldrich) and then dehydrated in gradient ethanol solutions followed by HDMS (hexamethyldisilazane, Sigma-Aldrich) for 15 min and subsequently mounted onto aluminum stubs, sputter-coated with platinum using Leica EM ACE600 vacuum coater, and imaged by SEM (Zeiss Crossbeam 340, Carl Zeiss AG, Oberkochen, Germany) with acceleration voltage of 2 kV. We also used Energy Dispersive X-ray Spectroscopy (EDS, X-max^N, Oxford instruments) with an acceleration voltage of 8 kV to study qualitative elemental and the local distributions of certain elements (Carbon and Nitrogen) in the sample. Focused Ion Beam (FIB)/SEM (Zeiss Crossbeam 340, Carl Zeiss AG, Oberkochen, Germany) and FIB/SEM/EDS were employed to investigate the cross-sectional structures of the membranes at high resolution (30 kV; 700 pA and 1.5 nA). Surface roughness was assessed by an Atomic Force Microscope (AFM, Nanosurf Flex-Axiom) at room temperature. A scanning area of 80 µm was chosen. Scan rates of 0.5–0.15 Hz were used during mapping with 512 points per scan.

Surface Wettability (Water Contact Angle)

The surface wettability or Water Contact Angle (WCA) of the membranes was determined with the sessile drop method using an automated contact angle system OCA20 with an image processing system as described previously (Doryab et al., 2020).

Elastic Modulus (Young's Modulus)

Uniaxial (1D) tensile test (BOSE 5500 system, ElectroForce, Eden Prairie, MN, USA) with a load capacity of 22 N at a rate of 0.01 mm/s until rupture was used to calculate Young's modulus of the membrane (in phase I). Young's modulus of the membrane in wet (phase II) condition was measured using our novel pressure-based technique integrated into our CIVIC system described in more detail in **Figure 1A**.

Porosity

We used the liquid displacement method to measure the 3D porosity of the interconnected three-dimensional (3D) pore network of the membranes. Briefly, membranes were submerged in ethanol (EtOH, $\geq$99% purity) for 24 h. Gravimetric analysis prior to and after soaking the membrane with EtOH revealed the volume of EtOH (V_{EtOH}) inside the pores ($V = m/\rho$; $m_{EtOH} =$ difference of mass prior to and after soaking; $\rho_{EtOH} = 0.789$ g cm^{-3}) and the volume of the dry membrane (V_m) [$m_m =$ mass of membrane prior to soaking; ρ_m is the volume-weighted density of PCL (1.145 g cm^{-3}) and gelatin (1.3 g cm^{-3})]. The empirical 3D porosity can then be calculated according to Equation (5).

$$Porosity = \frac{V_{EToH}}{V_{EToH} + V_m}. \tag{5}$$

To account for EtOH adsorption on and/or microporosity of PCL itself, the apparent porosity of the pure PCL membrane (9.3 $\pm$ 1.7%; according to Equation 5) was subtracted from the measured porosity of the PCL/gelatin membranes.

Moreover, one can estimate the upper limit of porosity from the chemical composition of the membrane. Assuming gelatin has been completely dissolved in the culture medium (PCL is insoluble), one finds a theoretical upper limit for porosity from the volume fraction of gelatin based on Equation (6), where V_g and V_{PCL} are the volume fraction of gelatin and PCL in the composite of PCL/gelatin, respectively, and ρ_g and ρ_{PCL} are the density of gelatin and PCL ($\rho_g = 1.30$ g cm^{-3} and $\rho_{PCL} = 1.45$ g cm^{-3}), respectively.

$$Theoretical\ Porosity = \frac{\frac{V_g}{\rho_g}}{\frac{V_g}{\rho_g} + \frac{V_{PCL}}{\rho_{PCL}}} \tag{6}$$

Cell Proliferation, Morphology, and Cell Viability

Cell proliferation was assessed from the known number of cells seeded on the membrane (day 0) and the cells counted based on DAPI-stained (cell nucleus) CLSM images at the end of the submerged cell culture conditions (day 6). Moreover,

cell proliferation was monitored indirectly with higher time-resolution by measuring cell viability in terms of a non-destructive metabolic activity assay (WST1, Roche, Mannheim, Germany), provided the metabolic activity of the cells is similar during the 6 days of cell growth. This test was performed on cell covered BETA membranes (1.3 cm^3) and Corning® Costar® Transwell® cell culture inserts (PET, 12-well, 3 µm pore), which was used as a commercial membrane to compare cell viability, cell number and morphology with that of the BETA membrane. Each membrane was incubated with 1 mL diluted WST1 reagent (1:15) at 37°C. After 15 min, 150 µL supernatant was transferred to a 96-well plate (4 times for each membrane) and absorbance was measured in a plate reader (Magellan™ Tecan) at 450 nm. All the results were normalized to the mean value of blank.

Lactate Dehydrogenase (LDH) Release

The cytotoxicity effect of the manufactured membranes was assessed by the detection of the release of lactate dehydrogenase (LDH; Roche Applied Science, Mannheim, Germany) from the cells, which indicates perforation of the cell membrane. According to the manufacturer's protocol, the determination of LDH activity was determined in the basal (and apical) medium by absorbance measurement at a wavelength of 492 nm. The LDH release is presented as the ratio of LDH dose (LDH concentration times medium volume) in the cell culture medium and the high control (cells treated with 2% [w/v] Triton X-100). Transwell inserts were used as a positive control since BETA membranes are more limited in supply than standard Transwell inserts. The LDH release for each membrane was normalized by the maximum possible LDH level (LDH contained in all cells).

PDMS-Leached in Cell Culture Medium

We fabricated PDMS films for studying the leaching of PDMS oligomers into the culture medium. Briefly, the elastomers and crosslinker (1:10, Sylgard 184, Dow Corning) were mixed and degassed under vacuum. After casting, the film was cured in an oven at 60°C overnight. The PDMS film (thickness: 5 µm) was then cut using a standard biopsy punch (size: 5.0 mm; Kai medical, Solingen, Germany). The membranes were washed with PBS (three times) and disinfected using EtOH 80% and UV before immersing in the Dulbecco's Modified Eagle Medium: Nutrient Mixture F-12 (DMEM/F12, 1:1 v/v, Gibco) supplemented with 10% FCS (Gibco), 1% (v/v) Pen/Strep (100 U mL^{-1}, Gibco), 1% L-glutamine (2 mM, Gibco). The PDMS punches and BETA membranes of the same size were soaked in 2 mL of culture medium for 2 days (the ratio of the surface area and the bulk volume of the membrane to the culture medium were 0.1 cm^2 mL^{-1} and 4.9 $\times$ 10^{-5} cm^3 mL^{-1}).

The PDMS- and BETA-incubated media containing leached compounds were used to investigate their effect on cell viability with the WST1 assay. For this, A549 cells (1.5 $\times$ 10^5 cells cm^{-2}) were cultured under submerged conditions in 12-well multiwell plates using PDMS- and BETA membrane-leached media for up to 4 days and repeatedly analyzed for viability (WST1). As a control, A549 cells were seeded on the bottom of the well plate.

Immunofluorescence

Cells were fixed in 4% paraformaldehyde (Sigma-Aldrich), washed with PBS and, permeabilized by 0.3% Triton X-100 (Sigma-Aldrich) in PBS at room temperature. To prevent any unspecific antibody binding, a blocking buffer (5% BSA and 0.1% TritonX-100) was added for 10 min. The cells were then incubated overnight at 4°C with Anti-E-Cadherin (mouse, 1:1,000; Invitrogen) and anti–ZO-1 monoclonal (mouse, 1:100; Invitrogen), in a blocking buffer (5% BSA and 0.1% TritonX-100). Cells were then incubated with secondary antibody Alexa Fluor® 488 goat anti-mouse IgG (1:500; Invitrogen) and Alexa Fluor® 555 goat anti-mouse IgG (1:500; Invitrogen). The F-actin cytoskeleton and cell nuclei were stained with Phalloidin 594 (1:40) and DAPI (1:100), respectively. The cells were then embedded in Glycergel (DAKO Schweiz AG, Baar, Switzerland). All cell images were acquired using a confocal laser scanning microscope (CLSM; LSM710, Carl Zeiss; Oberkochen, Germany) coupled to the Zen2009 software. For intensity quantification of particles, the images were recorded at five independent fields of view (region of interest: $134.95 \times 134.95\,\mu m$) for each sample. The rectangular tool (Fiji) was used to measure the mean fluorescence intensity of background-subtracted images.

TEER Measurement

Trans-epithelial electrical resistance (TEER) measurements of epithelial cells grown on the membrane were measured using the Millicell-ERS system (Millicell ERS-2, Millipore, USA). TEER is calculated by multiplying the cell-specific resistance (Ohm, Ω) and the effective surface area of the membrane (cm^2). The TEER value of the blank BETA membrane was determined as 78 ± 10 ($\Omega\ cm^2$), which was then subtracted from the cell-covered membrane TEER values.

Particokinetic Studies

For particle studies, we chose fluorescent amine-modified polystyrene (PS-NH$_2$) spheres, fluorescent orange (Sigma-Aldrich, St. Louis, USA), with a mean diameter of 100 and 1,000 nm for particle study (**Figure 4A**) since amine-functionalized surfaces (positively charged particles) are associated with higher cellular uptake and internalization as compared to neutral or negatively charged ones (Rothen-Rutishauser et al., 2006; Zhu et al., 2013). A549 cells were grown on the optimized BETA membrane until confluence (submerged conditions for 6 days) and left for acclimatization at the ALI for 1 day. Particles were then nebulized directly onto the cells [deposited mass dose: 2.1 $\mu g\ cm^{-2}$; surface area dose: 1.2 $cm^2\ cm^{-2}$ (100 nm particles); 0.12 $cm^2\ cm^{-2}$ (1,000 nm)] and incubate with the cells for 2 h under stretched or unstretched conditions.

For the unstretched experiments, the membranes were first put in special holders and placed in a 6-well plate which was then positioned in the aerosol-cell exposure chamber of a VITROCELL®Cloud 6 system (VITROCELL Systems, Waldkirch, Germany; aerosol exposed area: 146 cm^2, deposition factor: 0.97), followed by nebulization of 250 μL of particle suspensions (1.25 mg mL^{-1} in 0.3% NaCl) with subsequent aerosol sedimentation onto the cells with 3 min

as described by Lenz and colleagues (Lenz et al., 2014). Corning® Costar® Transwell® cell culture inserts (6-well, PET membrane with 3 μm pores) were also used to compare transepithelial translocation of particles with cells cultured on the BETA membrane under unstretched and stretched conditions. For stretch experiments, particles are delivered to the cells using the nebulizer integrated in the CIVIC as described above (**Figures 1A,B, 4A**) with a known delivery efficiency of 52% (Doryab et al., 2020). Subsequently, a physiologic cyclic mechanical stretch (10% linear at 0.33 Hz) corresponding to respiratory conditions during light exercise was applied to the cells for 2 h.

The fractional particle transport across the epithelial barrier was determined by quantitative fluorescence spectroscopy of the culture media in the basal compartment of both unstretched and stretched treatment using a plate reader (Safire2™, Tecan; excitation: 520 nm, emission: 540 nm). For normalization to the cell-delivered dose a standard curve of the particle suspension in cell culture medium basal medium volume prepared and measured for fluorescence intensity. For the measurement of quantitative cellular uptake of particles with CLSM, the samples were washed with PBS to remove free or weakly adsorbed particles from the apical side of the cell layer. Subsequently, the cells on the membranes were fixed in 4% paraformaldehyde for CLSM analysis. The CLSM images (z-stacks) were then recorded at five randomly selected fields of view for each sample ($n = 4$; region of interest: $134.95 \times 134.95\,\mu m$) and quantified for cumulative fluorescence intensity of z-stacks.

Statistical Analysis

All data were analyzed using GraphPad Prism 8.4 (GraphPad Software, La Jolla, CA, USA). The details of each statistical analysis were presented in the caption of the figures.

AUTHOR CONTRIBUTIONS

AD and OS designed the experiments, analyzed the data, and wrote the manuscript. AD manufactured and characterized the BETA membrane and performed all the cell experiments and particle and particokinetic studies. AD, OS, and AS modified the CIVIC bioreactor systems. AD and PS performed SEM, FIB-SEM, and EDS-SEM. SO assisted AD with particle study of the Transwell® insert under static conditions. JG, MT, TS, AH, CV, AA, and MR provided the input to data interpretation in their respective field of expertise and contributed to the writing of the manuscript. All authors contributed to the article and approved the submitted version.

SUPPLEMENTARY MATERIAL

Supplementary Figure 1 | The Water Contact Angle (WCA) of the PDMS and BETA membranes using an automated contact angle system OCA20 with an image processing system (mean ± SD).

Supplementary Figure 2 | SEM micrograph of bronchial epithelial 16HBE14o⁻ cells grown on the membrane (cultured 6 days submerged and 24 h ALI culture). (Left) Confluent cell layer scale bar of overview and the magnified insert is 25 and

2 µm, respectively. (Right) Pseudocolored cells (using the GNU Image Manipulation Program (GIMP 2.10.8) (http://www.gimp.org/), showing cracks between cells, which were induced due to dehydration of the samples for SEM. The scale bar is 10 µm.

Supplementary Figure 3 | No significant effect of 2 h physiologic stretch and particle exposure (diameter: 100 and 1,000 nm) on cell viability (WST1 assay;

A549 cells) was observed. The viability data were normalized by the corresponding value of the Transwell inserts (no stretch) (Data are reported as mean ± SD. $n = 3$; Two-way ANOVA with Sidak test).

Supplementary Video 1 | BETA membrane motion in the CIVIC bioreactor system when a cyclic mechanical stretch (linear strain: 10%; breathing/stretch frequency: 0.33 Hz) is applied to the membrane.

REFERENCES

Ainslie, G. R., Davis, M., Ewart, L., Lieberman, L. A., Rowlands, D. J., Thorley, A. J., et al. (2019). Microphysiological lung models to evaluate the safety of new pharmaceutical modalities: a biopharmaceutical perspective. *Lab Chip* 19, 3152–3161. doi: 10.1039/C9LC00492K

Annika Mareike Gramatke, I. L. H. (2014). Size and cell type dependent uptake of silica nanoparticles. *J. Nanomed. Nanotechnol.* 5:6. doi: 10.4172/2157-7439.1000248

Artzy-Schnirman, A., Lehr, C. M., and Sznitman, J. (2020). Advancing human *in vitro* pulmonary disease models in preclinical research: opportunities for lung-on-chips. *Expert Opin. Drug Deliv.* 17, 621–625. doi: 10.1080/17425247.2020.1738380

Artzy-Schnirman, A., Zidan, H., Elias-Kirma, S., Ben-Porat, L., Tenenbaum-Katan, J., Carius, P., et al. (2019). Capturing the onset of bacterial pulmonary infection in acini-on-chips. *Adv. Biosyst.* 3:1900026. doi: 10.1002/adbi.201900026

Bachler, G., Losert, S., Umehara, Y., von Goetz, N., Rodriguez-Lorenzo, L., Petri-Fink, A., et al. (2015). Translocation of gold nanoparticles across the lung epithelial tissue barrier: combining *in vitro* and *in silico* methods to substitute *in vivo* experiments. *Part. Fibre Toxicol.* 12:18. doi: 10.1186/s12989-015-0090-8

Barosova, H., Maione, A. G., Septiadi, D., Sharma, M., Haeni, L., Balog, S., et al. (2020). Use of EpiAlveolar lung model to predict fibrotic potential of multiwalled carbon nanotubes. *ACS Nano* 14, 3941–3956. doi: 10.1021/acsnano.9b06860

Benam, K. H., Dauth, S., Hassell, B., Herland, A., Jain, A., Jang, K.-J., et al. (2015). Engineered *in vitro* disease models. *Annu. Rev. Pathol. Mech. Dis.* 10, 195–262. doi: 10.1146/annurev-pathol-012414-040418

Bou Jawde, S., Takahashi, A., Bates, J. H. T., and Suki, B. (2020). An analytical model for estimating alveolar wall elastic moduli from lung tissue uniaxial stress-strain curves. *Front. Physiol.* 11:121. doi: 10.3389/fphys.2020.00121

Carter, S. D., Atif, A., Kadekar, S., Lanekoff, I., Engqvist, H., Varghese, O. P., et al. (2020). PDMS leaching and its implications for on-chip studies focusing on bone regeneration applications. *Organs Chip* 2:100004. doi: 10.1016/j.ooc.2020.100004

Cei, D., Doryab, A., Lenz, A., Schröppel, A., Mayer, P., Burgstaller, G., et al. (2020). Development of a dynamic *in vitro* stretch model of the alveolar interface with aerosol delivery. *Biotechnol. Bioeng.* 1–13. doi: 10.1002/bit.27600

de Souza Carvalho, C., Daum, N., and Lehr, C.-M. (2014). Carrier interactions with the biological barriers of the lung: advanced *in vitro* models and challenges for pulmonary drug delivery. *Adv. Drug Deliv. Rev.* 75, 129–140. doi: 10.1016/j.addr.2014.05.014

Ding, Y., Weindl, P., Lenz, A. G., Mayer, P., Krebs, T., and Schmid, O. (2020). Quartz crystal microbalances (QCM) are suitable for real-time dosimetry in nanotoxicological studies using VITROCELL®Cloud cell exposure systems. *Part. Fibre Toxicol.* 17, 1–20. doi: 10.1186/s12989-020-00376-w

Doryab, A., Amoabediny, G., and Salehi-Najafabadi, A. (2016). Advances in pulmonary therapy and drug development: lung tissue engineering to lung-on-a-chip. *Biotechnol. Adv.* 34, 588–596. doi: 10.1016/j.biotechadv.2016.02.006

Doryab, A., Tas, S., Taskin, M. B., Yang, L., Hilgendorff, A., Groll, J., et al. (2019). Evolution of bioengineered lung models: recent advances and challenges in tissue mimicry for studying the role of mechanical forces in cell biology. *Adv. Funct. Mater.* 29:1903114. doi: 10.1002/adfm.201903114

Doryab, A., Taskin, M. B., Stahlhut, P., Schröppel, A., Wagner, D. E., Groll, J., et al. (2020). Stretch experiments with pulmonary epithelial cells at the air-liquid interface. *Adv. Funct. Mater.* 2004707. doi: 10.1002/adfm.202004707

Edwards, Y. S., Sutherland, L. M., Power, J. H., Nicholas, T. E., and Murray, A. W. (1999). Cyclic stretch induces both apoptosis and secretion in rat alveolar type II cells. *FEBS Lett.* 448, 127–130. doi: 10.1016/S0014-5793(99)00357-9

Ehrhardt, C., Kneuer, C., Fiegel, J., Hanes, J., Schaefer, U., Kim, K.-J., et al. (2002). Influence of apical fluid volume on the development of functional intercellular junctions in the human epithelial cell line 16HBE14o⁻: implications for the use of this cell line as an *in vitro* model for bronchial drug absorption studies. *Cell Tissue Res.* 308, 391–400. doi: 10.1007/s00441-002-0548-5

Ehrmann, S., Schmid, O., Darquenne, C., Rothen-Rutishauser, B., Sznitman, J., Yang, L., et al. (2020). Innovative preclinical models for pulmonary drug delivery research. *Expert Opin. Drug Deliv.* 17, 463–478. doi: 10.1080/17425247.2020.1730807

Flory, A. L., Brass, D. A., and Shull, K. R. (2007). Deformation and adhesive contact of elastomeric membranes. *J. Polym. Sci. B Polym. Phys.* 45, 3361–3374. doi: 10.1002/polb.21322

Foroozandeh, P., and Aziz, A. A. (2018). Insight into cellular uptake and intracellular trafficking of nanoparticles. *Nanoscale Res. Lett.* 13:339. doi: 10.1186/s11671-018-2728-6

Guenat, O. T., and Berthiaume, F. (2018). Incorporating mechanical strain in organs-on-a-chip: lung and skin. *Biomicrofluidics* 12:042207. doi: 10.1063/1.5024895

Hall, J. E. (2016). *Guyton and Hall Textbook of Medical Physiology, 13th Edn.* London: Elsevier.

Hammerschmidt, S., Kuhn, H., Grasenack, T., Gessner, C., and Wirtz, H. (2004). Apoptosis and necrosis induced by cyclic mechanical stretching in alveolar type II cells. *Am. J. Respir. Cell Mol. Biol.* 30, 396–402. doi: 10.1165/rcmb.2003-0136OC

Hänninen, O., Brüske-Hohlfeld, I., Loh, M., Stoeger, T., Kreyling, W., Schmid, O., et al. (2010). Occupational and consumer risk estimates for nanoparticles emitted by laser printers. *J. Nanoparticle Res.* 12, 91–99. doi: 10.1007/s11051-009-9693-z

Heydarian, M., Yang, T., Schweinlin, M., Steinke, M., Walles, H., Rudel, T., et al. (2019). Biomimetic human tissue model for long-term study of neisseria gonorrhoeae infection. *Front. Microbiol.* 10:1740. doi: 10.3389/fmicb.2019.01740

Higuita-Castro, N., Nelson, M. T., Shukla, V., Agudelo-Garcia, P. A., Zhang, W., Duarte-Sanmiguel, S. M., et al. (2017). Using a novel microfabricated model of the alveolar-capillary barrier to investigate the effect of matrix structure on atelectrauma. *Sci. Rep.* 7:11623. doi: 10.1038/s41598-017-12044-9

Huh, D., Kim, H. J., Fraser, J. P., Shea, D. E., Khan, M., Bahinski, A., et al. (2013). Microfabrication of human organs-on-chips. *Nat. Protoc.* 8, 2135–2157. doi: 10.1038/nprot.2013.137

Huh, D., Matthews, B. D., Mammoto, A., Montoya-Zavala, M., Hsin, H. Y., and Ingber, D. E. (2010). Reconstituting organ-level lung functions on a chip. *Science* 328, 1662–1668. doi: 10.1126/science.1188302

Huh, D., Torisawa, Y., Hamilton, G. a., Kim, H. J., and Ingber, D. E. (2012). Microengineered physiological biomimicry: organs-on-chips. *Lab Chip* 12:2156. doi: 10.1039/c2lc40089h

ICRP (1994). Human respiratory tract model for radiological protection. A report of a Task Group of the International Commission on Radiological Protection. *Ann. ICRP* 24, 1–482.

Kreyling, W. G., Hirn, S., Möller, W., Schleh, C., Wenk, A., Celik, G., et al. (2014). Air–blood barrier translocation of tracheally instilled gold nanoparticles inversely depends on particle size. *ACS Nano* 8, 222–233. doi: 10.1021/nn403256v

Kreyling, W. G., Semmler-Behnke, M., Takenaka, S., and Möller, W. (2013). Differences in the biokinetics of inhaled nano- versus micrometer-sized particles. *Acc. Chem. Res.* 46, 714–722. doi: 10.1021/ar300043r

Kuehn, A., Kletting, S., de Souza Carvalho-Wodarz, C., Repnik, U., Griffiths, G., Fischer, U., et al. (2016). Human alveolar epithelial cells expressing tight junctions to model the air-blood barrier. *ALTEX* 33, 1–20. doi: 10.14573/altex.1511131

Lehmann, A. D., Daum, N., Bur, M., Lehr, C. M., Gehr, P., and Rothen-Rutishauser, B. M. (2011). An *in vitro* triple cell co-culture model with primary cells mimicking the human alveolar epithelial barrier. *Eur. J. Pharm. Biopharm.* 77, 398–406. doi: 10.1016/j.ejpb.2010.10.014

Lenz, A. G., Stoeger, T., Cei, D., Schmidmeir, M., Semren, N., Burgstaller, G., et al. (2014). Efficient bioactive delivery of aerosolized drugs to human pulmonary epithelial cells cultured in air–liquid interface conditions. *Am. J. Respir. Cell Mol. Biol.* 51, 526–535. doi: 10.1165/rcmb.2013-0479OC

Meindl, C., Stranzinger, S., Dzidic, N., Salar-Behzadi, S., Mohr, S., Zimmer, A., et al. (2015). Permeation of therapeutic drugs in different formulations across the airway epithelium *in vitro*. *PLoS ONE* 10:e0135690. doi: 10.1371/journal.pone.0135690

Nishiguchi, A., Singh, S., Wessling, M., Kirkpatrick, C. J., and Möller, M. (2017). Basement membrane mimics of biofunctionalized nanofibers for a bipolar-cultured human primary alveolar-capillary barrier model. *Biomacromolecules* 18, 719–727. doi: 10.1021/acs.biomac.6b01509

Paur, H.-R., Cassee, F. R., Teeguarden, J., Fissan, H., Diabate, S., Aufderheide, M., et al. (2011). *In-vitro* cell exposure studies for the assessment of nanoparticle toxicity in the lung—a dialog between aerosol science and biology. *J. Aerosol Sci.* 42, 668–692. doi: 10.1016/j.jaerosci.2011.06.005

Peters, A., Wichmann, H. E., Tuch, T., Heinrich, J., and Heyder, J. (1997). Respiratory effects are associated with the number of ultrafine particles. *Am. J. Respir. Crit. Care Med.* 155, 1376–1383. doi: 10.1164/ajrccm.155.4.9105082

Polio, S. R., Kundu, A. N., Dougan, C. E., Birch, N. P., Aurian-Blajeni, D. E., Schiffman, J. D., et al. (2018). Cross-platform mechanical characterization of lung tissue. *PLoS ONE* 13:e0204765. doi: 10.1371/journal.pone.0204765

Pope, C. A., Ezzati, M., and Dockery, D. W. (2009). Fine-particulate air pollution and life expectancy in the United States. *N. Engl. J. Med.* 360, 376–386. doi: 10.1056/NEJMsa0805646

Regehr, K. J., Domenech, M., Koepsel, J. T., Carver, K. C., Ellison-Zelski, S. J., Murphy, W. L., et al. (2009). Biological implications of polydimethylsiloxane-based microfluidic cell culture. *Lab Chip* 9:2132. doi: 10.1039/b903043c

Rothen-Rutishauser, B. M., Schürch, S., Haenni, B., Kapp, N., and Gehr, P. (2006). Interaction of fine particles and nanoparticles with red blood cells visualized with advanced microscopic techniques. *Environ. Sci. Technol.* 40, 4353–4359. doi: 10.1021/es0522635

Schaumann, F., Frömke, C., Dijkstra, D., Alessandrini, F., Windt, H., Karg, E., et al. (2014). Effects of ultrafine particles on the allergic inflammation in the lung of asthmatics: results of a double-blinded randomized cross-over clinical pilot study. *Part. Fibre Toxicol.* 11:39. doi: 10.1186/s12989-014-0039-3

Schmid, O., and Cassee, F. R. (2017). On the pivotal role of dose for particle toxicology and risk assessment: exposure is a poor surrogate for delivered dose. *Part. Fibre Toxicol.* 14:52. doi: 10.1186/s12989-017-0233-1

Schmid, O., Jud, C., Umehara, Y., Mueller, D., Bucholski, A., Gruber, F., et al. (2017). Biokinetics of aerosolized liposomal ciclosporin a in human lung cells *in vitro* using an air–liquid cell interface exposure system. *J. Aerosol Med. Pulm. Drug Deliv.* 30, 411–424. doi: 10.1089/jamp.2016.1361

Schmid, O., and Stoeger, T. (2016). Surface area is the biologically most effective dose metric for acute nanoparticle toxicity in the lung. *J. Aerosol Sci.* 99, 133–143. doi: 10.1016/j.jaerosci.2015.12.006

Stucki, A. O., Stucki, J. D., Hall, S. R. R., Felder, M., Mermoud, Y., Schmid, R. A., et al. (2015). A lung-on-a-chip array with an integrated bio-inspired respiration mechanism. *Lab Chip* 15, 1302–1310. doi: 10.1039/C4LC01252F

Takenaka, S., Möller, W., Semmler-Behnke, M., Karg, E., Wenk, A., Schmid, O., et al. (2012). Efficient internalization and intracellular translocation of inhaled gold nanoparticles in rat alveolar macrophages. *Nanomedicine* 7, 855–865. doi: 10.2217/nnm.11.152

Teeguarden, J. G., Hinderliter, P. M., Orr, G., Thrall, B. D., and Pounds, J. G. (2007). Particokinetics *in vitro*: dosimetry considerations for *in vitro* nanoparticle toxicity assessments. *Toxicol. Sci.* 95, 300–312. doi: 10.1093/toxsci/kfl165

Tenenbaum-Katan, J., Artzy-Schnirman, A., Fishler, R., Korin, N., and Sznitman, J. (2018). Biomimetics of the pulmonary environment *in vitro*: a microfluidics perspective. *Biomicrofluidics* 12:042209. doi: 10.1063/1.5023034

Vlahakis, N. E., Schroeder, M. A., Limper, A. H., and Hubmayr, R. D. (1999). Stretch induces cytokine release by alveolar epithelial cells *in vitro*. *Am. J. Physiol. Cell. Mol. Physiol.* 277, L167–L173. doi: 10.1152/ajplung.1999.277.1.L167

Wang, L., Sun, B., Ziemer, K. S., Barabino, G. A., and Carrier, R. L. (2010). Chemical and physical modifications to poly(dimethylsiloxane) surfaces affect adhesion of Caco-2 cells. *J. Biomed. Mater. Res. A* 93, 1260–1271. doi: 10.1002/jbm.a.32621

Wang, Z., Volinsky, A. A., and Gallant, N. D. (2014). Crosslinking effect on polydimethylsiloxane elastic modulus measured by custom-built compression instrument. *J. Appl. Polym. Sci.* 131:41050. doi: 10.1002/app.41050

Weibel, E. R. (1970). Morphometric estimation of pulmonary diffusion capacity. *Respir. Physiol.* 11, 54–75. doi: 10.1016/0034-5687(70)90102-7

Weibel, E. R. (2009). What makes a good lung? *Swiss Med. Wkly.* 139, 375–86. doi: 10.4414/smw.2009.12270

Winnik, F. M., and Maysinger, D. (2013). Quantum dot cytotoxicity and ways to reduce it. *Acc. Chem. Res.* 46, 672–680. doi: 10.1021/ar3000585

Young, B. M., Shankar, K., Allen, B. P., Pouliot, R. A., Schneck, M. B., Mikhaiel, N. S., et al. (2017). Electrospun decellularized lung matrix scaffold for airway smooth muscle culture. *ACS Biomater. Sci. Eng.* 3, 3480–3492. doi: 10.1021/acsbiomaterials.7b00384

Zhu, M., Nie, G., Meng, H., Xia, T., Nel, A., and Zhao, Y. (2013). Physicochemical properties determine nanomaterial cellular uptake, transport, and fate. *Acc. Chem. Res.* 46, 622–631. doi: 10.1021/ar300031y

11

An Inflamed Human Alveolar Model for Testing the Efficiency of Anti-Inflammatory Drugs *in vitro*

Barbara Drasler[1], Bedia Begum Karakocak[1], Esma Bahar Tankus[1], Hana Barosova[1], Jun Abe[2], Mauro Sousa de Almeida[1], Alke Petri-Fink[1,3] and Barbara Rothen-Rutishauser[1]*

[1] Institut Adolphe Merkle, Faculté des Sciences et de Médecine, Université de Fribourg, Fribourg, Switzerland, [2] Department of Oncology, Microbiology and Immunology, Faculty of Science and Medicine, University of Fribourg, Fribourg, Switzerland, [3] Département de Chimie, Faculté des Sciences et de Médecine, Université de Fribourg, Fribourg, Switzerland

Correspondence:
Barbara Rothen-Rutishauser
barbara.rothen@unifr.ch

A large number of prevalent lung diseases is associated with tissue inflammation. Clinically, corticosteroid therapies are applied systemically or via inhalation for the treatment of lung inflammation, and a number of novel therapies are being developed that require preclinical testing. In alveoli, macrophages and dendritic cells play a key role in initiating and diminishing pro-inflammatory reactions and, in particular, macrophage plasticity (M1 and M2 phenotypes shifts) has been reported to play a significant role in these reactions. Thus far, no studies with *in vitro* lung epithelial models have tested the comparison between systemic and direct pulmonary drug delivery. Therefore, the aim of this study was to develop an inflamed human alveolar epithelium model and to test the resolution of LPS-induced inflammation *in vitro* with a corticosteroid, methylprednisolone (MP). A specific focus of the study was the macrophage phenotype shifts in response to these stimuli. First, human monocyte-derived macrophages were examined for phenotype shifts upon exposure to lipopolysaccharide (LPS), followed by treatment with MP. A multicellular human alveolar model, composed of macrophages, dendritic cells, and epithelial cells, was then employed for the development of inflamed models. The models were used to test the anti-inflammatory potency of MP by monitoring the secretion of pro-inflammatory mediators (interleukin [IL]-8, tumor necrosis factor-α [TNF-α], and IL-1β) through four different approaches, mimicking clinical scenarios of inflammation and treatment. In macrophage monocultures, LPS stimulation shifted the phenotype towards M1, as demonstrated by increased release of IL-8 and TNF-α and altered expression of phenotype-associated surface markers (CD86, CD206). MP treatment of inflamed macrophages reversed the phenotype towards M2. In multicellular models, increased pro-inflammatory reactions after LPS exposure were observed, as demonstrated by protein secretion and gene expression measurements. In all scenarios, among the tested mediators the most pronounced anti-inflammatory effect of MP was observed for IL-8. Our findings demonstrate that our inflamed multicellular human lung model is a promising tool for the evaluation of anti-inflammatory potency of drug candidates *in vitro*. With the presented setup, our model allows a meaningful comparison of the systemic vs. inhalation administration routes for the evaluation of the efficacy of a drug *in vitro*.

Keywords: inflammation, lung, *in vitro*, multicellular models, macrophage phenotype, anti-inflammatory drugs, corticosteroids

INTRODUCTION

Lung inflammation plays an important role in the pathogenesis of a number of respiratory diseases, such as pneumonia, acute respiratory distress syndrome, or chronic inflammatory disorders such as asthma and chronic obstructive pulmonary disease (Johnson and Matthay, 2010; Roth, 2014). As the lung is the vital organ for gas exchange, excessive inflammation in the lung tissue can be life-threatening (Moldoveanu et al., 2009). Lung tissue inflammation, as well as the anti-inflammatory reactions, involve complex interactions between and among the immune cells and the structural lung cells (Nicod, 2005; Holt et al., 2008). The airways and the lung parenchyma contain dense networks of immune cells, e.g., dendritic cells and alveolar macrophages, which play a key role in regulating the body's immune responses (Holt et al., 2008). Dendritic cells are professional antigen-presenting cells (APCs) linking innate and adaptive immunity (Banchereau and Steinman, 1998; Cook and MacDonald, 2016). Another type of APCs, macrophages, are located in the apical part of the epithelium, and their main role is professional phagocytosis (Brain, 1988; Lehnert, 1992; Hussell and Bell, 2014). Macrophages and dendritic cells are capable of triggering rapid pro-inflammatory reactions in response to inhaled foreign materials, as well as bacterial, viral, and fungal infections through the release of pro-inflammatory mediators, such as tumor necrosis factor α (TNF-α), interleukin (IL)-1β, and IL-8, along with the increased release of reactive oxygen and nitrogen species (Condon et al., 2011; Laskin et al., 2011). In particular, macrophages also play a pivotal role in the resolution of alveolar inflammation (Frankenberger et al., 2005; Moldoveanu et al., 2009; Tu et al., 2017; Lu et al., 2018). The biological activity of macrophages is mediated by their phenotypically distinct subpopulations, i.e., the M1 and M2 phenotypes, which develop and shift in response to the mediators in their microenvironment. According to the basic dichotomic macrophage polarization classification, M1 macrophage polarization, the pro-inflammatory phenotype is stimulated by specific pathogens (Atri et al., 2018). The M1 phenotype is associated with the release of pro-inflammatory mediators, with the expression of toll-like receptors (TLR-2 and TLR-4) and co-stimulatory molecules, such as cluster of differentiation (CD) 86 (Martinez and Gordon, 2014). The activity of M1 macrophages is balanced by those with M2 phenotypes through the secretion of anti-inflammatory mediators (Martinez and Gordon, 2014). The M2 subset is stimulated with anti-inflammatory agents, such as steroids (Laskin et al., 2011; Wang et al., 2014; Jaroch et al., 2018; Desgeorges et al., 2019). The M2 phenotype is associated with expression of the mannose receptor-1 (CD206) as well as macrophage scavenger receptors (CD204 and CD163) (Gordon, 2003).

Due to the distinctive roles of macrophages in the lung, they have been proposed as the main cellular targets in the treatment of lung-inflammation-related disorders (Laskin et al., 2011). Clinically, immunosuppressant drugs, such as corticosteroids, among them methylprednisolone (MP), play an integral role in anti-inflammatory treatments of pulmonary diseases, particularly in asthma, acute lung injury, and acute respiratory distress syndrome (Silva et al., 2009; Barnes, 2011; Marik et al., 2011; Liu et al., 2013). The efficacy of corticosteroids in suppressing lung inflammation has been confirmed by both systemic administration and inhalation (Sethi and Singhal, 2008; Higham et al., 2015). MP has been shown to attenuate acute lung injury, induced with bacterial endotoxin lipopolysaccharide (LPS), via promoting macrophage polarization into the M2 subset (Tu et al., 2017). Although corticosteroids are widely used agents for the treatment of lung inflammation, strong systemic side effects such as respiratory tract infections, allergies, wound healing impairment, and bronchitis have been reported (Liu et al., 2013; Waljee et al., 2017). As a result, alternative anti-inflammatory therapies are currently being investigated (da Silva et al., 2017).

The role of macrophage phenotypes in lung inflammation and its resolution has been investigated extensively in murine models in vivo (Leite-Junior et al., 2008; Katsura et al., 2015; Florentin et al., 2018; Lu et al., 2018). The anti-inflammatory activity of corticosteroids in murine lung epithelia has also been investigated in vivo, both for the treatment of allergic asthma (Klaßen et al., 2017) and in order to determine their contribution to fetal lung maturation (Habermehl et al., 2011). On the other hand, based on the findings of clinical studies, it has been proposed that distinctive macrophage phenotype populations play an important role in anti-inflammatory treatment, e.g., in that of chronic obstructive pulmonary disease with poor response to corticosteroids (Barnes, 2011; Chana et al., 2014). Nevertheless, it should be noted that dendritic cells and the alveolar epithelium also contribute significantly to glucocorticoid-mediated immunosuppressive effects (Zach et al., 1993; Piemonti et al., 1999; Rozkova et al., 2006; Klaßen et al., 2017).

With respect to human lung models, mono- and multicellular models, primary or cell line-derived, have been developed to mimic human airway epithelia and the alveolar epithelial-endothelial tissue barrier (Hermanns et al., 2004; Steimer et al., 2005; Bur and Lehr, 2008; Haghi et al., 2015; Hittinger et al., 2016; Yonker et al., 2017; Costa et al., 2019; Artzy-Schnirman et al., 2020). These models have been employed in investigations of lung inflammation to study various lung diseases and disorders, such as cystic fibrosis (Castellani et al., 2018), chronic obstructive pulmonary disorder (Haghi et al., 2015; Zhou et al., 2019), and acute respiratory distress syndrome (Viola et al., 2019). Also, these models have been employed to investigate the safety and efficacy of aerosolized and dry powder formulations for pulmonary drug delivery (Hittinger et al., 2016), including that of steroid drugs (Bur and Lehr, 2008; Haghi et al., 2015). Finally, an in vitro human airway model differentiated from primary human bronchial cells has been proposed for pharmacokinetics studies (Rivera-Burgos et al., 2016). LPS is a major component of the outer membrane of Gram-negative bacteria, such as *Haemophilus influenzae*, which are considered one of the main causes of infectious lung diseases (King, 2012). For induction of inflammation, LPS is often used as a stimulus to investigate lung inflammation in vitro, to study the efficacy of drugs or vaccinations, or to elucidate the mechanisms of the pulmonary response to bacterial ligands (Knapp, 2009; Bisig et al., 2019;

Nova et al., 2019). To date, however, there have been no studies demonstrating a comparison of drug delivery approaches, i.e., systemic vs. direct pulmonary delivery of anti-inflammatory drugs, using 3D multicellular systems of human lung epithelial tissue *in vitro*.

Given this paucity and the high potential utility of such a comparative study, this study was aimed at the development of an inflamed, immunocompetent, multicellular human lung model, including macrophages and dendritic cells. The simultaneous presence of both immune cell types is important in the cellular interplay in response to exposure to an inflammatory mediator, such as the endotoxin LPS (Bisig et al., 2019; Nova et al., 2019). As a model cell type for human alveolar pneumocytes, the epithelial A549 cell line, isolated from a pulmonary adenocarcinoma, was used. A549 cells possess characteristics of squamous type II epithelial cells of the alveolar region; these cells carry lamellar bodies containing densely packed phospholipids, the constituents of the pulmonary surfactant (Shapiro et al., 1978), and release the surfactant upon exposure to air-liquid interface (ALI) (Blank et al., 2006). In this study, a widely used anti-inflammatory drug, the corticosteroid MP, was initially tested for its ability to induce macrophage phenotype shifts in primary human monocyte-derived macrophages (MDMs) from the pro-inflammatory (M1) towards the anti-inflammatory (M2) subset, and vice-versa. Then, a 3D multicellular human lung epithelial tissue barrier model composed of the same macrophage type along with an alveolar epithelial cell layer, and monocyte-derived dendritic cells (MDDCs) (Rothen-Rutishauser et al., 2005), was stimulated with LPS from either the basal or apical side, mimicking systemic or alveolar lumen-derived inflammation, respectively. These inflamed lung models were further treated with MP in the co-presence of the pro-inflammatory stimulus (LPS) applied from the opposite side of the human lung model, simulating either intravenous drug administration or aerosolized drug administration via inhalation. In the last step, the LPS was removed prior to the anti-inflammatory treatment, mimicking a lower degree of inflammation in the tissue, and the steroid therapy was applied via the respiratory route, i.e., onto the apical side of the tissue. We employed the adverse outcome pathway (AOP) concept for pulmonary fibrosis as it involves a strong inflammatory component. As a result, the focus herein is on so-called key event two (KE2), which is the release of pro-inflammatory cytokines (e.g., tumor necrosis factor-alpha [TNF-α], interleukin [IL]-1β, and IL-8) and the loss of alveolar barrier integrity (Labib et al., 2016; Vietti et al., 2016; Villeneuve et al., 2018).

Herein, we provide experimental evidence for suppression of pro-inflammatory reactions *in vitro* using a widely used anti-inflammatory drug, a corticosteroid MP. We discuss these reactions with respect to the macrophage phenotype shifts towards pro- and anti-inflammatory subsets. We demonstrate the responsiveness of our 3D human lung model to pro- and anti-inflammatory agents, both at the pro-inflammatory protein secretion and gene expression levels. The presented model may serve as a diseased human lung model for *in vitro* pre-clinical testing of the safety, potency, and efficacy of newly developed

anti-inflammatory formulations and also can serve as a diseased model to assess occupational exposures to all types of aerosols.

MATERIALS AND METHODS

Chemicals, Reagents, and Laboratory Conditions

All the chemical reagents were purchased from Sigma-Aldrich (Switzerland), while all cell culture reagents were purchased from Gibco and Thermo Fisher Scientific (Switzerland) unless stated otherwise. MilliQ water (ultrapure water of 18.2 MΩ.cm) was used in all the experiments. Methylprednisolone (MP; Cayman Chemical, Ann Arbor, MI, United States) powder was dissolved in absolute ethanol to 5 mg/mL. At every step during cell culture and exposure, cells were kept in an incubator under controlled conditions (humidified atmosphere, 37°C, 5% CO_2). Cell numbers were determined using an EVE^{TM} bench-top automated cell counter (Witec AG, Switzerland) with the trypan blue exclusion method (0.4% trypan blue solution in phosphate buffer saline [PBS]).

Isolation and Differentiation of Primary Human Peripheral Blood-Derived Immune Cells

Human MDMs and MDDCs were prepared from monocytes isolated from buffy coats provided by the Swiss Transfusion Center (Bern, Switzerland), as described previously (Barosova et al., 2020). In brief, isolated blood monocytes were cultured in 6-well tissue culture plates (Corning, FALCON®, United States) for six days at a density of 10^6 cells/mL in 3 mL Roswell Park Memorial Institute (RPMI)-1640 cell culture medium supplemented with 10% (v/v) fetal bovine serum (42G1189K), 2 mM L-glutamine, and penicillin-streptomycin (100 units/mL and 100 μg/mL, respectively), referred to as the complete cell culture medium (cRPMI). For MDM differentiation, 10 ng/mL of macrophage colony-stimulating factor (M-CSF) was added to cRPMI. MDDC differentiation was performed in the presence of 10 ng/mL of recombinant human interleukin 4 (IL-4) and 10 ng/mL of granulocyte-macrophage colony-stimulating factor (GM-CSF; all the factors were obtained from Milteny Biotec, Germany). Experiments involving primary monocyte isolation from human blood were approved by the committee of the Federal Office for Public Health Switzerland (reference number: 611-1, Meldung A110635/2) for the Adolphe Merkle Institute.

Macrophage Phenotype Shifts: Monoculture Experiments
Macrophage Challenge With Pro- and Anti-inflammatory Agents

After six days of MDMs differentiation, cRPMI containing the growth factor was aspirated and replaced with either 2.5 mL fresh cRPMI or cRPMI containing lipopolysaccharide (LPS; 1 μg/mL; isolated from *E. coli*, strain O55:B5, Sigma-Aldrich, Switzerland). After 24 h, cRPMI containing MP or vehicle was added to the cells (the summary of the treatments is presented in **Table 1**).

TABLE 1 | Treatments of the differentiated MDMs.

Sample Description	0 to 24 h	24 to 48 h
Untreated cells	cRPMI (3 mL)	cRPMI not changed
Negative control	cRPMI (2.5 mL)	Vehicle (0.5 mL)
LPS	cRPMI (2.5 mL) with LPS (1 μg/mL)	Vehicle (0.5 mL)
LPS + MP10	cRPMI (2.5 mL) with LPS (1 μg/mL)	MP (0.5 mL of 0.06 mM stock in cRPMI). Final concentration 0.01 mM
MP control	cRPMI (2.5 mL)	MP (0.5 mL of 0.06 mM stock in cRPMI). Final concentration 0.01 mM
IL-4+IL-13 (M2 control)	cRPMI with IL-4 and IL-13 (20 ng/mL)	Treatment not changed
Triton X-100 (positive control for LDH)	cRPMI (3 mL)	Triton X-100 (0.3 mL). Final concentration 0.2% (v/v)

Vehicle is a solution of absolute ethanol (0.005% in cRPMI; v/v).

Flow Cytometry

Immunostaining for cell surface protein markers

After stimulation of MDMs, supernatant and non-adherent cells were removed, centrifuged (500 RCF, 5 min), and kept at 4°C or −80°C until being subjected to a cell viability assay or enzyme-linked immunosorbent assay (ELISA), respectively. Adherent cells were gently washed with PBS and detached from the wells using a cell scraper (SARSTEDT, United States) in fresh PBS. Cells from two identically treated wells in a 6-well plate were pooled in flow cytometry tubes (FALCON® 5 mL Polystyrene Round-Bottom Tube, Corning, Switzerland), counted, centrifuged (5702R, Eppendorf; 500 RCF, 5 min), and resuspended in cold flow cytometry buffer (PBS with 1% BSA, 0.1% NaN3, 1 mM ethylenediaminetetraacetic acid [EDTA] at pH 7.4). Before antibody labeling, cells were incubated with Fc-receptor-blocking reagent (Miltenyi Biotec, Germany) according to the supplier's protocol. After incubation for 10 min, the suspensions were split into two separate flow cytometry tubes at a density of 1×10^6 cells/mL for staining or as unstained controls.

Cells were stained with Alexa Fluor 488 conjugated anti-human CD86 (B7-2) monoclonal antibody (clone IT2.2; at 1.25 μg/mL), and APC conjugated anti-human CD206 (MMR) monoclonal antibody (clone 19.2; at 3 μg/mL), as M1 and M2 macrophage markers, respectively, in cold flow cytometry buffer containing 2 μM 4,6-diamidino-2-phenylindole (DAPI; Sigma Aldrich, Switzerland) for dead cell exclusion. Both antibodies were obtained from eBioscience™ (Thermo Fisher Scientific, Switzerland). Additional untreated samples were prepared for fluorescence minus one control staining using OneComp™ ebeads compensation beads (Thermo Fisher Scientific, Switzerland) to set up the cytometer. After antibody labeling for 30 min at 4°C in the dark, the cells were washed with flow cytometry buffer (3 mL) and centrifuged (500 RCF, 5 min, 4°C). The cell pellet was resuspended with cold flow cytometry buffer and stored at 4°C until data acquisition (up to 2 h). Data were acquired using LSRFortessa (BD Biosciences, Switzerland) and analyzed using FlowJo software (Version 10.6.1, TreeStar, United States).

Cytokine Secretion

The amount of released pro-inflammatory mediators (IL-8, IL-1β, and TNF-α) was quantified using a DuoSet ELISA Development Kit (R&D Systems, Switzerland) according to the supplier's protocol. For IL-8, all the samples were diluted 1:4

(v/v) in reagent diluent for the measured values to remain within the detection limit of the instrument. TNF-α and IL-1β were measured in polystyrene high-binding surface 96-well plates (Corning®, Switzerland) without dilution. Standards and samples were run in triplicate. The concentrations of the cytokines released in the cell culture medium were calculated based on the standard curves and fitted with a four-parameter logistic (4PL) approach using GraphPad Prism 8 software (GraphPad Software Inc., San Diego, CA, United States).

Cell Viability/Membrane Rupture

Cell viability was evaluated by the lactate dehydrogenase (LDH; cytosolic enzyme) released in cRPMI, analyzed in triplicate using LDH cytotoxicity detection kit (Roche Applied Science, Mannheim, Germany) according to the manufacturer's protocol. The absorbance of the colorimetric product was determined spectrophotometrically (Benchmark Microplate reader, BioRad, Switzerland) at 490 nm with a reference wavelength of 630 nm with 30-s intervals for 10 measurements. The values were expressed as fold increase of slopes (0–5 min reaction) of the treated samples relative to those of untreated samples of the multicellular models.

MULTICELLULAR HUMAN LUNG MODEL ASSEMBLY

The multicellular models of human alveolar epithelial type II cell line A549, MDMs, and MDDCs were prepared as previously described (Barosova et al., 2020). In brief, A549 cells were maintained in cRPMI (passage number 5 to 25). A549 cells were seeded on transparent cell culture inserts (surface area of 4.2 cm^2, 3.0 μm pore diameter, high pore density, polyethylene terephthalate [PET] membranes for 6-well plates; Falcon, BD Biosciences, Switzerland) at a cell density of 28.0×10^4 cells/cm^2 in 2 mL of cRPMI at 58×10^4 cells/mL. The membrane inserts with cells were placed in tissue culture plates (6-well plates; Falcon, BD Biosciences, Switzerland) containing 3 mL of cRPMI and cultured for four days to form a confluent monolayer. For the multicellular model composition, membrane inserts with A549 cells were removed from the 6-well plates and placed in a sterile glass petri dish turned upside down. Cells that had grown through the pores on the basal side of the inserts were gently abraded with a cell scraper. MDDCs were pipetted onto the bottom side of the inserts: 300 μL of cell suspension in cRPMI at 98.0×10^4 cells/mL

(29.4 × 10^4 cells/insert, corresponding to a seeded cell density of 7 × 10^4 cells/cm^2) and incubated for 70 min at 37°C and 5% CO_2. Membrane inserts were placed back into 6-well plates containing 3 mL of pre-heated fresh cRPMI. Then, 2 mL of a MDM suspension at concentration 2.95 × 10^4 cells/mL in cRPMI was gently added on the top of the A549 cells on inserts (5.9 × 10^4 cells/insert, corresponding to 1.4 × 10^4 cells/cm^2). The assembled multicellular models were exposed for 24 h to air at the ALI to allow for surfactant production by the A549 cells. MDDCs and MDMs prepared from one buffy coat donor and A549 cells from an individual passage were used for each independent experiment. The A549 cell line was purchased from the American Tissue Type Culture Collection (ATCC®CCL-185^{TM}) and was authenticated using short tandem repeat (STR) profiling. Cells were regularly tested for the absence of mycoplasma.

Inflamed Model: Induction and Assessment of Pro-inflammatory Reactions

The assembled multicellular model was challenged with 1 μg/mL LPS for 48 h, from either apical or basal compartments. LPS stock (1 mg/mL in water) was diluted in cRPMI. Old cRPMI was aspirated from the bottom compartments in all samples. Then, either cRPMI (3 mL) with LPS was applied to the basal compartment, and nothing to the apical (approach 1), or fresh cRPMI was added to the basal compartment and 0.2 mL of cRPMI with LPS to the apical side, referred to as pseudo-ALI conditions (Endes et al., 2014) (approach 2).

Inflammatory Reactions
Secretion of pro-inflammatory mediators
After the LPS challenge, the concentration of IL-8, IL-1β, and TNF-α released in the cell culture medium in the basal compartment was quantified by ELISA, as described for the monoculture experiments.

Response at Gene Expression Levels
Upon collection of supernatants in the basal compartment, models were washed with PBS, and inserts with cells were cut out of the plastic holders. Half of each insert was incubated in RNA protection buffer (Qiagen, Germany). The cells were removed from the membranes by extensive vortexing and kept at 4°C for up to seven days (the other half was fixed for immunofluorescence staining). Then, RNA isolation was performed using ReliaPrep^{TM} RNA Miniprep Systems (Promega, Switzerland) according to the manufacturer's protocol. RNA concentrations in samples were analyzed with a NanoDrop 2000 spectrophotometer (Thermo Scientific, United States) and stored at −20°C. Complementary DNA (cDNA) was synthesized with the Omniscript RT system (Qiagen, Germany), Oligo dT (Microsynth, Switzerland), and RNasin Inhibitor (Promega, Switzerland). Reverse transcriptase reactions were performed in 10 μL volumes with an RNA concentration of 25 ng/μL (Omniscript RT, Qiagen) and Oligo dT primers (Qiagen). RNase inhibitor (0.25 μL; RNasin Plus RNase Inhibitor, Promega) was added to the reverse transcriptase reactions. A total of 2 μL of the tenfold diluted cDNA was used for real-time PCR in

reaction volumes of 10 μL with SYBR Green as reporter dye (Fast SYBR Green master mix, 7500 fast real-time PCR system, Applied Biosystems, United States). The mRNA levels were calculated using the double delta of cycle threshold (ΔΔCt) method, calculated based on the expression of a standard gene (glyceraldehyde-3-phosphate dehydrogenase; GAPDH) and the respective gene expressions in untreated cells. Primer sequences and database accession numbers are listed in the **Supplementary Material** (**Supplementary Table S1**).

Suppression of LPS-Induced Pro-inflammatory Reactions

To prepare inflamed cell-culture models, LPS was added either from the basal compartment or from the apical compartments and left to stand for 24 h, following the procedure described above. After the first 24 h, MP was added and left to stand for an additional 24 h while LPS was still present. In approach 1, the MP stock (13 mM in absolute ethanol) was diluted in PBS to the final concentrations of 10 and 100 μM, and 200 μL was applied directly to the apical side of the models. In approach 2, MP stock was diluted in the existing cRPMI in the basolateral compartment to the same final concentrations and left to stand for 24 h. For negative control samples, the vehicle, absolute ethanol, was added at a final concentration of 0.07% or 0.7% to gauge potential biological effects of the solvent alone for comparison with entirely untreated samples. LPS-treated samples were considered as the positive controls for the pro-inflammatory scenario. In parallel, the effects of MP treatments on non-inflamed models were tested following the same procedure as described in approaches 1 and 2, but without LPS in cRPMI. After treatment, the biological responses of the models were assessed by ELISA, real-time RT-qPCR, and confocal microscopy.

Suppression of Pro-inflammatory Reactions Upon LPS Removal

In approaches 3 and 4, inflamed models were established by a 24-h pre-challenge with LPS from the apical side at the pseudo-ALI (**Figure 1**). After 24 h, the apical sides were gently rinsed with PBS, and MP was added to the apical side at the pseudo-ALI for an additional 24 h. In approach 3, the basal cell culture medium was not changed before the MP treatment. In approach 4, the models were washed with PBS from both sides, and cRPMI in the basal compartment was refreshed. Positive controls ("LPS") and "MP only" controls were treated with the vehicle at the pseudo-ALI. Upon completion of the treatment, the biological response was assessed as described above.

Multicellular Model Visualization
Tissue morphology of both LPS-challenged and MP-treated models, immuno-fluorescently stained, was visualized via confocal laser scanning fluorescence microscopy (LSM).

Immunofluorescent Staining
Upon completion of the exposures, the models were washed with PBS, and half of the membrane inserts (the remaining half which was not used for real-time RT-qPCR) were fixed in 4%

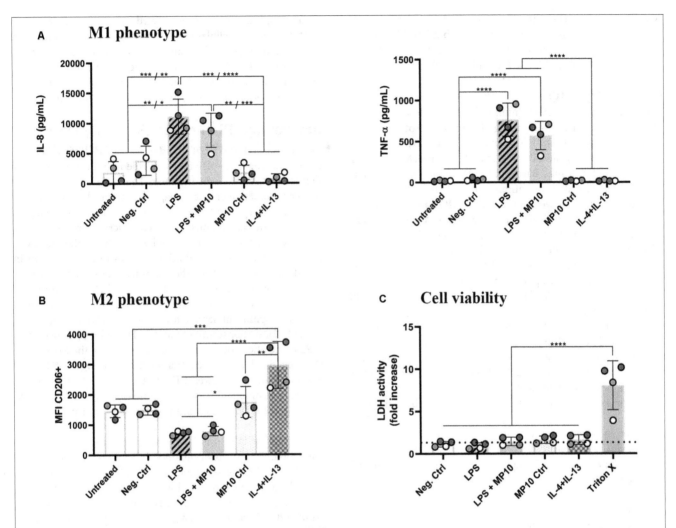

FIGURE 1 | Phenotype shift in macrophage monocultures upon exposure to pro- and anti-inflammatory stimuli. **(A)** Secretion of pro-inflammatory mediators (IL-8 and TNF-α; in pg/mL) in cell-culture medium in the basal compartment, assessed via ELISA. **(B)** Expression of CD206 surface marker (median fluorescence intensity), denoting M2 phenotype, assessed via flow cytometry analysis. The CD206 intensity histogram is shown in **Supplementary Figure S2**. **(C)** Cell viability of MDMs after all of the treatments, assessed via membrane rupture (LDH assay), presented as fold increase over untreated cells (the dotted line). The data is presented as the mean of the four biological repetitions ± standard deviation, whereas individual values from biological repetitions are presented as circles, color-coded for the data from the same biological repetitions (donors). Statistically significant differences among the groups (One-way ANOVA, Tukey's *post hoc*; α = 0.05): *p ≤ 0.05; **p ≤ 0.01; ***p ≤ 0.001, ****p ≤ 0.0001. Abbreviations: IL-8, interleukin 8; TNF-α, tumor necrosis factor α; MFI, median fluorescence intensity; CD206, cluster of differentiation 206, mannose receptor; IL-4+IL-13, interleukins 4 and 13 (both applied at 20 ng/mL for 48 h); LDH, lactate dehydrogenase; Pos. ctrl Triton X, positive control for LDH assay, i.e., cells exposed to 0.2% Triton X-100 (v/v; 24 h).

paraformaldehyde (in PBS, v/v) for 15 min, washed three-times with PBS and stored at 4°C until the staining procedure. Then, cells were permeabilized with 0.2% Triton X-100 (in PBS, v/v) for 15 min and washed (three-times with 0.1% w/v BSA in PBS). The models were immersed in a mixture of primary antibodies for 2 h: mouse mature macrophage marker monoclonal antibody (clone eBio25F9; eBioscience™; Thermo Fisher Scientific, Germany) at 5 μg/mL and rabbit anti-CD83 antibody (clone EPR22405, Abcam, Switzerland) at 10 μg/mL in 0.1% BSA in PBS. After washing (three-times with 0.1% BSA in PBS), the models were incubated for 2 h in a mixture of secondary antibodies: 20 μg/mL of goat anti-mouse polyclonal secondary antibody, Alexa 647 conjugated (ab150115, Abcam, United Kingdom), 9 μg/mL goat anti-rabbit DY 488 conjugated (AS09 633; Agisera, Sweden)

and 0.66 μM rhodamine-phalloidin (Thermo Fisher Scientific, Switzerland) in 0.1% BSA in PBS. After washing (three-times with 0.1% BSA in PBS), the inserts were incubated for an additional 10 min with 1 μg/mL DAPI (Sigma Aldrich, Switzerland) in 0.1% BSA in PBS. All the staining steps were performed in the dark at room temperature. After staining, the cells were washed with PBS, and half of the membranes were cut with a scalpel into two pieces. For optical analysis, both pieces of each sample were mounted in glycergel (DAKO Schweiz AG, Switzerland) to visualize both sides of the model.

Confocal Laser Scanning Microscopy

Visualization of the models was conducted with an inverted LSM Zeiss 710 microscope (Carl Zeiss, Switzerland) equipped with a

40x objective lens (EC Plan-Neofluar 40x/1.30 Oil DIC M27). Representative images (z-stacks) of both apical and basal sides were collected and were further processed using the ImageJ-based software Fiji [ImageJ, NIH, US (Schindelin et al., 2012)].

Barrier Integrity

The barrier integrity of the multicellular models was assessed via a permeability assay using fluorescein isothiocyanate-dextran solution (70 kDa; FITC-dextran). FITC-dextran (stock at 25 mg/mL in water) and EDTA (stock at 0.5 M in water) solutions were prepared in Hank's Balanced Salt Solution (HBSS) without Mg and Ca salts at 2 mg/mL and 10 mM, respectively. After exposure, the models were washed with HBSS and placed in 6-well plates containing 2 mL of HBSS in the basal compartment. First, 1 mL of HBSS buffer was added to the apical compartment of untreated, LPS-, and MP-exposed models, whereas 1 mL of 10 mM EDTA solution was added for positive control samples for barrier integrity disruption. Then, 1 mL of a 2 mg/mL FITC-dextran solution was added to the apical compartments of all the samples and incubated for 60 min (dark, 37°C). In parallel, a blank insert without cells but with HBSS and FITC-dextran was prepared as described above. After incubation, membrane inserts were immediately removed from the cell-culture plates. The supernatants of HBSS containing FITC-dextran were collected from the basal compartments with precise collected volumes noted for each sample. Samples were kept in the dark until the measurements. Fluorescence intensity was measured in triplicate in black 96-well plates using a microplate reader (Tristar LB 941, Berthold Technologies; using the following filters setup: λex/λem: 485/535 nm). Results were corrected with the supernatant volumes (i.e., fluorescence intensity per mL) and expressed as relative to the average fluorescence measured in blank samples.

Cell Viability/Membrane Rupture

Lactate dehydrogenase activity was measured in the basal cell culture medium of exposed models and analyzed in triplicate using the LDH cytotoxicity detection kit, as described for the monoculture experiments. Apical application of 0.2 mL Triton-X (0.2% in sterile-filtered ultrapure water) for 24 h served as a positive control. LDH values are presented as fold increase values relative to untreated cells.

Statistical Analysis

Statistical analysis was performed using GraphPad Prism 8 software (GraphPad Software Inc., San Diego, CA, United States). Parametric one-way analysis of variance (ANOVA; $\alpha = 0.05$) with post hoc Tukey's multiple comparison test was used to compare values among the different treatments. Statistically significant values among the treatments are shown as: $^*p \leq 0.05$; $^{**}p \leq 0.01$; $^{***}p \leq 0.001$, $^{****}p \leq 0.0001$.

RESULTS

The anti-inflammatory effects of MP were first tested on MDM monocultures with respect to the drug's priming potential to shift macrophage phenotypes towards the anti-inflammatory subset. In the multicellular human alveolar model, LPS-induced inflammation, triggered from apical and basal sides of the model, is demonstrated, followed by four experimental approaches of pro-inflammation induction and its suppression, mimicking various scenarios of lung inflammation and treatment in clinics.

Macrophage Phenotype Plasticity Upon Pro- and Anti-inflammatory Treatments

Alveolar macrophages play a pivotal role in both pro- and anti-inflammatory reactions in the lung. Therefore, in this study, a known phenomenon of macrophage phenotype plasticity, i.e., the shift from M1 (pro-inflammatory) to M2 (anti-inflammatory) and vice-versa, in response to their microenvironment was initially tested. MDMs were treated with LPS for the first 24 h, and MP was added for an additional 24 h while LPS was left in the system (Table 1). After the exposure, the secretion of pro-inflammatory cytokines was assessed via ELISA and expression of surface markers via flow cytometry. LPS stimulation induced statistically significant secretion of IL-8 and TNF-α (Figure 1A and Table 2), demonstrating that MDMs exhibit responsiveness to LPS stimulation. In contrast, the expression of the M1 marker CD86 remained unchanged (Supplementary Figure S2). LPS exposure resulted in lower CD206 expression than untreated cells, while a combined IL-4 + IL-13 treatment, which is known to induce M2 polarization, induced its significant upregulation (Figure 1B). Next, we tested whether treatment with MP during the latter half of LPS stimulation mitigates manifestation of M1 polarization. Treatment of inflamed MDMs with MP or vehicle alone did not induce secretion of pro-inflammatory cytokines, nor did it cause a phenotypic shift. In contrast, MP treatment of LPS-stimulated MDMs for 24 h resulted in decreased secretion of IL-8 and TNF-α (Figure 1A), while leaving the expression of CD86 and CD206 unchanged (Figure 1B and Supplementary Figure S2). Thus, MP inhibited the secretion of the tested pro-inflammatory markers (IL-8, TNF-α) but did not reprogram the MDM phenotype. None of the treatments used affected the viability of MDMs (Figure 1C and Supplementary Figure S2a). There are four individual repetitions representing the four blood donors. The gating strategy is presented in the Supplementary Material (Supplementary Figure S1).

LPS-Induced Inflamed Multicellular Human Lung Model

As the next step, we adapted a more complex lung model to investigate the orchestrated immune cell responses upon exposure to LPS with or without the presence of MP: multicellular models, composed of alveolar epithelial cells (A549) and immune cells (MDDCs and MDMs on basal and apical sides, respectively). The models were challenged with LPS for 48 h from either basal (approach 1) or apical (approach 2) sides. As inflammation in an epithelial tissue often leads to impaired epithelial barrier integrity, the permeability of the model to labeled dextran (70 kDa) was first assessed. LPS challenge from the basal side resulted in increased tissue permeability, demonstrated by the absence of significant differences compared

TABLE 2 | A summary of the pro-inflammatory reactions in monocultures and multicellular human lung models.

Treatment	MDMs			LPS or MP application / in vivo significance	Approach 1	Approach 2	Approach 3	Approach 4
	MP10 Ctrl	LPS	LPS + MP10	LPS / MP	Basal / blood-derived inflammation — Apical / pulmonary drug delivery	Apical / inflammation from the airways — Basal /systemic drug administration	Apical / inflammation from the airways — Apical / pulmonary drug delivery	Basal and apical / strong tissue inflammation — Apical / pulmonary drug delivery
Surface marker expression								
CD86	0	+	0	LPS / MP	—	—	+	NA
Pro-inflammatory mediators secretion								
IL-8	0	+++	++		++	+	++	+
TNF-α	0	+++	++		+	++	+	+
IL-1β	NA	NA	NA		+	++	+	+
Pro-inflammatory gene expression								
CXCL8					++	—	++	—
TNF					0	+	+	—
IL1B					0	+	++	—

to the positive control (EDTA-treated) models, indicating a disruption of barrier integrity (approach 1). In contrast, apical LPS application (approach 2) did not alter the permeability compared to untreated cells but there was statistical significance observed compared to the positive control models (**Figure 2A**). Neither of the treatments induced membrane rupture as assessed by LDH release in the basal cRPMI (**Figure 2B**). The morphology of the epithelial layer on the apical side of the insert was impaired in approach 1 and also slightly after the apical LPS challenge in approach 2. In contrast, the morphology of the basal sides of the inserts, i.e., at the side of MDDCs, was comparable with untreated cells for both approaches (**Figure 2C**).

LPS stimulation significantly increased the expression of pro-inflammatory mediators at protein and gene expression levels, irrespective of the approach used. In both approaches, LPS induced the secretion of IL-8, TNF-α, and IL-1β (the IL-1β secretion was statistically significant only in approach 2; **Figure 3A**). Accordingly, in both approaches, increased mRNA levels were observed compared to untreated cells, with the lowest difference observed for *IL1B* in approach 2 (**Figure 3B**). LPS-induced oxidative stress was evidenced with the onset of mitochondrial antioxidant superoxide dismutase-2 (*SOD2*) mRNA levels in both approaches (**Figure 3C**). The absence of pro-apoptotic reactions was evidenced by unaltered *FAS* mRNA expression levels in both the approaches after 48-h LPS treatments (**Figure 3D**).

Corticosteroids Suppress Pro-inflammatory Reactions in the Inflamed Model

Next, we examined whether the MP treatment of LPS-stimulated multicellular model leads to decreased production of pro-inflammatory factors IL-1 β, IL-8, and TNF-α, following four approaches of LPS and MP application. In approaches 1 and 2, MP treatment of inflamed models was performed in the presence of LPS. LPS and MP were applied either in the basal or the apical compartments (approach 1) or vice-versa (approach 2), respectively (**Figure 4**; left panel). Alternatively, in approaches 3 and 4, LPS was removed from the system before the application of MP. In approach 3, inflamed models were treated with MP while being in contact with LPS-conditioned medium, whereas the basal compartment was refilled with fresh medium in approach 4 (**Figure 4**; right panel). At the protein level, there was an overall trend of slightly reduced secretion of pro-inflammatory mediators (**Figure 5A**). Interestingly, however, the mRNA levels of all three factors were found to have dropped significantly 24 h after the addition of MP in approach 1, which generally induced higher expression of mRNA of the pro-inflammatory factors. A similar trend was observed when we treated the multicellular model using approach 2 (**Figure 5B**). The trends in pro-inflammatory mediator secretion were also observed in approaches 3 and 4 (**Figure 6A**), where LPS was removed before the apical application of MP (**Figure 4**; right panel). Reduced mRNA levels of pro-inflammatory mediators were observed upon

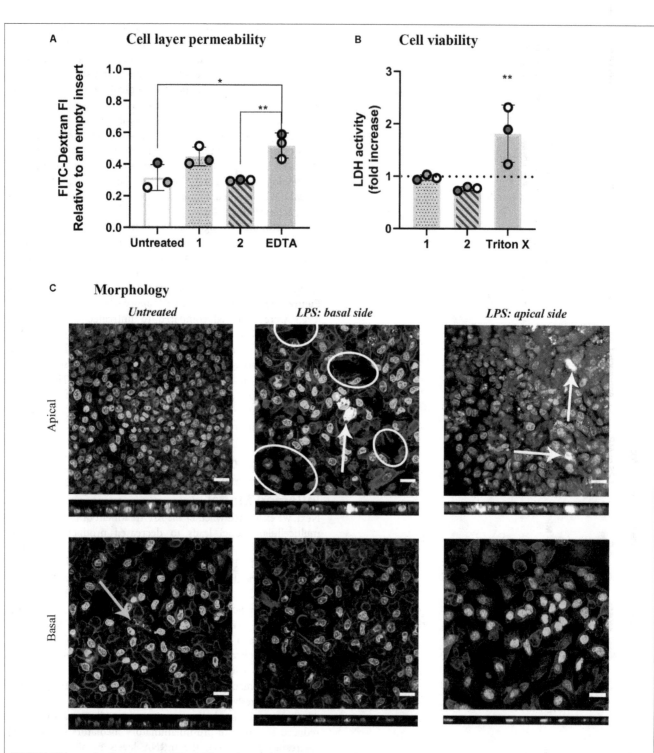

FIGURE 2 | The results of barrier permeability, viability, and morphology assessment of inflamed multicellular models after LPS challenge (1 μg/mL, 48 h) from either basal (approach 1) or apical compartment (approach 2). **(A)** Barrier permeability assessed via FITC-Dextran (70 kDa) permeability assay. The data is presented as fluorescence intensity of FITC-Dextran, measured in the basal compartment, normalized to the values of empty inserts, as the mean of three biological repetitions ± standard deviation. Individual values from biological repetitions are presented as circles, color-coded to represent the data from the same biological repetitions. EDTA (5 mM, 60 min) was used as a positive control for the barrier disruption analysis. **(B)** Cell viability assessed via a membrane rupture assay based on the LDH enzyme released in the cell culture medium of the basal compartment presented as fold increase over untreated cells (the dotted line). Positive control cells were apically exposed to Triton X-100 (0.2%; 24 h). Statistically significant differences among the groups (One-way ANOVA, Tukey's *post hoc*; α = 0.05) or to untreated cells (LDH assay): *$p \leq 0.05$; **$p \leq 0.01$. **(C)** Morphology, visualized via confocal laser scanning microscopy of apical and basal sides of the inserts, shown as XY and XZ projections. Immuno-fluorescence labeling: nuclei (cyan), cytoskeleton (magenta), MDMs (mature macrophage marker 25F9; white), MDDCs (CD 83; green). White ellipsoids point out the regions with epithelial barrier disruption. The white arrow denotes MDMs, whereas the green arrow denotes MDDCs. Scale bars are 20 μm.

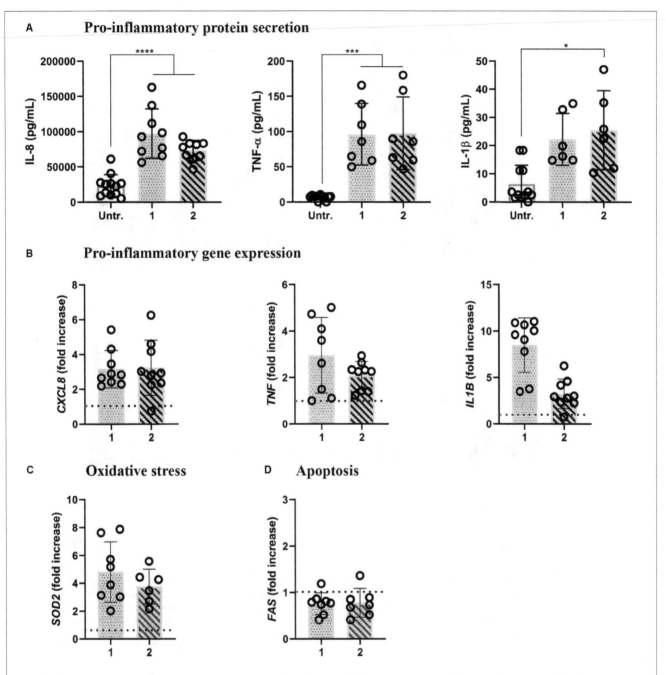

FIGURE 3 | Pro-inflammatory, oxidative stress, and apoptotic reactions in inflamed multicellular models upon LPS challenge (1 μg/mL, 48 h) from either basal (approach 1) or apical compartment (approach 2). **(A)** Secretion of pro-inflammatory mediators IL-8, TNF-α, and IL-1β (upper panel) and **(B)** the respective gene expressions (lower panel). The data for protein secretion are shown in pg/mL, measured in the basal compartment via ELISA. The data on gene expression, assessed via real-time RT-qPCR, is shown as a fold increase of mRNA calculated via the Δ ΔCt method, i.e., normalized to the expression of the housekeeping gene GAPDH and the expression of the gene of interest in the untreated samples. The dotted lines denote the mean values of the untreated cells. **(C)** Oxidative stress and **(D)** apoptotic gene expression levels, assessed via real-time RT-qPCR. Statistical analysis for ELISA was performed on pg/mL values using One-way ANOVA (Tukey's *post hoc*; α = 0.05). For gene expression, statistically significant differences compared to the untreated cells are shown. *$p \leq 0.05$; **$p \leq 0.01$; ***$p \leq 0.001$, ****$p \leq 0.0001$. Abbreviations: Untr., untreated models; IL-8, *CXCL8*, interleukin 8; TNF-α, *TNF*, tumor necrosis factor α; IL-1β, *IL1B*, interleukin1β; *SOD2*, superoxide dismutase; *FAS*, Fas cell surface death receptor.

exposure to MP for 24 h compared to positive controls ("LPS"; **Figure 4**), yet this was statistically significant for *CXCL8* in both approaches 3 and 4, *TNF* in approach 4 and *IL1B* in approach 3 (**Figure 6B**). Of the three mediators, MP treatment decreased the IL-8 level the most. A summary of results regarding pro-inflammatory mediator secretion and mRNA levels, along with the monoculture phenotype-associated endpoints, are presented in **Table 2**.

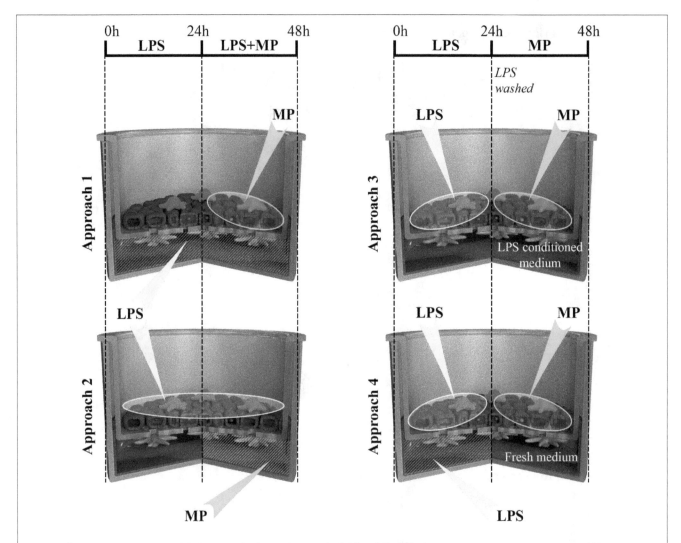

FIGURE 4 | Schematic representation of the four scenarios (approaches 1 to 4) of LPS and MP applications to the multicellular models. Multicellular human lung models, composed of alveolar epithelial cells (A549; red) and human monocyte-derived macrophages (MDMs; blue) and dendritic cells (MDDCs; green), were cultivated at the air-liquid interface conditions (ALI) for 24 h. Subsequently, the models were challenged with LPS (at time 0 h), followed by treatment with MP following four distinct approaches. **Approach 1**: LPS was applied in the basal compartment (1 µg/mL in 3 ml cRPMI), and after the first 24 h, MP was added to the apical side as a thin layer of liquid (i.e., at pseudo-ALI) at 10 or 100 µM, for an additional 24 h. **Approach 2**: LPS was added to the apical compartment at the pseudo-ALI for the first 24 h, and then MP was added in co-exposure from the basal compartment for the next 24 h. **Approach 3**: LPS, applied apically at the pseudo-ALI, was removed after 24 h, and the models were then exposed to the pre-conditioned medium during the MP treatment for an additional 24 h. **Approach 4**: Multicellular models were challenged with LPS both from the apical and basal compartment for 24 h. Then, LPS was removed from both the compartments, the model was washed, and a fresh cell-culture medium was applied during the MP treatment. Abbreviations: LPS, lipopolysaccharide; MP, methylprednisolone.

In all four approaches, the resolution of LPS-induced oxidative stress that had occurred in inflamed models (**Supplementary Figure S3**) was observed, as evidenced by increased levels of the mitochondrial antioxidant superoxide dismutase-2 (*SOD2*) compared to the positive control models ("LPS"; **Figure 4**). These trends were more pronounced in multicellular models treated through approaches 1 and 2, where LPS was applied for 48 h (**Supplementary Figure S3**). None of the treatments exerted notable effects on apoptotic gene expression levels (*FAS* mRNA levels; **Supplementary Figure S3b**). Morphology of the apical epithelial layer remained mostly unaffected after all of the treatments (**Figure 7**), similar to what was observed for untreated cells (**Figure 2C**); only in approaches 1 and 2 did the cell layer integrities appear to be slightly disrupted (**Figure 7A**). The morphological appearance remained unaltered after the apical or basal application of MP alone (**Figure 7D**) relative to the untreated counterparts (**Figure 2C**). These healthy models (in the absence of LPS) treated with MP alone served as a control to rule out the potential effects of MP alone. Exposure to MP at 100 µM both apically and basally did not induce changes in barrier integrity and cell viability (**Supplementary Figures S4a,b**). Levels of secreted IL-8, TNF-α, and IL-1β were lower than in the untreated cells, although the differences were not statistically significant. Similarly, the mRNA content

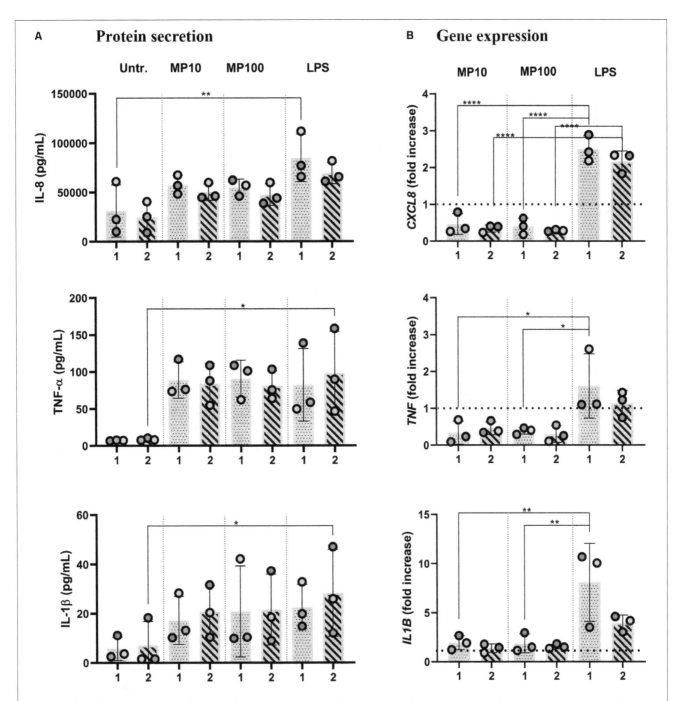

FIGURE 5 | Anti-inflammatory reactions after the addition of MP to inflamed multicellular models in the co-presence of LPS. The *x*-axis represents the number of the approach applied: approaches 1 and 2. Inflamed models were triggered with LPS from either basal (approach 1) or apical (approach 2) compartments for 24 h; then, MP was applied to the opposite compartment for an additional 24 h at 10 or 100 μM. **(A)** Secretion of pro-inflammatory mediators IL-8, TNF-α, and IL-1β and **(B)** the respective gene expressions. The data of protein secretion is shown in pg/mL, measured in the basal compartment via ELISA. The data on gene expression, assessed via real-time RT-qPCR, is shown as fold increase of mRNA calculated via the Δ ΔCt method, i.e., normalized to the expression of the housekeeping gene *GAPDH* and the expression of the gene of interest in the untreated samples. Dotted lines denote the mean value of untreated cells. Statistical analysis for ELISA was performed on pg/mL values using One-way ANOVA (Tukey's *post hoc*; α = 0.05). For gene expression, statistically significant differences to untreated cells are shown. *$p \leq 0.05$; **$p \leq 0.01$; ***$p \leq 0.001$, ****$p \leq 0.0001$. Abbreviations: Untr.: untreated models; MP10 and MP100: models treated with LPS (24 h) followed by methylprednisolone at 10 or 100 μM for an additional 24 h; LPS: positive control models, i.e., treated with LPS for 48 h.

was slightly reduced in all MP-treated samples, with the most pronounced effect observed for *CXCL8* (**Supplementary Figure S4c**). MP treatment resulted in a slight reduction in *SOD2*

mRNA levels in approaches 1 and 2 (**Supplementary Figure S4d**) while leading to a modest increase in the mRNA level of the apoptotic gene *FAS* (**Supplementary Figure S4e**). Given the small

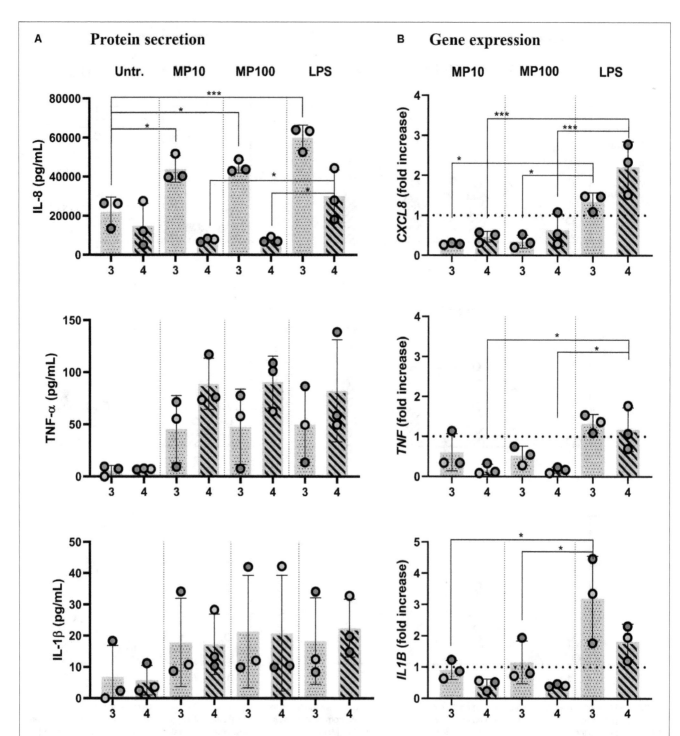

FIGURE 6 | Anti-inflammatory reactions after addition of MP to inflamed multicellular models upon removal of LPS. The x-axis represents the number of the approach applied: approaches 3 and 4. Inflamed models were triggered with LPS from the basal compartment (approach 3) or both sides (approach 4) for 24 h. Then, either LPS was removed from the apical side with the cRPMI left in during the apical MP treatment (approach 3) or cRPMI was removed, and inserts were thoroughly washed before MP application (approach 4) for an additional 24 h, at 10 or 100 μM MP. **(A)** Secretion of pro-inflammatory mediators IL-8, TNF-α, and IL-1β and **(B)** the respective gene expressions. The data of protein secretion is shown in pg/mL, measured in the basal compartment via ELISA. The data on gene expression, assessed via real-time RT-qPCR, is shown as fold increase of mRNA calculated via the Δ ΔCt method, i.e., normalized to the expression of the housekeeping gene *GAPDH* and the expression of the gene of interest in the untreated samples. The dotted lines denote the mean value of untreated cells. Statistical analysis for ELISA was performed on pg/mL values using One-way ANOVA (Tukey's *post hoc*; α = 0.05). For gene expression, statistically significant differences to untreated cells are shown. $*p \leq 0.05$; $**p \leq 0.01$; $***p \leq 0.001$. Abbreviations: Untr., untreated models; MP10 and MP100, models treated with LPS (24 h) followed by methylprednisolone at 10 or 100 μM for additional 24 h; LPS, positive control models, i.e., treated with LPS for 24 h, then washed accordingly and treated with the vehicle instead of MP.

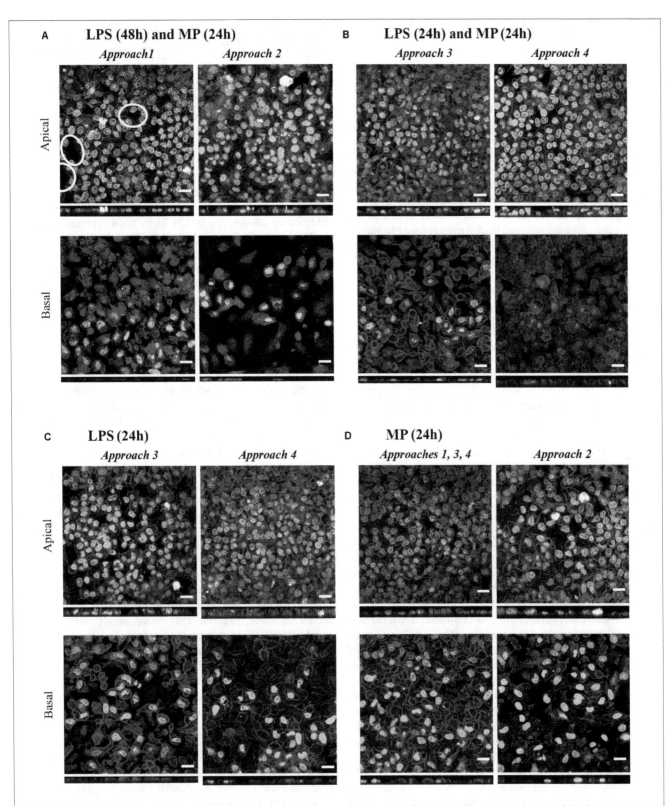

FIGURE 7 | Confocal microscopy images representing the tissue morphology upon exposures to LPS+MP, and LPS or MP alone for 24 h. Multicellular models were treated with **(A)** LPS (24 h + 24 h) and MP at 100 μM from either apical (approach 1) or basal (approach 2) compartments, with **(B)** LPS (24 h) and MP at 100 μM (24 h) corresponding to approaches 3 and 4, respectively **(C)** LPS (24 h) corresponds to the positive controls in approaches 3 and 4. **(D)** MP control tissues, treated only with MP at 100 μM (24 h) from either apical (approaches 1, 3, 4) or basal (approach 2) compartments. Confocal laser scanning microscopy of apical and basal sides of the inserts, shown as XY and XZ projections. Immuno-fluorescence labeling: nuclei (cyan), cytoskeleton (magenta), MDMs (mature macrophage marker 25F9; white), MDDCs (CD 83; green). White ellipsoids point out the regions with epithelial barrier disruption. Scale bars are 20 μm.

degree of differences, however, we considered these effects as biologically insignificant.

DISCUSSION

In this study, we present a multicellular human lung model and the resolution of LPS-induced inflammation *in vitro* using a corticosteroid drug, MP. Four experimental approaches to pro-inflammation induction and its suppression are presented, mimicking various scenarios of lung inflammation and treatment in clinics. As alveolar macrophages are the main actors in the induction and resolution of pro-inflammatory reactions in the tissue, we discuss the anti-inflammatory effects of MP considering its priming potential to shift macrophage phenotypes towards the anti-inflammatory subset and with the potential to reduce pro-inflammatory reactions *in vitro* (**Table 2**).

Pro-inflammatory Reactions and Impaired Alveolar Barrier Integrity in Inflamed Models

Initially, we used a previously established multicellular model of the human alveolar epithelium (Bisig et al., 2019; Barosova et al., 2020) to induce an inflammatory model via a 48-h challenge with LPS. The LPS was applied either from the basal side of the models simulating a systemically derived alveolar inflammation or from the apical side mimicking the source of the tissue inflammation derived from inhaled stimulants. Microbial products such as LPS are a widely used pro-inflammatory stimulus in *in vitro* assays because of their prominent activity to stimulate innate immune responses (Rosadini and Kagan, 2017). The primary mechanism of LPS-induced response begins through its action towards the toll-like receptor 4 (TLR-4), which is present on both of the immune cell types within the model, i.e., macrophages and dendritic cells (Visintin et al., 2001; Fekete et al., 2012). Upon activation of TLR-4, the onset of the nuclear factor kappa B (NF-kB) signaling pathway results in an increase in the secretion of pro-inflammatory cytokines and chemokines, such as the main actor of central inflammation, TNF-α, and interleukins, e.g., IL-1 (Beutler, 2000; Nova et al., 2019). As LPS-induced macrophage phenotype shifts towards M1 have been observed (Wang et al., 2014; Lu et al., 2018; Orecchioni et al., 2019), we employed LPS as the pro-inflammatory stimulus in both the macrophage monocultures and multicellular experiments.

The onset of pro-inflammatory reactions of both the mono- and multicellular models upon LPS challenge can be explained by the high expression of TLR-4 in mononuclear cells (Beutler and Rietschel, 2003; Lawrence and Natoli, 2011), i.e., MDMs and MDDCs. Additionally, the CD14 receptor present in these cells is also involved in the extracellular binding of LPS, which contributes to the initiation of the NF-kB signaling cascade (Beutler, 2000; Lu et al., 2008). Stimulation of MDM monocultures with LPS induced secretion of pro-inflammatory mediators (IL-8, TNF-α) depleted the mannose receptor (CD206) expression (**Figure 1**) and slightly increased CD86 expression, which are established markers of M2 and M1 activation, respectively (Lawrence and Natoli, 2011; Smith et al., 2016). It

is important to note that the classical division into distinctive macrophage phenotypes has been questioned in multiple studies, which have proposed that cells adopt a mixed phenotype depending on the stimuli present in their microenvironment, rather than polarization into two distinctive phenotypes (Smith et al., 2016; Atri et al., 2018; Orecchioni et al., 2019). M-CSF, used for monocytes differentiation into macrophages, is also very effective in polarizing macrophages towards the M2 phenotype (Fleetwood et al., 2007; Orecchioni et al., 2019). In fact, by the time we removed the M-CSF from the MDM differentiation culture, the cells were already skewed towards the M2 phenotype, and the addition of LPS might not have been a strong enough stimulus to trigger surface marker expression alterations. The addition of interferon-γ to LPS likely has a synergistic effect of facilitating skewing towards the M1 phenotype along with LPS, as was observed in parallel experiments (data not shown) and in previous reports (Müller et al., 2017; Orecchioni et al., 2019). In this study, however, we focused on LPS-challenged MDMs to compare the onset and suppression of pro-inflammatory reactions between a 2D monoculture setting and more realistic exposures in 3D models.

It should be noted that in *in vivo* settings, macrophages and dendritic cells both respond to microbial danger signals by secretion of inflammatory cytokines and interact with the alveolar epithelial cells as well as one another (Banchereau and Steinman, 1998; Beutler and Rietschel, 2003; Gordon, 2003; Fekete et al., 2012; Cook and MacDonald, 2016). Therefore, *in vitro* multicellular models simulate *in vivo* settings more faithfully than do 2D monocultures (Fitzgerald et al., 2015), as they enable an interplay between the three relevant cell types of alveolar epithelial tissue to take place *in vitro* (Rothen-Rutishauser et al., 2005; Blank et al., 2007). In addition to the immune cells in the model, epithelial cells themselves are also responsive to a pro-inflammatory stimulus, such as LPS (Guillot et al., 2004). LPS stimulation of monocultures of A549 cells results in increased pro-inflammatory marker secretion (IL-8, TNF-α) and the respective gene expression (CXCL8 and TNFA). However, the pro-inflammatory response is significantly lower as compared to that in the co-culture model including immune cells (Bisig et al., 2019; Barosova et al., 2020). Indeed, we observed more pronounced pro-inflammatory reactions in the inflamed multicellular alveolar models, regardless of the side of LPS application, relative to their untreated counterparts (**Figure 3**). However, it is important to note that stressor-induced inflammation in a tissue is a highly complex process involving a combination of events. According to the recently proposed adverse outcome pathway (AOP) framework (Villeneuve et al., 2018), the pro-inflammatory reactions observed in our experiments can be classified as part of the second general key event (KE2): increased pro-inflammatory mediators and a loss of the alveolar barrier integrity (Villeneuve et al., 2018) due to tight junction disruption (Chignard and Balloy, 2000; Eutamene et al., 2005). The latter was observed in the multicellular model upon 48 h of basal LPS exposure (approach 1; **Figure 2A**). Reduced barrier integrity upon basal LPS challenge (approach 1) was also confirmed by the change in the morphological appearance of the multicellular models.

In essence, distinctive patches of ruptured tissue were observed on the apical side of the inserts, whereas the confluency of the apical cell layer in approach 2 was comparable to untreated cells (**Figure 2C**). As we have shown earlier that tight junctions in A549 appear irregularly (Hilton et al., 2019) we did not perform a tight junction staining but assessed the barrier integrity by a permeability assay using FITC-dextran. This suggests that the cytokines released by the MDDCs, present on the basal side of the multicellular model, may affect tight junctions in the epithelial barrier via the release of pro-inflammatory cytokines (Prakash et al., 2014; Agrawal, 2017) and it seems that MDMs are more effective at resolving the inflammation. Consequently, the epithelial permeability is enhanced, which, in *in vivo* settings, allows for infiltration of immune cells at the site of infection/inflammation (Martin et al., 1997). Our observations thus suggest that our inflamed multicellular model can mimic a combination of inflammation-distinctive features in the human lung tissue.

Oxidative and apoptotic reactions are other hallmarks of LPS-induced tissue inflammation (Mukhopadhyay et al., 2006; Ma et al., 2010; Nova et al., 2019). Expression of an oxidative stress-related gene, a mitochondrial antioxidant, manganese-dependent superoxide dismutase (MnSOD) SOD2 was upregulated in the LPS-challenged multicellular models as compared to untreated cells (**Figure 2C**). This result is in line with observations of LPS-challenged monocytes, macrophage cell lines, and primary cells *in vitro*, where SOD2 upregulation is associated with the NF-kB pathway activation (Sharif et al., 2007; Widdrington et al., 2018). Another reason for the increased SOD2 expression can be attributed to MDDCs (Jin et al., 2010). In our untreated multicellular models, MDDCs induced by GM-CSF and IL-4 remain in their immature state, with the ability to take up and process antigen (Fekete et al., 2012). When the models are stimulated with LPS, MDDCs undergo their maturation process, which is accompanied by a 28-fold upregulation of SOD2 in 24 h (Jin et al., 2010). Activation of the Fas-mediated apoptosis pathway has been reported to play a key role in inflammation-induced damage of the alveolar epithelium (Ma et al., 2010). In our study, we did not observe a statistically significant upregulation of FAS mRNA levels, nor was there any increase in cell membrane rupture as a measure of cell viability in either multicellular models or monoculture (**Figures 1C, 2B**, and **Supplementary Figure S2a**). This was nevertheless expected, as we had chosen a sub-cytotoxic LPS concentration based on our previous studies (Bisig et al., 2019).

Anti-inflammatory Reactions Induced With Corticosteroids

In the next step of the study, we treated the inflamed monocultures and multicellular models with a known anti-inflammatory therapy, corticosteroids. Corticosteroids exert anti-inflammatory activity through their binding to corticosteroid hormone receptors, and this process operates via several molecular mechanisms (Barnes, 2011). When corticosteroids bind to glucocorticoid receptors (GR), which are expressed in almost all cell types, the resulting GR-glucocorticoid complex

can take either of two paths: (i) the activated GR complex upregulates the expression of anti-inflammatory proteins the nucleus or (ii) the GR complex represses the expression of pro-inflammatory cytokines and chemokines, or their mRNA degradation (Barnes, 2011).

In the monoculture experiments, we investigated the effect of MP on the priming of inflamed MDMs towards the anti-inflammatory M2 phenotype, as has been reported for MP and other corticosteroids in ex vivo and *in vitro* human and *in vivo* animal studies (Frankenberger et al., 2005; Tu et al., 2017; Desgeorges et al., 2019; Xie et al., 2019). We observed decreased IL-8 and TNF-α secretions and CD86 expression, together with increased CD206 expression, relative to that of LPS-treated cells, albeit without statistical significance among the two groups (**Figure 1** and **Supplementary Figure S2**; **Table 2**). Thus, these findings suggest that MP inhibits the secretion of pro-inflammatory mediators but does not appear to reprogram the MDM phenotype. A possible reason for the absence of more pronounced differences in cellular phenotypes upon MP treatment in our study is that LPS was not removed from the medium before the MP treatment in order to make the environment comparable with approaches 1 and 2 of the multicellular system. However, as discussed above, the M1/M2 paradigm should not be perceived as two distinctive sub-populations, but rather as a continuum of macrophage polarization states (Edholm et al., 2017; Tu et al., 2017). Therefore, our findings on the increased percentage of M2-associated surface markers accompanied by decreased M1 markers present a valid observation, and suggest that MP helped to balance the macrophage population by shifting them towards the anti-inflammatory phenotype.

Furthermore, in multicellular models, the efficiency of MP in dampening pro-inflammatory reactions was confirmed in models in all of the four different experimental settings applied herein. Overall, the reduction of inflammation compared to the positive controls ("LPS") was comparable among the four approaches (summarized in **Table 2**). Consistent trends were observed in the resolution of LPS-induced inflammation by MP (**Figure 5**). Analogous to the monoculture data (**Figures 1A,B**), the absence of a potent anti-inflammatory effect can be attributed to the simultaneous presence of LPS during the anti-inflammatory treatment. Our findings suggest that the multicellular model recapitulated the effect of MP treatment observed in the monocellular culture of MDMs (summarized in **Table 2**), but potentially with delayed kinetics. In fact, the *in vivo* immunosuppressive properties of corticosteroids, including MP, are primarily associated with their influence on macrophages and T lymphocytes (Coutinho and Chapman, 2011), yet their immunosuppressive effect on dendritic cells and alveolar epithelial cells should not be neglected (Zach et al., 1993; Piemonti et al., 1999; Rozkova et al., 2006; Klaßen et al., 2017). Therefore, it is vital to use an immunocompetent multicellular lung model, i.e., one including immune cells along with epithelial cells, to achieve a realistic assessment of the anti-inflammatory and immunosuppressive actions of corticosteroids. Namely, by applying LPS in the basal compartment and the drug at the apical side (approach 1), we mimicked a systemic inflammation caused by blood-derived danger signals and an anti-inflammatory treatment via inhalation. Vice versa, in approach 2, alveolar inflammation was mimicked by applying LPS apically and MP in the basal compartment, simulating an intravenous steroid therapy (**Figure 4**). Our findings of reduced pro-inflammation in approaches 1 and 2 suggest that MP can be used as an anti-inflammatory drug to model corticosteroid therapy of severe alveolar inflammation in the absence of other treatments that facilitate the resolution of inflammation (such as an antibiotic-based bacteria elimination).

Having demonstrated that a reduction of pro-inflammatory reactions can be assessed *in vitro* in the presence of the stimulus, we developed this test system further by reducing the inflammation. With these *in vitro* conditions, we simulated *in vivo* settings involving pre- or concurrent therapy with agents other than corticosteroids (approaches 3 and 4; **Figure 4**). Similar trends in the reduction of secretion of the pro-inflammatory mediators and their respective mRNA levels (**Figure 6**) were observed as in the MP treatments following the previous two approaches (**Figure 5** and **Table 2**). The mildly disrupted cell layer integrities in approaches 1 and 2 (**Figure 7A**) can be attributed to the extended LPS challenge (48 vs. 24 h), as similar disintegration of the apical cell layer was observed for the positive control models, i.e., those treated with LPS for 48 h (**Figure 2C**), and less disintegration was observed after 24 h (**Figure 7B**). Overall, inflamed models treated with MP presented higher cell-layer integrity than positive control samples (LPS), especially those following approach 3 (**Figures 2C, 7**). This was expected, however, as MP has been demonstrated to lead to complete resolution of *in vivo* and *in vitro* mechanical and histological lung alterations in mice (Silva et al., 2009). Furthermore, a minimal reduction of pro-inflammatory reactions in healthy tissues was observed upon treatment with MP for all the pro-inflammatory mediators (**Supplementary Figure S4c**). A possible explanation for this is that the assembly of the immunocompetent multicellular human lung model itself triggers a certain amount of pro-inflammatory response, which can then be further reduced with an anti-inflammatory drug. This is indeed consistent with the common side effects of steroid drugs, which can also affect untargeted, healthy cells and tissues (Waljee et al., 2017).

We observed high variations, especially in the cytokine secretion data upon treatment with MP (**Figures 5A, 6A, Supplementary Figure S4c**). This can be explained by biological variations of the immune cell source. First, for each experiment, i.e., for each biological replicate, human blood-derived monocytes were isolated from a different blood donor. Second, the medical history of blood donors cannot be revealed due to ethical reasons; thus, it was unknown whether the patient had an ongoing inflammation and/or treatment at the time of blood sampling. Therefore, we consider that the high variations in our results reflect the variability in donors and not the poor robustness of our model.

The anti-inflammatory activity of MP appeared to be independent of the doses tested. In approaches 1, 3, and 4, MP was applied at the pseudo-ALI in concentrations of 10

and 100 μM, whereas in approach 2, MP was diluted with 1.2 mL of cRPMI, with the same final concentrations of 10 and 100 μM. We set two main criteria for the development of our *in vitro* system: (i) the pro-inflammatory reactions fall within a comparable range irrespective of the side of LPS application (as explained under inflamed model) (Bisig et al., 2019; Barosova et al., 2020), and (ii) MP is applied at a clinically relevant dose (Vichyanond et al., 1989) which is high enough to promote anti-inflammatory reactions in an *in vitro* system without causing adverse effects on the tissues. Overall, the concentrations tested in the study (10 or 100 μM) are in the range of MP concentrations evaluated in human bronchioalveolar fluid upon intravenous drug administration, i.e., 2000 ng/mL [corresponding to 5.2 μM (Vichyanond et al., 1989)] and are in line with the doses tested in the *in vivo* and *in vitro* study of the effects of MP on mice macrophage polarization (Tu et al., 2017).

Clinical Significance

In a clinical setting, MP is predominantly administered intravenously or orally (Kinoshita et al., 2017; Meduri et al., 2018), while other corticosteroid drugs, such as budesonide and formoterol, have proven clinical benefits when inhaled (Barnes, 2011). However, the aim of this study was not to evaluate the action of MP by itself but rather to show the responsiveness of the model to corticosteroid treatment *in vitro*. The purpose of this study was to develop a versatile *in vitro* system to test newly developed drugs, including nanoparticle-based candidates, for the treatment of lung inflammation.

In all of the tested approaches to LPS and MP applications, an efficient reduction of pro-inflammatory reactions was observed at both the protein secretion and gene expression levels (**Table 2**). The authors recommend assessment of the suppression of pro-inflammatory reactions at the gene expression level for inclusion in the endpoint assessment because the decrease in these reactions was more evident than the changes in the secretion of pro-inflammatory factors. In particular, IL-8 (*CXCL8*) yielded the most significant differences among the tested markers (**Table 2**). Our model provides a flexible choice of the scenarios to test novel drug candidates, depending on the research question. For example, if testing the efficiency of a systemically administered drug is the aim, approach 2 can be employed (**Figure 4**). This approach also showed the most pronounced reduction of pro-inflammatory reactions at both protein secretion and gene expression levels (**Table 2**). In contrast, to test candidates for pulmonary drug delivery, approaches 1, 3, and 4 can be followed. Furthermore, a decrease in barrier integrity was observed for the basal application of LPS for 48 h (approach 1). Therefore, where the AOP framework for inflammation and fibrosis (Villeneuve et al., 2018; Halappanavar et al., 2020) is applied, the use of approach 1 is recommended. When a newly developed therapy is envisaged in a combined treatment with, for example, antibiotics, approach 3 or 4 can be employed to test the anti-inflammatory activities of the candidate when the source of inflammation (bacteria) is removed from the microenvironment. Another advantage of the multiple approaches adopted in our study is that the action of the tested drug in respiratory and systemic delivery models can be compared using approaches 1 and 2, respectively. The advantage of creating such a model is that the interplay between the representative cell types is now in an *in vitro* human lung setting, which successfully mimics several key aspects of an *in vivo* setting.

Depending on the stimulus of interest and the research question, additional cell types can also be added to the model, or part of the model elements can be replaced with a relevant type. For the purpose of this study to showcase the responsiveness of the model, A549 have been selected as the epithelial cell type as they are the most widely used cell lines in human respiratory research. An important feature of A549-based model is that surfactant is secreted at the apical surface when cultivated at the air-liquid interface, a key feature to recapitulate *in vivo* conditions in the model. The A549 cell model also has been used to assess the biokinetic distribution of apically administered liposomal Ciclosporin A, and the data was in agreement with the clinically observed pharmacokinetics profile (Schmid et al., 2017). Thus, this model offers a reliable and relevant *in vitro* platform to study the effects of aerosolized substances. Furthermore, depending on the research question and availability of cells the epithelial cells can be replaced for instance with bronchial cells such as the bronchial cell line 16HBE14o-, or with primary alveolar type I-like cells (Lehmann et al., 2011). Importantly, the choice of immune cells is also versatile. Epithelial cells can be co-cultured with other immune cells, such as natural killer cells (Roth et al., 2017). Immune cells such as macrophages can be replaced with differentiated macrophage-like cells (THP-1), and mast cells and/or endothelial cells can be included in similar models (Klein et al., 2013). Additionally, inclusion of polymorphonuclear cells, such as neutrophils, is foreseen, which would, for instance, enable exploration of neutrophil transepithelial migration. However, the importance of other barriers and immune cells needs to be explored in future studies.

An interesting future application of the presented model could be to compare the responsiveness of the model triggered with LPS with the reactions upon stimulation with other inflammatory agents derived from organic dust, such as mold spores (mold antigens). The latter model resembles, for example, a specific respiratory syndrome such as hypersensitivity pneumonitis or extrinsic allergic alveolitis (Riario Sforza and Marinou, 2017) where MP has been used as one of the main treatment drugs (Buchvald et al., 2011).

In conclusion, we have established an *in vitro* human 3D multicellular alveolar epithelial model that is responsive to both pro-inflammatory stimulation and anti-inflammatory treatment. Responses of the model correlated well with phenotypic shifts of macrophages, highlighting their importance in the faithful reproduction of *in vivo* settings. Supported by the use of permeable membranes, our new model also enables the assessment of the permeability of agents through the barrier. Further development is aimed at coupling our multicellular human lung models with an aerosolization system to assess the efficiency of nebulized compounds. Given that a large number of researchers are currently exploring novel anti-inflammatory formulations, and in particular nanoparticle-based candidates intended for administration via inhalation, we anticipate that our "inflammable" human lung model will serve as a versatile and realistic toolkit for efficient evaluation of the efficiency and safety of various drug candidates.

ETHICS STATEMENT

The work involving primary monocytes isolated from human blood was approved by the committee of the Federal Office for Public Health Switzerland (reference number: 611-1, Meldung A110635/2) for the Adolphe Merkle Institute. Written informed consent for participation was not required for this study in accordance with the national legislation and the institutional requirements.

AUTHOR CONTRIBUTIONS

BD designed and planned the study, carried out majority of the experiments, analyzed and interpreted the data, and finally drafted the manuscript. BK and ET supported the planning and execution of the tissue culture experiments, and BK also supported the writing process of the main text. HB assisted with monocyte isolation and multicellular model experiments. JA provided expert knowledge on flow cytometry. MS provided lab support with the real-time RT-PCR experiments. AP-F and BR-R were involved in the planning and technical advisory of the study and critically revised the manuscript draft for important intellectual content and approved publication of the content. All authors contributed to the article and approved the submitted version.

ACKNOWLEDGMENTS

The authors would like to thank Dr. Miguel Spuch-Calvar for the multicellular human lung model scheme in **Figure 4**.

REFERENCES

Agrawal, A. (2017). Dendritic cell-airway epithelial cell cross-talk changes with age and contributes to chronic lung inflammatory diseases in the elderly. *Int. J. Mol. Sci.* 18:1206. doi: 10.3390/ijms18061206

Artzy-Schnirman, A., Lehr, C.-M., and Sznitman, J. (2020). Advancing human in vitro pulmonary disease models in preclinical research: opportunities for lung-on-chips. *Expert Opin. Drug Deliv.* 17, 621–625. doi: 10.1080/17425247.2020.1738380

Atri, C., Guerfali, F. Z., and Laouini, D. (2018). Role of human macrophage polarization in inflammation during infectious diseases. *Int. J. Mol. Sci.* 19:1801. doi: 10.3390/ijms19061801

Banchereau, J., and Steinman, R. M. (1998). Dendritic cells and the control of immunity. *Nature* 392, 245–252. doi: 10.1038/32588

Barnes, P. J. (2011). Glucocorticosteroids: current and future directions. *Br. J. Pharmacol.* 163, 29–43. doi: 10.1111/j.1476-5381.2010.01199.x

Barosova, H., Drasler, B., Petri-Fink, A., and Rothen-Rutishauser, B. (2020). Multicellular human alveolar model composed of epithelial cells and primary immune cells for hazard assessment. *J. Vis. Exp.* 6:e61090. doi: 10.3791/61090

Beutler, B. (2000). Tlr4: central component of the sole mammalian LPS sensor. *Curr. Opin. Immunol.* 12, 20–26. doi: 10.1016/S0952-7915(99)00046-1

Beutler, B., and Rietschel, E. T. (2003). Innate immune sensing and its roots: the story of endotoxin. *Nat. Rev. Immunol.* 3, 169–176. doi: 10.1038/nri1004

Bisig, C., Voss, C., Petri-Fink, A., and Rothen-Rutishauser, B. (2019). The crux of positive controls - Pro-inflammatory responses in lung cell models. *Toxicol. Vitro* 54, 189–193. doi: 10.1016/j.tiv.2018.09.021

Blank, F., Rothen-Rutishauser, B., and Gehr, P. (2007). Dendritic cells and macrophages form a transepithelial network against foreign particulate antigens. *Am. J. Respir. Cell Mol. Biol.* 36, 669–677. doi: 10.1165/rcmb.2006-0234OC

Blank, F., Rothen-Rutishauser, B. M., Schurch, S., and Gehr, P. (2006). An optimized *in vitro* model of the respiratory tract wall to study particle cell interactions. *J. Aerosol. Med.* 19, 392–405. doi: 10.1089/jam.2006.19.392

Brain, J. D. (1988). Lung macrophages: how many kinds are there? What do they do? *Am. Rev. Respir. Dis.* 137, 507–509. doi: 10.1164/ajrccm/137.3.507

Buchvald, F., Petersen, B. L., Damgaard, K., Deterding, R., Langston, C., Fan, L. L., et al. (2011). Frequency, treatment, and functional outcome in children with hypersensitivity pneumonitis. *Pediatr. Pulmonol.* 46, 1098–1107. doi: 10.1002/ppul.21479

Bur, M., and Lehr, C. M. (2008). Pulmonary cell culture models to study the safety and efficacy of innovative aerosol medicines. *Expert Opin. Drug Deliv.* 5, 641–652. doi: 10.1517/17425247.5.6.641

Castellani, S., Di Gioia, S., di Toma, L., and Conese, M. (2018). Human cellular models for the investigation of lung inflammation and mucus production in cystic fibrosis. *Anal. Cell. Pathol.* 2018:3839803. doi: 10.1155/2018/3839803

Chana, K. K., Fenwick, P. S., Nicholson, A. G., Barnes, P. J., and Donnelly, L. E. (2014). Identification of a distinct glucocorticosteroid-insensitive pulmonary macrophage phenotype in patients with chronic obstructive pulmonary disease. *J. Allergy Clin. Immunol.* 133, 207.e1–e11–216.e1–e11. doi: 10.1016/j.jaci.2013.08.044

Chignard, M., and Balloy, V. (2000). Neutrophil recruitment and increased permeability during acute lung injury induced by lipopolysaccharide. *Am. J. Physiol. Lung. Cell Mol. Physiol.* 279, L1083–L1090. doi: 10.1152/ajplung.2000.279.6.L1083

Condon, T. V., Sawyer, R. T., Fenton, M. J., and Riches, D. W. H. (2011). Lung dendritic cells at the innate-adaptive immune interface. *J. Leukoc. Biol.* 90, 883–895. doi: 10.1189/jlb.0311134

Cook, P. C., and MacDonald, A. S. (2016). Dendritic cells in lung immunopathology. *Semin. Immunopathol.* 38, 449–460. doi: 10.1007/s00281-016-0571-3

Costa, A., de Souza Carvalho-Wodarz, C., Seabra, V., Sarmento, B., and Lehr, C. M. (2019). Triple co-culture of human alveolar epithelium, endothelium and macrophages for studying the interaction of nanocarriers with the air-blood barrier. *Acta Biomater.* 91, 235–247. doi: 10.1016/j.actbio.2019.04.037

Coutinho, A. E., and Chapman, K. E. (2011). The anti-inflammatory and immunosuppressive effects of glucocorticoids, recent developments and mechanistic insights. *Mol. Cell. Endocrinol.* 335, 2–13. doi: 10.1016/j.mce.2010.04.005

da Silva, A. L., Cruz, F. F., Rocco, P. R. M., and Morales, M. M. (2017). New perspectives in nanotherapeutics for chronic respiratory diseases. *Biophys. Rev.* 9, 793–803. doi: 10.1007/s12551-017-0319-x

Desgeorges, T., Caratti, G., Mounier, R., Tuckermann, J., and Chazaud, B. (2019). Glucocorticoids shape macrophage phenotype for tissue repair. *Front. Immunol.* 10:1591. doi: 10.3389/fimmu.2019.01591

Edholm, E.-S., Rhoo, K. H., and Robert, J. (2017). Evolutionary aspects of macrophages polarization. *Results Probl. Cell Differ.* 62, 3–22. doi: 10.1007/978-3-319-54090-0_1

Endes, C., Schmid, O., Kinnear, C., Mueller, S., Camarero-Espinosa, S., Vanhecke, D., et al. (2014). An in vitro testing strategy towards mimicking the inhalation of high aspect ratio nanoparticles. *Part. Fibre Toxicol.* 11:40. doi: 10.1186/s12989-014-0040-x

Eutamene, H., Theodorou, V., Schmidlin, F., Tondereau, V., Garcia-Villar, R., Salvador-Cartier, C., et al. (2005). LPS-induced lung inflammation is linked to increased epithelial permeability: role of MLCK. *Eur. Respir. J.* 25, 789–796. doi: 10.1183/09031936.05.00064704

Fekete, T., Szabo, A., Beltrame, L., Vivar, N., Pivarcsi, A., Lanyi, A., et al. (2012). Constraints for monocyte-derived dendritic cell functions under inflammatory conditions. *Eur. J. Immunol.* 42, 458–469. doi: 10.1002/eji.201141924

Fitzgerald, K. A., Malhotra, M., Curtin, C. M., Brien, F. J. O., and O'Driscoll, C. M. (2015). Life in 3D is never flat: 3D models to optimise drug delivery. *J. Control. Release* 215, 39–54. doi: 10.1016/j.jconrel.2015.07.020

Fleetwood, A. J., Lawrence, T., Hamilton, J. A., and Cook, A. D. (2007). Granulocyte-macrophage colony-stimulating factor (CSF) and macrophage CSF-Dependent macrophage phenotypes display differences in cytokine profiles and transcription factor activities: implications for CSF blockade in inflammation. *J. Immunol.* 178, 5245–5252. doi: 10.4049/jimmunol.178.8.5245

Florentin, J., Coppin, E., Vasamsetti, S. B., Zhao, J., Tai, Y.-Y., Tang, Y., et al. (2018). Inflammatory macrophage expansion in pulmonary hypertension depends upon mobilization of blood-borne monocytes. *J. Immunol.* 200, 3612–3625. doi: 10.4049/jimmunol.1701287

Frankenberger, M., Haussinger, K., and Ziegler-Heitbrock, L. (2005). Liposomal methylprednisolone differentially regulates the expression of TNF and IL-10 in human alveolar macrophages. *Int. Immunopharmacol.* 5, 289–299. doi: 10.1016/j.intimp.2004.09.033

Gordon, S. (2003). Alternative activation of macrophages. *Nat. Rev. Immunol.* 3, 23–35. doi: 10.1038/nri978

Guillot, L., Medjane, S., Le-Barillec, K., Balloy, V., Danel, C., Chignard, M., et al. (2004). Response of human pulmonary epithelial cells to lipopolysaccharide involves Toll-like receptor 4 (TLR4) dependent signaling pathways: evidence for an intracellular compartmentalization of TLR4. *J. Biol. Chem.* 279, 2712–2718. doi: 10.1074/jbc.M305790200

Habermehl, D., Parkitna, J. R., Kaden, S., Brügger, B., Wieland, F., Gröne, H. J., et al. (2011). Glucocorticoid activity during lung maturation is essential in mesenchymal and less in alveolar epithelial cells. *Mol. Endocrinol.* 25, 1280–1288. doi: 10.1210/me.2009-0380

Haghi, M., Hittinger, M., Zeng, Q., Oliver, B., Traini, D., Young, P. M., et al. (2015). Mono- and cocultures of bronchial and alveolar epithelial cells respond differently to proinflammatory stimuli and their modulation by salbutamol and budesonide. *Mol. Pharm.* 12, 2625–2632. doi: 10.1021/acs.molpharmaceut.5b00124

Halappanavar, S., van den Brule, S., Nymark, P., Gaté, L., Seidel, C., Valentino, S., et al. (2020). Adverse outcome pathways as a tool for the design of testing strategies to support the safety assessment of emerging advanced materials at the nanoscale. *Part. Fibre Toxicol.* 17:16. doi: 10.1186/s12989-020-00344-4

Hermanns, M. I., Unger, R. E., Kehe, K., Peters, K., and Kirkpatrick, C. J. (2004). Lung epithelial cell lines in coculture with human pulmonary microvascular endothelial cells: development of an alveolo-capillary barrier in vitro. *Lab. Invest.* 84, 736–752. doi: 10.1038/labinvest.3700081

Higham, A., Booth, G., Lea, S., Southworth, T., Plumb, J., and Singh, D. (2015). The effects of corticosteroids on COPD lung macrophages: a pooled analysis. *Respir. Res.* 16:98. doi: 10.1186/s12931-015-0260-0

Hilton, G., Barosova, H., Petri-Fink, A., Rothen-Rutishauser, B., and Bereman, M. (2019). Leveraging proteomics to compare submerged versus air-liquid interface carbon nanotube exposure to a 3D lung cell model. *Toxicol. In Vitro* 54, 58–66. doi: 10.1016/j.tiv.2018.09.010

Hittinger, M., Mell, N. A., Huwer, H., Loretz, B., Schneider-Daum, N., and Lehr, C.-M. (2016). Autologous Co-culture of primary human alveolar macrophages and epithelial cells for investigating aerosol medicines. Part II: evaluation of IL-10-loaded microparticles for the treatment of lung inflammation. *Altern. Lab. Anim.* 44, 349–360. doi: 10.1177/026119291604400405

Holt, P. G., Strickland, D. H., Wikstrom, M. E., and Jahnsen, F. L. (2008). Regulation of immunological homeostasis in the respiratory tract. *Nat. Rev. Immunol.* 8, 142–152. doi: 10.1038/nri2236

Hussell, T., and Bell, T. J. (2014). Alveolar macrophages: plasticity in a tissue-specific context. *Nat. Rev. Immunol.* 14, 81–93. doi: 10.1038/nri3600

Jaroch, K., Jaroch, A., and Bojko, B. (2018). Cell cultures in drug discovery and development: the need of reliable in vitro-in vivo extrapolation for pharmacodynamics and pharmacokinetics assessment. *J. Pharm. Biomed. Anal.* 147, 297–312. doi: 10.1016/j.jpba.2017.07.023

Jin, P., Han, T. H., Ren, J., Saunders, S., Wang, E., Marincola, F. M., et al.

(2010). Molecular signatures of maturing dendritic cells: implications for testing the quality of dendritic cell therapies. *J. Transl. Med.* 8:4. doi: 10.1186/1479-5876-8-4

Johnson, E. R., and Matthay, M. A. (2010). Acute lung injury: epidemiology, pathogenesis, and treatment. *J. Aerosol Med. Pulm. Drug Deliv.* 23, 243–252. doi: 10.1089/jamp.2009.0775

Katsura, Y., Harada, N., Harada, S., Ishimori, A., Makino, F., Ito, J., et al. (2015). Characteristics of alveolar macrophages from murine models of OVA-induced allergic airway inflammation and LPS-induced acute airway inflammation. *Exp. Lung Res.* 41, 370–382. doi: 10.3109/01902148.2015.1044137

King, P. (2012). *Haemophilus influenzae* and the lung (*Haemophilus* and the lung). *Clin. Transl. Med.* 1:10. doi: 10.1186/2001-1326-1-10

Kinoshita, Y., Ishii, H., Kushima, H., Watanabe, K., and Fujita, M. (2017). High-dose steroid therapy for acute respiratory distress syndrome lacking common risk factors: predictors of outcome. *Acute Med. Surg.* 5, 146–153. doi: 10.1002/ams2.321

Klaßen, C., Karabinskaya, A., Dejager, L., Vettorazzi, S., Van Moorleghem, J., Lühder, F., et al. (2017). Airway epithelial cells are crucial targets of glucocorticoids in a mouse model of allergic asthma. *J. Immunol.* 199, 48–61. doi: 10.4049/jimmunol.1601691

Klein, S. G., Serchi, T., Hoffmann, L., Blömeke, B., and Gutleb, A. C. (2013). An improved 3D tetraculture system mimicking the cellular organisation at the alveolar barrier to study the potential toxic effects of particles on the lung. *Part. Fibre Toxicol.* 10:31. doi: 10.1186/1743-8977-10-31

Knapp, S. (2009). LPS and bacterial lung inflammation models. *Drug Discov. TodayDis. Models* 6, 113–118. doi: 10.1016/j.ddmod.2009.08.003

Labib, S., Williams, A., Yauk, C. L., Nikota, J. K., Wallin, H., Vogel, U., et al. (2016). Nano-risk Science: application of toxicogenomics in an adverse outcome pathway framework for risk assessment of multi-walled carbon nanotubes. *Part Fibre Toxicol.* 13:15. doi: 10.1186/s12989-016-0125-9

Laskin, D. L., Sunil, V. R., Gardner, C. R., and Laskin, J. D. (2011). Macrophages and tissue injury: agents of defense or destruction? *Annu. Rev. Pharmacol. Toxicol.* 51, 267–288. doi: 10.1146/annurev.pharmtox.010909.105812

Lawrence, T., and Natoli, G. (2011). Transcriptional regulation of macrophage polarization: enabling diversity with identity. *Nat. Rev. Immunol.* 11, 750–761. doi: 10.1038/nri3088

Lehmann, A. D., Daum, N., Bur, M., Lehr, C. M., Gehr, P., and Rothen-Rutishauser, B. M. (2011). An in vitro triple cell co-culture model with primary cells mimicking the human alveolar epithelial barrier. *Eur. J. Pharm. Biopharm.* 77, 398–406. doi: 10.1016/j.ejpb.2010.10.014

Lehnert, B. E. (1992). Pulmonary and thoracic macrophage subpopulations and clearance of particles from the lung. *Environ. Health Perspect.* 97, 17–46. doi: 10.1289/ehp.929717

Leite-Junior, J. H., Garcia, C. S., Souza-Fernandes, A. B., Silva, P. L., Ornellas, D. S., Larangeira, A. P., et al. (2008). Methylprednisolone improves lung mechanics and reduces the inflammatory response in pulmonary but not in extrapulmonary mild acute lung injury in mice. *Crit. Care Med.* 36, 2621–2628. doi: 10.1097/CCM.0b013e3181847b43

Liu, D., Ahmet, A., Ward, L., Krishnamoorthy, P., Mandelcorn, E. D., Leigh, R., et al. (2013). A practical guide to the monitoring and management of the complications of systemic corticosteroid therapy. *AllergyAsthmaClin. Immunol.* 9:30. doi: 10.1186/1710-1492-9-30

Lu, H. L., Huang, X. Y., Luo, Y. F., Tan, W. P., Chen, P. F., and Guo, Y. B. (2018). Activation of M1 macrophages plays a critical role in the initiation of acute lung injury. *Biosci. Rep.* 38:BSR20171555. doi: 10.1042/bsr20171555

Lu, Y.-C., Yeh, W.-C., and Ohashi, P. S. (2008). LPS/TLR4 signal transduction pathway. *Cytokine* 42, 145–151. doi: 10.1016/j.cyto.2008.01.006

Ma, X., Xu, D., Ai, Y., Ming, G., and Zhao, S. (2010). Fas inhibition attenuates lipopolysaccharide-induced apoptosis and cytokine release of rat type II alveolar epithelial cells. *Mol. Biol. Rep.* 37, 3051–3056. doi: 10.1007/s11033-009-9876-9

Marik, P. E., Meduri, G. U., Rocco, P. R. M., and Annane, D. (2011). Glucocorticoid treatment in acute lung injury and acute respiratory distress syndrome. *Crit. Care Clin.* 27, 589–607. doi: 10.1016/j.ccc.2011.05.007

Martin, L. D., Rochelle, L. G., Fischer, B. M., Krunkosky, T. M., and Adler, K. B. (1997). Airway epithelium as an effector of inflammation: molecular regulation of secondary mediators. *Eur. Respir. J.* 10, 2139–2146. doi: 10.1183/09031936.97.10092139

Martinez, F. O., and Gordon, S. (2014). The M1 and M2 paradigm of macrophage activation: time for reassessment. *F1000Prime Rep.* 6:13. doi: 10.12703/p6-13

Meduri, G. U., Siemieniuk, R. A. C., Ness, R. A., and Seyler, S. J. (2018). Prolonged low-dose methylprednisolone treatment is highly effective in reducing duration of mechanical ventilation and mortality in patients with ARDS. *J. Intensive Care* 6:53. doi: 10.1186/s40560-018-0321-9

Moldoveanu, B., Otmishi, P., Jani, P., Walker, J., Sarmiento, X., Guardiola, J., et al. (2009). Inflammatory mechanisms in the lung. *J. Inflammation Res.* 2, 1–11.

Mukhopadhyay, S., Hoidal, J. R., and Mukherjee, T. K. (2006). Role of TNFα in pulmonary pathophysiology. *Respir. Res.* 7:125. doi: 10.1186/1465-9921-7-125

Müller, E., Christopoulos, P. F., Halder, S., Lunde, A., Beraki, K., Speth, M., et al. (2017). Toll-Like receptor ligands and Interferon-γ synergize for induction of antitumor M1 macrophages. *Front. Immunol.* 8:1383. doi: 10.3389/fimmu.2017.01383

Nicod, L. P. (2005). Lung defences: an overview. *Eur. Respi. Rev.* 14, 45–50. doi: 10.1183/09059180.05.00009501

Nova, Z., Skovierova, H., and Calkovska, A. (2019). Alveolar-capillary membrane-related pulmonary cells as a target in endotoxin-induced acute lung injury. *Int. J. Mol. Sci.* 20:831. doi: 10.3390/ijms20040831

Orecchioni, M., Ghosheh, Y., Pramod, A. B., and Ley, K. (2019). Macrophage polarization: different gene signatures in M1(LPS+) vs. Classically and M2(LPS-) vs. alternatively activated macrophages. *Front. Immunol.* 10:1084. doi: 10.3389/fimmu.2019.01084

Piemonti, L., Monti, P., Allavena, P., Sironi, M., Soldini, L., Leone, B. E., et al. (1999). Glucocorticoids affect human dendritic cell differentiation and maturation. *J. Immunol.* 162, 6473–6481.

Prakash, S., Agrawal, S., Vahed, H., Ngyuen, M., BenMohamed, L., Gupta, S., et al. (2014). Dendritic cells from aged subjects contribute to chronic airway inflammation by activating bronchial epithelial cells under steady state. *Mucosal Immunol.* 7, 1386–1394. doi: 10.1038/mi.2014.28

Riario Sforza, G. G., and Marinou, A. (2017). Hypersensitivity pneumonitis: a complex lung disease. *Clin. Mol. Allergy* 15:6. doi: 10.1186/s12948-017-0062-7

Rivera-Burgos, D., Sarkar, U., Lever, A. R., Avram, M. J., Coppeta, J. R., Wishnok, J. S., et al. (2016). Glucocorticoid clearance and metabolite profiling in an in vitro human airway epithelium lung model. *Drug Metab. Dispos.* 44, 220–226. doi: 10.1124/dmd.115.066365

Rosadini, C. V., and Kagan, J. C. (2017). Early innate immune responses to bacterial LPS. *Curr. Opin. Immunol.* 44, 14–19. doi: 10.1016/j.coi.2016.10.005

Roth, M. (2014). [Fundamentals of chronic inflammatory lung diseases (asthma. COPD, fibrosis)]. *Ther. Umsch.* 71, 258–261. doi: 10.1024/0040-5930/a000510

Roth, M., Usemann, J., Bisig, C., Comte, P., Czerwinski, J., Mayer, A. C. R., et al. (2017). Effects of gasoline and ethanol-gasoline exhaust exposure on human bronchial epithelial and natural killer cells in vitro. *Toxicol. In Vitro* 45(Pt 1), 101–110. doi: 10.1016/j.tiv.2017.08.016

Rothen-Rutishauser, B. M., Kiama, S. G., and Gehr, P. (2005). A three-dimensional cellular model of the human respiratory tract to study the interaction with particles. *Am. J. Respir. Cell Mol. Biol.* 32, 281–289. doi: 10.1165/rcmb.2004-0187OC

Rozkova, D., Horvath, R., Bartunkova, J., and Spisek, R. (2006). Glucocorticoids severely impair differentiation and antigen presenting function of dendritic cells despite upregulation of Toll-like receptors. *Clin. Immunol.* 120, 260–271. doi: 10.1016/j.clim.2006.04.567

Schindelin, J., Arganda-Carreras, I., Frise, E., Kaynig, V., Longair, M., Pietzsch, T., et al. (2012). Fiji: an open-source platform for biological-image analysis. *Nat. Methods* 9, 676–682. doi: 10.1038/Nmeth.2019

Schmid, O., Jud, C., Umehara, Y., Mueller, D., Bucholski, A., Gruber, F., et al. (2017). Biokinetics of aerosolized liposomal ciclosporin a in human lung cells in vitro using an air-liquid cell interface exposure system. *J. Aerosol Med. Pulm. Drug Deliv.* 30, 411–424. doi: 10.1089/jamp.2016.1361

Sethi, G. R., and Singhal, K. K. (2008). Pulmonary diseases and corticosteroids. *Indian J. Pediatr.* 75, 1045–1056. doi: 10.1007/s12098-008-0209-0

Shapiro, D. L., Nardone, L. L., Rooney, S. A., Motoyama, E. K., and Munoz, J. L. (1978). Phospholipid biosynthesis and secretion by a cell line (A549) which resembles type II alveolar epithelial cells. *Biochim. Biophys. Acta Lipids Lipid Metab.* 530, 197–207. doi: 10.1016/0005-2760(78)90005-X

Sharif, O., Bolshakov, V. N., Raines, S., Newham, P., and Perkins, N. D. (2007). Transcriptional profiling of the LPS induced NF-κB response in macrophages. *BMC Immunol.* 8:1. doi: 10.1186/1471-2172-8-1

Silva, P. L., Garcia, C. S. N. B., Maronas, P. A., Cagido, V. R., Negri, E. M., Damaceno-Rodrigues, N. R., et al. (2009). Early short-term versus prolonged low-dose methylprednisolone therapy in acute lung injury. *Eur. Respir. J.* 33, 634–645. doi: 10.1183/09031936.00052408

Smith, T. D., Tse, M. J., Read, E. L., and Liu, W. F. (2016). Regulation of macrophage polarization and plasticity by complex activation signals. *Integrat. Biol.* 8, 946–955. doi: 10.1039/c6ib00105j

Steimer, A., Haltner, E., and Lehr, C. M. (2005). Cell culture models of the respiratory tract relevant to pulmonary drug delivery. *J. Aerosol Med. Depos. Clear. Effects Lung* 18, 137–182. doi: 10.1089/jam.2005.18.137

Tu, G. W., Shi, Y., Zheng, Y. J., Ju, M. J., He, H. Y., Ma, G. G., et al. (2017). Glucocorticoid attenuates acute lung injury through induction of type 2 macrophage. *J. Transl. Med.* 15:181. doi: 10.1186/s12967-017-1284-7

Vichyanond, P., Irvin, C. G., Larsen, G. L., Szefler, S. J., and Hill, M. R. (1989). Penetration of corticosteroids into the lung - evidence for a difference between methylprednisolone and prednisolone. *J. Allergy Clin. Immunol.* 84, 867–873. doi: 10.1016/0091-6749(89)90381-3

Vietti, G., Lison, D., and van den Brule, S. (2016). Mechanisms of lung fibrosis induced by carbon nanotubes: towards an adverse outcome pathway (AOP). *Part. Fibre Toxicol.* 13:11. doi: 10.1186/s12989-016-0123-y

Villeneuve, D. L., Landesmann, B., Allavena, P., Ashley, N., Bal-Price, A., Corsini, E., et al. (2018). Representing the process of inflammation as key events in adverse outcome pathways. *Toxicol. Sci.* 163, 346–352. doi: 10.1093/toxsci/kfy047

Viola, H., Chang, J., Grunwell, J. R., Hecker, L., Tirouvanziam, R., Grotberg, J. B., et al. (2019). Microphysiological systems modeling acute respiratory distress syndrome that capture mechanical force-induced injury-inflammation-repair. *Apl. Bioengin.* 3:41503. doi: 10.1063/1.5111549

Visintin, A., Mazzoni, A., Spitzer, J. H., Wyllie, D. H., Dower, S. K., and Segal, D. M. (2001). Regulation of toll-like receptors in human monocytes and dendritic cells. *J. Immunol.* 166, 249–255. doi: 10.4049/jimmunol.166.1.249

Waljee, A. K., Rogers, M. A. M., Lin, P., Singal, A. G., Stein, J. D., Marks, R. M., et al. (2017). Short term use of oral corticosteroids and related harms among adults in the United States: population based cohort study. *BMJ* 357:j1415. doi: 10.1136/bmj.j1415

Wang, N., Liang, H., and Zen, K. (2014). Molecular mechanisms that influence the macrophage m1-m2 polarization balance. *Front. Immunol.* 5:614. doi: 10.3389/fimmu.2014.00614

Widdrington, J. D., Gomez-Duran, A., Pyle, A., Ruchaud-Sparagano, M.-H., Scott, J., Baudouin, S. V., et al. (2018). Exposure of monocytic cells to lipopolysaccharide induces coordinated endotoxin tolerance. Mitochondrial biogenesis, mitophagy, and antioxidant defenses. *Front. Immunol.* 9:2217. doi: 10.3389/fimmu.2018.02217

Xie, Y., Tolmeijer, S., Oskam, J. M., Tonkens, T., Meijer, A. H., and Schaaf, M. J. M. (2019). Glucocorticoids inhibit macrophage differentiation towards a pro-inflammatory phenotype upon wounding without affecting their migration. *Dis. Models Mech.* 12:dmm037887. doi: 10.1242/dmm.037887

Yonker, L. M., Mou, H., Chu, K. K., Pazos, M. A., Leung, H., Cui, D., et al. (2017). Development of a primary human co-culture model of inflamed airway mucosa. *Sci. Rep.* 7:8182. doi: 10.1038/s41598-017-08567-w

Zach, T. L., Herrman, V. A., Hill, L. D., and Leuschen, M. P. (1993). Effect of steroids on the synthesis of complement C3 in a human alveolar epithelial cell line. *Exp. Lung Res.* 19, 603–616. doi: 10.3109/01902149309031731

Zhou, T., Hu, Y., Wang, Y., Sun, C., Zhong, Y., Liao, J., et al. (2019). Fine particulate matter (PM2.5) aggravates apoptosis of cigarette-inflamed bronchial epithelium in vivo and vitro. *Environ. Pollut.* 248, 1–9. doi: 10.1016/j.envpol.2018.11.054

12

Poloxamer 188 Attenuates Ischemia-Reperfusion-Induced Lung Injury by Maintaining Cell Membrane Integrity and Inhibiting Multiple Signaling Pathways

Shih-En Tang[1,2], Wen-I Liao[3], Hsin-Ping Pao[4], Chin-Wang Hsu[5], Shu-Yu Wu[1], Kun-Lun Huang[1,2] and Shi-Jye Chu[2]*

[1]Institute of Aerospace and Undersea Medicine, National Defense Medical Center, Taipei, Taiwan, [2]Department of Internal Medicine, Tri-Service General Hospital, National Defense Medical Center, Taipei, Taiwan, [3]Department of Emergency Medicine, Tri-Service General Hospital, National Defense Medical Center, Taipei, Taiwan, [4]The Graduate Institute of Medical Sciences, National Defense Medical Center, Taipei, Taiwan, [5]Department of Emergency and Critical Medicine, Wan Fang Hospital, Taipei Medical University, Taipei, Taiwan

*Correspondence:
Shi-Jye Chu
d1204812@mail.ndmctsgh.edu.tw

Background: Poloxamer 188 (P188) possesses anti-inflammatory properties and can help to maintain plasma membrane function. P188 has been reported to exert beneficial effects in the treatment of various disorders. However, the effects of P188 in ischemia/reperfusion (IR)-induced acute lung injury have not been examined.

Methods: We investigated the ability of P188 to attenuate IR-induced acute lung injury in rats and hypoxia/reoxygenation (HR) injury in murine epithelial cells. Isolated perfused rat lungs were exposed to 40 min ischemia followed by 60 min reperfusion to induce IR injury.

Results: IR led to lung edema, increased pulmonary arterial pressure, promoted lung tissue inflammation and oxidative stress, and upregulated the levels of TNF-α, IL-6 and CINC-1, and increased Lactic dehydrogenase (LDH) activity in bronchoalveolar lavage fluid. IR also downregulated the levels of inhibitor of κB (IκB-α), upregulated nuclear factor (NF)-κB (NF-κB), and promoted apoptosis in lung tissues. P188 significantly suppressed all these effects. *In vitro*, P188 also exerted a similar effect in murine lung epithelial cells exposed to HR. Furthermore, P188 reduced the number of propidium iodide-positive cells, maintained cell membrane integrity, and enhanced cell membrane repair following HR.

Conclusion: We conclude that P188 protects against lung IR injury by suppressing multiple signaling pathways and maintaining cell membrane integrity.

Keywords: acute lung injury, ischemia-reperfusion, poloxamer 188, hypoxia/reoxygenation, membrane integrity

INTRODUCTION

The nonionic triblock co-polymer poloxamer 188 (P188; molecular weight 8.4 kDa; also known as Pluronic® F68) consists of two hydrophilic side-chains attached to a central polyoxypropylene molecule. P188 has been shown to reduce cell membrane damage and cell injury in various *in vivo* and *in vitro* models (Moloughney and Weisleder, 2012; Zarrintaj et al., 2020), and employed as an antithrombotic drug, a rheological agent in sickle cell disease, and an emulsifying agent in artificial blood (Moloughney and Weisleder, 2012; Zarrintaj et al., 2020). Most importantly, P188 has been demonstrated to exert plasma membrane-sealing properties, which enhance the repair of skeletal muscle cells, cardiac myocytes, neurons, fibroblasts, and corneal endothelial cells after a variety of insults (Moloughney and Weisleder, 2012). P188 also protected neurons from injury induced by spinal cord compression, excitotoxicity, traumatic brain injury, and acute intracranial hemorrhage (Bao et al., 2012; Wang et al., 2015; Paleo et al., 2020). Furthermore, several studies have indicated that P188 can protect against intestinal, muscle, myocardial, cerebral, and hepatic ischemia-reperfusion (IR) injury, and prolong the survival of cardiac, renal, and skin allografts (Forman et al., 1992; Hunter et al., 2010; Yildirim et al., 2015; Bartos et al., 2016). P188 has been suggested to exert these protective effects by intercalating with lipid bilayers to restore the integrity of damaged plasma membranes, and also by protecting cells against apoptosis and oxidative stress (Moloughney and Weisleder, 2012; Gu et al., 2013).

Lung transplantation is the only effective therapy for patients with advanced lung disease (Laubach and Sharma, 2016). Exposure of the donor lung to ischemia for up to several hours is unavoidable during the transplantation procedure, and the severity of lung malfunctions correlates with the duration of ischemia. Early reestablishment of the blood supply to the lung limits the severity of ischemia. However, reperfusion of the transplanted lung can induce an intense inflammatory response and cellular alterations that further exaggerate tissue injury and cause cell death, and these changes may subsequently result in permeability lung edema (Kalogeris et al., 2012; Laubach and Sharma, 2016). Even with the enormous improvements in lung transplantation procedures, IR-induced lung injury remains the major cause of primary graft dysfunction and early recipient death after lung transplantation. IR-induced lung injury also contributes to the progression to chronic lung allograft dysfunction (Laubach and Sharma, 2016).

The pathogenesis of IR-induced lung injury involves a spectrum of pathological processes that result in the activation of inflammatory response genes. For example, alveolar epithelial cells exposed to IR release inflammatory cytokines, and this response is subsequently magnified that result in plasma membrane disruption (Laubach and Sharma, 2016). Damaged alveolar resident cells are observed in experimental models of lung IR and human lungs with acute respiratory distress syndrome (Kalogeris et al., 2012; Laubach and Sharma, 2016). Thus, it is reasonable to speculate that cell injury and repair contribute to the pathogenesis of IR-induced lung injury (Cong et al., 2017).

Loss of plasma membrane integrity induces various downstream inflammatory events and exacerbates cell injury during IR and represents a major pathogenic mechanism that leads to lung edema and epithelial cell death (Kalogeris et al., 2012). A previous study showed that P188 reduced ventilator-induced lung injury in isolated perfused rat lungs by restoring plasma membrane integrity and protecting alveolar resident cells from stress-induced necrosis (Plataki et al., 2011). In addition,

P188 has been reported to possess anti-inflammatory properties (Moloughney and Weisleder, 2012). Strategies that maintain or restore the integrity of cell membranes exposed to IR and suppress the associated inflammatory response may represent a potential treatment approach for IR-induced injury. In this study, we examined the effect of P188 on IR-induced lung injury and explored the mechanisms by which P188 maintains cell membrane integrity and inhibits the inflammatory response.

MATERIALS AND METHODS

Isolated Perfused Rat Lung Model

Sprague-Dawley male rats weighing 350 ± 20 g were handled according to the guidelines of the National Institutes of Health; all animal experiments were approved by the Animal Review Committee of the National Defense Medical Center (Permit Number: IACUC-18-218). Rat lungs were isolated and perfused in the chest as previously described (Chu et al., 2002; Wu et al., 2015; Wu et al., 2017). Briefly, after tracheotomy, the rats were ventilated with air containing 5% CO_2 at 60 breaths/min at a tidal volume of 3 ml with a positive end-expiratory pressure of 1 cm H_2O. A sternotomy was performed, heparin was injected into the right ventricle, and approximately 10 ml intracardiac blood was collected. The pulmonary artery was cannulated, and a drainage cannula was placed in the left ventricle. The cannulae were connected to the perfusion circuit and perfused with physiological salt solution (119 mM NaCl, 4.7 mM KCl, 1.17 mM $MgSO_4$, 22.6 mM $NaHCO_3$, 1.18 mM KH_2PO_4, 1.6 mM $CaCl_2$, 5.5 mM glucose, 50 mM sucrose) containing 4% bovine serum albumin. The 10 ml collected blood was added to the perfusate and subsequently mixed with the physiological salt solution as a perfusate for the isolated lungs. The roller pump (Minipuls 2; Gilson Medical Electronic, Middleton, WI, United States) was maintained at a flow rate of 8–10 ml/min. In situ isolated rat lungs were placed on an electronic scale to monitor real-time changes in lung weight. Left atrial pressure, which indicates pulmonary venous pressure (PVP), and the pulmonary artery pressure (PAP) were constantly recorded through the side arm of the cannula using pressure transducers (Gould Instruments, Cleveland, OH, United States).

Microvascular Permeability Assay

K_f, an indicator of microvascular permeability to water was estimated from the change in lung weight due to elevated venous pressure, as described previously (Wu et al., 2015; Wu et al., 2017). K_f was designated as the initial weight gain rate (g min^{-1}) divided by the PVP (10 cmH_2O) and lung weight, and expressed in units of g min^{-1} cm $H_2O^{-1} \times 100$ g.

Determination of Lung Weight/Body Weight and Wet/Dry Weight Ratios

After IR, the right lung was removed from the hilar region and LW was computed to determine the LW/BW ratio. A part of the right upper lobe of the lung was harvested from each rat, weighed, and placed in an oven at 60°C for 48 h. The dry weight was determined, and the W/D lung weight ratio was calculated.

Total Cell Counts, LDH Activity, and Levels of Protein, Cytokine-Induced Neutrophil Chemoattractant-1, Interleukin-6, and Tumor Necrosis Factor-α in Bronchoalveolar Lavage Fluid

BALF was analyzed to determine total cell count, protein content (Bicinchoninic Acid Protein Assay Kit; Pierce, Rockford, IL, United States), and Lactic dehydrogenase (LDH) activity (LDH Detection Kit, Roche Applied Science, Indianapolis, IN, United States). The levels of TNF-α, IL-6 and CINC-1 in BALF were measured using commercial ELISA kits (R&D Systems Inc., Minneapolis, MN, United States), as instructed by the manufacturer.

Determination of Malondialdehyde Level and Protein Carbonyl Content in Lung Tissues

The levels of MDA and protein carbonyl contents in right upper lung lobe ere determined as described previously (Liao et al., 2017; Wu et al., 2017) using the Carbonyl Content Assay Kit (Abcam, Cambridge, MA, United States) and Lipid Peroxidation (MDA) Assay Kit (Abcam) following the manufacturer's instructions.

Western Blotting

Prepared right middle lung lobe or cellular protein lysates containing 30 μg protein were separated by 10% SDS polyacrylamide gel electrophoresis and immunoblotting was performed as previously described (Liao et al., 2017; Hung et al., 2019). The membranes were probed with a β-actin antibody as a loading control (1:10,000; Sigma Chemical Company, St. Louis, MO, United States) and primary antibodies against B-cell lymphoma (Bcl)-2 (1:200; Santa Cruz Biotechnology, Dallas, Texas, United States), nuclear factor (NF)-κB (NF-κB) p65, phospho-NF-κB p65, inhibitor of NF-κB (IκB)-α, cleaved caspase-3 (1:1,000; Cell Signaling Technology, Danvers, MA, United States) or Lamin B1 (1:1,000; Abcam). All data are presented as the ratio of the target protein to the reference protein (β-actin).

Immunohistochemical Analyses

Immunohistochemical staining to identify myeloperoxidase (MPO) and Ly6G was performed as previously described (Tang et al., 2019). Briefly, paraffin-embedded right lower lung lobe sections were deparaffinized, endogenous peroxidase activity was quenched using 3% H_2O_2 in 100% methanol for 15 min, and immunostaining was performed using the rabbit polyclonal antibody against MPO (1:100; Cell Signaling Technology) and rabbit polyclonal antibody against Ly6G (1:300, Biorbyt, UK).

Pathological Evaluation

Paraffin sections of right lower lung lobe were stained with hematoxylin-eosin (H&E) to evaluate the extent of lung injury. The average number of polymorphonuclear neutrophils in the interstitium was determined from 10 different high-power fields (×400) by two investigators who were blinded to the groups. Semiquantitative grading of lung injury was performed as previously described (Wu et al., 2015; Liao et al., 2017). Briefly, within each field, lung injury was scored based on 1) infiltration or aggregation of neutrophils in the airspace or vessel wall, and 2) the thickness of the alveolar wall. Each assessment was graded on the following four-point scale: 0, 1, 2, or 3, for no, mild, moderate, or severe injury. The two scores were summed and recorded as the lung injury score for that section.

Terminal Deoxynucleotidyl Transferase dUTP Nick End Labeling Assay of Lung Tissue

Paraffin-embedded lung tissue sections (5 mm-thick) were subjected to the TUNEL assay using the FragELTM DNA Fragmentation Detection Kit and Fluorescent-TdT Enzyme (Merck Millipore, Darmstadt, Germany) following the manufacturer's instructions. TUNEL-positive nuclei were identified by fluorescence microscopy.

Study Protocol

A total of 24 rat lungs were randomized to the following groups: control (0.9% NaCl, $n = 6$), P188 alone (1 mg/ml, $n = 6$), I/R alone ($n = 6$), or IR with P188 (1 mg/ml, $n = 6$). P188 was added to the reservoir containing 20 ml perfusate. IR was induced in the deflated lungs by stopping ventilation and perfusion for 40 min ischemia. After ischemia, perfusion and ventilation were continued for 60 min. The dose of P188 (Pluronic F-68; Sigma-Aldrich) was based on a previous study (Plataki et al., 2011).

Cell Culture and Hypoxia/Reoxygenation Injury

Mouse alveolar type II epithelial (MLE-12) cells (American Type Culture Collection, Manassas, VA, United States) were cultured in DMEM/F-12 medium (Sigma-Aldrich) containing 10% fetal bovine serum, penicillin (100 U/mL), and streptomycin (10 μg/ml) in a humidified atmosphere containing 5% CO_2 and 95% air (Pao et al., 2019). The cells were pretreated with saline, ammonium pyrrolidinedithiocarbamate 2 μM (PDTC, NF-κB specific inhibitor), or 1 mg/ml P188 (Plataki et al., 2011), then subjected to hypoxia (1% O_2, 5% CO_2, 94% N_2) for 3 h, followed by reoxygenation (5% CO_2, 95% air) for 2 h. Control cells were maintained under normoxic conditions without hypoxic stimulus. The cell supernatants were collected and assayed for chemokine (C-X-C motif) ligand 1 (CXCL1) using a mouse CXCL1 ELISA kit (R&D, Inc., Minneapolis, MN, United States).

Measurement of Hydrogen Peroxide, Superoxide Dismutase and Glutathione in the Lung Tissue and Cells

The GSH levels were assessed using fluorometric glutathione detection assay kit (ab 65322, Abcam, Cambridge, MA, United States). H_2O_2 concentrations were measured using Hydrogen Peroxide Assay Kit (ab102500, Abcam). SOD activity was determined using a colorimetric

Superoxide Dismutase Activity Assay Kit (ab65354; Abcam). All experiments were performed following the instructions of the manufacturer with each kit.

Assessment of Cell Membrane Integrity Using Propidium Iodide

Propidium iodide (PI) is an impermeable nucleic acid dye that emits bright red fluorescence when it binds to DNA and RNA following cell membrane injury.

Following HR, the cells were stained with 200 µL of PI (1 mg/ml solution of PI diluted 1:3,000 in PBS) for 30 min, washed extensively in PBS for 3 min, fixed with 4% paraformaldehyde for 20 min, counterstained with 4′,6-diamidino-2-phenylindole (DAPI) to identify nuclei, and imaged using a fluorescence microscope.

Measurements of Mitochondrial Membrane Potential (MMP)

The MMP of MLE-12 cells was assessed using the JC-1 Mitochondrial Membrane Potential Assay Kit (Abcam) according to the manufacturer's instructions. Briefly, the cells were incubated with 10 µmol/L JC-1 dye for 20 min at 37°C, washed twice with 1× dilution buffer, and imaged using a fluorescence microscope at excitation/emission wavelengths of 535/595 nm (green) and 485/535 nm (red).

Cell Wounding and Repair Assays

MLE-12 cells were preincubated in medium with or without P188 (1 mg/ml) before HR. Fluorescent dextran (FDx, 2.5 mg/ml; Sigma-Aldrich) was added and monolayers were then exposed to HR. Cells were allowed to repair for 2 min, and then washed and incubated with PI-containing medium. The number of FDx- and PI-positive cells per × 20 view field was counted. Cells with green cytoplasmic dextran fluorescence were considered wounded but healed, whereas cells with red PI-fluorescent nuclei were considered wounded but permanently injured. The percentage of wounded and repaired cells was presented (Plataki et al., 2011).

Data Analysis

Data are presented as mean ± SD and were analyzed using GraphPad Prism 5 for Windows (GraphPad Software, San Diego, CA, United States). Multiple group comparisons were performed using one-way ANOVA and the *post-hoc* Bonferroni test. LWG and PAP were assessed using repeated-measures two-way ANOVA followed by the *post-hoc* Bonferroni test. Statistical significance was defined as a *p*-value of 0.05 or less.

RESULTS

Poloxamer 188 Reduces the Severity of Ischemia/Reperfusion-Induced Pulmonary Edema

IR induced a significant increase in lung weight over 60 min; however, P188 treatment suppressed this effect (**Figure 1A**). IR

also led to a significantly higher K_f, W/D ratio, LW/BW ratio, and concentration of protein in bronchoalveolar lavage fluid (BALF) after 60 min reperfusion ($p < 0.05$, **Figures 1B–E**). P188 treatment significantly reduced all these IR-induced increases in a dose-dependent manner.

Poloxamer 188 Suppresses the Increase in PAP (ΔPAP) in Ischemia/ Reperfusion-Induced Lung Injury

PAP remained steady during the 100 min observation period in the control group. IR led to a sudden, initial increase in PAP, and PAP subsequently decreased after reperfusion (**Supplementary Figure 1**). In lungs exposed to IR, PAP was significantly higher at 60 min after reperfusion than at baseline. However, treatment with P188 significantly suppressed the IR-induced increase in PAPin a dose-dependent manner ($p < 0.05$; **Supplementary Figure 1**).

Poloxamer 188 Suppresses the Increases in Tumor Necrosis Factor-α, Cytokine-Induced Neutrophil Chemoattractant-1 and Interleukin-6 Levels, LDH Activity, and Total Cell Counts in Bronchoalveolar Lavage Fluid During Ischemia/Reperfusion-Induced Lung Injury

IR significantly increased the concentrations of TNF-α, CINC-1, and IL-6, LDH activity, and the total cell count in BALF after 60 min reperfusion ($p < 0.05$; **Figure 2**). However, P188 significantly attenuated these IR-induced effects.

Poloxamer 188 Attenuates the Increases in the Oxidative Stress in Ischemia/ Reperfusion Lung Tissue

IR significantly increased MDA level, protein carbonyl content, the production of H_2O_2, and decreased SOD activity and GSH levels in the lung tissues after 60 min reperfusion ($p < 0.05$, **Figures 3A–E**). However, treatment with P188 (1 mg/ml) significantly suppressed these IR-induced effects.

Poloxamer 188 Attenuates the Increases in Neutrophil Infiltration in Ischemia/ Reperfusion Lung Tissue

IR significantly increased the number of MPO and Ly6G (neutrophil marker) -positive cells in the lung tissues after 60 min reperfusion. However, treatment with P188 (1 mg/ml) significantly suppressed these IR-induced effects (**Figure 3F**).

Poloxamer 188 Attenuates Histopathological Changes in Ischemia/ Reperfusion Lung Tissue

IR induced histological abnormalities in the lung tissues, including enhanced neutrophil infiltration and obvious

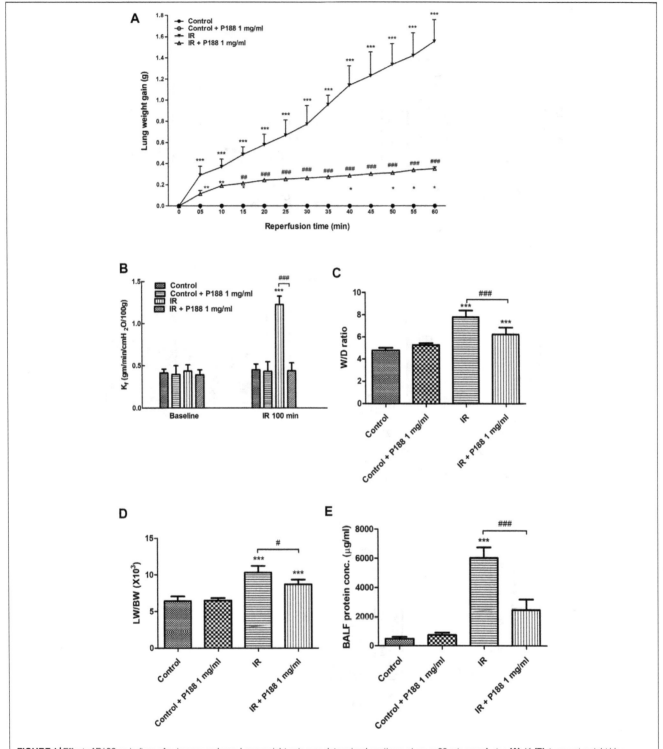

FIGURE 1 | Effect of P188 on indices of pulmonary edema. Lung weight gain was determined continuously over 60 min reperfusion **(A)**. K$_f$ **(B)**, lung wet weight/dry weight (W/D) ratio **(C)**, lung weight/body weight (LW/BW) ratio **(D)**, and protein concentration in bronchoalveolar lavage fluid (BALF) **(E)** were measured after 60 min reperfusion. Data are mean ± SD (6 rats per group); ***$p < 0.001$, compared with the control group; #$p < 0.05$, ##$p < 0.01$, ###$p < 0.001$, compared with the IR group.

widening of the interalveolar walls. Treatment with P188 (1 mg/ml) attenuated the severity of these abnormalities after 60 min reperfusion (**Figure 4A**). Furthermore, treatment with P188 (1 mg/ml) also significantly lessened the lung injury scores (**Figure 4B**) and neutrophil infiltration (**Figure 4C**) in lungs exposed to IR.

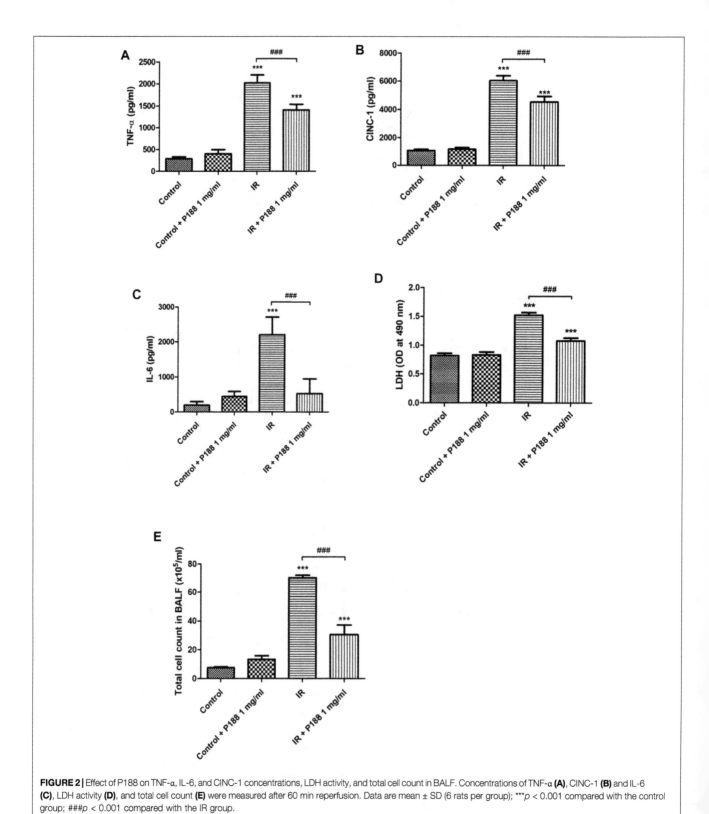

FIGURE 2 | Effect of P188 on TNF-α, IL-6, and CINC-1 concentrations, LDH activity, and total cell count in BALF. Concentrations of TNF-α **(A)**, CINC-1 **(B)** and IL-6 **(C)**, LDH activity **(D)**, and total cell count **(E)** were measured after 60 min reperfusion. Data are mean ± SD (6 rats per group); ***$p < 0.001$ compared with the control group; ###$p < 0.001$ compared with the IR group.

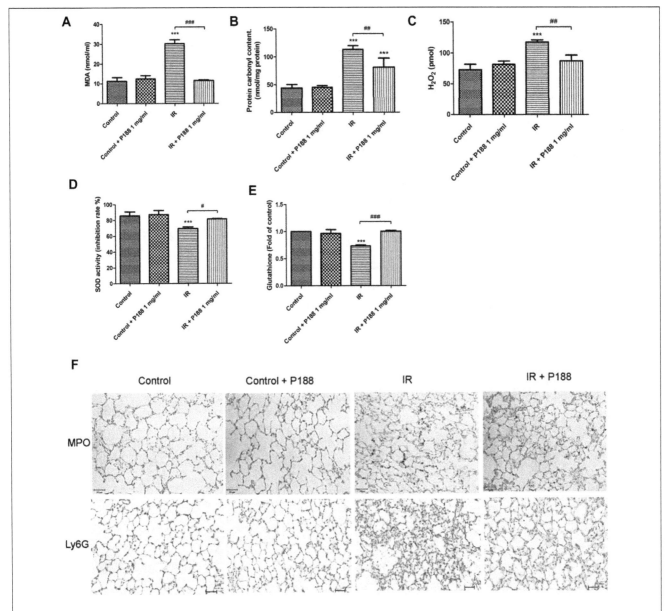

FIGURE 3 | Effect of P188 on oxidative stress and the number of MPO and Ly6G -positive cells in lung tissues. Quantification of the MDA level **(A)**, carbonyl content **(B)**, H_2O_2 concentrations **(C)**, SOD activity **(D)**, and GSH levels **(E)** in the lung tissue were performed after 60 min reperfusion. **(F)** Immunohistochemical stainings of MPO and Ly6G were performed after 60 min reperfusion. Representative images (×200 magnification) are shown. Scale bar = 50 μm. Data are mean ± SD (6 rats per group); ***$p < 0.001$ compared with the control group; #$p < 0.05$, ##$p < 0.01$, ###$p < 0.001$ compared with the IR group.

Poloxamer 188 Inhibits DNA Fragmentation, Cleaved Caspase-3, and Downregulation of Bcl-2 in Ischemia/Reperfusion Lung Tissue

The number of TUNEL-positive cells (**Figure 5A**) and the protein levels of cleaved caspase-3 (**Figure 5B**) were significantly higher, and the protein level of Bcl-2 was significantly lower (**Figure 5C**) in the lungs of the IR group after 60 min reperfusion compared to the control group. However, treatment with P188 significantly attenuated the severity of these apoptosis-related changes in lungs exposed to IR.

Poloxamer 188 Attenuates Activation of the NF-κB Pathway in Ischemia/Reperfusion Lung Tissue

Western blot analysis of lung tissues indicated that IR significantly increased the nuclear level of NF-κB p65 and significantly decreased the cytoplasmic level of IκB-α after 60 min reperfusion (**Figures 5D,E**), indicating that IR activated the NF-κB pathway. However, treatment with P188 (1 mg/ml) significantly inhibited these effects.

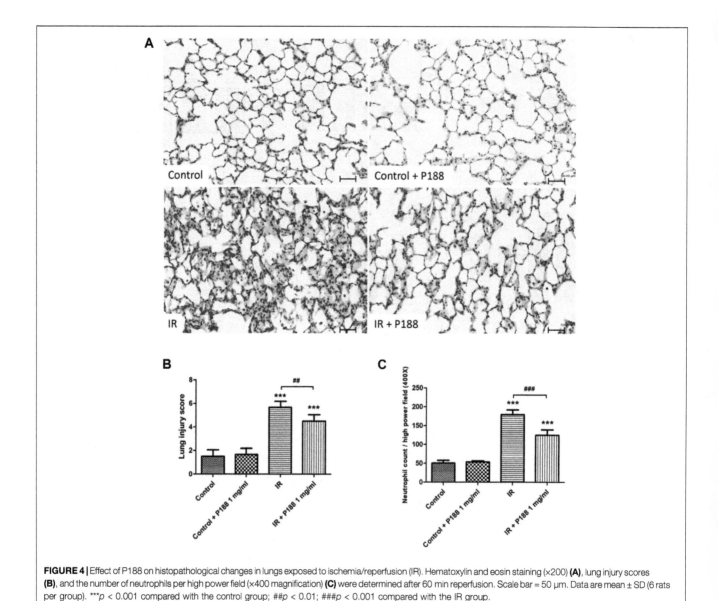

FIGURE 4 | Effect of P188 on histopathological changes in lungs exposed to ischemia/reperfusion (IR). Hematoxylin and eosin staining (×200) **(A)**, lung injury scores **(B)**, and the number of neutrophils per high power field (×400 magnification) **(C)** were determined after 60 min reperfusion. Scale bar = 50 μm. Data are mean ± SD (6 rats per group). ***$p < 0.001$ compared with the control group; ##$p < 0.01$; ###$p < 0.001$ compared with the IR group.

Poloxamer 188 Attenuates Hypoxia/ Reoxygenation Injury in MLE-12 Cells

The protective effects of P188 on HR injury were examined using MLE-12 cells (**Figure 6**). HR increased phosphorylation of NF-κB and cleaved caspase-3 protein expression, decreased IκB-α and BCL-2 protein expression, and upregulated CXCL-1 levels at 2 h after H/R (**Figures 6A–E**). However, P188 (1 mg/ml) significantly inhibited these HR-induced effects.

Poloxamer 188 Attenuates Oxidative Stress in MLE-12 Cells Exposed to Hypoxia/ Reoxygenation

HR increased the production of H_2O_2, and decreased SOD activity and GSH levels at 2 h after HR. However, P188 (1 mg/ml) significantly inhibited these HR-induced effects (**Figures 6F–H**).

PDTC Reduces Hypoxia/Reoxygenation Injury in MLE-12 Cells

The protective effects of PDTC on HR injury were examined using MLE-12 cells (**Supplementary Figure 2**). PDTC decreased phosphorylation of NF-κB, increased IκB-α expression, and reduced CXCL-1 levels at 2 h after HR (**Supplementary Figures 2A–D**).

Poloxamer 188 Attenuates the Depolarization of MMP in MLE-12 Cells Exposed to Hypoxia/Reoxygenation

MMP was determined using the probe JC-1, which easily enters cells and normal mitochondria. At high MMP, JC-1 forms red fluorescent aggregates. At low MMP, JC-1 is present as a green fluorescent monomer. JC-1 exhibited red fluorescence in control

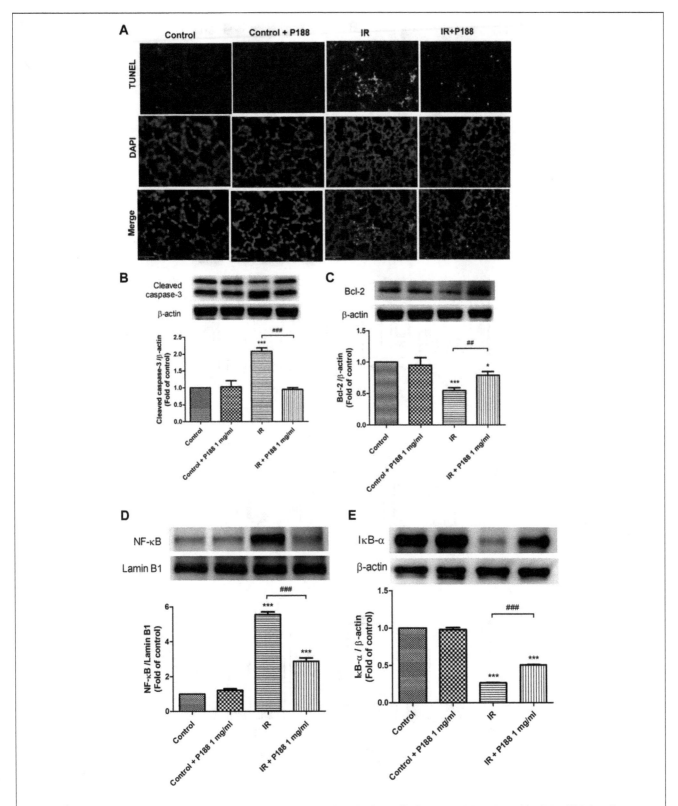

FIGURE 5 | Effect of P188 on DNA fragmentation, expression of cleaved caspase-3 and Bcl-2, and NF-κB activation during ischemia/reperfusion (IR)-induced lung injury. **(A)** TUNEL assay of lung tissue. **(B–E)** Western blot analysis of cleaved caspase-3 **(B)**, Bcl-2 **(C)**, nuclear NF-κB p65 **(D)**, and cytoplasmic IκB-α **(E)** protein expressions in lung tissues. Lamin B1 and β-actin were used as loading controls for nuclear and cytoplasmic proteins, respectively. Representative blots are shown. Data are mean ± SD (6 rats per group); *$p < 0.05$, ***$p < 0.001$ compared with the control group; ##$p < 0.05$, ###$p < 0.001$ compared with the IR group.

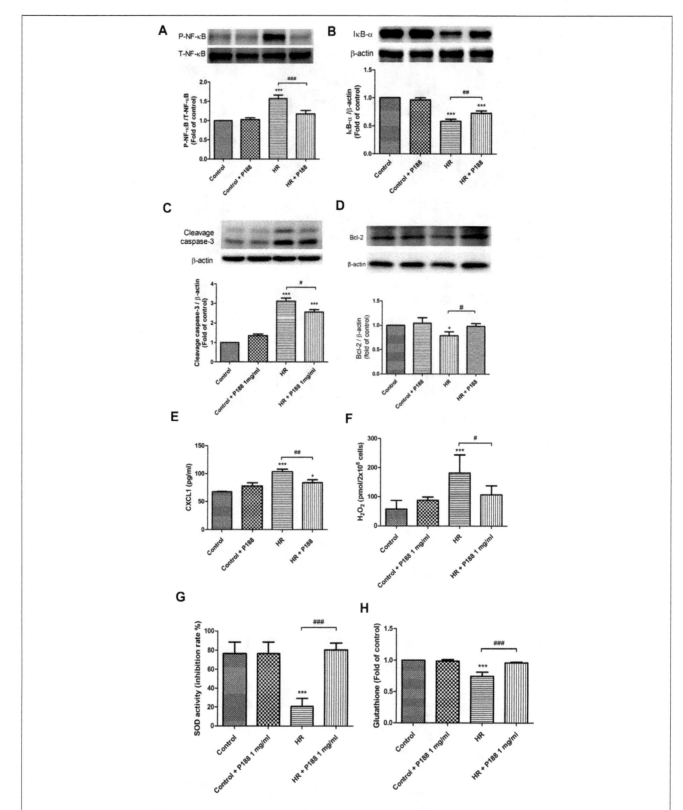

FIGURE 6 | Effect of P188 on hypoxia/reoxygenation (HR) injury in MLE-12 cells. NF-κB phosphorylation **(A)**, IκB-α degradation **(B)**, cleaved caspase-3 **(C)** and Bcl-2 **(D)** protein expression, CXCL-1 **(E)**, hydrogen peroxide (H_2O_2) **(F)**, superoxide dismutase (SOD) **(G)**, and glutathione (GSH) **(H)** levels were measured at 2 h after HR. β-actin served as the loading control. A representative blot is shown. Data are mean ± SD ($n = 6$ per group); *$p < 0.05$, ***$p < 0.001$ compared with the control group. #$p < 0.05$, ##$p < 0.01$, ###$p < 0.001$ compared with the HR group.

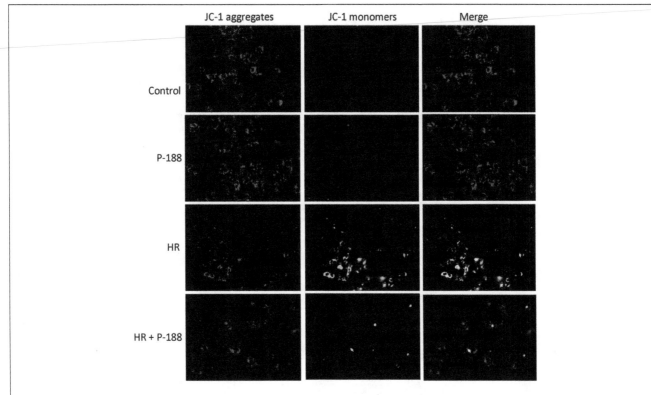

FIGURE 7 | Effect of P188 on depolarization of mitochondrial membrane potential in MLE-12 cells exposed to hypoxia/reoxygenation (HR). Red JC-1 dimers indicate normal mitochondrial membrane potential. Green JC-1 monomers reflect depolarization of mitochondrial membrane potential. The red dimers and green monomers co-localized. Experiments were repeated three times each.

MLE-12 cells, indicating normal MMP. Exposure of MLE-12 cells to HR resulted in MMP depolarization, as indicated by increased levels of green fluorescence in JC-1 stained cells. However, P188 treatment blocked HR-induced MMP depolarization, as confirmed by higher levels of red fluorescence and lower levels of green fluorescence compared to cells exposed to HR alone (**Figure 7**).

Poloxamer 188 Maintains Cell Membrane Integrity in MLE-12 Cells Exposed to Hypoxia/Reoxygenation

Propidium iodide (PI, red fluorescence) labelling was used to detect cell membrane disruption and DAPI counterstaining (blue fluorescence) was used to visualize cell nuclei. No obvious PI staining was detected in the control cells, whereas HR significantly increased the number of PI-positive cells (**Figure 8**). However, P188 reduced the number of PI-positive cells in cells exposed to HR.

Poloxamer 188 Enhances Cell Membrane Repair After Hypoxia/Reoxygenation Injury in MLE-12 Cells

As shown in **Figure 9**, in the presence of P188, there were significantly fewer wound fluorescently labeled cells (FDx and PI). The percentage of FDx-labeled cells relative to the total

number of labeled cells was significantly greater in the HR + P188 group, indicating that more cells repaired when P188 was added.

DISCUSSION

This study demonstrates that administration of P188 exerts a protective effect against IR-induced injury in rat lungs. P188 decreased lung edema by reducing vascular permeability, PAP, the LW/BW and W/D lung weight ratios, LWG, and the protein levels and LDH activity in BALF. P188 treatment also suppressed IR-induced production of pro-inflammatory cytokines and free radicals, reduced the influx of pulmonary neutrophils, and attenuated apoptosis and tissue damage. In addition, P188 inhibited IR-induced activation of the NF-κB signaling pathway. *In vitro* experiments showed that P188 decreased the levels of phosphorylated NFκB p65 and CXCL-1, apoptosis, oxidative stress, and increased the level of IκB-α in MLE-12 cells exposed to HR. Furthermore, P188 inhibited MMP depolarization, maintained membrane integrity, and promoted cell repair *in vitro*. The ability of P188 to attenuate these abnormalities implies P188 may have potential as an adjunct treatment to reduce IR-induced lung injury during lung transplantation.

The protective ability of P188 to insert into membranes may represent an attractive strategy to maintain membrane integrity

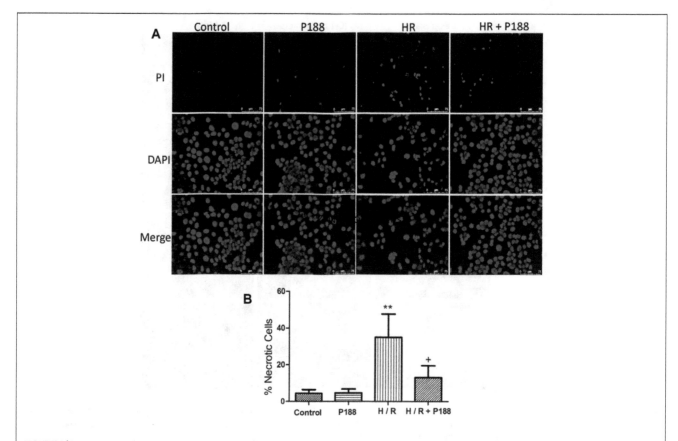

FIGURE 8 | P188 protects against hypoxia/reoxygenation (HR)-induced MLE-12 cell death. **(A)** Representative fluorescence images of MLE-12 cells stained with propidium iodide (red color) and counterstained with DAPI (blue color). **(B)** Percentage of necrotic cells exposed to HR. Data are mean ± SD (n = 6 experiments under each condition). $**p < 0.01$ compared with the control group; $\#p < 0.05$ compared with the HR group.

(Moloughney and Weisleder, 2012). We used PI to assess membrane integrity *in vitro*. When cell membrane integrity is disrupted, PI can penetrate into cells, bind to DNA and RNA and emit red fluorescence; thus, only necrotic cells produce red fluorescence. In the current study, P188 reduced the number of PI-positive cells following HR, indicating P188 maintained cell membrane integrity.

In addition to its membrane-resealing effects, the membrane surfactant P188 may also exert protective effects via other mechanisms. Firstly, under pathologic situations such as acute lung IR, epithelial barrier disruption alters pulmonary vascular permeability, increases penetration of proteins into alveolar regions, and leads to lung edema. Our results indicate that P188 prevented the increase in vascular permeability induced by IR. Similarly, P188 protected against increased vascular permeability in rats exposed to injurious ventilation and prevented extravasation of lung fluid in rats subjected to hemorrhagic shock (Zhang et al., 2009; Plataki et al., 2011).

P188 has been proven to exert anti-inflammatory effects in several experimental models, such as reperfusion injury during prolonged hypotensive resuscitation, acute myocardial infarction, and bleomycin toxicity (Justicz et al., 1991; Tan and Saltzman, 1999; Zhang et al., 2009). Oxidative stress is well-recognized to play a vital role in the pathogenesis of IR injury (Ferrari and Andrade, 2015; Hsu et al., 2015; Wu et al., 2015). Oxidative stress

can induce epithelial and endothelial damage, increase vascular permeability, enhance neutrophil infiltration, and promote formation of edema in the lungs (Ferrari and Andrade, 2015). Numerous studies have indicated that inhibition of oxidative stress represents an effective therapeutic approach in animal models of IR lung injury (Bao et al., 2012; Ferrari and Andrade, 2015). Our results demonstrate that P188 can also reduce oxidative stress in IR lung tissues and MLE-12 epithelial cells exposed to HR. A previous investigation showed that P188 significantly blocked lipid peroxidation of hippocampal and cerebellar neurons induced by Fe^{2+} and H_2O_2 (Marks et al., 2001). In addition, P188 also decreased lipid peroxidation in the spinal cords of G93ASOD1 transgenic mice (Riehm et al., 2018). Insertion of the hydrophobic polypropylene block of P188 into cell membranes may possibly reduce lipid peroxidation (Inyang et al., 2020). Therefore, inhibition of lipid peroxidation may partly explain the ability of P188 to protect against IR-induced lung injury.

IR dramatically increases the number of rolling and adherent leukocytes, which are primarily neutrophils (Kalogeris et al., 2012; Laubach and Sharma, 2016; Liao et al., 2017). Neutrophils secrete a host of inflammatory mediators that contribute to tissue damage. Indeed, depletion of neutrophils significantly reduced IR-induced tissue injury (Kalogeris et al., 2012; Laubach and Sharma, 2016). In this study, P188 decreased

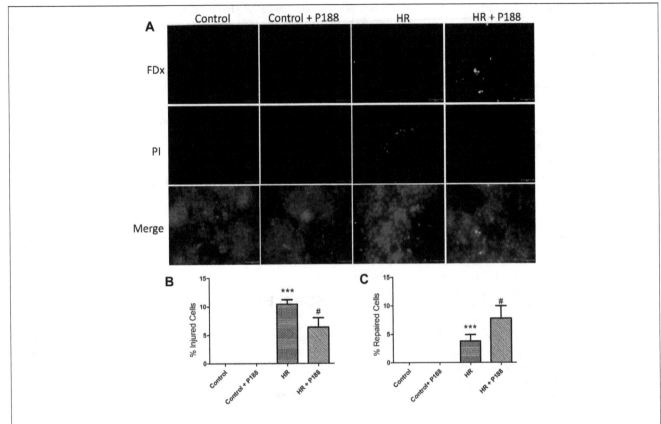

FIGURE 9 | (A) P188 enhances cell membrane repair after hypoxia/reoxygenation (HR) injury in MLE-12 cells. Representative fluorescence images of cells exposed to HR in the presence or absence of P188. Cells with green cytoplasmic dextran (FDx) fluorescence were considered wounded but healed, whereas cells with red propidium iodide (PI) fluorescent nuclei were considered wounded but permanently injured. Images were merged with DAPI nuclear counterstain (blue). **(B)** Percentage of injured cells per field. **(C)** Percentage of repaired cells per field. Scale bar shows 100 μm. Data are mean ± SD (n = 6 plates). ***$p < 0.001$ compared with the control group; #$p < 0.05$ compared with the HR group.

neutrophil infiltration into IR lung tissues, as indicated by lower numbers of neutrophils and MPO-positive cells. These observations are comparable with reports that P188 reduced neutrophil migration and adherence, prevented neutrophil transfer to inflammatory sites, and attenuated the release of proteolytic enzymes from neutrophils in *in vitro* studies and animal models (Lane and Lamkin, 1984, 1986; Babbitt et al., 1990; Tan and Saltzman, 1999).

Apoptosis plays a crucial role in IR-induced lung injury (Ng et al., 2005). Membrane injury induced by IR can promote cell death. Disruption of membrane integrity initiates a variety of downstream events that result in secondary cellular injury. Conversely, inactivation of apoptotic signaling pathways can attenuate IR lung injury (Ng et al., 2005; Hsu et al., 2015; Liao et al., 2017). In the current study, P188 reduced the levels of apoptosis in the lung tissues after IR, as indicated by decreased expression of cleaved caspase-3, reduced numbers of TUNEL-positive cells, and increased Bcl-2 expression. P188 also significantly decreased the number of PI-positive epithelial cells and apoptosis after HR *in vitro*. Similarly, P188 markedly decreased the numbers of TUNEL-positive and PI-positive neuronal cells after mechanical and IR injury, reduced lysosomal membrane permeabilization-mediated cell apoptosis

in vitro and *in vivo*, and decreased caspase activity induced by hemorrhagic shock (Serbest et al., 2005; Serbest et al., 2006; Zhang et al., 2009; Gu et al., 2013; Wang et al., 2017; Dong et al., 2019).

Assessment of mitochondrial membrane potential using the dual-emission dye JC-1 provides an earlier indicator of cell death than TUNEL or PI staining. Low mitochondrial potential was observed in MLE-12 epithelial cells exposed to HR. However, P188 attenuated the reduction in mitochondrial membrane potential in cells exposed to HR. Several investigators recently reported that P188 acts directly on the mitochondria to prevent mitochondrial outer membrane permeabilization, reduce mitochondrial dysfunction and inhibit mitochondrial-dependent death pathways in models of neuronal injury (Shelat et al., 2013; Luo et al., 2015; Wang et al., 2017). Thus, lung cells that do not directly break down in response to IR may subsequently undergo apoptosis. This study demonstrates that the ability of P188 to repair the initial membrane injury caused by IR not only prevented lung cells from acute death, but also inhibited the secondary events that lead to late cell death.

The transcription factor NF-κB modulates the production of various pro-inflammatory cytokines and chemokines. When IκB is degraded, active NF-κB translocates into the nucleus, and enhances the transcription of pro-inflammatory cytokines such as TNF-α and

CINC-1, which exacerbate lung injury by inducing production of additional pro-inflammatory cytokines and promoting leukocyte infiltration. Previous experiments demonstrated that activation of NF-κB plays an important role in IR-induced lung injury (Hsu et al., 2015; Wu et al., 2015; Liao et al., 2017). This study clearly showed that P188 significantly suppressed IR-induced activation of NF-κB, which decreased the production of proinflammatory cytokines and reduced infiltration of leukocytes. Furthermore, investigation of the direct effects of P188 on alveolar epithelial cells showed that P188 significantly inhibited degradation of IκBα, phosphorylation of NF-κB p65, and the production of KC in MLE-12 epithelial cells subjected to HR. In addition, PDTC (NF-κB specific inhibitor) also provided similar effects in HR-exposed MLE-12 cells. These results corroborate a previous study, which showed that P188 suppressed the NF-κB signaling pathway in a mouse model of intracerebral hemorrhage (Wang et al., 2015).

The literature suggests that P188 exerts medical benefits in the treatment of various disorders. P188 is also widely available and easy to manufacture [2]. Numerous pharmacological approaches to reduce I/R lung injury have proven largely ineffective in clinical settings (Laubach and Sharma, 2016). The use of P188 may represent an alternative simple, safe therapeutic approach. To the best of our knowledge, this is the first study to show that P188 significantly attenuates IR-induced acute lung injury. We administered P188 at the onset of ischemia, thus P188 may be suitable as an adjunct during lung transplantation procedures. However, future studies are required to address the value of administering P188 after I/R has occurred.

In summary, this study demonstrates that P188 can protect against IR-induced lung injury *in vivo* and *in vitro* via mechanisms involving maintenance of plasma membrane integrity and inhibition of multiple signaling pathways. P188 has potential as an effective adjunct to reduce IR-induced injury during lung transplantation.

ETHICS STATEMENT

The animal study was reviewed and approved by Animal Review Committee of the National Defense Medical Center (Permit Number: IACUC-18-218).

AUTHOR CONTRIBUTIONS

S-JC and S-ET participated in research design. H-PP and S-YW conducted experiments. W-IL and C-WH performed data analysis. S-ET, K-LH, and S-JC contributed to the writing of the manuscript.

SUPPLEMENTARY MATERIAL

Supplementary Figure 1 | Effect of P188 on pulmonary artery pressure (ΔPAP). Change in pulmonary artery pressure (ΔPAP) from baseline was measured continuously during 60 min reperfusion. Data are mean ± SD (6 rats per group); ***$p < 0.001$ compared with the control group; ###$p < 0.001$ compared with the IR group.

Supplementary Figure 2 | Effect of ammonium pyrrolidinedithiocarbamate (PDTC) on hypoxia/reoxygenation (HR) injury in MLE-12 cells. NF-κB phosphorylation, IκB-α degradation, and CXCL-1 level were measured at 2 h after HR. NF-κB was detected using **(A)** immunofluorescence staining and **(B)** Western blotting. β-actin served as the loading control. Representative blot and image are shown. Data are mean ± SD ($n = 6$ per group); *$p < 0.05$, **$p < 0.01$, ***$p < 0.001$ compared with the control group. #$p < 0.05$, ##$p < 0.01$, ###$p < 0.001$ compared with the HR group.

REFERENCES

Babbitt, D. G., Forman, M. B., Jones, R., Bajaj, A. K., and Hoover, R. L. (1990). Prevention of Neutrophil-Mediated Injury to Endothelial Cells by Perfluorochemical. *Am. J. Pathol.* 136 (2), 451–459.

Bao, H.-J., Wang, T., Zhang, M.-Y., Liu, R., Dai, D.-K., Wang, Y.-Q., et al. (2012). Poloxamer-188 Attenuates TBI-Induced Blood-Brain Barrier Damage Leading to Decreased Brain Edema and Reduced Cellular Death. *Neurochem. Res.* 37 (12), 2856–2867. doi:10.1007/s11064-012-0880-4

Bartos, J. A., Matsuura, T. R., Tsangaris, A., Olson, M., McKnite, S. H., Rees, J. N., et al. (2016). Intracoronary Poloxamer 188 Prevents Reperfusion Injury in a Porcine Model of ST-Segment Elevation Myocardial Infarction. *JACC Basic Transl Sci.* 1 (4), 224–234. doi:10.1016/j.jacbts.2016.04.001

Chu, S.-J., Chang, D.-M., Wang, D., Chen, Y.-H., Hsu, C.-W., and Hsu, K. (2002). Fructose-1,6-diphosphate Attenuates Acute Lung Injury Induced by Ischemia-Reperfusion in Rats. *Crit. Care Med.* 30 (7), 1605–1609. doi:10.1097/00003246-200207000-00034

Cong, X., Hubmayr, R. D., Li, C., and Zhao, X. (2017). Plasma Membrane Wounding and Repair in Pulmonary Diseases. *Am. J. Physiol. Lung Cel Mol Physiol* 312 (3), L371–L391. doi:10.1152/ajplung.00486.2016

Dong, H., Qin, Y., Huang, Y., Ji, D., and Wu, F. (2019). Poloxamer 188 Rescues MPTP-Induced Lysosomal Membrane Integrity Impairment in Cellular and Mouse Models of Parkinson's Disease. *Neurochem. Int.* 126, 178–186. doi:10.1016/j.neuint.2019.03.013

Ferrari, R. S., and Andrade, C. F. (2015). Oxidative Stress and Lung Ischemia-Reperfusion Injury. *Oxidative Med. Cell Longevity* 2015, 1–14. doi:10.1155/2015/590987

Forman, M. B., Ingram, D. A., and Murray, J. J. (1992). Role of Perfluorochemical Emulsions in the Treatment of Myocardial Reperfusion Injury. *Am. Heart J.* 124 (5), 1347–1357. doi:10.1016/0002-8703(92)90422-r

Gu, J.-H., Ge, J.-B., Li, M., Xu, H.-D., Wu, F., and Qin, Z.-H. (2013). Poloxamer 188 Protects Neurons against Ischemia/reperfusion Injury through Preserving Integrity of Cell Membranes and Blood Brain Barrier. *PLoS One* 8 (4), e61641. doi:10.1371/journal.pone.0061641

Hsu, H.-H., Wu, S.-Y., Tang, S.-E., Wu, G.-C., Li, M.-H., Huang, K.-L., et al. (2015). Protection against Reperfusion Lung Injury via Aborgating Multiple Signaling Cascades by Trichostatin A. *Int. Immunopharmacology* 25 (2), 267–275. doi:10.1016/j.intimp.2015.02.013

Hung, K.-Y., Liao, W.-I., Pao, H.-P., Wu, S.-Y., Huang, K.-L., and Chu, S.-J. (2019). Targeting F-Box Protein Fbxo3 Attenuates Lung Injury Induced by Ischemia-Reperfusion in Rats. *Front. Pharmacol.* 10, 583. doi:10.3389/fphar.2019.00583

Hunter, R. L., Luo, A. Z., Zhang, R., Kozar, R. A., and Moore, F. A. (2010). Poloxamer 188 Inhibition of Ischemia/reperfusion Injury: Evidence for a Novel Anti-adhesive Mechanism. *Ann. Clin. Lab. Sci.* 40 (2), 115–125.

Inyang, E., Abhyankar, V., Chen, B., and Cho, M. (2020). Modulation of *In Vitro* Brain Endothelium by Mechanical Trauma: Structural and Functional Restoration by Poloxamer 188. *Sci. Rep.* 10 (1), 3054. doi:10.1038/s41598-020-59888-2

Justicz, A. G., Farnsworth, W. V., Soberman, M. S., Tuvlin, M. B., Bonner, G. D., Hunter, R. L., et al. (1991). Reduction of Myocardial Infarct Size by Poloxamer 188 and Mannitol in a Canine Model. *Am. Heart J.* 122 (3 Pt 1), 671–680. doi:10.1016/0002-8703(91)90510-o

Kalogeris, T., Baines, C. P., Krenz, M., and Korthuis, R. J. (2012). Cell Biology of Ischemia/reperfusion Injury. *Int. Rev. Cel Mol Biol* 298, 229–317. doi:10.1016/

B978-0-12-394309-5.00006-7

Lane, T., and Lamkin, G. (1986). Increased Infection Mortality and Decreased Neutrophil Migration Due to a Component of an Artificial Blood Substitute. *Blood* 68 (2), 351–354. doi:10.1182/blood.v68.2.351.351

Lane, T., and Lamkin, G. (1984). Paralysis of Phagocyte Migration Due to an Artificial Blood Substitute. *Blood* 64 (2), 400–405. doi:10.1182/blood.v64.2.400.400

Laubach, V. E., and Sharma, A. K. (2016). Mechanisms of Lung Ischemia-Reperfusion Injury. *Curr. Opin. Organ. Transplant.* 21 (3), 246–252. doi:10.1097/MOT.0000000000000304

Liao, W.-I., Wu, S.-Y., Wu, G.-C., Pao, H.-P., Tang, S.-E., Huang, K.-L., et al. (2017). Ac2-26, an Annexin A1 Peptide, Attenuates Ischemia-Reperfusion-Induced Acute Lung Injury. *Int. J. Mol. Sci.* 18 (8), 1771. doi:10.3390/ijms18081771

Luo, C., Li, Q., Gao, Y., Shen, X., Ma, L., Wu, Q., et al. (2015). Poloxamer 188 Attenuates Cerebral Hypoxia/Ischemia Injury in Parallel with Preventing Mitochondrial Membrane Permeabilization and Autophagic Activation. *J. Mol. Neurosci.* 56 (4), 988–998. doi:10.1007/s12031-015-0568-8

Marks, J. D., Pan, C.-y., Bushell, T., Cromie, W., and Lee, R. C. (2001). Amphiphilic, Tri-block Copolymers Provide Potent, Membrane-targeted Neuroprotection. *FASEB j.* 15 (6), 1107–1109. doi:10.1096/fj.00-0547fje10.1096/fsb2fj000547fje

Moloughney, J. G., and Weisleder, N. (2012). Poloxamer 188 (P188) as a Membrane Resealing Reagent in Biomedical Applications. *Recent Pat Biotechnol.* 6 (3), 200–211. doi:10.2174/1872208311206030200

Ng, C. S. H., Wan, S., and Yim, A. P. (2005). Pulmonary Ischaemia-Reperfusion Injury: Role of Apoptosis. *Eur. Respir. J.* 25 (2), 356–363. doi:10.1183/09031936.05.00030304

Paleo, B. J., Madalena, K. M., Mital, R., McElhanon, K. E., Kwiatkowski, T. A., Rose, A. L., et al. (2020). Enhancing Membrane Repair Increases Regeneration in a Sciatic Injury Model. *PLoS One* 15 (4), e0231194. doi:10.1371/journal.pone.0231194

Pao, H.-P., Liao, W.-I., Wu, S.-Y., Hung, K.-Y., Huang, K.-L., and Chu, S.-J. (2019). PG490-88, a Derivative of Triptolide, Suppresses Ischemia/reperfusion-Induced Lung Damage by Maintaining Tight junction Barriers and Targeting Multiple Signaling Pathways. *Int. Immunopharmacol* 68, 17–29. doi:10.1016/j.intimp.2018.12.058

Plataki, M., Lee, Y. D., Rasmussen, D. L., and Hubmayr, R. D. (2011). Poloxamer 188 Facilitates the Repair of Alveolus Resident Cells in Ventilator-Injured Lungs. *Am. J. Respir. Crit. Care Med.* 184 (8), 939–947. doi:10.1164/rccm.201104-0647OC

Riehm, J. J., Wang, L., Ghadge, G., Teng, M., Correa, A. M., Marks, J. D., et al. (2018). Poloxamer 188 Decreases Membrane Toxicity of Mutant SOD1 and Ameliorates Pathology Observed in SOD1 Mouse Model for ALS. *Neurobiol. Dis.* 115, 115–126. doi:10.1016/j.nbd.2018.03.014

Serbest, G., Horwitz, J., and Barbee, K. (2005). The Effect of Poloxamer-188 on Neuronal Cell Recovery from Mechanical Injury. *J. Neurotrauma* 22 (1), 119–132. doi:10.1089/neu.2005.22.119

Serbest, G., Horwitz, J., Jost, M., and Barbee, K. A. (2006). Mechanisms of Cell Death and Neuroprotection by Poloxamer 188 after Mechanical Trauma. *FASEB j.* 20 (2), 308–310. doi:10.1096/fj.05-4024fje

Shelat, P. B., Plant, L. D., Wang, J. C., Lee, E., and Marks, J. D. (2013). The Membrane-Active Tri-block Copolymer Pluronic F-68 Profoundly Rescues Rat Hippocampal Neurons from Oxygen-Glucose Deprivation-Induced Death through Early Inhibition of Apoptosis. *J. Neurosci.* 33 (30), 12287–12299. doi:10.1523/JNEUROSCI.5731-12.2013

Tan, J., and Saltzman, W. M. (1999). Influence of Synthetic Polymers on Neutrophil Migration in Three-Dimensional Collagen Gels. *J. Biomed. Mater. Res.* 46 (4), 465–474. doi:10.1002/(sici)1097-4636(19990915)46:4<465::aid-jbm4>3.0.co;2-n

Tang, S.-E., Liao, W.-I., Wu, S.-Y., Pao, H.-P., Huang, K.-L., and Chu, S.-J. (2019). The Blockade of Store-Operated Calcium Channels Improves Decompression Sickness in Rats. *Front. Physiol.* 10, 1616. doi:10.3389/fphys.2019.01616

Wang, J. C., Bindokas, V. P., Skinner, M., Emrick, T., and Marks, J. D. (2017). Mitochondrial Mechanisms of Neuronal rescue by F-68, a Hydrophilic Pluronic Block Co-polymer, Following Acute Substrate Deprivation. *Neurochem. Int.* 109, 126–140. doi:10.1016/j.neuint.2017.04.007

Wang, T., Chen, X., Wang, Z., Zhang, M., Meng, H., Gao, Y., et al. (2015). Poloxamer-188 Can Attenuate Blood-Brain Barrier Damage to Exert Neuroprotective Effect in Mice Intracerebral Hemorrhage Model. *J. Mol. Neurosci.* 55 (1), 240–250. doi:10.1007/s12031-014-0313-8

Wu, G.-C., Liao, W.-I., Wu, S.-Y., Pao, H.-P., Tang, S.-E., Li, M.-H., et al. (2017). Targeting of Nicotinamide Phosphoribosyltransferase Enzymatic Activity Ameliorates Lung Damage Induced by Ischemia/reperfusion in Rats. *Respir. Res.* 18 (1), 71. doi:10.1186/s12931-017-0557-2

Wu, S.-Y., Tang, S.-E., Ko, F.-C., Wu, G.-C., Huang, K.-L., and Chu, S.-J. (2015). Valproic Acid Attenuates Acute Lung Injury Induced by Ischemia-Reperfusion in Rats. *Anesthesiology* 122 (6), 1327–1337. doi:10.1097/ALN.0000000000000618

Yıldırım, T., Eylen, A., Lule, S., Erdener, S. E., Vural, A., Karatas, H., et al. (2015). Poloxamer-188 and Citicoline Provide Neuronal Membrane Integrity and Protect Membrane Stability in Cortical Spreading Depression. *Int. J. Neurosci.* 125 (12), 941–946. doi:10.3109/00207454.2014.979289

Zarrintaj, P., Ramsey, J. D., Samadi, A., Atoufi, Z., Yazdi, M. K., Ganjali, M. R., et al. (2020). Poloxamer: A Versatile Tri-block Copolymer for Biomedical Applications. *Acta Biomater.* 110, 37–67. doi:10.1016/j.actbio.2020.04.028

Zhang, R., Hunter, R. L., Gonzalez, E. A., and Moore, F. A. (2009). Poloxamer 188 Prolongs Survival of Hypotensive Resuscitation and Decreases Vital Tissue Injury after Full Resuscitation. *Shock* 32 (4), 442–450. doi:10.1097/SHK.0b013e31819e13b1

13

Kinetic Analysis of Label-Free Microscale Collagen Gel Contraction using Machine Learning-Aided Image Analysis

Cameron Yamanishi[1,2], Eric Parigoris[1,2] and Shuichi Takayama[1,2]*

[1] Wallace H. Coulter Department of Biomedical Engineering, Georgia Institute of Technology, Atlanta, GA, United States,
[2] The Parker H. Petit Institute of Bioengineering and Bioscience, Georgia Institute of Technology, Atlanta, GA, United States

*Correspondence:
Shuichi Takayama
takayama@gatech.edu

Pulmonary fibrosis is a deadly lung disease, wherein normal lung tissue is progressively replaced with fibrotic scar tissue. An aspect of this process can be recreated *in vitro* by embedding fibroblasts into a collagen matrix and providing a fibrotic stimulus. This work expands upon a previously described method to print microscale cell-laden collagen gels and combines it with live cell imaging and automated image analysis to enable high-throughput analysis of the kinetics of cell-mediated contraction of this collagen matrix. The image analysis method utilizes a plugin for FIJI, built around Waikato Environment for Knowledge Analysis (WEKA) Segmentation. After cross-validation of this automated image analysis with manual shape tracing, the assay was applied to primary human lung fibroblasts including cells isolated from idiopathic pulmonary fibrosis patients. In the absence of any exogenous stimuli, the analysis showed significantly faster and more extensive contraction of the diseased cells compared to the healthy ones. Upon stimulation with transforming growth factor beta 1 (TGF-β1), fibroblasts from the healthy donor showed significantly more contraction throughout the observation period while differences in the response of diseased cells was subtle and could only be detected during a smaller window of time. Finally, dose-response curves for the inhibition of collagen gel contraction were determined for 3 small molecules including the only 2 FDA-approved drugs for idiopathic pulmonary fibrosis.

Keywords: pulmonary fibrosis, collagen contraction, fibroblasts, phenotypic assay, aqueous two-phase systems, machine learning

INTRODUCTION

Pulmonary fibrosis is a deadly lung disease, characterized by an aberrant wound healing response (Ahluwalia et al., 2014). Healthy lung parenchyma is progressively replaced with fibrotic scar tissue, reducing patients' lung capacity and often leading to death. Although progress has been made in understanding disease mechanisms, treatment options are limited to merely slowing the decline of lung function (Maher and Strek, 2019). Part of the difficulty in studying pulmonary fibrosis arises from the complex interplay between different cell types, mechanics, genetics, and the microenvironment (Ahluwalia et al., 2014; Barkauskas and Noble, 2014; Borensztajn et al., 2014; Betensley et al., 2016). Phenotypic assays, which can measure more holistic responses than gene or protein expression assays, are an important, complementary set of tools to understand cell and tissue processes (Yamanishi et al., 2019).

One of the classic phenotypic assays for pulmonary fibrosis is the collagen gel contraction assay (Bell et al., 1979). In this assay, fibroblasts are embedded into a collagen gel, which is detached from the surface of its container – usually a microplate well. Activated fibroblasts remodel the collagen gel, macroscopically shrinking the gel in a process similar to wound closure. Despite the assay's utility and reliability in cell lines, the behavior of primary lung fibroblasts can be more subtle and difficult to detect (Campbell et al., 2012; Cui et al., 2016; Jin et al., 2019). These differences arise, as primary cells have variable initial states and sensitivities to stimulation. Primary cells present additional challenges, as they have limited growth capacity. Furthermore, the throughput has previously been low, as the collagen gel contraction assay traditionally requires the user to manually detach each gel from the edges of the well with a pipet tip (Bell et al., 1979). Measurement of the contracting area has also been manual, with pictures taken daily and images traced by hand (**Figure 1A**). While some collagen contraction assays have been adapted to a 96-well format (Kondo et al., 2004; Mohan and Bargagna-Mohan, 2016; Zhang et al., 2019), these higher-throughput assays have not been universally adopted due to challenges of manual detachment and image analysis. While several techniques have been developed for automated segmentation of label-free spheroid images (Rodday et al., 2011; Chen et al., 2014), these multicellular structures generally have high contrast compared to the media; cell-laden hydrogels have lower contrast, thereby requiring more modern image analysis algorithms.

To address these issues, we explore methods to increase the throughput of the assay and incorporate high frequency imaging. Our lab has previously developed a high-throughput collagen microgel bioprinting technique that does not require manual gel detachment and demonstrated its effectiveness with cell lines (Moraes et al., 2013). In this assay, evaporation of the small microgel during the gelation process is prevented by mixing the collagen and cells with an aqueous solution of dextran (DEX), which forms an aqueous two-phase system (ATPS) with an aqueous solution of polyethylene glycol (PEG). Collagen mostly remains within the DEX phase as it gels (Singh and Tavana, 2018), while the PEG phase provides an aqueous buffer, containing the collagen and limiting evaporation. This approach may be applicable to a variety of other hydrogel systems, however, our work here focuses on collagen. In this study, we extend the ATPS collagen bioprinting technique through automated imaging and image analysis (**Figure 1B**) to examine contraction kinetics of normal vs. diseased primary human lung fibroblasts, particularly in the context of anti-fibrotic drugs. Furthermore, this high frequency of sampling aids in distinguishing the more subtle differences in primary cells, compared to the cell lines used in our initial proof of concept study (Moraes et al., 2013).

MATERIALS AND METHODS

Cell Culture

Normal human lung fibroblasts (NHLF, lot 0000655309, 56 year-old male) and idiopathic pulmonary fibrosis human lung fibroblasts (IPF, lot 0000627840, 52 year-old male) were purchased from Lonza (Walkersville, MD). These primary cells were cultured in complete Fibroblast Growth Medium (FGM-2,

Lonza) and used from passages 2–5. For collagen gel contraction assays, cells were passaged into FGM-2, without serum (FGM-SF), then seeded into collagen gels the following day where they were collected at ~75% confluence.

Collagen Microgel Contraction Assay

Collagen microgel contraction assays were seeded as previously described (Moraes et al., 2013). 96-well round bottom microplates were filled with 100 μL per well of 6% (w/w) PEG, MW 35,000 (Sigma) dissolved in serum-free DMEM (Gibco) with 10% distilled water (Gibco) to adjust for osmotic pressure. This plate was warmed to 37°C in a 5% CO_2 incubator. A collagen-dextran mixture was prepared on ice, consisting of 6% (w/w) DEX T500 (Sigma), 2 mg/mL Type I bovine skin collagen (Advanced Biomatrix), and 5 mM NaOH (Sigma) to neutralize the collagen. This mixture was mixed by pipetting up and down on ice, with care taken to avoid introducing bubbles. The mixture was kept on ice while cells were prepared for seeding. Cells were washed with PBS (Gibco), then trypsinized with 0.05% Trypsin (Gibco). After the cells lifted, they were quickly diluted in FGM-SF and centrifuged at 200 × g, 5 min, room temperature. After aspirating the supernatant, cells were resuspended in 1 mL FGM-SF and counted. Appropriate volumes of resuspended cells were centrifuged again and resuspended in DMEM. The cells were then mixed 1:1 with the collagen mixture to generate a 1 mg/mL collagen, 3% DEX solution. The collagen-DEX-cell suspension was transferred to a 96-well plate for seeding, where the DEX-cell suspension would be seeded into the wells containing PEG, as in **Figure 1B**.

Liquid Handling and Imaging

As in our previous publication (Moraes et al., 2013), a Cybio FeliX liquid handler (Analytik Jena) was used to prepare collagen microgel plates (see **Supplementary File** for liquid handler script).

Collagen microgels were incubated and imaged using an Incucyte S3 (Sartorius) in-incubator microscope system. The Incucyte S3 performs auto-focus on each well of the microplate. 4x brightfield images were acquired at 1 h intervals for 2 days, then at 6 h intervals for the next 6 days.

Drug Response Studies

Cell-laden collagen microgels were stimulated with or without 10 ng/mL TGF-β1 (R&D Systems) and anti-fibrotic drugs: nintedanib (Selleck Chem), pirfenidone (Selleck Chem), and the focal adhesion kinase inhibitor PF 431396 (Tocris) at specified concentrations. These collagen microgels were imaged over 8 days to monitor contraction. To determine the half maximal inhibitory concentration (IC50), the area under the curve (AUC) of the area over time graph was calculated for each individual gel as a parameter of overall contractility. These values were normalized, such that a gel with no contraction would have a normalized AUC of 100%. These contraction responses were fit

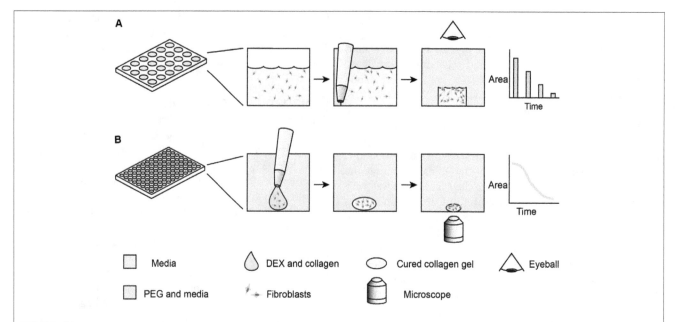

FIGURE 1 | Comparison of standard collagen contraction assay with high-throughput ATPS method presented here. **(A)** Overview of traditional collagen contraction assay in a 24-well plate. After seeding fibroblasts in a collagen matrix, the gels are individually detached from the well and imaged at discrete time intervals. **(B)** In the ATPS collagen contraction assay, DEX and collagen droplets containing fibroblasts are mixed with PEG and media in 96-well plates. This creates a microgel in the center of the well, thereby eliminating the need for individual gel removal from the wall. The PEG and DEX solutions are then washed out, and then imaged every 2 h with an Incucyte microscope.

to sigmoidal curves using the scipy module in python (Virtanen et al., 2020), using Eq. 1:

$$Response = A + \frac{100 - A}{1 + 10^{(\log(x) - \log(C)) * B}} \quad (1)$$

where A is the extent of contraction in the control condition, B is the Hill Coefficient, and C is the IC50.

Image Processing

Collagen microgel areas were quantified using three methods: manual, Incucyte, and trainable WEKA segmentation. For manual quantification, gel perimeters were traced using ImageJ and areas were measured. For Incucyte quantification, images were segmented using the built-in Incucyte 2019A segmentation software from the Spheroid Module. In the trainable WEKA segmentation plugin from FIJI (ImageJ) (Arganda-Carreras et al., 2017), 1–10 representative microgel images were annotated and used to train the classifier. We wrote a new plugin (see **Supplementary File**) to iterate through a folder of images exported from the Incucyte 2019A software, apply the WEKA classifier, run quality checks, measure areas, and generate a .csv file containing areas, well positions, and times. Further analyses were performed using the pandas module in python (McKinney, 2010).

Statistical Analysis

For the comparison between manual and algorithm measurements of gel areas, the Pearsons correlation coefficient was calculated. The differences between gel contraction for +/− TGF-β1 conditions at the indicated time points were analyzed

using multiple *t*-tests with a Bonferroni correction and a 95% confidence interval. Lastly, standard deviations for parameter estimates of the IC50 values in the drug dose response studies were acquired from the covariance matrix of the model fit (scipy.optimize.curve_fit module in Python).

RESULTS

Validation and Optimization of Machine Learning Image Processing

To quantify collagen microgel area, we initially examined the built-in Incucyte segmentation software. However, the software performed poorly with microplate imperfections (i.e., – plate scratches) and gels at early time points, when they are relatively translucent (data not shown). We next examined WEKA Trainable Segmentation, a machine learning plugin included in the open source image processing program, FIJI (ImageJ). **Figure 2** shows the process for training the WEKA Segmentation classifier. After loading an image sequence into FIJI and selecting Trainable WEKA Segmentation, the background area is manually identified with the cursor and marked as Class 1. Gel areas are similarly marked as Class 2. After training a classifier, additional annotations can be added to revise the classifier until it performs adequately. Once a satisfactory classifier has been found, it is saved for future use (**Figures 2A–C**).

To analyze large sets of images exported from the Incucyte in-incubator microscope, a FIJI plugin was written (**Supplementary File**). This plugin uses the built-in Trainable WEKA Segmentation plugin to apply the saved classifier to each

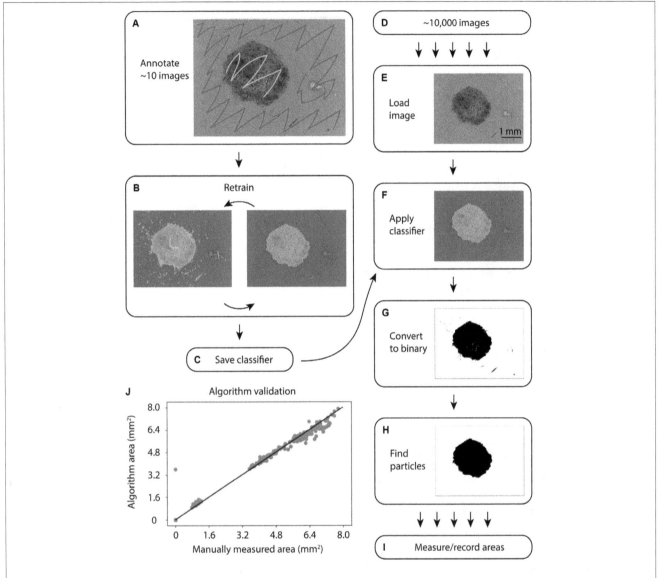

FIGURE 2 | Overview of WEKA segmentation. **(A)** First, the training set of ~10 images is annotated, clearly indicating the collagen gel and microwell plate background. **(B)** The classifier is retrained until it performs adequately. **(C)** After ensuring appropriate performance, the classifier is saved. **(D)** Approximately 10,000 images are acquired from the Incucyte microscopy system. **(E)** Images are loaded into FIJI and **(F)** the classifier created in **(A–C)** is applied. **(G)** The images are converted to binary and **(H)** particles are selected. **(I)** Finally, the area of each gel is measured and recorded. **(J)** Correlation plot of WEKA Segmentation and manual area annotation, showing a linear relationship.

image in a directory, as in **Figures 2D–I**. Following classification, the image was converted to binary and the largest particle was found using the built-in particles function. Areas and metadata were then recorded.

During initial testing on an Intel™ Core® i7-7700 CPU at 3.60 GHz, classification of a single image took 15 s. Further exploration revealed that smaller training sets enabled faster classification. The iterative training process in **Figure 2** allowed for fine-tuning small training sets to achieve accurate segmentation without sacrificing speed.

To validate the automated image analysis algorithm, 300 images of microgels from early and late time points were manually annotated for comparison of area measurements.

A strong correlation of 0.990 (Pearsons) with manual area measurements was achieved (**Figure 2J**).

Collagen Microgel Contractions Kinetics

We examined the performance of the ATPS collagen microgel contraction assay with NHLF and IPF responses to TGF-β1 stimulation at a high dose (10 ng/mL) using our automated seeding, washing, and image processing system. The NHLF had both slower baseline contraction and slower TGF-β1 activated contraction compared to IPF, as expected. However, we only tested cells from one patient of each category, so conclusions about biological differences between patients are not justified from this study alone. TGF-β1 induced a moderate increase in

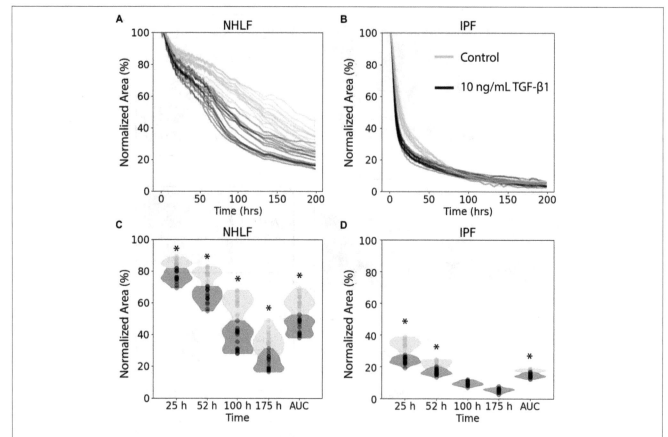

FIGURE 3 | Collagen microgel contraction kinetics and use of an aggregate statistic to distinguish contraction behavior depending on imaging timepoint.
(A) Normalized area of collagen gels over time for NHLF and **(B)** IPF cells. Each line represents an individual gel. Orange curves are for control samples, and black curves are for cells stimulated with 10 ng/ml TFG-β1. **(C)** Contraction of NHLF and **(D)** IPF cells in response to stimulation with 10 ng/mL TGF-β1. The ability to discern a difference in response depends on the timepoint at which measurements are made. However, the area under the curve more readily and consistently reflects these differences. $n = 15$ per condition. *$p < 0.05$ between the +/− TGF-β1 conditions on multiple t-tests with a Bonferroni correction.

the rate of contraction for both cell types, as shown in **Figure 3**. **Figures 3A,B** show the area of each collagen gel (NHLF and IPF, respectively) as it contracts over time, normalized to that gel's initial area. The same data is shown again in **Figures 3C,D**, but with violin plots to convey the distribution. For the NHLF cells, multiple t-tests with Bonferroni correction indicated significant differences with a 95% confidence interval between groups (presence or absence of TGF-β1) at each of the selected time points – 25, 52, 100, and 175 h, as well as using the area under the curve aggregated data. However, the IPF cells only showed significantly different responses to TGF-β1 at the early time points (25 and 52 h) and with the area under the curve.

Examination of Anti-fibrotic Drugs

We next assessed the ability of known anti-fibrotic drugs to inhibit contraction of collagen microgels. Using a concentration range of 32 nM to 500 μM, we analyzed the dynamic contraction of collagen microgels with NHLF and IPF cells, both with and without 10 ng/mL TGF-β1. For these studies, we selected the two FDA-approved fibrosis therapeutics, nintedanib (pan-kinase inhibitor) and pirfenidone (mechanism still unclear). Additionally, we examined the focal adhesion kinase (FAK)

inhibitor, PF 431396 (**Figures 4A–D** and **Supplementary Figures 1–3**).

Dose response curves were fit for normalized area measurements at each time point (**Supplementary Figure 4**). In comparison to the high variance seen at individual time points, dose response curves for area under the curve measurements incorporated kinetic data, generating narrower standard deviations of the parameter estimate for IC50, as seen in **Figure 4E**. The IC50 values for each drug and cell condition are shown for AUC measurements in **Figure 4E** and for each individual time point in **Supplementary Figure 4**. The IC50 values for AUC measurements are also listed in **Supplementary Table 1**. Both the FAK inhibitor (PF 431396) and nintedanib showed efficacy across the cell and stimulation type, while pirfenidone did not achieve 50% effect within the range of concentrations tested.

DISCUSSION

In this work, we added automated image acquisition and analysis to our group's prior development of an ATPS collagen microgel contraction assay (Moraes et al., 2013). We also analyzed normal

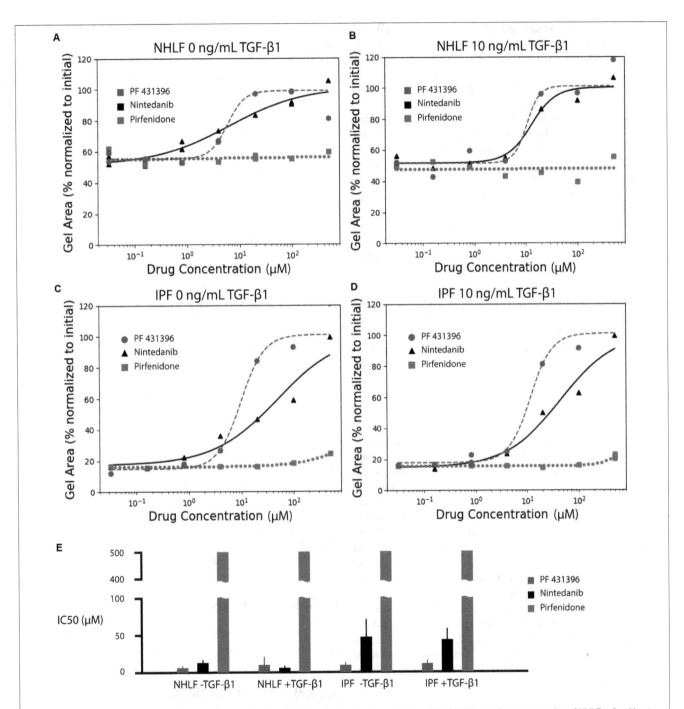

FIGURE 4 | Effect of anti-fibrotic drugs (nintedanib and pirfenidone) and focal adhesion kinase inhibitor (PF 431396) on collagen contraction of NHLF cells without **(A)** and with **(B)** 10 ng/mL TGF-β1, and IPF cells without **(C)** and with **(D)** 10 ng/mL TGF-β1. The fitted parameters for IC50 are plotted in **(E)**. Error bars are the standard deviation of the parameter estimate.

and diseased primary human lung fibroblasts, whereas we had previously analyzed only fibroblast immortalized cell lines. Our previous work focused on the miniaturization of the ATPS collagen microgel contraction assay, opening the possibility for more effective mass transport of agonists and antagonists to the cells (Moraes et al., 2013). The addition of automated imaging and subsequent analysis in this report enabled higher throughput,

as well as kinetic analysis of the collagen microgel contraction. Due to the translucent properties of the collagen microgels, the built-in image analysis software in the Incucyte was unable to accurately detect the collagen gels. This shortcoming was addressed by implementing WEKA Segmentation through a custom Jython plugin for FIJI. The WEKA Segmentation reliably yielded measurements matching those found by manually tracing

---

the outlines of the collagen gels, indicating that the WEKA Segmentation was a sufficient tool for image processing. The automated image acquisition and analysis enabled an order of magnitude higher frequency of imaging compared to the standard daily measurement. This temporal analysis unveiled the rapid initial contraction seen in IPF-sourced fibroblasts.

For downstream analysis, it is useful to aggregate the data from an individual contraction time course into a single metric. Although some individual time points are useful to detect the increased contraction in response to TGF-β1, much of the kinetic information is lost. Therefore, we used the area under the curve to aggregate the rate of contraction for each individual gel into a single metric.

Consistent with literature reports (Jin et al., 2019), pirfenidone has little effect below 500 μM, but mildly inhibits contraction at 500 μM in all conditions (**Supplementary Figure 1**). Previous examinations of pirfenidone to modulate fibroblast behavior *in vitro* have required concentrations of 500 μM or higher to see statistically significant suppression of α-SMA and collagen (Nakayama et al., 2008; Conte et al., 2014). However, 500 μM was selected as the high concentration for these studies due to the requirement for high concentrations of dimethyl sulfoxide (DMSO) necessary to achieve pirfenidone concentrations above 500 μM. In this study, the DMSO concentration was kept at 0.1%. None of the concentrations of pirfenidone tested in this study produced a half maximal inhibition of contraction (**Figure 4**).

In contrast, nintedanib exhibits a dose-dependent inhibition of contraction in all cell conditions tested (**Supplementary Figure 2**). Areas of collagen microgels were normalized to their initial area. Interestingly, the inhibition of microgel contraction was largely independent of TGF-β1 for both NHLF and IPF. After a rapid initial contraction, the area reduction dramatically slowed after ~1 day in culture for both cell types (Rangarajan et al., 2016). Our study is the only *in vitro* study to obtain IC50 values for nintedanib in NHLF and IPF cells with and without TGF-β1 in side-by-side studies. We do note that in the few *in vitro* studies that do report IC50, that those values were lower – 144 nM for inhibition of α-SMA in IPF cells (Wollin et al., 2014) and a conference abstract that notes 73 nM for inhibition of PDGF-stimulated collagen gel contraction with NHLF (Wollin et al., 2016). IC50, however, is not a fundamental constant but rather a convenient, assay-specific measure of potency. Thus, comparison of values across different experiments must be made with caution (Kalliokoski et al., 2013).

Lastly, the focal adhesion kinase (FAK) inhibitor, PF 431396, inhibited contraction at concentrations above 4 μM for all cell types, as shown in **Supplementary Figure 3**. Although FAK inhibition is not a widely used drug target due to many off-target effects, this experiment does corroborate previous reports indicating that NHLF contraction of collagen gels requires FAK stimulation (Liu et al., 2010; Epa et al., 2015).

These are, to our knowledge, the first reports of dose response for inhibition of TGF-β1 stimulated collagen gel contraction of primary human fibroblasts by pirfenidone, nintedanib, and PF 431396. While these results nicely demonstrate the technical capabilities, this proof-of-concept drug comparison study is limited with regards to biological conclusions by the small number of replicates and cells from just two donors.

CONCLUSION

We have extended the ATPS microgel contraction assay with live-cell imaging to uncover differential phenotypic behavior of primary cells, whereas our previous methods were limited to cell lines. Because contraction is a time-dependent process, a higher sampling frequency (e.g., every hour vs. the more common every 12–24 h) can provide richer information. We assessed and optimized an automated image segmentation algorithm using WEKA machine learning to measure the areas of 10,000 collagen gel images with high temporal resolution. The assay provides added convenience and throughput, making it appropriate for secondary screening assays and dose response studies. Lastly, we report dose response characteristics for two FDA approved drugs: nintedanib, pirfenidone, as well as the FAK inhibitor, PF 431396 with healthy and diseased primary human fibroblasts, each with and without TGF-β1 activation. The calculated IC50 values confirm previous reports of lower potency for pirfenidone relative to nintedanib. This assay could provide useful phenotypic data to aid secondary and tertiary drug screens, as well as high-throughput information about primary cell behavior in basic research on fibroblast contraction.

AUTHOR CONTRIBUTIONS

CY and ST conceptualized the project idea. CY performed experiments. All authors contributed to writing the manuscript.

ACKNOWLEDGMENTS

We thank Prof. Louise Hecker for helpful discussions.

REFERENCES

Ahluwalia, N., Shea, B. S., and Tager, A. M. (2014). New therapeutic targets in idiopathic pulmonary fibrosis. Aiming to rein in runaway wound-healing responses. *Am. J. Respir. Crit. Care Med.* 190, 867–878. doi: 10.1164/rccm.201403-0509PP

Arganda-Carreras, I., Kaynig, V., Rueden, C., Eliceiri, K. W., Schindelin, J.,

Cardona, A., et al. (2017). Trainable weka segmentation: a machine learning tool for microscopy pixel classification. *Bioinformatics* 33, 2424–2426. doi: 10.1093/bioinformatics/btx180

Barkauskas, C. E., and Noble, P. W. (2014). Cellular mechanisms of tissue fibrosis. 7. New insights into the cellular mechanisms of pulmonary fibrosis. *Am. J. Physiol. Cell Physiol.* 306, C987–C996. doi: 10.1152/ajpcell.00321.2013

Bell, E., Ivarsson, B., and Merrill, C. (1979). Production of a tissue-like structure by contraction of collagen lattices by human fibroblasts of different proliferative potential in vitro. *Proc. Natl. Acad. Sci. U.S.A.* 76, 1274–1278. doi: 10.1073/pnas. 76.3.1274

Betensley, A., Sharif, R., and Karamichos, D. (2016). A systematic review of the role of dysfunctional wound healing in the pathogenesis and treatment of idiopathic pulmonary fibrosis. *J. Clin. Med.* 6:2. doi: 10.3390/jcm6010002

Borensztajn, K., Crestani, B., and Kolb, M. (2014). Idiopathic pulmonary fibrosis: from epithelial injury to biomarkers-insights from the bench side. *Respiration* 86, 441–452. doi: 10.1159/000357598

Campbell, J. D., McDonough, J. E., Zeskind, J. E., Hackett, T. L., Pechkovsky, D. V., Brandsma, C. A., et al. (2012). A gene expression signature of emphysema-related lung destruction and its reversal by the tripeptide GHK. *Genome Med.* 4:67. doi: 10.1186/gm367

Chen, W., Wong, C., Vosburgh, E., Levine, A. J., Foran, D. J., and Xu, E. Y. (2014). High-throughput image analysis of tumor spheroids: A user-friendly software application to measure the size of spheroids automatically and accurately. *J. Vis. Exp.* e51639. doi: 10.3791/51639

Conte, E., Gili, E., Fagone, E., Fruciano, M., Iemmolo, M., and Vancheri, C. (2014). Effect of pirfenidone on proliferation, TGF-β-induced myofibroblast differentiation and fibrogenic activity of primary human lung fibroblasts. *Eur. J. Pharm. Sci.* 58, 13–19. doi: 10.1016/j.ejps.2014. 02.014

Cui, H., Banerjee, S., Xie, N., Ge, J., Liu, R. M., Matalon, S., et al. (2016). MicroRNA-27a-3p is a negative regulator of lung fibrosis by targeting myofibroblast differentiation. *Am. J. Respir. Cell Mol. Biol.* 54, 843–852. doi: 10.1165/rcmb. 2015-0205OC

Epa, A. P., Thatcher, T. H., Pollock, S. J., Wahl, L. A., Lyda, E., Kottmann, R. M., et al. (2015). Normal human lung epithelial cells inhibit transforming growth factor-β induced myofibroblast differentiation via prostaglandin E2. *PLoS One* 10:e0135266. doi: 10.1371/journal.pone.0135266

Jin, J., Togo, S., Kadoya, K., Tulafu, M., Namba, Y., Iwai, M., et al. (2019). Pirfenidone attenuates lung fibrotic fibroblast responses to transforming growth factor-β1. *Respir. Res.* 20, 1–14. doi: 10.1186/s12931-019-1093-z

Kalliokoski, T., Kramer, C., Vulpetti, A., and Gedeck, P. (2013). Comparability of mixed IC_{50} Data - a statistical analysis. *PLoS One* 8:e61007. doi: 10.1371/journal. pone.0061007

Kondo, S., Kagami, S., Urushihara, M., Kitamura, A., Shimizu, M., Strutz, F., et al. (2004). Transforming growth factor-β1 stimulates collagen matrix remodeling through increased adhesive and contractive potential by human renal fibroblasts. *Biochim. Biophys. Acta Mol. Cell Res.* 1693, 91–100. doi: 10. 1016/j.bbamcr.2004.05.005

Liu, F., Mih, J. D., Shea, B. S., Kho, A. T., Sharif, A. S., Tager, A. M., et al. (2010). Feedback amplification of fibrosis through matrix stiffening and COX-2 suppression. *J. Cell Biol.* 190, 693–706. doi: 10.1083/jcb.201004082

Maher, T. M., and Strek, M. E. (2019). Antifibrotic therapy for idiopathic pulmonary fibrosis: time to treat. *Respir. Res.* 20:205. doi: 10.1186/s12931-019-1161-4

McKinney, W. (2010). "Data structures for statistical computing in python," in *Proceedings of the. 9th Python Sicence*, Vol. 445, Austin, TX, 51–56. doi: 10. 25080/Majora-92bf1922-00a

Mohan, R., and Bargagna-Mohan, P. (2016). *The Use of Withaferin A to Study Intermediate Filaments*, 1st Edn. Amsterdam: Elsevier Inc.

Moraes, C., Simon, A. B., Putnam, A. J., and Takayama, S. (2013). Aqueous two-phase printing of cell-containing contractile collagen microgels. *Biomaterials* 34, 9623–9631. doi: 10.1016/j.biomaterials.2013.08.046

Nakayama, S., Mukae, H., Sakamoto, N., Kakugawa, T., Yoshioka, S., Soda, H., et al. (2008). Pirfenidone inhibits the expression of HSP47 in TGF-β1-stimulated human lung fibroblasts. *Life Sci.* 82, 210–217. doi: 10.1016/j.lfs.2007.11.003

Rangarajan, S., Kurundkar, A., Kurundkar, D., Bernard, K., Sanders, Y. Y., Ding, Q., et al. (2016). Novel mechanisms for the antifibrotic action of nintedanib. *Am. J. Respir. Cell Mol. Biol.* 54, 51–59. doi: 10.1165/rcmb.2014-0445OC

Rodday, B., Hirschhaeuser, F., Walenta, S., and Mueller-Klieser, W. (2011). Semiautomatic growth analysis of multicellular tumor spheroids. *J. Biomol. Screen.* 16, 1119–1124. doi: 10.1177/1087057111419501

Singh, S., and Tavana, H. (2018). Collagen partition in polymeric aqueous two-phase systems for tissue engineering. *Front. Chem.* 6:379. doi: 10.3389/fchem. 2018.00379

Virtanen, P., Gommers, R., Oliphant, T. E., Haberland, M., Reddy, T., Cournapeau, D., et al. (2020). SciPy 1.0: fundamental algorithms for scientific computing in Python. *Nat. Methods* 17, 261–272. doi: 10.1038/s41592-019-0686-2

Wollin, L., Maillet, I., Quesniaux, V., Holweg, A., and Ryffel, B. (2014). Antifibrotic and anti-inflammatory activity of the tyrosine kinase inhibitor nintedanib in experimental models of lung fibrosiss. *J. Pharmacol. Exp. Ther.* 349, 209–220. doi: 10.1124/jpet.113.208223

Wollin, L., Schuett, J., Ostermann, A., and Herrmann, F. (2016). "The effect of nintedanib on platelet derived growth factor-stimulated contraction of human primary lung fibroblasts," in *Proceedings of the American Thoracic Society International Conference Abstracts A73. LUNG FIBROSIS: NEW DIRECTIONS TO INFORM THE FUTURE*, (New York, NY: American Thoracic Society).

Yamanishi, C., Robinson, S., and Takayama, S. (2019). Biofabrication of phenotypic pulmonary fibrosis assays. *Biofabrication* 11:032005. doi: 10.1088/1758-5090/ ab2286

Zhang, T., Day, J. H., Su, X., Guadarrama, A. G., Sandbo, N. K., Esnault, S., et al. (2019). Investigating fibroblast-induced collagen gel contraction using a dynamic microscale platform. *Front. Bioeng. Biotechnol.* 7:196. doi: 10.3389/ fbioe.2019.00196

14

Pulmonary Deposition of Radionucleotide-Labeled Palivizumab

Anushi E. Rajapaksa[1,2,3]*, Lien Anh Ha Do[1,4], Darren Suryawijaya Ong[1,4], Magdy Sourial[5], Duncan Veysey[6], Richard Beare[7,8], William Hughes[1], William Yang[1], Robert J. Bischof[9,10], Amarin McDonnell[11], Peter Eu[12], Leslie Y. Yeo[11]*, Paul V. Licciardi[1,4]† and Edward K. Mulholland[1,2,13]†

[1] New Vaccines, Murdoch Children's Research Institute, Parkville, VIC, Australia, [2] Neonatal Research, Royal Children's Hospital, Parkville, VIC, Australia, [3] Newborn Research, Royal Women's Hospital, Parkville, VIC, Australia, [4] Department of Paediatrics, University of Melbourne, Parkville, VIC, Australia, [5] Animal Model Unit, The Royal Children's Hospital, Parkville, VIC, Australia, [6] Nuclear Imaging, The Royal Children's Hospital, Parkville, VIC, Australia, [7] Developmental Imaging, Murdoch Children's Research Institute, Parkville, VIC, Australia, [8] Department of Medicine, Monash University, Melbourne, VIC, Australia, [9] The Ritchie Centre, Hudson Institute of Medical Research, Clayton, VIC, Australia, [10] School of Health and Life Sciences, Federation University, Berwick, VIC, Australia, [11] School of Engineering, Royal Melbourne Institute of Technology, Melbourne, VIC, Australia, [12] Department of Cancer Imaging, Peter MacCallum Cancer Centre, Parkville, VIC, Australia, [13] Department of Disease Control, London School of Tropical Medicine and Hygiene, London, United Kingdom

*Correspondence:
Anushi E. Rajapaksa
anushi.rajapaksa@mcri.edu.au
Leslie Y. Yeo
leslie.yeo@rmit.edu.au

†These authors have contributed equally to this work

Objective: Current prevention and/or treatment options for respiratory syncytial virus (RSV) infections are limited as no vaccine is available. Prophylaxis with palivizumab is very expensive and requires multiple intramuscular injections over the RSV season. Here we present proof-of-concept data using nebulized palivizumab delivery as a promising new approach for the prevention or treatment of severe RSV infections, documenting both aerosol characteristics and pulmonary deposition patterns in the lungs of lambs.

Design: Prospective animal study.

Setting: Biosecurity Control Level 2-designated large animal research facility at the Murdoch Children's Research Institute, Melbourne, Australia.

Subjects: Four weaned Border-Leicester/Suffolk lambs at 5 months of age.

Interventions: Four lambs were administered aerosolized palivizumab conjugated to Tc-99m, under gaseous anesthesia, using either the commercially available AeroNeb Go® or the investigational HYDRA device, placed in-line with the inspiratory limb of a breathing circuit. Lambs were scanned in a single-photon emission computed tomography (SPECT/CT) scanner in the supine position during the administration procedure.

Measurements and Main Results: Both the HYDRA and AeroNeb Go® produced palivizumab aerosols in the 1–5 µm range with similar median (geometric standard deviation and range) aerosol droplet diameters for the HYDRA device (1.84 ± 1.40 µm, range = 0.54–5.41 µm) and the AeroNeb Go® (3.07 ± 1.56 µm, range = 0.86–10 µm). Aerosolized palivizumab was delivered to the lungs at 88.79–94.13% of the total aerosolized amount for all lambs, with a small proportion localized to either the trachea or stomach. No difference between devices were found. Pulmonary deposition ranged from 6.57 to 9.25% of the total dose of palivizumab loaded in the devices, mostly in the central right lung.

Conclusions: Aerosolized palivizumab deposition patterns were similar in all lambs, suggesting a promising approach in the control of severe RSV lung infections.

Keywords: respiratory syncytial virus, lamb model, prophylactic, monoclonal antibody, palivizumab, nebulization

INTRODUCTION

Respiratory syncytial virus (RSV) is the leading pathogen causing lower respiratory tract infections (O'Brien et al., 2019), and has been responsible for up to 199,000 deaths worldwide in children under 5 years old annually (Nair et al., 2010). Since 2013, the World Health Organization has designated protection against severe RSV disease as a high priority, particularly for infants <6 months of age, preterm infants, and infants with underlying comorbidities. There is no vaccine available, and palivizumab, a humanized monoclonal antibody (mAb) against RSV F protein, is currently the only licensed preventive product but is costly, limited in effectiveness and requires monthly intramuscular injections.

Inhaled delivery is one approach to provide pain- and needle-free administration of palivizumab. It also offers the advantage of delivering the mAb immediately and directly to the respiratory tract and lung, potentially providing a rapid clinical benefit for the prevention and/or treatment of severe RSV infection. Our recently developed acoustic nebulizer, HYDRA (HYbriD Resonant Acoustics) (Rezk et al., 2016) allows for fast and effective aerosol delivery of mAbs (Cortez-Jugo et al., 2015) and other large biological molecules such as DNA (Rajapaksa et al., 2014) to the respiratory surface *via* inhalation. Using a lamb model, we compare the deposition of aerosolized palivizumab to the lungs using the HYDRA or the commercially-available AeroNeb Go® (now marketed as Innospire Go by Philips Respironics) vibrating mesh nebulizer as a proof-of-concept approach for the prevention and/or treatment of severe RSV disease.

MATERIALS AND METHODS

Laser diffraction (Spraytec®, Malvern Instruments, Malvern, UK) was employed to determine the aerodynamic diameter (D_{ae}) of the aerosols produced using the HYDRA or the AeroNeb Go® (Aerogen, Galway, Ireland), from which the median aerosol size (D_{v50}) was calculated from a volume-based size distribution. The geometric standard deviation (GSD) was manually calculated using standard methodology (Finlay, 2019).

The lamb study was approved by the Murdoch Children's Research Institute (MCRI) Animal Ethics Committee. Experiments were designed and reported with reference to the ARRIVE (Animal Research: Reporting of *in vivo* Experiments) guidelines (Kilkenny et al., 2010). Four month-old lambs were given 60 mg of palivizumab (Synagis®, AbbVie, Illinois, USA) at 10 mg/ml, conjugated to a radiotracer technetium-99m (Tc-99m; Global Medical Solutions, Tullamarine, Australia). ^{99m}TcO$_4$-palivizumab was prepared by a ligand exchange method using glucoheptonate and tin chloride (SnCl$_2$). Briefly, 1 ml of palivizumab (100 mg/ml) was diluted in 1 ml water for injection, then incubated at room temperature with 150 µl of 2-mercaptoethanol for 20 min, before purification through a PD-10 size exclusion column (30,000 MWCO). To this purified

eluent, 100 µl of glucoheptonate/SnCl$_2$ stock (0.2 M glucoheptonate, 0.002 M SnCl$_2$) solution was added and mixed. Roughly, 0.5 MBq of ^{99m}TcO$_4$ was then added to the palivizumab/glucoheptonate solution and incubated for 30 min at room temperature. Purity was checked using the iTLC-SG method in water, before final dilution of the conjugate to 10 ml (10 mg/ml palivizumab).

Palivizumab aerosols were delivered *via* an endotracheal tube (Smiths Medical, Minnesota, USA) to spontaneously breathing lambs (n = 2 lambs for each device) under anesthesia placed in prone position. Pulmonary deposition was mapped using single-photon emission computed tomography and computed tomography (SPECT/CT) using a Symbia Intevo 16 scanner (Siemens, Munich, Germany).

Lambs were placed in the prone position for this procedure. SPECT portions of the scans were performed using the following SPECT parameters: 128 × 128 matrix, 1.23× zoom, Tc-99m NMG camera pre-set, 25 s per view for 64 views using a 180° detector rotation and continuous scan mode. CT portions of the scans were performed following topogram Scout view and imaged at 20mA and 80kV. Image slices of 3 mm thickness were reconstructed using a I50s Medium Sharp kernel with a lung window. Pre- and post-delivery radioactive counts were measured to determine efficiency of the aerosolized palivizumab administration. Briefly, for the SPECT/CT analysis, lung structure segmentation was performed using morphological watersheds with manually placed seeds applied to the gradient of the CT image. Regional distribution of pulmonary deposition was determined by voxelwise summation within each lung structure. The efficiency of palivizumab delivery to lambs relative to the total palivizumab prepared and the efficiency of palivizumab delivery to the lungs relative to the whole body are presented as geometric means (%). A RSV neutralization assay (Do et al., 2019) was used to determine the bioactivity of palivizumab before and after aerosolization.

RESULTS

Efficiency of palivizumab conjugation to Tc-99m was >90% (**Table 1**). The median aerosol droplet diameter for palivizumab were similar for both the HYDRA device (1.84 ± 1.40 µm, range = 0.54–5.41 µm) and the AeroNeb Go® (3.07 ± 1.56 µm, range = 0.86–10

TABLE 1 | Conjugation efficiency of palivizumab conjugated to technetium-99m (Tc-99m).

Lamb	Device	% palivizumab deposited in lungs	
		Reading 1	Reading 2
1	AeroNeb Go®	98.51	98.33
2	AeroNeb Go®	97.94	91.75
3	HYDRA	94.83	90.32
4	HYDRA	99.09	98.41

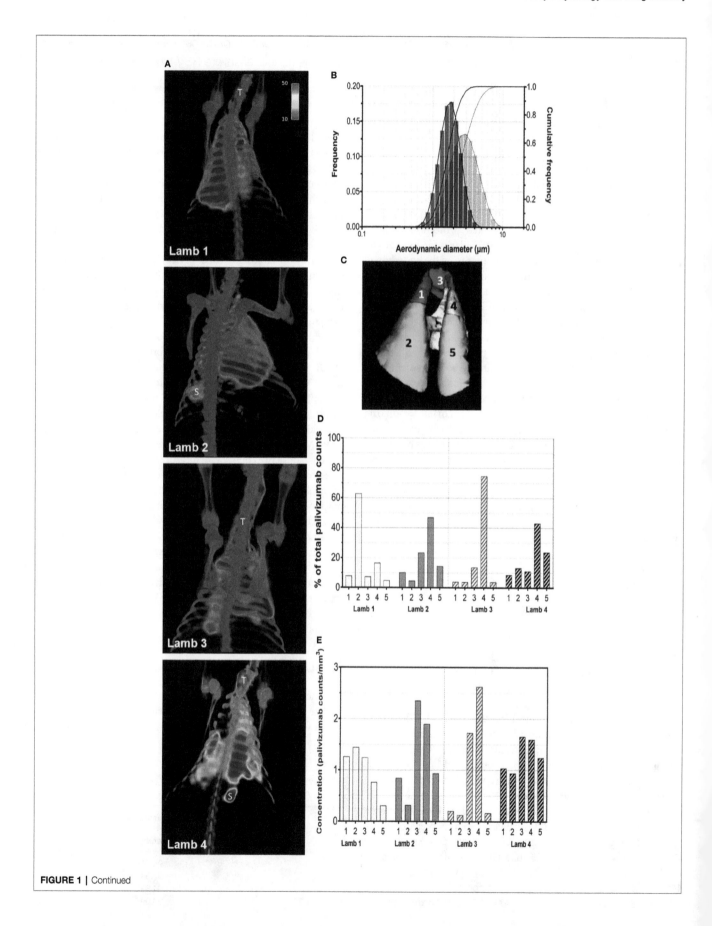

FIGURE 1 | Continued

FIGURE 1 | Aerosolization and pulmonary deposition of palivizumab in lambs. **(A)** Reconstructed SPECT/CT images are shown for lambs 1 and 2 administered palivizumab using AeroNeb Go® and lambs 3 and 4 using the HYDRA device. The trachea (T) and stomach (S) were also visible in some deposition images. **(B)** Volume frequencies of the palivizumab aerosol size at given aerodynamic diameters for the AeroNeb Go® (light bars, dotted lines) and HYDRA device (dark bars, solid lines). **(C)** Lungs were segmented into left apical (1), left caudal (2), right apical (3), right middle (4), and right caudal (5) lobes as shown. **(D)** Regional deposition patterns of aerosolized palivizumab in individual lambs relative to the whole lung. **(E)** Concentration of palivizumab aerosols (counts/mm³) are shown within individual lobes. Values on the intensity scale correspond to palivizumab density (counts per voxel).

μm) nebulizers, producing palivizumab aerosols in the 1–5 μm range that is optimal for deep lung deposition (**Figure 1A**). The RSV neutralizing activity of conjugated palivizumab before and after aerosolization was similar to native palivizumab and comparable between the devices (**Table 2**).

Analyses of pulmonary deposition data from the SPECT/CT images showed the percentage of total aerosolized palivizumab delivered to the lambs (relative to that loaded to the devices) ranged from 6.57 to 9.25% (**Table 2** and **Figure 1B**). A large percentage of the palivizumab aerosols (88.79–94.13%) was deposited in the lungs (**Table 1**) with only a small proportion localized to either the trachea or stomach. A similar level of deposition was found for both devices (**Table 2**). Regional deposition bias was demonstrated towards the left lung for lamb 1 and the right lung for all other lambs, with deposition detected across all five lung segments (**Figures 1C–E**; see also the **Supplementary Videos**).

DISCUSSION

This is the first study, to our knowledge, to explore the pulmonary deposition of aerosolized palivizumab. We used SPECT/CT as it is superior to planar imaging by providing a three-dimensional assessment of aerosol deposition, allowing determination of intrapulmonary distribution and precise anatomical regional measurements. We were able to accurately visualize palivizumab deposition in the lungs of all four lambs regardless of the aerosolization device employed, providing proof-of-concept for aerosol delivery of a RSV-specific mAb to the potential sites of RSV replication.

Both the AeroNeb Go® and HYDRA devices showed similar aerosol deposition in the lungs relative to the whole body, without detriment to the palivizumab activity. The HYDRA can potentially generate smaller particle size distributions

without the requirement of a mesh but we used a slightly reduced nebulization rate compared with Aeroneb Go® for large biomolecules such as palivizumab.

While significant loss of palivizumab due to deposition in the endotracheal tube was observed, we do not expect the tube to have any impact on the differences observed. In three lambs, we noticed a depositional bias towards the right lung, with two of these lambs showing higher deposition efficiency in the right upper lobes in contrast to the other lamb which had higher deposition in the lower left lobe. Several factors may explain the difference observed in lamb 1: (1) maintaining procedural anesthesia while receiving brief periods of manual ventilation and (2) scheduling differences with the BALF procedure (2 weeks earlier due to technical difficulties) could have induced fluid bias to the right lung. A possible explanation might be that the infusion of saline into the lung cavity during BALF collection promoted increased humidity in the respiratory tract, which has been shown to alter aerosol size and movement patterns (Cheng, 2014). As such the humid conditions of the right lung may have attracted more aerosols into the respective lobes.

Targeting the lungs is proving to be an effective strategy as this is the site of RSV infection (Davis et al., 2007). Recently, an anti-RSV nanobody ALX-0171 at 0.3 mg/kg dose was aerosolized using the AeroNeb Solo® system; whereby 11% of the therapeutic nanobody was delivered to the lungs of RSV-infected lambs leading to reductions in both RSV lesions and viral antigen expression (Mora et al., 2018). In our study, the concentration of palivizumab delivered to the lungs as a single dose (~0.57–0.85 mg/ml) was 2–4 fold greater than that shown previously to neutralize RSV activity *in vitro* (Carlin et al., 1999). Aerosolized palivizumab also appeared to cause low-level inflammatory responses in the lung following delivery (data not shown) but interpretation of this finding is difficult as we did not have a control lamb without aerosolized palivizumab. Future studies are therefore necessary to fully document these effects.

Conventional delivery of palivizumab *via* intramuscular (IM) injection takes 3–5 days to achieve the dose in serum needed to protect against RSV infections (Sáez-Llorens et al., 1998). Rapid airway delivery of palivizumab may have substantial therapeutic benefits for high-risk infants and may provide more targeted control of RSV nosocomial infections in neonatal intensive care units (NICU) compared to IM palivizumab previously used for this purpose (Abadesso et al., 2004).

Despite the small sample size, this proof-of-concept study provides important data on the feasibility of pulmonary delivery and neutralizing bioactivity of palivizumab directly to the potential site of infection. This concept could also be tested on the new extended half-life RSV F mAb product (nirsevimab) that has recently been granted Breakthrough Therapy Designation by the US Food and Drug Administration (FDA). The lungs of a lamb constitute a

TABLE 2 | Efficiency of aerosolized palivizumab delivery using the AeroNeb Go® and HYDRA devices.

Lamb	Device	NAb ED₅₀ titre (Mean ± SD)	% palivizumab delivered to lamb	% palivizumab deposited in lungs
1	AeroNeb Go®	11.35 ± 0.1[a]	8.8	88.79
2	AeroNeb Go®		9.25	91.86
3	HYDRA	11.39 ± 0.1[a]	ND[b]	94.13
4	HYDRA		6.57	92.51

Data shown for individual lambs.
NAb, neutralizing antibody; ED50, titre of antibody that neutralises 50% of RSV infection; [a]Mean (± SD) NAb titre of native palivizumab stock (15.45 ± 0.3); [b]ND, not determined due to failure in taking pre-aerosolization measurements in one portion of the SPECT scanner.

highly translational model that shares many key features with that of a human infant, including structure and function. Determining the effect of inhaled palivizumab on RSV disease as well as the optimal inhaled dose/schedule necessary to prevent the potential emergence of RSV resistant strains are important next steps in the evaluation of this novel delivery strategy.

Demonstrating the efficacy of regional lung deposition of aerosolized palivizumab in a relevant model of human RSV infection would be valuable to explore its therapeutic potential. If successful, this strategy could be translated to high-burden settings where 99% of RSV-related deaths occur.

ETHICS STATEMENT

The animal study was reviewed and approved by the Murdoch Children's Research Institute (MCRI) Animal Ethics Committee.

AUTHOR CONTRIBUTIONS

AR conceived the study design, obtained ethics approval, performed the experimental procedures, collected and processed the samples, and prepared the first draft of the manuscript. LD

contributed to the design of the study, performed the experimental procedures, and critically revised the manuscript. MS, RBi, and DS assisted with sample collection. DS, MS, RBe, DV, RBi, WY, WH, and AM performed the experimental procedures and critically revised the manuscript. PE and LY contributed to and critically revised the manuscript. AR, LD, DS, RBe, DV, and PL were involved in the data analysis. PL and KM conceived the design of the study and critically revised the manuscript. All authors contributed to the article and approved the submitted version.

ACKNOWLEDGMENTS

The authors thank Rebecca Sutton for her technical assistance on lamb management, and Kera Pethybridge and Ellie Wright for her technical assistance on nuclear imaging. This study is supported by a Jack Brockhoff Foundation Early Career Research Grant and a National Health and Medical Research Council (NHMRC) Early Career Fellowship (GNT1123030) awarded to AR, and the Victorian Government's Operational Infrastructure Support Program. PL is supported by an NHMRC Career Development Fellowship (GNT1165084).

REFERENCES

Abadesso, C., Almeida, H.II, Virella, D., Carreiro, M. H., and Machado, M. C. (2004). Use of palivizumab to control an outbreak of syncytial respiratory virus in a neonatal intensive care unit. *J. Hosp. Infect.* 58, 38–41. doi: 10.1016/j.jhin.2004.04.024

Carlin, D., Pfarr, D. S., Young, J. F., Woods, R., Koenig, S., Johnson, S., et al. (1999). A Direct Comparison of the Activities of Two Humanized Respiratory Syncytial Virus Monoclonal Antibodies: MEDI-493 and RSHZl9. *J. Infect. Dis.* 180, 35–40. doi: 10.1086/314846

Cheng, Y. S. (2014). Mechanisms of pharmaceutical aerosol deposition in the respiratory tract. *AAPS PharmSciTech* 15, 630–640. doi: 10.1208/s12249-014-0092-0

Cortez-Jugo, C., Qi, A., Rajapaksa, A., Friend, J. R., and Yeo, L. Y. (2015). Pulmonary monoclonal antibody delivery via a portable microfluidic nebulization platform. *Biomicrofluidics* 9, 052603. doi: 10.1063/1.4917181

Davis, I. C., Lazarowski, E. R., Chen, F.-P., Hickman-Davis, J. M., Sullender, W. M., and Matalon, S. (2007). Post-Infection A77-1726 Blocks Pathophysiologic Sequelae of Respiratory Syncytial Virus Infection. *Am. J. Respiratory Cell Mol. Biol.* 37, 379–386. doi: 10.1165/rcmb.2007-0142OC

Do, L. A. H., Tse, R., Nathanielsz, J., Anderson, J., Ong, D. S., Chappell, K., et al. (2019). An Improved and High Throughput Respiratory Syncytial Virus (RSV) Micro-neutralization Assay. *J. Visualized Experiments* 143. doi: 10.3791/59025

Finlay, W. H. (2019). "Particle size distributions," in *The Mechanics of Inhaled Pharmaceutical Aerosols 2nd edition.* (London: Elsevier).

Kilkenny, C., Browne, W. J., Cuthill, I. C., Emerson, M., and Altman, D. G. (2010). Improving bioscience research reporting: the ARRIVE guidelines for reporting animal research. *PloS Biol.* 8, e1000412–e1000412. doi: 10.1371/journal.pbio.1000412

Mora, A., Detalle, L., Gallup, J. M., Van Geelen, A., Stohr, T., Duprez, L., et al. (2018). Delivery of ALX-0171 by inhalation greatly reduces respiratory syncytial virus disease in newborn lambs. *mAbs* 10, 778–795. doi: 10.1080/19420862.2018.1470727

Nair, H., Nokes, D. J., Gessner, B. D., Dherani, M., Madhi, S. A., Singleton, R. J., et al. (2010). Global burden of acute lower respiratory infections due to respiratory syncytial virus in young children: a systematic review and meta-analysis. *Lancet* 375, 1545–1555. doi: 10.1016/S0140-6736(10)60206-1

O'Brien, K. L., Baggett, H. C., Brooks, W. A., Feikin, D. R., Hammitt, L. L., Higdon, M. M., et al. (2019). Causes of severe pneumonia requiring hospital admission in children without HIV infection from Africa and Asia: the PERCH multi-country case-control study. *Lancet* 394, 757–779. doi: 10.1016/S0140-6736(19)30721-4

Rajapaksa, A. E., Ho, J. J., Qi, A., Bischof, R., Nguyen, T.-H., Tate, M., et al. (2014). Effective pulmonary delivery of an aerosolized plasmid DNA vaccine via surface acoustic wave nebulization. *Respiratory Res.* 15, 1–12. doi: 10.1186/1465-9921-15-60

Rezk, A. R., Tan, J. K., and Yeo, L. Y. (2016). HYbriD Resonant Acoustics (HYDRA). *Adv. Mater.* 28, 1970–1975. doi: 10.1002/adma.201504861

Sáez-Llorens, X., Castaño, E., Null, D., Steichen, J., Sánchez, P. J., Ramilo, O., et al. (1998). Safety and pharmacokinetics of an intramuscular humanized monoclonal antibody to respiratory syncytial virus in premature infants and infants with bronchopulmonary dysplasia. *Pediatr. Infect. Dis. J.* 17, 787–791. doi: 10.1097/00006454-199809000-00007

miR-4456/CCL3/CCR5 Pathway in the Pathogenesis of Tight Junction Impairment in Chronic Obstructive Pulmonary Disease

Weiwei Yu[1†], Ting Ye[2†], Jie Ding[3], Yi Huang[1], Yang Peng[1], Qin Xia[1*] and Zhang Cuntai[1*]

[1]Department of Geriatric Medicine, Tongji Hospital, Tongji Medical College, Huazhong University of Science and Technology, Wuhan, China, [2]Department of Clinical Nutrition, Tongji Hospital, Tongji Medical College, Huazhong University of Science and Technology, Wuhan, China, [3]Urology Department of Xin Hua Hospital, Xin Hua Hospital Affliated to Shanghai Jiao Tong University, Shanghai, China

*Correspondence:
Qin Xia
804112953@qq.com
Zhang Cuntai
ctzhang0425@163.com

[†]These authors have contributed equally to this work.

Background: Cigarette smoke exposure (CSE) is a major cause of chronic obstructive pulmonary disease (COPD). The smoke disrupts cell-cell adhesion by inducing epithelial barrier damage to the tight junction (TJ) proteins. Even though the inflammatory mechanism of chemokine (C-C motif) ligand 3 (CCL3) in COPD has gained increasing attention in the research community, however, the underlying signaling pathway, remains unknown.

Objectives: To identify the relationship of CCL3 in the pathogenesis of tight junction impairment in COPD and the pathway through which CSE causes damage to TJ in COPD via CCL3, both *in vivo* and *in vitro*.

Methods: We screened the inflammatory factors in the peripheral blood mononuclear cells (PBMCs) from healthy controls and patients at each GOLD 1-4 stage of chronic obstructive pulmonary disease. RT-PCR, western blot, and ELISA were used to detect the levels of CCL3, ZO-1, and occludin after Cigarette smoke exposure. Immunofluorescence was applied to examine the impairment of the TJs in 16-HBE and A549 cells. The reverse assay was used to detect the effect of a CCR5 antagonist (DAPTA) in COPD. In the CSE-induced COPD mouse model, H&E staining and lung function tests were used to evaluate the pathological and physical states in each group. Immunofluorescence was used to assess the impairment of TJs in each group. ELISA and RT-PCR were used to examine the mRNA or protein expression of CCL3 or miR-4456 in each group.

Results: The *in vivo* and *in vitro* results showed that CCL3 expression was increased in COPD compared with healthy controls. CCL3 caused significant injury to TJs through its C-C chemokine receptor type 5 (CCR5), while miR-4456 could suppress the effect of CCL3 on TJs by binding to the 3′-UTR of CCL3.

Abbreviations: CCL3, chemokine (C-C motif) ligand 3; CCR5, C-C chemokine receptor type 5; COPD, chronic obstructive pulmonary disease; CSE, cigarette smoke exposure; GOLD, Global Initiative for Chronic Obstructive Lung Disease; MIP-1α, macrophage inflammatory protein-1α; PBMC, Peripheral blood mononuclear cells; ZO-1, zona occludens-1

Conclusion: miR-4456/CCL3/CCR5 pathway may be a potential target pathway for the treatment of COPD.

Keywords: tight junctions, miR-4456, C-C chemokine receptor type 5, chemokine (C-C motif) ligand 3, chronic obstructive pulmonary disease

INTRODUCTION

COPD is characterized by progressive, poorly reversible airflow obstruction associated with an abnormal inflammatory response to environmental exposure. Tobacco smoking causes a self-maintaining inflammatory process that is considered as a critical factor in the pathophysiology of COPD (Barnes et al., 2015). Inhaled tobacco smoke first reaches the airway epithelium, which represents a highly regulated barrier (Hammad and Lambrecht 2015). Epithelial physical barriers are maintained by various intercellular junctions. The tight junctions (TJs), which are comprised of the interacting proteins such as occludin, ZO-1 and claudins (Zihni et al., 2016; Buckley and Turner 2018). Occludin is found at TJs and involved in the formation, maintenance, and function of TJs (Furuse et al., 1993; Zihni et al., 2016), and claudins are tightly bound to the cell membrane and are important components of TJs (Ruffer and Gerke 2004; Zihni et al., 2016). ZO-1 is also critiacl component of the TJs, where it plays roles in signal transduction at the cell-cell junction (Itoh et al., 1997; Zihni et al., 2016). Numerous studies have shown that the TJs of airway epithelium are involved in the pathogenesis of COPD (Roscioli et al., 2017). For instance, Smoking may considerably disturb epithelial junctions by inducing structural changes in the airways of patients with COPD, such as mucous hyperplasia (Gohy et al., 2016). Therapeutic strategies that attenuate TJ damage during inflammation and/or support TJs restoration have been shown to improve the clinical outcomes in COPD patients (Wittekindt 2017). Smoking causes the delocalization of ZO-1 and occludin from the cell-cell boundaries and a subsequent loss of epithelial integrity (Azghani 1996; Mankertz et al., 2000; Olivera et al., 2010; Yadav et al., 2013). Nevertheless, the underlying mechanisms of how TJs were damaged thus causing barrier dysfunction are still not fully understood.

CCL3, also known as macrophage inflammatory protein-1α (MIP-1α), is a monocyte and macrophage chemoattractant (Larsson 2008). There existed evidence that CCL3 levels increase in bronchial epithelial cells of COPD patients (Villanueva and Llovet 2011). CCL3 is also potentially an important genetic regulator of T-lymphocytes, macrophages, and chemoattractants for mononuclear cells (Larsson 2008). CCR5, the receptor of CCL3, was reported to increase the numbers of macrophages and T-cells in the lungs of patients with COPD, And the inhibition of CCR5 was considered as a viable treatment to reduce the inflammatory response COPD (Wang and He 2012; Costa et al., 2016; Ravi, Plumb et al., 2017). The expression level of CCR5 in inflammatory cells from induced sputum was potentially associated with COPD severity (Wang and He 2012). CCL3 also played an important role in promoting the TJs injury in lung epithelial by binding to CCR5 (Polianova et al., 2005; Camargo et al., 2009; Li et al., 2016; Ahmad et al., 2019). The upregulation of CCL3 might facilitate the recruitment of macrophages into the airways since CCR1 and CCR5, the receptors for CCL3, participate together in macrophage recruitment (Ravi et al., 2014). Using a CCR5 antagonist could attenuate aberrant immune responses (Ahmad et al., 2019), thus protecting against ischemia-reperfusion injury (Li et al., 2016) while overexpressing CCR5 will lead to enhance IL-2 production by T cells (Camargo et al., 2009). The exact regulatory mechanism of CCL3 and CCR5 in COPD pathogenesis remained unkown.

There have been studies showing the dysregulation and role of microRNAs (miRNAs) in COPD. Van Pottelberge et al. reported that 34 miRNAs were differentially expressed between never-smokers and current smokers without airflow limitation, and eight of them was significantly lower in current-smokers with COPD (Van Pottelberge et al., 2011). Another study showed that miRNA-34c is associated with emphysema severity in COPD (Francis et al., 2014). Moreover, miRNAs have been shown to regulate transforming growth factor (TGF)-β, Wnt, and focal adhesion pathways, thus suggesting that they might also involved in the pathogenesis of COPD (Ezzie et al., 2012). In human bronchial airway epithelium, the expression of miRNAs was largely affected by smoking, among them, most miRNAs were down-regulated in current smokers (Schembri et al., 2009). In the epithelial cells of intestine and urethra, miRNAs exhibited vital roles in the barrier function of intestinal epithelial cells and urethra epithelial cells (Ikemura et al., 2014; Chung et al., 2018). Specifically, many genes that associated with epithelial TJ barrier permeability such as occludin, tumor necrosis factor (TNF)-α, and HIF1α (Ikemura et al., 2014; Kar et al., 2017) were regulated. miR-21 might regulate intestinal epithelial TJ permeability through the PTEN/PI3K/Akt signaling pathway (Zhang et al., 2015).

Therefore, we hypothesized that specific microRNAs played key roles in the epithelial TJ of COPD by modulating the CCL3/CCR5 axis. The aim of the present study was to elucidate the role and miRNAs regulation mechanism of CCL3 in the pathogenesis of tight junction impairment correlated COPD. The present study also investigated the relationship between miRNA and epithelial TJ and found the target miR-4456, which could regulate the CCL3/CCR5-induce impairment of TJ in COPD.

MATERIALS AND METHODS

Study Subjects

COPD patients were categorized according to the GOLD (Vogelmeier et al., 2017). Peripheral blood mononuclear cells (PBMCs) were obtained from subjects with normal lung function

TABLE 1 | Clinical characteristics of the subjects involved in the studies.

Characteritics	NS	GOLD1	GOLD2	GOLD3	GOLD4
Number of subjects	8	9	9	10	12
Age (years)	63.2 ± 11.2	61.1 ± 13.2	64.5 ± 15.8	68.3 ± 12.2	62.3 ± 10.5
Sex, male (female)	7 (1)	8 (1)	7 (2)	8 (2)	10 (2)
Pack-years	0	15.3 ± 4.5*	34.8 ± 9.5**	32.5 ± 4.7**	32.5 ± 4.7**
FEV1 (% predicted)	90.3 ± 6.2	63.7 ± 5.3	54.2 ± 5.3*	43.4 ± 3.5**	41.1 ± 2.5**
FEV1/FVC (%)	83.4 ± 5.9	62.3 ± 7.3	50.9 ± 4.9*	40.1 ± 2.1**	38.4 ± 3.1**

**Notes: Values are expressed as mean ± SD. *p < 0.05, p < 0.01, * compared with NS. Abbreviations: NS, no smoke; FEV1 (% predicted), forced expiratory volume in 1 s as percentage of percentage of predicated value; FVC, forced vital capacity.

[non-smokers (NS); eight subjects] and 40 patients with mild to severe COPD (stage 1, nine subjects; stage 2, nine subjects; stage 3, 10 subjects; and stage 4, 12 subjects). The participants had no history of allergy (negative IgE tests) or asthma, did not use inhaled or oral corticosteroids, and had no exacerbations for >3 months prior to study inclusion.

The ethics committee of Tongji Hospital, Tongji Medical College of Huazhong University of Science and Technology approved this study, and informed written consent was obtained from all subjects (Ethical consent for clinical trials. No:WDWHTZKJTJ-0123566). The clinical features of the patients and healthy controls are shown in **Table 1**.

PBMCs Isolation and RNA Extraction

PBMCs were isolated from venous blood by density gradient centrifugation using Ficoll-Paque PLUS (GE Healthcare, Uppsala, Sweden) and suspended in QIAzol lysis reagent (Qiagen, Dusseldorf, Germany). Total RNA was extracted using the miRNeasy Mini Kit (Qiagen) according to the manufacturer's procedure. RNA integrity was determined by formaldehyde denaturing gel electrophoresis.

Human Cytokine Array

Protocol followed manual instructions from R&D Systems Europe, Ltd., Human Cytokine Array (#ARY005B). Briefly, cell lysates of PBMCs were diluted and incubated overnight with either array. The array was washed to remove unbound proteins followed by incubation with a cocktail of biotinylated detection antibodies and with streptavidin-HRP antibodies. Captured signal corresponded to the amount of bound phosphorylated protein. The R software (version 3.2.0) was used for further cluster analysis.

Cell Culture and CSE Treatment

The 16-HBE cell line was purchased from the American Type Culture Collection (ATCC, Manassas, VA, United States). A549 cells were kindly provided by D.C. Shuyuan Yeh (University of Rochester, Rochester, NY, United States). The human bronchial epithelial cells BEpic (CS1028Hu01) and human alveolar epithelial cells (CS1093Hu01) were purchased from Wuhan Cloud-Clone Co., Ltd. (Wuhan, China). The cells were cultured in F-12K medium added with 10% fetal bovine serum (GIBCO, Invitrogen Inc., Carlsbad, CA, United States) (Marcos-Vadillo and Garcia-Sanchez 2016a; Marcos-Vadillo and Garcia-Sanchez 2016b). Before experimentation, cell viability was

evaluated by Trypan blue staining (mean viability 95 ± 0.6% for brushed cells and 93 ± 1.6% for Lonza cells). CSE was freshly prepared on the day of the experiment. In brief, the smoke generated from two burning cigarettes (Red Roses Label; tar, 13 mg; nicotine, 1.3 mg) without filters was sucked under a constant flow rate (50 ml/10 s) into a syringe and then bubbled into a tube containing 10 ml of serum-free DMEM medium. The CSE solution was sterilized using a 0.22 μm filter (Millipore, Bedford, MA, United States), and the pH was adjusted to 7.4. This CSE solution was considered as 100% CSE. The cells were treated with 0 and 1% CSE concentrations for 24 h, respectively. The cells treated with 0 and 1% CSE were the control and CSE treatment groups, respectively. Cells pretreated with DAPTA (0.1 mM) served as CSE + DAPTA treatment group. After treatment of CSE, the cells were washed with serum free RPMI and were treated with DAPTA at the indicated concentrations for 6 h at 37 C, 5% CO2. Cultures were washed two times to remove unabsorbed DAPTA. The dosage of DAPTA was based on the literature (Polianova, Ruscetti et al., 2005). There were three wells in each group.

RT-PCR Analysis

Total RNA (1 μg) was subjected to reverse transcription using the Superscript III transcriptase (Invitrogen, Grand Island, NY, United States). Quantitative real-time PCR (qRT-PCR) was conducted using a Bio-Rad CFX96 system with SYBR green to determine the mRNA expression levels of a gene of interest. Expression levels were normalized to the expression of β-actin. miRNAs were isolated using the PureLink® miRNA kit. Briefly, 50 ng of RNA was processed for poly-A addition by adding one unit of polymerase with 1 mM ATP in 1× RT buffer at 37°C for 10 min in 10 μl, and heat inactivating at 95°C for 2 min. Next, 50 mM of anchor primer was added to a total of 12.5 μl and incubated at 65°C for 5 min. cDNA synthesis was performed by adding 2 μl of 5× RT buffer, 2 μl of 10 mM dNTP, and 1 μl of reverse transcriptase was added to a total of 20 μl, and the sample was incubated at 42°C for 1 h. Quantitative real-time PCR (qRT-PCR) was conducted using a Bio-Rad CFX96 system with SYBR green to determine the mRNA expression level of a gene of interest. The expression levels were normalized to the expression of 5S RNA and/or U6.

Western Blotting

The cells were lysed in RIPA buffer. Proteins (30 μg) were separated by 8–10% SDS/PAGE and transferred onto PVDF membranes (Millipore, Billerica, MA, United States). After blocking, the membranes were incubated with the appropriate dilutions of specific primary antibodies against ZO-1 (1:200, cat#: pa5-28858, Thermo Fisher Scientific, Rochester, NY, United States) occludin (1:200, cat#: ab216327, Abcam, Cambridge, MA, United States), Claudin (1:200, cat#: ab180158, Abcam, Cambridge, MA, United States), CCL3 (1: 1000, cat#: ab229900, Abcam, Cambridge, MA, United States), and CCR5 (1:200, cat#: ab110103, Abcam, Cambridge, MA, United States). The blots were next incubated with HRP-conjugated secondary antibodies (1; 1000, cat#: a12004-1, Gepigentek, Farmingdale, NY, United States) and visualized using the ECL system.

ELISA

Analysis of the CCL3 levels was carried out based on the enzyme-linked immunosorbent assay with the Human CCL3 Quantikine ELISA Kit (cat#: SMA00, R&D, Minneapolis United States) according to the manufacturer's instructions.

Transepithelial Electrical Resistance (TER) Measurement

The 16HBE or A549 cells were seeded in the upper chamber of a Transwell tissue culture plate (12 mm diameter, 0.4 μm pore size, Costar, Corning Inc., Corning, NY, United States) and allowed to reach confluence. The basolateral and apical sides of the filters were exposed to CCL3 (10 mg/ml) when indicated. The TER of the cells grown on filters was measured after 7 days, with an epithelial volt-ohm meter (Endohm; World Precision Instruments, Sarasota, FL, United States). To explore the rapid effect of CCL3 on the TER, the volt-ohm meter was coupled to an A/N converter (World Precision Instruments, Sarasota, FL, United States), and the TER measurement was monitored using Powerlab software (Chart for Windows, v4.0, AD Instruments, Sydney, Australia) with an acquisition frequency of 2 Hz. The background electrical resistance attributed to fluid and a blank Transwell filter were subtracted from the measured TER. The TER measurements were normalized by the area of the monolayer and given as cm^2. Untreated 16HBE cells have been reported to have a TER around $600 \, \Omega \cdot cm^2$ (Yuan et al., 2020), while A549 cells have been reported to have a TER around $175 \, \Omega \cdot cm^2$ (Albano et al., 2020).

Animal Studies

C57BL/6 mice, 6–8 weeks old, weighing 18–25 g, were obtained from Tongji Medical Laboratory Animal Center (Wuhan, China). All animals were housed in an environment with a temperature of $22 \pm 1°C$, relative humidity of $50 \pm 1\%$, and a light/dark cycle of 12/12 h. All animal studies (including the mice euthanasia procedure) were carried out in compliance with the regulations and guidelines of Huazhong University institutional animal care and conducted according to the AAALAC and the IACUC guidelines (Animal Ethical consent No:SYXK2017-0023).

The C57BL/6 mice were randomized into following groups ($n = 8$ for each group): 1) control group: exposed to normal air, then

subcutaneously injected with PBS, $10 \, ml \, kg^{-1}$, 2) CCL3 group: exposed to normal air, then subcutaneously injected with CCL3 (cat#: csb-ap001221monthsnth, $200 \, ng \, kg^{-1}$, $0.01 \, mg \, ml^{-1}$ dissolved in normal saline, CUSABIO, Wuhan, China) for 6 weeks, 3) CSE group: inhalation of CS for up to 12 weeks as previously described (Li et al., 2018a; Li et al., 2018b), and each exposure lasted for 75 min, 4) CSE + DAPTA group: mice were chronically exposed to CS for 12 weeks, then subcutaneously injected with DAPTA (cat#: ab120810, Abcam, Cambridge, MA, United States; $l0 \, \mu g \, kg^{-1}$, $0.01 \, mg \, ml^{-1}$ dissolved in normal saline) 15 min before the first CS-exposure on each day, starting at 6 weeks (Li et al., 2016). 5) CSE + miR-4456 group and CSE + miR-NC group: mice were chronically exposed to CS for 12 weeks, then 120 nM/kg miR-4456 agomir or miR-NC was injected via the tail vein weekly over the next four weeks. The mice were sacrificed on day 56 following CSE/CCL3 administration. The sequence of agomir-miR-4456 was: cucuggaaucaucaugucacaga (double-stranded); the sequence of the miR-NC was: uucuccgaa cgugucacgu (double-stranded). Lung tissues were harvested, quick-frozen in liquid nitrogen and stored at −80 C immediately for further analysis.

Lung Function Measurement

The modeling efficiency was evaluated by lung function, including airway resistance, elasticity, static compliance. Lung function was evaluated as previously described (Zhuang, Huang et al., 2016; (Irvin and Bates 2003). The rats undergoing non-invasive pulmonary function were monitored by whole-body barometric plethysmography (WBP; EMKA Technologies, Paris, France). Rats were placed in a plethysmograph chamber, and a 10 min accommodation was allowed before analysis. Respiratory parameters were recorded while the rats were unrestrained, and the respiratory frequency (F) and tidal volume (TV) were analyzed by emka Technologies iox2 software.

H&E Staining

The whole lungs were fixed in 4% neutral buffered paraformaldehyde and embedded in paraffin. Tissues were cut into 5 μm sections and analyzed using H&E staining.

Bronchoalveolar Lavage

Following lung mechanical measurements, the animals were detached from the ventilator and sacrificed by exsanguination (inferior vena cava and descending aorta dissection). The left main bronchus was temporarily ligated, and the right lung was lavaged with three aliquots of 2.5 ml of normal saline. Bronchoalveolar lavage fluid (BALF) was withdrawn and immediately centrifuged at 300 ×g for 10 min at 4°C. The supernatant was collected and stored at −80°C, while the cell pellet was resuspended in 1 ml of normal saline. Total protein concentration in BALF was measured using a colorimetric protein assay according to the manufacturer's instructions (Bio-Rad Laboratories Inc., Hercules, CA, United States). Bovine serum albumin was used to create standard curves.

Immunofluorescence Microscopy

The cells were first fixed in 100% methanol for 5 min at room temperature and then incubated with 1% BSA in Ca^{2+}– and

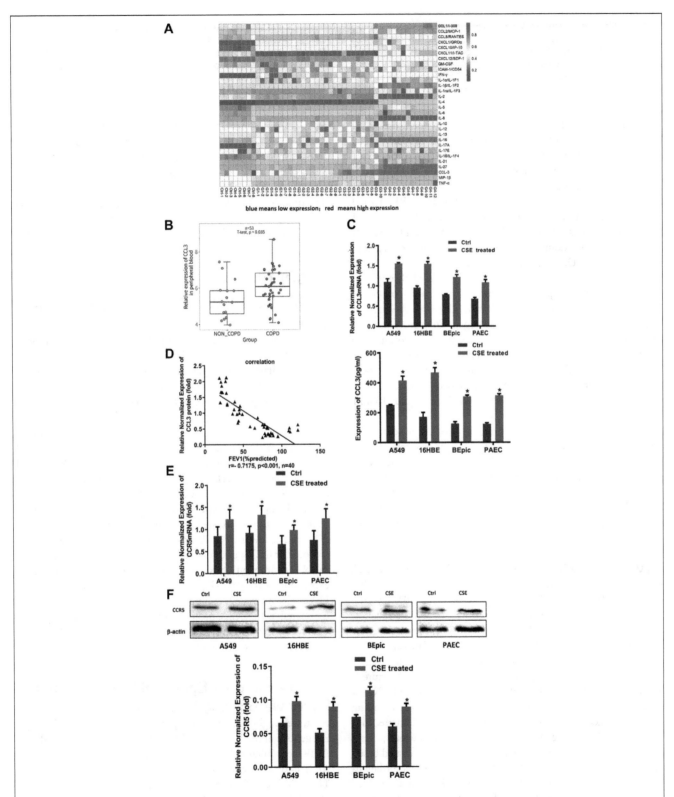

FIGURE 1 | Higher expression of CCL3 in the supernatants of PBMCs cells **(A)** Human Cytokine Array for the parallel determination of relative levels of cytokines and chemokines in the supernatants of PBMCs cells. Downregulated proteins are shown in blue, and upregulated proteins are shown in red, as the mean of all specimens included (*n* = 48). non-smokers: Ctrl-1 to Ctrl-8, GOLD 1:G1-1 to G1-9, GOLD2: G2-1 to G2-9, GOLD3:G3-1 to G3-10, GOLD4:G4-1 to G4-12 **(B)** Expression of CCL3 in no-COPD and COPD patients in the human GEO database (*n* = 53) **(C)** Real-time PCR assays were performed in 16HBE, A549, BEpic, and PAEC cells to detect CCL3 mRNA expression before and after CSE treatment. *n* = 3, *p < 0.05, vs. the control group (left panel). The expression levels were normalized to

(Continued)

FIGURE 1 | the expression of GAPDH. ELISA assays were performed in 16HBE, A549, BEpic, and PAEC cells to detect CCL3 protein expression before and after CSE treatment. $n = 3$, *$p < 0.05$, vs. the control group (right panel) **(D)** Correlation between FEV1 (%predicted) and CCL3 expression in patients with COPD. $r = 0.7175$, $p < 0.001$, $n = 40$ **(E)** Real-time PCR assays were performed in 16HBE, A549, BEpic, and PAEC cells to detect CCR5 mRNA expression before and after CSE treatment. *$p < 0.05$, vs. the control group **(F)** Western blot assays were performed in 16HBE, A549, BEpic, and PAEC cells to detect CCR5 protein expression before and after CSE treatment. $n = 3$, *$p < 0.05$, vs. the control group. The expression levels were normalized to the expression of β-actin.

Mg^{2+}–free PBS (PBS(−)) for 1 h at room temperature. After incubation for 2 h with ZO-1 antibody (1:100, cat#:pa5-28858, Thermo Fisher, Waltham, MA, USA) or occludin antibody (1: 100, ab216327, Abcam, Cambridge, MA, United States) for 1 h at 37 C, washed with PBS(−), the cells were incubated for 1 h with Alexa Fluor 488-conjugated secondary antibodies HRP (1:2000, cat#:ab205718, Abcam, Cambridge, MA, United States) or H&L (1:2000, cat#:ab150077, Abcam, Cambridge, MA, United States). The results were examined with a fluorescence microscope (Olympus BX51; Olympus, Tokyo, Japan).

Mouse lungs in the thoracic cages were infused through the trachea with 60% optimal cutting temperature compound (Tissue-Tek; Miles Laboratories, Elkhart, IN, United States) in PBS, removed, and frozen in liquid nitrogen. The tissues were cut into 10 μm-thick frozen sections using a cryostat. For immunofluorescence staining, the lungs were fixed with ice-cold 95% ethanol, followed by 100% acetone at room temperature for 1 min, and then washed three times in PBS. Cultured cells were fixed with 3% formaldehyde for 15 min, followed by 0.1% Triton X-100 for 3 min at room temperature, and washed three times in PBS. After soaking in PBS containing 3% BSA, the sections were incubated with primary antibodies in a moist chamber for 1 h. They were washed three times with PBS and incubated for 30 min with secondary antibodies and 4,6-diamino-2-phenylindole for nuclear staining. The samples were washed with PBS and observed under a fluorescence microscope (Olympus BX51; Olympus, Tokyo, Japan).

Cytokine Levels in Lung Tissue Using ELISA

Frozen lung tissue sections were homogenized with a buffer containing 50 mM HEPES (pH 7.5), 150 nM NaCl, 10% glycerol, 1% Triton X-100, 1 mM EDTA, 1.5 mM $MgCl_2$, and a cocktail of protease and phosphatase inhibitors at a 1:1000 concentration. The samples were centrifuged at 10,000 ×g for 10 min. The supernatant was collected, and total protein concentration was estimated using a colorimetric protein assay according to the manufacturer's instructions. Protein levels of interleukin IL-6, IL-18 and TNF- α were determined in lung tissue homogenates using ELISA, according to the manufacturer's protocol (DuoSet ELISA; R&D Systems, Inc., Minneapolis, MN, United States) and normalized to the total protein content of lung homogenates. Oxidative stress was evaluated based on the levels of SOD, CAT, and GSH-Px using ELISA, according to the manufacturer's protocol (DuoSet ELISA; R&D Systems, Inc., Minneapolis, MN, United States) and normalized to the total protein content of lung homogenates.

Statistical Analysis

Data are expressed as means ± standard deviations from at least three sets of independent experiments performed in triplicate

(n = 3/experiment). The data were checked for normal distribution using the Kolmogorov-Smirnov test and were log-transformed to normalize their distribution when needed. Statistical analyses involved Student's t-test, one-way ANOVA, and the log-rank (Mantel-Cox) test with SPSS 22 (IBM Corp, Armonk, NY, United States) or GraphPad Prism 6 (GraphPad Software, Inc., La Jolla, CA, United States). $p < 0.05$ was considered statistically significant.

RESULTS

Higher Expression of CCL3 in the PBMCs of COPD

It was well established that PBMCs had a crucial role in COPD.(Bahr et al., 2013). We first screened the inflammatory factors (Inflammatory Factors kits, Roche) in the PBMCs; the level of CCL3 was significantly higher in patients with COPD GOLD 3–4 stage compared with the NS and COPD GOLD 1–2 stage (**Figure 1A**). Consistantly, the analysis form the human GEO database also showed a significantly higher expression of CCL3 in COPD compared with non-COPD ($p = 0.0304$, $n = 53$; **Figure 1B**). We then treated alveolar epithelial cells (A549 cells), bronchial epithelial cells (16HBE cells), and primary cells (BEpic and PAEC) with CSE and found that CSE evoked a significantly up-regulation expression of the CCL3 mRNA ($p < 0.05$; **Figure 1C**, upper) as well as its protein expression ($p < 0.05$) (**Figure 1C**, lower). We also measured the CCR5 expression, the receptor of CCL3, and found that CSE could also prompt CCR5 mRNA expression ($p < 0.05$; **Figure 1E**) and CCR5 protein expression ($p < 0.05$) (**Figure 1F**). **Figure 1D** revealed that the FEV1 (% predicted) of patients with COPD was negatively correlated with CCL3 protein expression ($p < 0.001$, $n = 40$). Taken together, these results suggested that CSE could promote the expression of CCL3 and CCR5 in COPD.

CCL3 Promotes Epithelial Tight Junction Injury *via* Binding With CCR5

Next, we sought to evaluate the potential roles of CCL3 in COPD. Exogenous application of CCL3 (10 mg/ml) in both 16HBE and A549 cells obviously reduced the epithelial TJs injury when compared with control cells (**Figure 2A**) and decreased the TER (**Figure 2B**). Moreover, CCL3 decreased the expression of ZO-1 and occludin, but not claudin, at both the mRNA and protein levels in a concentration-dependent manner ($p < 0.05$) (**Figures 2C,D**). Previous studies have shown that the expression of CCR5, the critical receptor of CCL3 is higher in patients vs. normal individuals, with the clinical stage (Costa et al., 2016)). We then examined whether CSE induces TJs injury

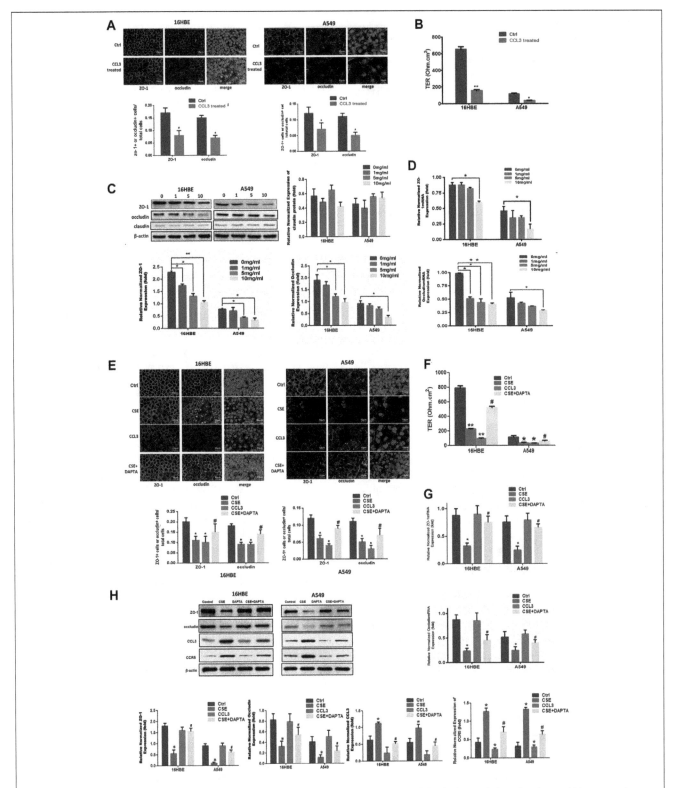

FIGURE 2 | CCL3 promotes epithelial tight junction injury by binding with CCR5 **(A)** Tight junction proteins ZO-1 (red), occludin (green), and merged (blue + orange) were stained in 16HBE cells (left panel) and A549 cells (right panel) by immunofluorescence. Presented as means ± standard error. $n = 3$, *$p < 0.05$, vs. the control group. Data are representative of three independent experiments. Scale bar = 10 μm **(B)** Transepithelial electrical resistance (TER) after CCL3 treatment (10 mg/ml), as a cell function test 7 days after plating the airway epithelial cells on coated permeable filters. Presented as means ± standard error. $n = 3$, *$p < 0.05$, vs. the control group **(C)** Western blot analysis to detect protein expression of ZO-1, claudin and occludin in 16HBE cells and A549 cells using different concentrations of CCL3. $n = 3$, *$p < 0.05$, vs. the control group, **$p < 0.01$, vs. the control group (CCL3: 0 ng/ml). The expression levels were normalized to the expression of β-actin (left panel). $n = 3$ **(D)**

(Continued)

FIGURE 2 | Real-time PCR assays of ZO-1 (upper) and occludin (lower) mRNA expression in 16HBE cells and A549 cells using different concentrations of CCL3. $n = 3$, $^*p < 0.05$, vs. the Ctrl group, $^{**}p < 0.01$, vs. the control group. Protein expression was normalized to GAPDH **(E)** Tight junction proteins ZO-1 (red), occludin (green) and merged (blue and orange) were stained by immunofluorescence in the four groups: 1) Ctrl (PBS:10 mg ml^{-1}), 2) CSE (10 mg ml^{-1}), 3) CCL3 (CCL3 10 mg ml^{-1}), and 4) CSE (10 mg ml^{-1})+DAPTA (0.1 mg ml^{-1}) in 16HBE cells (left panel) and A549 cells (right panel). Presented as means ± standard error. $n = 3$, $^*p < 0.05$, vs. the control group. #$p < 0.05$, vs. the CSE group. Data are representative of three independent experiments. Scale bar = 10 μm **(F)** TER in the four groups same as Fig3E in 16HBE cells (left panel) and A549 cells (right panel). The results are shown as a function test on 7 days after plating the airway epithelial cells on coated permeable filters. Presented as means ± standard error. $n = 3$,$^*p < 0.05$, vs. the control group, $^{**}p < 0.01$, vs. the control group, #$p < 0.05$, vs. the CSE group **(G)** Real-time PCR assays to detect ZO-1 mRNA (upper panel) and occludin mRNA (lower panel) expression in 16HBE cells and A549 cells in four groups same as Fig3E. $n = 3$,$^*p < 0.05$, vs. the control group, #$p < 0.05$, vs. the CSE group. The expression levels were normalized to the expression of GAPDH (left panel) **(H)** Western blot analysis to detect ZO-1protein, occludin protein, CCL3 protein and CCR5 protein expression in 16HBE cells and A549 cells in four group same as Fig3E. Protein expression levels were normalized to β-actin expression. $n = 3$, $^*p < 0.05$, vs. the control group, #$p < 0.05$, vs. the CCL3 group. Protein expression was normalized to β-actin.

through the CCR5 receptor in 16HBE and A549 cells. We found that CCR5 antagonist (DAPTA, ab120810, 0.1 mM) significantly reduced the CSE-induced TJs injury (**Figures 2E,F**). Mechanically, DAPTA hampered the CSE reduced expression of ZO-1, occludin, CCL3 and CCR5 in these cells (**Figures 2G,H**). The increased expression level of CCL3 and CCR5, inversly, were inhibited by DAPTA. Together, our data suggest that CCL3 and CSE promote epithelial tight junction injury via binding with CCR5.

MiR-4456 Is an Upstream Signal for CCL3-Induced TJ Injury

Recent evidences have highlighted an emerging role for miRNAs as the crucial regulators of epithelial barrier functions (Neudecker et al., 2017; Zhu et al., 2018). We then examined whether miRNAs were involved in the CCL3 dependent TJs injury. We first identified six candidate miRNAs (miR-5002, miR-4456, miR-2355, miR-6501, miR-4687 and miR-7847) that might suppress CCL3 expression through its 3'UTR target by searching multiple databases (TargetScan, miRDB, and microRNA.org). We examined the overexpression effects of these miRNAs on CCL3 expression in 16HBE and A549 cell lines. We found miR-4456 overexpression led to a significant decrease of CCL3 in both cell lines (**Figure 3A**). Furthermore, the miR-4456 inhibitor (5 nM, MIN0000090, Qiagen) increased CCL3 mRNA in both cell lines (**Figure 3A**). In very severe COPD, the expression of mir-4456 was lower than that of the normal control group, but there was no significant difference between patients with mild and moderate COPD (**Figure 3B**). Cells pretreated with miR-4456 significantly correlated with the effect of CSE on the expression of ZO-1, occludin, CCL3 and CCR5 protein (**Figure 3C**). Besides, we examined miR-4456 and CCL3 expression in blood samples of GOLD3-4 stage COPD and found a significant positive correlation ($r = 0.426$, $p = 0.0337$) between miR-4456 expression and CCL3 expression in 22 specimens (**Figure 3D**). So we further investigated the correlation of miR-4456 and CCL3 expression in very severe COPD tissues ($n = 76$, **Supplementary Figure S1** and **Supplementary Table S1**), which showed a significant negative correlation ($r = -0.8813$, $p < 0.0001$), indicating a potential suppressive role of miR-4456 in the progression of severe COPD. We then applied an immunofluorescence assay to examine the effect of miR-4456 in TJs, and found that miR-4456 significantly suppressed the destruction of TJs induced by

CSE. Morever, overexpression of miR-4456 with CCL3 could not suppress the destruction, indicating that miR-4456 improved the CSE induced TJs injury through a CCL3 dependent way in 16HBE cells and A549 cells (**Figures 3E,F**). Together, these results demonstrated that miR-4456 could improve TJ injury by downregulating CCL3 expression.

MiR-4456 Suppresses CCL3 Expression via the 3'UTR

To further dissect the molecular mechanisms through which miR-4456 decreased CCL3 expression, we identified one predicted miRNA-responsive-element that matched the seed sequence of miR-4456 in the 3'UTR of the CCL3 gene (**Figure 4A**). We inserted a 359 bp fragment from the CCL3 3'UTR with the predicted miR-4456 target site into a dual-luciferase reporter backbone (psiCHECK™-2) downstream of the Renilla luciferase open reading frame (ORF). Simultaneously, we also included a mutated version at the predicted target site (**Figure 4B**). As expected, the luciferase assay revealed that depletion of miR-4456 significantly increased luciferase activity in 16HBE cells, while the addition of miR-4456 markedly decreased luciferase activity in A549 cells transfected with wild type TR4 3'UTR. However, these effects could not be observed when the mutant CCL3 3'UTR was transfected into these cells (**Figure 4C**), suggesting that miR-4456 could directly and specifically regulate CCL3 expression through binding to the CCL3 3'UTR.

In vivo Mice Studies Confirmed the Role of CCL3 and miR-4456 in COPD

Because cigarette smoke (CS) was critical to the pathogenesis of COPD, we then accessed the expression of CCL3 in a mouse model of CS-induced COPD. The mouse developed an emphysematous phenotype after 24 weeks of CSE, showing enlargement of the air spaces accompanied by the destruction of the alveolar architecture (**Figure 5A**, upper). To quantify the presence and severity of emphysema, we determined the enlargement of alveolar spaces by measuring the mean linear intercept (Lm). Compared with air-control mice (25.2 ± 1.8 μm), significant alveolar space enlargement was observed in mice exposed to CS (38.9 ± 4.6 μm); CCL3 had a similar effect to that of CSE (37.4 ± 3.6 μm), and DAPTA could reverse the effect of CCL3 (27.5 ± 3.9 μm) (**Figure 5A**, lower). We next detected the

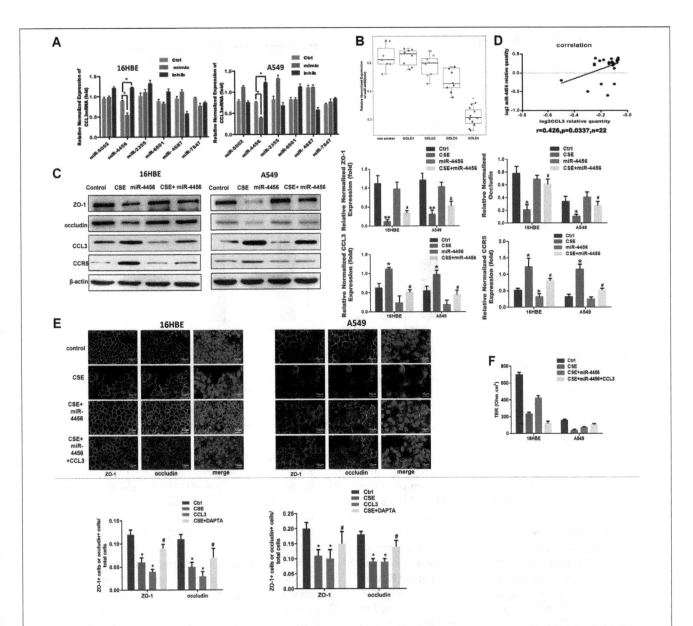

FIGURE 3 | Identification of miR-4456 as an upstream signal of CCL3 induced-tight junction injury (A) Real-time PCR screen in 16-HBE cells (left panel) and A549 cells (right panel) for miRNAs that could target CCL3 mRNA. CCL3 mRNA expression levels were normalized to GAPDH expression. n = 3, *p < 0.05, vs. the control group. The expression levels were normalized to the expression of GAPDH (B) Baseline expression of miR-4456 according to COPD grade. *p < 0.05 vs. the non-smoker group ((n = 48. non-smokers:8, GOLD 1:9, GOLD2: 9, GOLD3:10, GOLD4:12) (C) Western blot analysis of ZO-1, occludin, CCL3, and CCR5 protein expression in the four groups: 1) Control (PBS 10 mg ml⁻¹), 2) CSE (10 mg ml⁻¹), 3) miR-4456, and 4) CSE (10 mg ml⁻¹)+miR-4456 mimics in 16HBE cells and A549 cells. n = 3, **p < 0.01, vs. the control group, *p < 0.05, vs. the control group, #p < 0.05, vs. the CSE group. Protein expression was normalized to β-actin (D) Correlation analysis of miR-4456 and CCL3 mRNA levels by Pearson correlation coefficient from a total of 22 COPD peripheral blood samples (n = 22) (E) Tight junction proteins ZO-1 (red), occludin (green) and merged (blue + orange) were stained by immunofluorescence in the four groups: 1) Control (PBS 10 mg ml⁻¹), 2) CSE (10 mg ml⁻¹), 3) CSE (10 mg ml⁻¹)+miR4456, and 4) CSE (10 mg ml⁻¹)+miR4456 mimics + CCL3 (10 mg ml⁻¹) in 16HBE cells (left panel) and A549 cells (right panel). Presented as means ± standard error. n = 3, *p < 0.05, vs. the control group, **p < 0.01, vs. the control group, #p < 0.05, vs. the CSE group, Δp < 0.05, vs. the CSE + miR-4456 group. Data are representative of three independent experiments. Scale bar = 10 μm (F) TER in the four groups same as Figure-3E is shown as a function test on 7 days after plating the airway epithelial cells on coated permeable filters. Presented as means ± standard error. n = 3, *p < 0.05, vs. the control group, **p < 0.01, vs. the control group, #p < 0.05, vs. the CSE group, Δp < 0.05, vs. the CSE + miR-4456 mimics group.

mouse lung function: the airway resistance of the CSE or CCL3 groups was significantly increased compared to the control group, while elasticity and compliance was increased, and total protein concentrations were elevated. Those changes induced by CSE could be reversed by DAPTA. (**Figure 5B**). **Figure 5C** showed

that CSE and CCL3 increased the IL-18 and TNF-α levels compared with the controls and decreased SOD, CAT, and GSH-Px levels (all p < 0.05). Only IL-18 was decreased by DAPTA compared with the CSE group (p < 0.05), IL-6 was not influenced by CSE or CCL3. Furthermore, there was

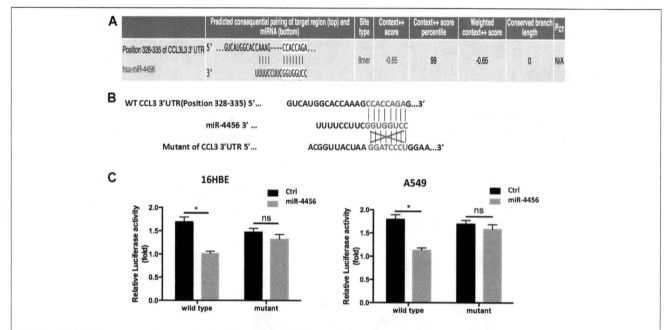

FIGURE 4 | miR-4456 suppresses CCL3 expression through 3'UTR of CCL3 **(A,B)** The predicted duplex formation between wild human type (WT) CCL3 3'-UTR and human miR-4456 **(C)** luciferase assays were performed to detect the regulation of miR-4456 on WT and mutant CCL3-3'UTR. Assays were performed on CCL3-wt.3'UTR ± miR-4456, or CCL3-mut.3'UTR ± miR-4456 in 16-HBE cells (left panel) and A549 cells (right panel). Data are represented as the mean ± standard deviation. $n = 3$, *$p < 0.05$, compared to controls.

significant epithelial TJ injury in the CSE and CCL3 groups compared with the control group, while DAPTA could reverse the effect of CSE in mice (**Figure 5D**). Accordingly, CSE or CCL3 decreased the mRNA expression of ZO-1 and occludin, while DAPTA partly abolished this effect (**Figure 5E**). Similar effects were observed at the protein level by western blotting (**Figure 5F**). Consistent with the results in COPD patients, we found that CCL3 and CCR5 mRNAs were significantly upregulated in the lung of mice after CSE treatment when compared with air-control mice, while DAPTA could reverse the effect of CSE in mice, and similar results were also found in the blood of the mice (**Figures 5G,H**). Similarly, there was a significant decrease in miR-4456 mRNA expression in blood and lung tissues of mice exposed to CS, but DAPTA could not reverse the effect of CSE to miR-4456 (**Figure 5I**). CSE or CCL3 decreased the protein expression of ZO-1 and occludin, while miR-4456 partly blocked the effect of CSE (**Figures 5J,K**).

Taken together, our results from the *in vivo* mouse model were consistent with that of the *in vitro* cell line studies, demonstrating that CCL3 promoted epithelial TJ injury through the miR-4456-CCL3-CCR5 pathway.

DISCUSSION

The lung tissues of patients with COPD are affected by the local immune and inflammatory environment, but the systemic immune and inflammatory environment also play a role in the development of COPD. Studies have proved that PBMCs had a crucial role in COPD (Bahr et al., 2013, Tan, Xuan et al., 2016). We demonstrated that CCL3 was a significantly increased

inflammatory cytokine in the PBMCs from patients with severe COPD. CCL3 downregulated the expression of ZO-1 and occludin, thus inducing severe injury of TJs both *in vivo* and *in vitro*. CSE could upregulate the mRNA and protein level of CCL3, while CCR5 antagonist DAPTA could reverse this effect of CSE. Furthermore, miR-4456 could suppress the effects of CCL3 on TJs by binding to the CCL3 3'-UTR. Our results demonstrated that CSE induced injury to airway epithelium TJs via the miR-4456/CCL3/CCR5 pathway.

The loss of lung function in patients with COPD and emphysema is associated with a high percentage of CD4[+] and CD8[+] T lymphocytes that express receptors CCR5 and CXCR3, but not CCR3 or CCR4 (both markers of T helper one cells) (Grumelli et al., 2004). Previous studies showed that CCR1 and CCR5 acted together with CCL3 to play a role in COPD. Since using CCR1 antagonists could not treat COPD (Kerstjens et al., 2010), we thus applied CCR5 antagonist in our research. Previous studies have shown that CCR3/CCR5 expression was correlated with COPD severity (Freeman et al., 2007). Chronic CSE significantly increased CCR5 expression, and the number and extent of peribronchial lymphoid follicles (Bracke et al., 2007). It could also induce airspace enlargement in wild-type mice. Conversely, inflammatory cells in BALF and peribronchial lymphoid follicles were all significantly attenuated, and airspace enlargement was reduced in CCR5 knockout (KO) mice (Bracke et al., 2007). Still, CCR5 deficiency did not affect CSE-induced airway wall remodeling (Bracke et al., 2007). The follow-up studies showed that CCL3/CCR5 contributed to increased numbers of macrophages and T-cells in the lungs of patients with COPD (Ravi et al., 2014; Costa et al., 2016). Recently, it has been suggested that IL-8 overexpression increased the expression of CCL3 and reduced the expression of Claudin 18 and

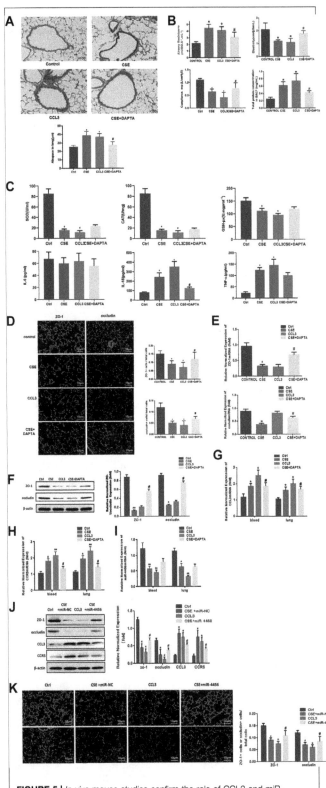

FIGURE 5 | *In vivo* mouse studies confirm the role of CCL3 and miR-4456 in COPD **(A)** H&E staining confirms the macroscopic appearance of pulmonary tissue in the four groups: 1) Control (Ctrl), 2) CSE, 3) CCL3, and 4) CSE + DAPTA. Quantification of the alveolar space is in the lower panels. $n = 8$, *$p < 0.05$, vs. the control group, #$p < 0.05$, vs. the CSE group **(B)** Airway resistance, Elasticity, Compliance, and total BALF proteins were detected in *(Continued)*

F11r, inducing damage to the epithelial organization and leading to leaky TJs (Reynolds et al., 2018). These results showed that CCL3/CCR5 specifically caused lung damage through persistent inflammation and damaged TJs, but not lung remodeling. Our results demonstrated that CCL3 induced significant injury to TJs through its receptor CCR5, which was in accordance with previous CCL3/CCR5 studies in COPD. Furthermore, CSE could upregulate the expression of CCL3 mRNA and protein, and CCR5 antagonist DAPTA could reverse the effect of CSE both *in vivo* and *in vitro*.

It was well established that miRNAs were relevant to the pathogenesis of COPD (Ezzie et al., 2012). A previous study has shown that in human bronchial airway epithelium, miRNA expression was affected by smoking, since most miRNAs were found to be downregulated in current-smokers (Schembri et al., 2009). Exosomal miRNAs released from macrophages could lead to a series of events in recipient alveolar epithelial cells, resulting in impairment of tight junction barrier integrity and mitochondrial bioenergetics (Zhang et al., 2020). These changes in the alveolar microenvironment increased the susceptibility to lung infection and injury (Yuan et al., 2019). Nevertheless, those exosomal miRNAs were not assessed in the present study. Growing evidence indicated that lung epithelial damage resulted in impairment of the tight junction barrier, which disrupted homeostasis of the tissue microenvironment.

FIGURE 5 | the four groups same as Figure 5A $n = 8$, *$p < 0.05$, vs. the control group, #$p < 0.05$, vs. the CSE group **(C)** Inflammatory and oxidative stress markers in the four groups same as Figure 5A $n = 8$, *$p < 0.05$, vs. the control group, #$p < 0.05$, vs. the CSE group **(D)** Tight junction proteins ZO-1 merge (red and blue), and occludin merge (green and blue) were stained using immunofluorescence in the four groups same as Figure 5A. Data are representative of three independent experiments. Scale bar = 10 μm $n = 8$, *$p < 0.05$, vs. the control group, #$p < 0.05$, vs. the CSE group **(E)** Real-time PCR assays were performed in the blood and lung to detect ZO-1 and occludin mRNA before and after CSE treatment in the four groups same as Figure 5A. Data are represented as the mean ± standard deviation. $n = 8$, *$p < 0.05$, vs. the control group. #$p < 0.05$, vs. the CSE group. The expression levels were normalized to the expression of GAPDH, $n = 3$ **(F)** Western blot for ZO-1 and occludin protein expression in the four groups same as Figure 5A $n = 8$, *$p < 0.05$, vs. the control group, **$p < 0.01$, vs. the control group, #$p < 0.05$, vs. the CSE group. Protein expression was normalized to β-actin **(G)** Real-time PCR assays were performed in the whole blood and lung to detect CCL3 mRNA expression in four groups same as Figure 5A. Data are represented as the mean ± standard deviation. $n = 8$, *$p < 0.05$, vs. the control group, #$p < 0.05$, vs. the CSE group. The expression levels were normalized to the expression of GAPDH **(H)** Real-time PCR assays were performed in the whole blood and lung to detect CCR5 mRNA expression in four groups same as Figure 5A. Data are represented as the mean ± standard deviation. $n = 8$, *$p < 0.05$, vs. the control group, **$p < 0.01$, vs. the control group, #$p < 0.05$, vs. the CSE group. The expression levels were normalized to the expression of GAPDH **(I)** Real-time PCR assays were performed in the whole blood and lung to detect miR-4456 expression in four groups same as Figure 5A. Data are represented as the mean ± standard deviation. $n = 8$, *$p < 0.05$, vs. the control group, **$p < 0.01$, vs. the control group. The expression levels were normalized to the expression of 5S RNA and/or U6 **(J)** Western blot for ZO-1 and occludin protein expression in the four groups: 1) Control (Ctrl), 2) CSE, 3) CCL3, and 4) CSE + miR-4456. $n = 8$, *$p < 0.05$, vs. the control group, #$p < 0.05$, vs. the CSE group. Protein expression was normalized to β-actin **(K)** Tight junction proteins ZO-1 merge (red and blue), and occludin merge (green and blue) were stained using immunofluorescence in the four groups same as Figure 5J. Data are representative of three independent experiments. Scale bar = 10 μm $n = 8$, *$p < 0.05$, vs. the control group, #$p < 0.05$, vs. the CSE group.

The junctional adaptor protein ZO-1 was reported to have a central regulatory role in epithelial barrier formation (Nazli et al., 2010; Fernandes et al., 2018). Taking advantage of the data from multiple databases (TargetScan, miRDB, and microRNA.org), we screened miRNAs and found that miR-4456 could suppress the effect of CCL3/CCR5 on TJs through binding to the $3'$-UTR of CCL3. In addition, there was a significant decrease in miR-4456 mRNA expression both in lung tissues from CS-exposed mice. In this study, we showed that the crosstalk between PBMCs and lung epithelial cells impaired epithelial barrier integrity through miR-4456/CCL3/CCR5/ZO-1 and occludin. The present study suggested that targeting miR-4456 might be of therapeutic value to enhance lung epithelial barrier in COPD, and miR-4456 mRNA might be an indicator of the severity of inflammation in COPD. Future investigation should be done to further understand the roel of miR-4456 in the pathogenesis and immune regulation of COPD.

There were very few effective disease-modifying treatments for COPD, and most treatments were merely symptomatic treatments (Barnes 2018). Identification of new mechanisms that could suppress the inflammatory response in COPD was urgently needed for the development of better therapies. Importantly, since we found that CCL3 can promote TJ injury via CCR5, and miR-4456 can suppress CCL3 both *in vivo* and *in vitro*, thus targeting these genes might lead to novel therapies for COPD. Nevertheless, there were probably hundreds of miRNAs that are upregulated or downregulated in COPD (Ezzie et al., 2012; Osei et al., 2015; Sato et al., 2015; Szymczak et al., 2016; Conickx et al., 2017; Keller et al., 2018), and the aim of the present study was only to examine those that could modulate the CCL3/CCR5 axis. In addition, although A549 cells were used to study alveolar epithelial cells (Akram et al., 2013; Mortaz et al., 2017; Somborac-Bacura et al., 2018), they were malignant cells that might not reflect reality. Future studies should be done to examine a wide panel of miRNAs, and also to deline at the effects of circulating miRNAs vs. those of miRNAs produced locally in the lungs. Furthermore, larger sample size and patients with different stages required to be explored, since in our study, the correlation of miR-4456 and CCL3 expression in Stage 3–4 COPD was contradictory with two different sample size, which might resulte from small sample size or flexible expression of miRNAs in the peripheral blood of different stages.

CONCLUSION

MiR-4456 played an important role in the epithelial TJs impairment of COPD. miR-4456/CCL3/CCR5 was a potential therapeutic pathway for the treatment of COPD.

ETHICS STATEMENT

The studies involving human participants were reviewed and approved by the Ethics Committee of Tongji Hospital, Tongji Medical College of Huazhong University of Science and Technology. The patients/participants provided their written informed consent to participate in this study. The animal study was reviewed and approved by Huazhong University Institutional Animal Care.

AUTHOR CONTRIBUTIONS

WY is responsible for the experiments and article writing. JD is responsible for the project design. YH and YP are responsible for the animal experiments. TY is responsible for the molecular biology experiments. YH is responsible for the cell experiments. YP and TY are responsible for assisting the data processing and picture modification. QX and CC is responsible for the final modification of the manuscript.

ACKNOWLEDGMENTS

We thank Prof. Shu yuan Yeh for supplying A549 cells.

REFERENCES

Ahmad, S. F., Ansari, M. A., Nadeem, A., Bakheet, S. A., Alotaibi, M. R., Alasmari, A. F., et al. (2019). DAPTA, a C-C chemokine receptor 5 (CCR5) antagonist attenuates immune aberrations by downregulating Th9/Th17 immune responses in BTBR T(+) Itpr3tf/J mice. *Eur. J. Pharmacol.* 846, 100–108. doi:10.1016/j.ejphar.2019.01.016

Akram, K. M., Lomas, N. J., Spiteri, M. A., and Forsyth, N. R. (2013). Club cells inhibit alveolar epithelial wound repair via TRAIL-dependent apoptosis. *Eur. Respir. J.* 41 (3), 683–694. doi:10.1183/09031936.00213411

Albano, G. D., Moscato, M., Montalbano, A. M., Anzalone, G., Gagliardo, R., Bonanno, A., et al. (2020). Can PBDEs affect the pathophysiologic complex of epithelium in lung diseases? *Chemosphere* 241, 125087. doi:10.1016/j.chemosphere.2019.125087

Azghani, A. O. (1996). Pseudomonas aeruginosa and epithelial permeability: role of virulence factors elastase and exotoxin A. *Am. J. Respir. Cell Mol. Biol.* 15 (1), 132–140. doi:10.1165/ajrcmb.15.1.8679217

Bahr, T. M., Hughes, G. J., Armstrong, M., Reisdorph, R., Coldren, C. D., Edwards, M. G., et al. (2013). Peripheral blood mononuclear cell gene expression in chronic obstructive pulmonary disease. *Am. J. Respir. Cell Mol. Biol.* 49 (2), 316–323. doi:10.1165/rcmb.2012-0230OC

Barnes, P. J., Burney, P. G. J., Silverman, E. K., Celli, B. R., Vestbo, J., Wedzicha, J. A., et al. (2015). Chronic obstructive pulmonary disease. *Nat. Rev. Dis. Primers* 1, 15076. doi:10.1038/nrdp.2015.76

Barnes, P. J. (2018). Targeting cytokines to treat asthma and chronic obstructive pulmonary disease. *Nat. Rev. Immunol.* 18 (7), 454–466. doi:10.1038/s41577-018-0006-6

Bracke, K. R., D'Hulst, A. I., Maes, T., Demedts, I. K., Moerloose, K. B., Kuziel, W. A., et al. (2007). Cigarette smoke-induced pulmonary inflammation, but not airway remodelling, is attenuated in chemokine receptor 5-deficient mice. *Clin. Exp. Allergy.* 37 (10), 1467–1479. doi:10.1111/j.1365-2222.2007.02808.x

Buckley, A., and Turner, J. R. (2018). Cell biology of tight junction barrier regulation and mucosal disease. *Cold Spring Harb Perspect. Biol.* 10 (1), a029314. doi:10.1101/cshperspect.a029314

Camargo, J. F., Quinones, M. P., Mummidi, S., Srinivas, S., Gaitan, A. A., Begum, K., et al. (2009). CCR5 expression levels influence NFAT translocation, IL-2 production, and subsequent signaling events during T lymphocyte activation. *J. Immunol.* 182 (1), 171–182. doi:10.4049/jimmunol.182.1.171

Chung, H. K., Wang, S. R., Xiao, L., Rathor, N., Turner, D. J., Yang, P., et al. (2018). α4 coordinates small intestinal epithelium homeostasis by regulating stability of HuR. *Mol. Cell Biol.* 38 (11), e00631–17. doi:10.1128/MCB.00631-17

Conickx, G., Avila Cobos, F., van den Berge, M., Faiz, A., Timens, W., Hiemstra, P. S., et al. (2017). microRNA profiling in lung tissue and bronchoalveolar lavage of cigarette smoke-exposed mice and in COPD patients: a translational approach. *Sci. Rep.* 7 (1), 12871. doi:10.1038/s41598-017-13265-8

Costa, C., Traves, S. L., Tudhope, S. J., Fenwick, P. S., Belchamber, K. B., Russell, R. E., et al. (2016). Enhanced monocyte migration to CXCR3 and CCR5 chemokines in COPD. *Eur. Respir. J.* 47 (4), 1093–1102. doi:10.1183/13993003.01642-2015

Ezzie, M. E., Crawford, M., Cho, J. H., Orellana, R., Zhang, S., Gelinas, R., et al. (2012). Gene expression networks in COPD: microRNA and mRNA regulation. *Thorax.* 67 (2), 122–131. doi:10.1136/thoraxjnl-2011-200089

Fernandes, S. M., Pires, A. R., Matoso, P., Ferreira, C., Nunes-Cabaco, H., Correia, L., et al. (2018). HIV-2 infection is associated with preserved GALT homeostasis and epithelial integrity despite ongoing mucosal viral replication. *Mucosal Immunol.* 11 (1), 236–248. doi:10.1038/mi.2017.44

Francis, S. M. S., Davidson, M. R., Tan, M. E., Wright, C. M., Clarke, B. E., Duhig, E. E., et al. (2014). MicroRNA-34c is associated with emphysema severity and modulates SERPINE1 expression. *BMC Genomics.* 15, 88. doi:10.1186/1471-2164-15-88

Freeman, C. M., Curtis, J. L., and Chensue, S. W. (2007). CC chemokine receptor 5 and CXC chemokine receptor 6 expression by lung CD8+ cells correlates with chronic obstructive pulmonary disease severity. *Am. J. Pathol.* 171 (3), 767–776. doi:10.2353/ajpath.2007.061177

Furuse, M., Hirase, T., Itoh, M., Nagafuchi, A., Yonemura, S., Tsukita, S., et al. (1993). Occludin: a novel integral membrane protein localizing at tight junctions. *J. Cell Biol.* 123 (6 Pt 2), 1777–1788. doi:10.1083/jcb.123.6.1777

Gohy, S. T., Hupin, C., Pilette, C., and Ladjemi, M. Z. (2016). Chronic inflammatory airway diseases: the central role of the epithelium revisited. *Clin. Exp. Allergy.* 46 (4), 529–542. doi:10.1111/cea.12712

Grumelli, S., Corry, D. B., Song, L. Z., Song, L., Green, L., Huh, J., et al. (2004). An immune basis for lung parenchymal destruction in chronic obstructive pulmonary disease and emphysema. *PLoS Med.* 1 (1), e8. doi:10.1371/journal.pmed.0010008

Hammad, H., and Lambrecht, B. N. (2015). Barrier epithelial cells and the control of type 2 immunity. *Immunity* 43 (1), 29–40. doi:10.1016/j.immuni.2015.07.007

Ikemura, K., Iwamoto, T., and Okuda, M. (2014). MicroRNAs as regulators of drug transporters, drug-metabolizing enzymes, and tight junctions: implication for intestinal barrier function. *Pharmacol. Ther.* 143 (2), 217–224. doi:10.1016/j.pharmthera.2014.03.002

Irvin, C. G., and Bates, J. H. T. (2003). Measuring the lung function in the mouse: the challenge of size. *Respir. Res.* 4, 4. doi:10.1186/rr199

Itoh, M., Nagafuchi, A., Moroi, S., and Tsukita, S. (1997). Involvement of ZO-1 in cadherin-based cell adhesion through its direct binding to alpha catenin and actin filaments. *J. Cell Biol.* 138 (1), 181–192. doi:10.1083/jcb.138.1.181

Kar, S., Bali, K. K., Baisantry, A., Geffers, R., Samii, A., and Bertalanffy, H. (2017). Genome-wide sequencing reveals MicroRNAs downregulated in cerebral cavernous malformations. *J. Mol. Neurosci.* 61 (2), 178–188. doi:10.1007/s12031-017-0880-6

Keller, A., Fehlmann, T., Ludwig, N., Kahraman, M., Laufer, T., Backes, C., et al. (2018). Genome-wide MicroRNA expression profiles in COPD: early predictors for cancer development. *Genomics Proteomics Bioinformatics* 16 (3), 162–171. doi:10.1016/j.gpb.2018.06.001

Kerstjens, H. A., Bjermer, L., Eriksson, L., Dahlstrom, K., and Vestbo, J. (2010). Tolerability and efficacy of inhaled AZD4818, a CCR1 antagonist, in moderate to severe COPD patients. *Respir. Med.* 104 (9), 1297–1303. doi:10.1016/j.rmed.2010.04.010

Larsson, K. (2008). Inflammatory markers in COPD. *Clin. Respir. J.* 2 (Suppl. 1), 84–87. doi:10.1111/j.1752-699X.2008.00089.x

Li, L., Zhi, D., Shen, Y., Liu, K., Li, H., and Chen, J. (2016). Effects of CC-chemokine receptor 5 on ROCK2 and P-MLC2 expression after focal cerebral ischaemia-reperfusion injury in rats. *Brain Inj.* 30 (4), 468–473. doi:10.3109/02699052.2015.1129557

Li, D., Wang, J., Sun, D., Gong, X., Jiang, H., Shu, J., et al. (2018a). Tanshinone IIA sulfonate protects against cigarette smoke-induced COPD and down-regulation of CFTR in mice. *Sci. Rep.* 8 (1), 376. doi:10.1038/s41598-017-18745-5

Li, X., Michaeloudes, C., Zhang, Y., Wiegman, C. H., Adcock, I. M., Lian, Q., et al. (2018b). Mesenchymal stem cells alleviate oxidative stress-induced mitochondrial dysfunction in the airways. *J. Allergy Clin. Immunol.* 141 (5), 1634–1645.e5. doi:10.1016/j.jaci.2017.08.017

Mankertz, J., Tavalali, S., Schmitz, H., Mankertz, A., Riecken, E. O., Fromm, M., et al. (2000). Expression from the human occludin promoter is affected by tumor necrosis factor alpha and interferon gamma. *J. Cell Sci.* 113 (Pt 11), 2085–2090.

Marcos-Vadillo, E., and Garcia-Sanchez, A. (2016a). Cell culture techniques: corticosteroid treatment in A549 human lung epithelial cell. *Methods Mol. Biol.* 1434, 169–183. doi:10.1007/978-1-4939-3652-6_12

Marcos-Vadillo, E., and Garcia-Sanchez, A. (2016b). Protocol for lipid-mediated transient transfection in A549 epithelial lung cell line. *Methods Mol. Biol.* 1434, 185–197. doi:10.1007/978-1-4939-3652-6_13

Mortaz, E., Alipoor, S. D., Movassaghi, M., Varahram, M., Ghorbani, J., Folkerts, G., et al. (2017). Water-pipe smoke condensate increases the internalization of *Mycobacterium* Bovis of type II alveolar epithelial cells (A549). *BMC Pulm. Med.* 17 (1), 68. doi:10.1186/s12890-017-0413-7

Nazli, A., Chan, O., Dobson-Belaire, W. N., Ouellet, M., Tremblay, M. J., Gray-Owen, S. D., et al. (2010). Exposure to HIV-1 directly impairs mucosal epithelial barrier integrity allowing microbial translocation. *PLoS Pathog.* 6 (4), e1000852. doi:10.1371/journal.ppat.1000852

Neudecker, V., Yuan, X., Bowser, J. L., and Eltzschig, H. K. (2017). MicroRNAs in mucosal inflammation. *J. Mol. Med. (Berl)* 95 (9), 935–949. doi:10.1007/s00109-017-1568-7

Olivera, D., Knall, C., Boggs, S., and Seagrave, J. (2010). Cytoskeletal modulation and tyrosine phosphorylation of tight junction proteins are associated with mainstream cigarette smoke-induced permeability of airway epithelium. *Exp. Toxicol. Pathol.* 62 (2), 133–143. doi:10.1016/j.etp.2009.03.002

Osei, E. T., Florez-Sampedro, L., Timens, W., Postma, D. S., Heijink, I. H., and Brandsma, C. A. (2015). Unravelling the complexity of COPD by microRNAs: it's a small world after all. *Eur. Respir. J.* 46 (3), 807–818. doi:10.1183/13993003.02139-2014

Polianova, M. T., Ruscetti, F. W., Pert, C. B., and Ruff, M. R. (2005). Chemokine receptor-5 (CCR5) is a receptor for the HIV entry inhibitor peptide T (DAPTA). *Antivir. Res.* 67 (2), 83–92. doi:10.1016/j.antiviral.2005.03.007

Ravi, A. K., Khurana, S., Lemon, J., Plumb, J., Booth, G., Healy, L., et al. (2014). Increased levels of soluble interleukin-6 receptor and CCL3 in COPD sputum. *Respir. Res.* 15, 103. doi:10.1186/s12931-014-0103-4

Ravi, A. K., Plumb, J., Gaskell, R., Mason, S., Broome, C. S., Booth, G., et al. (2017). COPD monocytes demonstrate impaired migratory ability. *Respir. Res.* 18 (1), 90. doi:10.1186/s12931-017-0569-y

Reynolds, C. J., Quigley, K., Cheng, X., Suresh, A., Tahir, S., Ahmed-Jushuf, F., et al. (2018). Lung defense through IL-8 carries a cost of chronic lung remodeling and impaired function. *Am. J. Respir. Cell Mol. Biol.* 59 (5), 557–571. doi:10.1165/rcmb.2018-0007OC

Roscioli, E., Jersmann, H. P., Lester, S., Badiei, A., Fon, A., Zalewski, P., et al. (2017). Zinc deficiency as a codeterminant for airway epithelial barrier dysfunction in an *ex vivo* model of COPD. *Int. J. Chron. Obstr. Pulm. Dis.* 12, 3503–3510. doi:10.2147/COPD.S149589

Ruffer, C., and Gerke, V. (2004). The C-terminal cytoplasmic tail of claudins 1 and 5 but not its PDZ-binding motif is required for apical localization at epithelial and endothelial tight junctions. *Eur. J. Cell Biol.* 83 (4), 135–144. doi:10.1078/0171-9335-00366

Sato, T., Baskoro, H., Rennard, S. I., Seyama, K., and Takahashi, K. (2015). MicroRNAs as therapeutic targets in lung disease: prospects and challenges. *Chronic Obstr. Pulm. Dis.* 3 (1), 382–388. doi:10.15326/jcopdf.3.1.2015.0160

Schembri, F., Sridhar, S., Perdomo, C., Gustafson, A. M., Zhang, X., Ergun, A., et al. (2009). MicroRNAs as modulators of smoking-induced gene expression changes in human airway epithelium. *Proc. Natl. Acad. Sci. U S A.* 106 (7), 2319–2324. doi:10.1073/pnas.0806383106

Somborac-Bacura, A., Rumora, L., Novak, R., Rasic, D., Dumic, J., Cepelak, I., et al. (2018). Differential expression of heat shock proteins and activation of mitogen-activated protein kinases in A549 alveolar epithelial cells exposed to cigarette smoke extract. *Exp. Physiol.* 103 (12), 1666–1678. doi:10.1113/EP087038

Szymczak, I., Wieczfinska, J., and Pawliczak, R. (2016). Molecular background of miRNA role in asthma and COPD: an updated insight. *Biomed. Res. Int.* 2016, 7802521. doi:10.1155/2016/7802521

Van Pottelberge, G. R., Mestdagh, P., Bracke, K. R., Thas, O., van Durme, Y. M.,

Joos, G. F., et al. (2011). MicroRNA expression in induced sputum of smokers and patients with chronic obstructive pulmonary disease. *Am. J. Respir. Crit. Care Med.* 183 (7), 898–906. doi:10.1164/rccm.201002-0304OC

Villanueva, A., and Llovet, J. M. (2011). Targeted therapies for hepatocellular carcinoma. *Gastroenterology* 140 (5), 1410–1426. doi:10.1053/j.gastro.2011.03.006

Vogelmeier, C. F., Criner, G. J., Martinez, F. J., Anzueto, A., Barnes, P. J., Bourbeau, J., et al. (2017). Global strategy for the diagnosis, management, and prevention of chronic obstructive lung disease 2017 report. GOLD executive summary. *Am. J. Respir. Crit. Care Med.* 195 (5), 557–582. doi:10. 1164/rccm.201701-0218PP

Wang, F., and He, B. (2012). CCR1 and CCR5 expression on inflammatory cells is related to cigarette smoking and chronic obstructive pulmonary disease severity. *Chin. Med. J. (Engl)* 125 (23), 4277–4282. doi:10.3760/cma.j.issn. 0366-6999.2012.23.021

Wittekindt, O. H. (2017). Tight junctions in pulmonary epithelia during lung inflammation. *Pflugers Arch.* 469 (1), 135–147. doi:10.1007/s00424-016-1917-3

Yadav, U. C., Naura, A. S., Aguilera-Aguirre, L., Boldogh, I., Boulares, H. A., Calhoun, W. J., et al. (2013). Aldose reductase inhibition prevents allergic airway remodeling through PI3K/AKT/GSK3beta pathway in mice. *PLoS One* 8 (2), e57442. doi:10.1371/journal.pone.0057442

Yuan, H. S., Xiong, D. Q., Huang, F., Cui, J., and Luo, H. (2019). MicroRNA-421 inhibition alleviates bronchopulmonary dysplasia in a mouse model via targeting Fgf10. *J. Cell Biochem.* 120 (10), 16876–16887. doi:10.1002/jcb.28945

Yuan, W-Y., Li, L-Q., Chen, Y-Y., Zhou, Y-J., Bao, K-F., Zheng, J., et al. (2020). Frontline Science: two flavonoid compounds attenuate allergic asthma by regulating epithelial barrier via G protein-coupled estrogen receptor: probing a possible target for allergic inflammation. *J. Leukoc. Biol.* 108 (1), 59–71. doi:10.1002/JLB.3HI0220-342RR

Zhang, L., Shen, J., Cheng, J., and Fan, X. (2015). MicroRNA-21 regulates intestinal epithelial tight junction permeability. *Cell Biochem. Funct.* 33 (4), 235–240. doi:10.1002/cbf.3109

Zhang, N., Nan, A., Chen, L., Li, X., Jia, Y., Qiu, M., et al. (2020). Circular RNA circSATB2 promotes progression of non-small cell lung cancer cells. *Mol. Cancer* 19 (1), 101. doi:10.1186/s12943-020-01221-6

Zhu, A. X., Finn, R. S., Edeline, J., Cattan, S., Ogasawara, S., Palmer, D., et al. (2018). Pembrolizumab in patients with advanced hepatocellular carcinoma previously treated with sorafenib (KEYNOTE-224): a non-randomised, open-label phase 2 trial. *Lancet Oncol.* 19 (7), 940–952. doi:10.1016/S1470-2045(18)30351-6

Zihni, C., Mills, C., Matter, K., and Balda, M. S. (2016). Tight junctions: from simple barriers to multifunctional molecular gates. *Nat. Rev. Mol. Cel Biol.* 17 (9), 564–580. doi:10.1038/nrm.2016.80

16

Lian Hua Qing Wen Capsules, a Potent Epithelial Protector in Acute Lung Injury Model, Block Proapoptotic Communication between Macrophages and Alveolar Epithelial Cells

Qi Li[1†], Qingsen Ran[1†], Lidong Sun[1], Jie Yin[1,2], Ting Luo[1], Li Liu[1], Zheng Zhao[1], Qing Yang[1], Yujie Li[1], Ying Chen[1], Xiaogang Weng[1], Yajie Wang[1], Weiyan Cai[1] and Xiaoxin Zhu[1*]

[1] Institute of Chinese Materia Medica, China Academy of Chinese Medical Sciences, Beijing, China, [2] School of Chinese Materia Medica, Capital Medical University, Beijing, China

*Correspondence:
Xiaoxin Zhu
zhuxiaoxin@icmm.ac.cn

†These authors have contributed equally to this work and share first authorship

Besides pathogen evading, Acute Lung Injury (ALI), featuring the systematic inflammation and severe epithelial damages, is widely believed to be the central non-infectious factor controlling the progression of infectious diseases. ALI is partly caused by host immune responses. Under the inspiration of unsuccessful treatment in COVID-19, recent insights into pathogen–host interactions are leading to identification and development of a wide range of host-directed therapies with different mechanisms of action. The interaction unit consisting of macrophages and the alveolar epithelial cells has recently revealed as the therapeutic basis targeting ALI. Lian Hua Qing Wen capsule is the most effective and commonly-used clinical formula in treating respiratory infection for thousands of years in China. However, little is known about its relevance with ALI, especially its protective role against ALI-induced alveolar tissue damages. Aiming to evaluate its contribution in antibiotics-integrating therapies, this study pharmacologically verified whether LHQW could alleviate lipopolysaccharide (LPS)-induced ALI and explore its potential mechanisms in maintaining the physiology of macrophage-epithelial unit. In ALI mouse model, the pathological parameters, including the anal temperature, inflammation condition, lung edema, histopathological structures, have all been systematically analyzed. Results consistently supported the effectiveness of the combined strategy for LHQW and low-dose antibiotics. Furthermore, we established the macrophages-alveolar epithelial cells co-culture model and firstly proved that LHQW inhibited LPS-induced ER stress and TRAIL secretion in macrophages, thereby efficiently protected epithelial cells against TRAIL-induced apoptosis. Mechanistically, results showed that LHQW significantly deactivated NF-κB and reversed the SOCS3 expression in inflammatory macrophages. Furthermore, we proved that the therapeutic effects of LHQW were highly dependent on

JNK-AP1 regulation. In conclusion, our data proved that LHQW is an epithelial protector in ALI, implying its promising potential in antibiotic alternative therapy.

Keywords: Lian Hua Qing Wen capsule, acute lung injury, macrophages and epithelial cells, endoplasmic reticulum stress, tumor necrosis factor-related apoptosis-inducing ligand

INTRODUCTION

Acute lung injury (ALI), characterized by increased alveolar epithelial and lung epithelial permeability, followed by alveolar flooding and systematic inflammation, was considered as a common pathological mechanism and happened in most infectious diseases (Quartin et al., 2009). ALI is often manifested as one of the most important mechanisms, which involves various tissues damage and eventually leads to multiple organ dysfunction (Oflazoglu et al., 2018). Notably, among all the pathological processes within the ALI network, recent studies have found that aberrant macrophage activation followed by disturbed phenotypic switch are all closely linked with pathological changes in the development of ALI. They promote the lung inflammation and tissue damage, as well as the damage of pulmonary vascular permeability, resulting in pulmonary edema, are all closely linked with pathological changes in the development of ALI (Gordon, 2005; Imai et al., 2008). Therefore, it is of great importance to confirm the relationship between ALI and tissue damage induced by macrophages, so as to provide new revelation in the treatment strategies of the respiratory infectious diseases system.

Disappointedly, in contrast to the essential roles of macrophages in ALI, drugs targeting macrophages regulation and tissue protection under inflammatory conditions are rarely mentioned at present. The treatment of pulmonary infectious diseases still focused on pathogen inhibition, frequently resulting in the upgrading of drug resistance and failure of treatment. This therapeutic dilemma has greatly inspired current researchers. Instead of simply pathogen eliminating, accumulating evidences have highlighted strategies focusing on immune-relevant mechanisms as represented by macrophage regulation and immunological balance remodeling of ALI. Particularly, coronavirus disease 2019, (COVID-19) is rampant spreading all over the world. Due to the poorly understanding about this novel virus and the lacking of specific anti-virus drugs it has become the biggest threat for clinicians in the world(Li and De Clercq, 2020). The lacking drugs of direct inhibition to the pathogen and non-pathogen treatment strategies have mostly contributed to an overwhelming threat of COVID-19. Hopefully, like a beam lightening the darkness, the traditional Chinese medicine (TCM), specialized in immune correcting and tissue protection under inflammatory conditions, plays decisive role in the pandemic controlling, which put another evidence for the importance and effectiveness of non-pathology-killing strategies against infectious respiratory diseases.

In ALI conditions, the pathogenesis of tissue damage, which can be seen as the indicator of pathological progress, is related to inflammatory reaction, cell apoptosis, necrosis and death. Particularly, tumor necrosis factor related apoptosis-inducing ligand (TRAIL) displays core role in regulating these processes and then contribute to pathological damage. Pathologically, the activation of proapoptotic and pro-necroptotic pathways, which can result in a structural disruption of the airway, is a major hallmark of pathological process controlled by TRAIL. In addition, TRAIL can also induce the disruption of the alveolar epithelial barrier by cell death, which significantly contributes to worsened unspecific tissue injury and disease severity in ALI (Tabas, 2010; Alessandri et al., 2013; Condamine et al., 2014; Huang et al., 2015). Recent reports further suggested that TRAIL expression is mediated by ERS, which is linked to CHOP, a popular marker for assessment of ERS. A number of investigators have reported that suppression of ER stress markedly reduced the LPS-induced lung injury. Mechanically, ERS-induced TRAIL expression is mediated by the JNK/AP-1 signaling pathway, nevertheless the production of TRAIL induced by ERS was negatively controlled by SOCS3 through inhibiting phosphorylation of c-Jun *via* the JNK pathway.

Lian Hua Qing Wen capsules (LHQW) is the most effective and commonly-used clinical formula in treating respiratory infection for thousands of years in China. It has approved by China Food and Drug Administration (CFDA). LHQW is composed of 11 herbs including Forsythia suspensa (Thunb.) Vahl (Lianqiao); Lonicera japonica Thunb. (Jinyinhua); Honey-fried Ephedra sinica Stapf (Mahuang); Prunus armeniaca L. (Kuxingren); Isatis tinctoria L. (Banlangen); Dryopteris crassirhizoma Nakai (Mianmaguanzhong); Houttuynia cordata Thunb. (Yuxingcao); Pogostemon cablin Benth. (Guanghuoxiang); Rheum palmatum L. (Dahuang), Rhodiola crenulata (Hook.f. & Thomson) H.Ohba (Hongjingtian); and Glycyrrhiza glabra L. (Gancao); along with menthol (Bohenao) and a traditional Chinese mineral medicine, Gypsum Fibrosum (Shigao). Chemically, a total of 61 compounds were unambiguously or tentatively identified and divided into flavonoids, phenylpropanoids, anthraquinones, triterpenoids, iridoids, and

---

Abbreviations: ALI, acute lung injury; AP-1, activator protein 1; AV-PI, annexin V-propidium iodide; BALF, bronchoalveolar lavage fluid; Caspase3, cysteine-requiring aspartate protease 3; CHOP, DNA damage inducible transcript 3; DEX, dexamethasone; ELISA, enzyme-linked immunosorbent assay; ERS, endoplasmic reticulum stress; HPA cell, human pulmonary alveolar epithelial cells; ICAM1, intercellular adhesion molecule 1; IFN, interferon; IKB-α, inhibitor of nuclear factor kappa-B kinase-α; IKK, inhibitor of nuclear factor kappa-B kinase; IL-1β, interleukin 1 beta; IL-6, interleukin 6; JNK, c-Jun N-terminal kinase; LHQW, Lian Hua Qing Wen capsule; LPS, lipopolysaccharide; MTT, methyl thiazolyl tetrazolium; NC, negative control; P-65, RELA proto-oncogene; PMA, phorbol-12-myristate-13-acetate; PS, penicillin-streptomycin; SOCS3, suppressor of cytokine signaling 3; THP1 cell, human acute monocytic leukemia cell line; TM, tunicamycin; TNF-α, tumor necrosis factor alpha; TRAIL, tumor necrosis factor-related apoptosis-inducing ligand; TUNEL, terminal-deoxynucleotidyl transferase-mediated nick end labeling; VCAM1, vascular cell adhesion molecule 1.

other types by ultrahigh-performance liquid chromatography coupled with diode array detection and quadrupole time-of-flight mass spectrometry analysis (Jia et al., 2015). Pharmacologically, the activities of individual components have been partially revealed (**Table 1**). Pharmacological studies of LHQW have shown that it has a clear inhibitory effect on the growth and spread of pulmonary infectious pathogens (Dong et al., 2014). Strikingly, LHQW capsule have shown therapeutic effects on inhibiting the COVID-19 based on its ability in significantly improving fever and cough symptoms in confirmed pneumonia patients. Recent clinical studies showed that disappearance rate of fever was 85.7% (57.1% in the control group), and the disappearance rate of cough was 46.7% (5.6% in the control group) after LHQW treatment.

The previous research of ALI were concentrated in direct killing for pathogens clearance. However, it lacked the evaluation and mechanism disclosure to the tissue damage in ALI. Based on the deficiencies, our studies showed a comprehensive understanding of LHQW. It is of great significance to expand the field and deepen the treatment thinking in treating respiratory infectious diseases. Our studies previously showed that LHQW can effectively ameliorate LPS-induced lung inflammation. In this current research, we focused on the core mechanism of pathological damages. We also evaluate the efficacy and potential molecular mechanism of LHQW in tissue protection and physiological reconstruction in the treatment of ALI. Importantly, the results of this study can provide some reference value for the treatment of ALI in humans.

MATERIALS AND METHODS

Reagents

LianHuaQingWen capsules (LHQW) were from Shijiazhuang Yiling Pharmaceutical Co., Ltd. (Shijiazhuang, China, batch number: B1509001). DEX was from Li Sheng Pharmaceutical Inc. (TianJin, China). PS was obtained from Solarbio (Beijing, China), LPS (Escherichia coli 055: B5) and PMA were from Sigma (St. Louis, MO, USA). RPMI-1640 and Dulbecco's minimum essential medium (DMEM) were from Gibco (Grand Island, NY, USA). Heat-inactivated fetal calf serum was obtained from HyClone (Logan, UT, USA). Methyl thiazolyl tetrazolium (MTT) and dimethyl sulfoxide (DMSO) were from Amresco (Solon, OH, USA). Annexin V-propidium iodide (AV-PI) was from BD Biosciences (Franklin Lakes, NJ, USA). Caspase3 and Bradford protein assay kits were from Beyotime (Shanghai, China). Primary antibodies against phospho-JNK (#4671), total-JNK (#9258), phospho-p65 (#3033), phospho-IKK (#2697), total-IKK (#2682), IKB-α

(#11930), and GRP78 (#3177S) were from Cell Signaling (Danvers, MA, USA); CHOP (ab11419), DR5 (ab199357), and SOCS3 (ab16030) were from Abcam (Cambridge, UK); β-actin (66009-1) and GAPDH (60004-1) were from Proteintech (Rosemont, IL, USA); total-p65 (sc33020), ICAM1 (sc-8439), and VCAM1 (sc-1504) were from Santa Cruz Biotechnology (Dallas, TX, USA); and Na,K ATPase (-369) was from Millipore (Burlington, MA, USA). Enzyme-linked immunosorbent assay (ELISA) kits for TRAIL, tumor necrosis factor (TNF)-α, interleukin (IL)-1β, and IL-6 were purchased from DAKEWEI (Shenzhen, China). All other chemical reagents meet the reagent specification standards.

Sample Preparation

The powder of LHQW capsules (0.4 g) was accurately weighed and extracted with 60% methanol-water (v/v) solution (20 ml) in an ultrasonic water bath for 30 min at room temperature. The supernatant solution was diluted with the same amount of water and then centrifuged for 10 min at 14,000 r/min. All the obtained solutions were filtered through 0.22 μm syringe filter before the UPLC analysis.

Animal Model of ALI and Experimental Groups

A total of 100 ICR male mice (6–8 weeks old, 18–20 g weight) were purchased from Si Bei Fu (Beijing, China). All mice were kept in an environment of 24°C ± 1°C and 65% humidity, under a 12-h light cycle for 3 days before starting the experiments. Water and food were available ad libitum. All experiments were carried out according to the guidelines for proper conduct of animal experiments published by the Science Council of Beijing, as well as the ARRIVE (Animal Research: Reporting of *In Vivo* Experiments) guidelines for animal research.

For each experiment, age-and weight-matched groups of mice were used. After the last drug treatment, mice were anesthetized with 4% chloral hydrate (0.4 g.kg⁻¹) for 20 min and placed in the supine position on the surgical board(the statement of the use of chloral hydrate was described as following: It is undeniable that the application of chloral hydrate possesses potential risks and serious adverse effects during operative anesthesia, which include, but not limited to, post-operative ileus.). The route of administration was intraperitoneal injection. Then the trachea was exposed by a cervical incision. The whole courses were supported by ventilator. Control mice were instilled with saline, and others were treated with LPS (5 mg·kg⁻¹). All of the above processes were performed on a ventilator. The mice were treated daily for one week prior to the LPS administration. Additionally, the operations were carefully monitored and under strict

---

TABLE 1 | Effects of the components from Lian Hua Qing Wen capsule (LHQW) capsule.

Component	Effect	Reference
Flavonoids	Preventing Carcinogen Metabolic Activation, anti-oxidative Activity	(Li, 2003)
Phenylpropanoids	Anticancer, antiviral, anti-inflammatory, wound healing, and antibacterial	(Korkina et al., 2011)
Anthraquinones	Inhibit cellular proliferation, induce apoptosis, and prevent metastasis.	(Huang et al., 2007)
Triterpenoids	Defend against signal transducer, and activate transcription and angiogenesis	(Petronelli et al., 2009)
Iridoids	Anti-mutagenic, antispasmodic, anti-tumor, antiviral, immunomodulation	(Yamazaki et al., 1994)

experimental control. The anesthesia-only control group and sham-operative group were both set to avoid interference from chloral hydrate -induced unintended adverse effects. During and after the surgery, we also paid much attention to the living conditions of mice once the chloral hydrate was administrated and such post-operative care were maintained until the mice were recovered from anesthesia. For example, we put the mice on the heating pad, which set to keep the body temperature at 37°C. Besides, for the mice receiving operations, their cages were covered with soft cotton pads to prevent the unintended injury.

LHQW and dexamethasone (DEX) were suspended in 0.5% (w/v) carboxymethylcellulose solution and orally administered *via* gavage once daily (300, 600, and 1,200 mg.kg^{-1}) from day 0 to day 7. Penicillin-streptomycin (PS) was injected intramuscular once daily (10, 2.5 ml.kg^{-1}).

Cell Culture and Cell Viability Assay

All cells were maintained in culture medium supplemented with 10% fetal bovine serum (Gibco) at 37°C in a humidified incubator (5% CO_2) (SANYO, Osaka, Japan), with HPAepic and THP-1 cells in RPMI-1640 medium and RAW 264.7 cells in DMEM medium. MTT assay was used to detect living conditions of cells at 450 nm with a microplate reader. HPAepic were purchased in National Infrastructure of Cell line Resource. (According to the information provided by the company, HPAepic cells were not directly isolated from human tissues by us. Also, they were not the primary cells cultured by any companies. Instead, they were immortalized cell line and can be stably passaged *in vitro*).

Detection of Wet/Dry Weight of Lung Tissues and Anal Temperature

The measurement was performed at room temperature of 24.0°C. The Anal temperatures of the mice were measured by using a digital, blunt-tipped stem thermometer(SH series), with Vaseline smearing on it, 2 h after surgery. According to the manufacturer`s instruction, half the length of the blunt-tipped stem was staying in the anus for 30 s and final temperatures were recorded when the temperature remains unchanged for 10 s. After the mice were euthanized, the lungs were removed and the wet weight was determined. The lung tissue was placed in an oven at 60°C for 48 h to obtain the dry weight. The ratio of the wet lung to the dry lung was calculated to assess tissue edema. (The arrive-guidelines of experimental-procedures were shown in **Table 2**).

Alveolar Lavage and Alveolar Macrophage Preparation

Mice were firstly anesthetized with 4% chloral hydrate (0.4 g.kg-1) (intraperitoneal injection) for 20 min 24 h after surgery. After that, the trachea was fully exposed and can be clearly visualized. Then the lungs were lavaged three times with 1 ml saline each time. Alveolar lavage was centrifuged at 135 rcf ·min^{-1} for 5 min, the pellet on the bottom was resuspended by 1 ml 1640 medium, after that the cell suspension was put in 6 well plate and then incubated 30 min in 37°C in a humidified incubator (5% CO_2). Pulmonary macrophages were isolated by the adherent method. The numbers of macrophages counting were counted under a microscope at 40×

TABLE 2 | Arrive-guidelines of experimental-procedures.

Procedures	Euthanasia
Method of euthanasia	Anesthesia methods (The mice were maintained in a specific pathogen-free animal care holding room. It was evaluated monthly to monitor the colony for pathogen exposure. In addition, colony animals identified for euthanasia were monitored for pathogen exposure. Mice were housed in polycarbonate (19.56 cm × 30.91 cm × 14.92 cm) ventilated cages. Cages were changed twice weekly. The animal holding room was maintained under environmental conditions of 22 ± 1°C, relative humidity of 50% ± 10%, 20 air changes/h, and a 12:12-h light:dark cycle. Mice received pelleted rodent diet and water ad libitum.)
Pharmacological agent	Drug formulation was liquid, the dose was 1.2 g.kg-1, the concentration was 10% chloral hydrate (10g chloral hydrate in 100 ml 0.9% saline), the administration method was intraperitoneal injection
Any measures taken to reduce pain and distress before or during euthanasia	Every anesthetized mice was placed in dorsal recumbency on a specialized mouse board with heating elements. This board was placed on top of a 37°C heated recirculating water pad. rectal body temperature was monitored continuously.
Tissues collected post-euthanasia and timing of collection	Lung tissues were collected. Timing of collection was when the animal lost its righting reflex, stopped moving, or appeared to be unconscious.

magnification. The measurement of cell infiltration in BALF were measured by Cell-Counting Kit-8 (CCK-8) assays.

RNA Extraction and Reverse Transcription Polymerase Chain Reaction (RT-PCR)

Total RNA was extracted from lungs using TRIzol reagent (Invitrogen, Carlsbad, CA, USA), and single-strand cDNA was synthesized from total RNA using a Thermoscript RT-PCR synthesis kit (Thermo Fisher Scientific, Waltham, MA USA) according to the manufacturer's instructions. The glyceraldehyde-3-phosphate dehydrogenase (GAPDH) gene was used as an internal control for normalization. Gene transcription levels were detected with real-time PCR (AB7500, Applied Biosystems, Foster City, CA, USA) using the specific primers, Primer name and sequence were listed as:

GAPDH (Mus musculus):

Forward-5'-CAAGGTCATCCATGACAACTTTG-3';

Reverse-5'-GTCCACCACCCTGTTGCTGTAG-3'

CHOP (Mus musculus):

Forward-5'-AAGTCTAAGGCACTGAGCGTATC-3';

Reverse-5'-TTCCAGGAGGTGAAACATAGGTA-3'

TRAIL (Mus musculus):

Forward-5'-GGATGAGGATTTCTGGGACT-3';

Reverse-5'-CTGCCACTTTCTGAGGTCTT-3'

Dual Luciferase Gene Reporter Assay

Briefly, 30 μl of the cell lysates were extracted and transferred into 96-well plates (Gronier, 655075). Subsequently, the samples were reacted with the substrates for firefly and Renilla luciferase according to the manufacturer's instruction (Promega, Madison, WI, USA). Then, a Veritas Microplate Luminometer (Turner Biosystems, Sunnyvale, CA, USA) was used to sequentially detect the activities of firefly (Photinus pyralis) and Renilla (Renilla reniformis) luciferases. The final results were calculated as the fluorescence intensity of firefly luciferase corrected by the Renilla luciferase fluorescence intensity.

Protein Extraction and Western Blot

Lung tissues were homogenized and lysed using lysis buffer containing protease inhibitor phenylmethylsulfonyl fluoride (PMSF). Protein concentrations were measured using a bicinchoninic acid assay kit. Total sample was separated by 10% sodium dodecyl sulfate-polyacrylamide gel electrophoresis (SDS-PAGE) and then blotted to polyvinylidene fluoride (PVDF) membranes (Merck Millipore, IPVH00010). Membranes were blocked for 2 h at room temperature with 5% bovine serum albumin (BSA). Next, incubate with primary antibodies overnight at 4°C. Horseradish peroxidase-conjugated antibodies against mouse and rabbit were used as secondary antibodies. After extensive washing, blots were developed with an enhanced chemiluminescent plus assay kit (Thermo Scientific), developed on X-ray film, and analyzed by ImageJ software (National Institutes of Health, Bethesda, MD, USA).

ELISA Assay

The levels of soluble TRAIL, monocyte chemoattractant protein 1 (MCP1), TNF-α, IL-1β, and IL-6 in the broncho alveolar lavage fluid (BALF) were determined using ELISA kits (R&D Systems, Minneapolis, MN, USA) according to the manufacturer's instructions. ELISA data were obtained in duplicate from at least three independent experiments.

Cell Apoptosis Detection

The supernatant of THP1 cells treated with PMA and LHQW for 24 h in 6-well plates was transferred to HPA cells (3 × 10^5/ml). After 24 h, the HPA cells were dissociated by trypsin for apoptosis detection. Caspase3 and AV-PI assays were performed according to the manufacturer's instructions. Protein concentrations in Caspase3 assay were measured using a bradford protein assay kit according to the manufacturer's specification.

Histopathologic Evaluation of the Lung Tissue

Lungs were clipped at the trachea, perfused with 4% paraformaldehyde (PFA), removed, and fixed for 24 h in 4% PFA. Lungs were embedded in paraffin (ASP200S, Leica, Wetzlar, Germany) and cut into 5-μm thick sections. Sections were stained with TUNEL (Takara Biomedicals, Tokyo, Japan) or NKAα1 (clone C464.6, EMD Millipore, Burlington, MA, USA) after antigen retrieval with 10 mM sodium citrate at 95°C for 20 min according to the manufacturer's instructions. Analyses were performed with ImageJ software.

Statistical Analysis

Data were analyzed using SPSS 20.0 (IBM, Armonk, NY, USA). Values were presented as mean ± standard deviation.

Comparisons among groups were performed using Student's t tests or one-way analysis of variance. In all cases, $P < 0.05$ was considered statistically significant.

RESULTS

Chemical Compounds of LHQW

UPLC was performed to identify the chemical compounds of each herb contained in LHQW. The 12 main active ingredient chemical compositions were as follows: Salidroside (1701.25 μg.g^{-1}), Chlorogenic acid (2,492.15 μg.g^{-1}), Forsythoside E (1620.78 μg.g^{-1}), Cryptochlorogenic acid (1,851.64 μg.g^{-1}), Amygdalin (1,455.39 μg.g^{-1}), Sweroside (813.18 μg.g^{-1}), Hyperin (151.73 μg.g^{-1}), Rutin (121.17 μg.g^{-1}), Forsythoside A (2,536.34 μg.g^{-1}), Phillyrin (1521.45 μg.g^{-1}), Rhein (1102.06 μg.g^{-1}), Glycyrrhizic acid (1,680.43 μg.g^{-1}) (Jia et al., 2015).

LHQW Significantly Protected Lungs From Inflammatory Damage and Decreased Antibiotic Need in an LPS-Induced ALI Model

To evaluate the pharmacodynamics of LHQW, we first measured anal temperature. Compared to the NC group, the anal temperature in the ALI model group decreased to 25.3°C, which was significantly increased after LHQW and PS 10 ml.kg-1 treatment. Notably, there was a synergistic effect of LHQW 1,200 mg.kg-1 combined with PS 2.5 ml.kg-1 compared with PS 2.5 ml.kg-1 alone (**Figure 1A**). Because of the importance of edema for ALI progression and prognosis, we assessed the wet and dry weights for lungs and the ratio. After LPS injection, the ratio was increased nearly 3-fold, but this was significantly attenuated with LHQW and PS 10 ml.kg^{-1} treatment. We also observed a significant increasing in the ratio after LHQW 1,200 mg.kg^{-1} combined with PS 2.5 ml.kg-1 compared with PS 2.5 ml.kg-1 alone (**Figure 1B**). Furthermore, LHQW combined with PS (2.5 or 10 ml.kg-1) treatment were having similar effects. To assess the chemotactic ability of infiltrated cells, MCP1 concentration in BALF was measured by ELISA after LPS treatment. The concentration of MCP1 decreased significantly in mice treated with LHQW. Subsequently, LHQW 1200 mg.kg-1 also had a synergistic effect of PS 2.5 ml.kg-1 compared with PS 2.5 ml.kg-1 alone (**Figure 1C**).

The total infiltrated cells in BALF, which is an indicator of the lung inflammatory response. The numbers were obviously increased by LPS; however, this increase was significantly reduced by LHQW and PS 10 ml.kg-1 treatment. Consistent with our hypothesis, total infiltrated cell numbers were also decreased by at least 2-fold after LHQW 1200 mg.kg-1 combined with PS 2.5 ml.kg-1 compared with PS 2.5 ml.kg-1 alone (**Figures 1D–F**). Alveolar epithelial Na,K ATPases drive the clearance of excess edema fluid, and passive activity of Na,K ATPase in the lung leads to edema due to an imbalance of fluid and salt (Peteranderl et al., 2016). Notably, Na,K ATPase activity was significantly decreased by LPS, but this was reversed by

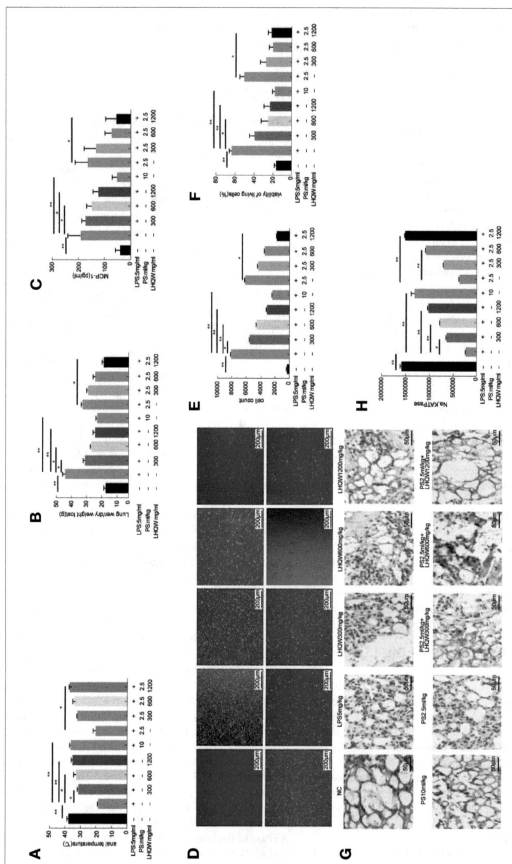

FIGURE 1 | Lian Hua Qing Wen capsule (LHQW) significantly protected lung tissue from inflammatory damage and functioned synergistically with antibiotics in an lipopolysaccharide (LPS)-induced Acute Lung Injury (ALI) model. At 24 h after the last drug treatment, all mice were anesthetized with 4% chloral hydrate (0.4 g.kg⁻¹) and placed in the supine position on the surgical board. Control mice were instilled with saline, and others were treated with LPS (5 mg·kg-1). All of the above processes were performed on a ventilator. **(A)** Effects of LHQW on anal temperature. **(B)** Effects of LHQW on lung wet/dry ratio. **(C)** Effect of LHQW on MCP1 secretion. **(D–F)** Effects of LHQW on the measurement of infiltrated cells in BALF were measured with CCK-8 and microscope assays(40x). Lung tissue from ALI model mice were fixed in 4% PFA, then 3-5-μm sections were prepared after paraffin embedding. All sections were subjected to immunohistochemistry. **(G, H)** Effects of LHQW on the degree of edema by measuring Na, K ATPase levels in lung tissue (200x). The data was presented as the mean ± S.E.M.; n = 8 mice per group; *P < 0.05, **P < 0.01 vs. the LPS group.

LHQW and PS 10 ml.kg-1. Moreover, LHQW 600, 1,200 mg.kg-1 worked synergistically with PS 2.5 ml.kg-1 to enhance Na,K ATPase activity (**Figures 1G, H**). Collectively, these results demonstrate that LHQW significantly protected lung tissue from inflammatory damages and decreased the required antibiotics dose in an LPS-induced ALI mouse model. LHQW may have a role in decreasing antibiotic abuse and resistance.

LHQW Inhibited the Expression and Secretion of Inflammatory Molecules and Dampened Inflammatory Responses by Targeting Macrophages *In Vitro* Study

We next measured activity of the transcription factor nuclear factor (NF-κB) (Hamid et al., 2011; Oeckinghaus et al., 2011). We first evaluated the impact of LHQW on NF-κB with dual luciferase reporter gene assays in RAW 264.7 cells. The results clearly showed that LPS-induced macrophages had increased fluorescence intensity in cells transfected with the NF-κB-dependent luciferase reporter construct, subsequently, which was significantly reversed by LHQW (**Figure 2A**). Additionally, the expression of phospho-P65, phospho-IKK, and IKB-α in THP1 cells were detected by western blot. Expression of phospho-P65 and phospho-IKK were significantly upregulated, while IKB-α was obviously downregulated after LPS treatment. These changes were clearly reversed with LHQW treatment (**Figures 2B, C**). Furthermore, we prepared VCAM1 and ICAM1 antibodies (Yang et al., 2015) for western blot analysis in THP1 cells and detected obviously increased expression of both proteins in response to LPS. Both increases were significantly downregulated after LHQW 1,200 mg.kg-1 treatment and VCAM1 was more markedly downregulated than ICAM1 (**Figures 2D, E**).

ELISA assays were performed to assess the concentrations of TNF-α, IL-1β, and IL-6 in BALF. All three pro-inflammatory cytokines were obviously increased in response to LPS (**Figure 2F**). However, we detected marked decreases in TNF-α, IL-1β, and IL-6 concentrations after LHQW 1200 mg.kg-1 and PS 10 ml.kg-1 treatment. TNF-α and IL-1β concentrations were also decreased by LHQW (600 or 1,200 mg.kg-1) combined with PS 2.5 ml.kg-1, and IL-6 concentration was decreased observably by LHQW (1200 mg.kg-1) combined with PS 2.5 ml.kg-1 compared with PS 2.5 ml.kg-1 alone. The expression levels of Phospho-P65, VCAM1, and ICAM1 were consistent with *in vitro* evidence in alveolar macrophages (**Figures 2G, H**). Taken together, these results show that LHQW inhibited the expression and secretion of inflammatory molecules and dampened inflammatory responses by targeting macrophages *in vitro* studies.

LHQW Alleviated LPS-Induced ERS and Inhibited TRAIL Expression in Macrophages *In Vitro*

To detect the ERS markers CHOP and GRP78, we first prepared CHOP primers (**Table 1**) for reverse-transcription PCR. CHOP expression in LPS-induced THP1 cells was clearly upregulated;

however, there was a 5-fold change with LHQW 500 µg/kg treatment. We also measured CHOP and GRP78 in western blot analyses, which obviously upregulated CHOP and GRP78 expression in response to LPS. Both ERS markers were dramatically downregulated by at least 1-fold change after LHQW treatment. Consistent results were obtained in the alveolar macrophages (**Figures 3A1, D–G**). These results demonstrate that LHQW is a candidate for alleviating LPS-induced ERS.

Next, we performed additional reverse-transcription PCR assays and found that and test TRAIL transcription was decreased by LHQW (300, 600 mg.kg-1) treatment compared with LPS-induced THP1 cells (**Figure 3A2**). To measure TRAIL secretion, we performed ELISA assays by using supernatant of THP1 cells and BALF from mice. Both *in vitro* and *in vivo*, TRAIL secretion was clearly upregulated after LPS induction compared with the NC group, but this was dramatically downregulated by LHQW treatment. We hypothesized that TRAIL secretion might be closely related with ERS in macrophages. The ERS inhibitor PBA was used to test this in THP1 cells. There was no significant difference in the response to PBA between the LHQW and LPS groups (**Figures 3B, C**). To identify the specificity of LHQW for an effect on TRAIL, we detected Death Receptor 5 (DR5), the ligand of TRAIL (Liu, et al.) We prepared DR5 antibody for western blot assay in HPA cells that had been treated with supernatant from THP1 cells. DR5 expression was essentially unchanged in response to LPS and LHQW treatment (**Figures 3H, I**). Overall, these results show that LHQW alleviated LPS-induced ERS and TRAIL expression in macrophages *in vitro* and *in vivo*.

LHQW Significantly Protected Alveolar Epithelial Cells Against TRAIL-Induced Apoptosis in a Macrophage-Epithelial Co-Cultural Model

Crosstalk between macrophages and epithelial cells eventually leads to disease progression and complications (Peteranderl et al., 2016). Firstly, MTT assays showed that LHQW increased the cell counting of HPA cells in the macrophage-epithelial co-cultural model (**Figure 4A**). AV-PI reagents were added to cells prior to flow cytometry. There were no significant differences in numbers of necrotic epithelial cells (AV⁻PI⁺). TM, which promotes ERS, significantly increased the mean number of HPA cells in early apoptosis (AV⁺PI⁻), which was significantly reduced by LHQW treatment (**Figure 4B**). Next, Capase3 kits were used to determine the mechanism by which LHQW inhibited apoptosis. Mechanistically, caspase3 activity levels were highly consistent with the AV-PI results (**Figure 4C**). To further confirm the antiapoptotic ability of LHQW, TUNEL staining was performed. We observed increased numbers of apoptotic cells in response to LPS 5 mg.kg-1 compared with the NC and VACANT (with no surgery) groups. As expectedly, dramatic reductions in apoptosis were observed after LHQW, PS10 ml.kg-1, and DEX 5 mg.kg-1 treatment (**Figure 4D**). LHQW effectively protected alveolar epithelial cells against TRAIL-induced apoptosis in a macrophage-epithelial co-cultural model.

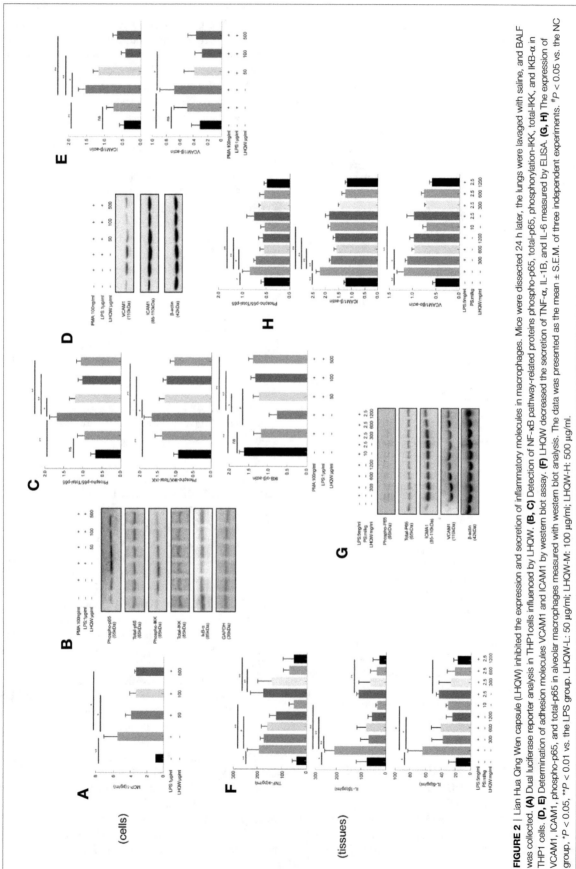

FIGURE 2 | Lian Hua Qing Wen capsule (LHQW) inhibited the expression and secretion of inflammatory molecules in macrophages. Mice were dissected 24 h later, the lungs were lavaged with saline, and BALF was collected. **(A)** Dual luciferase reporter analysis in THP1cells influenced by LHQW. **(B, C)** Detection of NF-κB pathway-related proteins phospho-p65, total-p65, phosphorylation-IKK, total-IKK, and IKB-α in THP1 cells. **(D, E)** Determination of adhesion molecules VCAM1 and ICAM1 by western blot analysis. **(F)** LHQW decreased the secretion of TNF-α, IL-1B, and IL-6 measured by ELISA. **(G, H)** The expression of VCAM1, ICAM1, phospho-p65, and total-p65 in alveolar macrophages measured with western blot analysis. The data was presented as the mean ± S.E.M. of three independent experiments. #P < 0.05 vs. the NC group, *P < 0.05, **P < 0.01 vs. the LPS group. LHQW-L: 50 μg/ml; LHQW-M: 100 μg/ml; LHQW-H: 500 μg/ml.

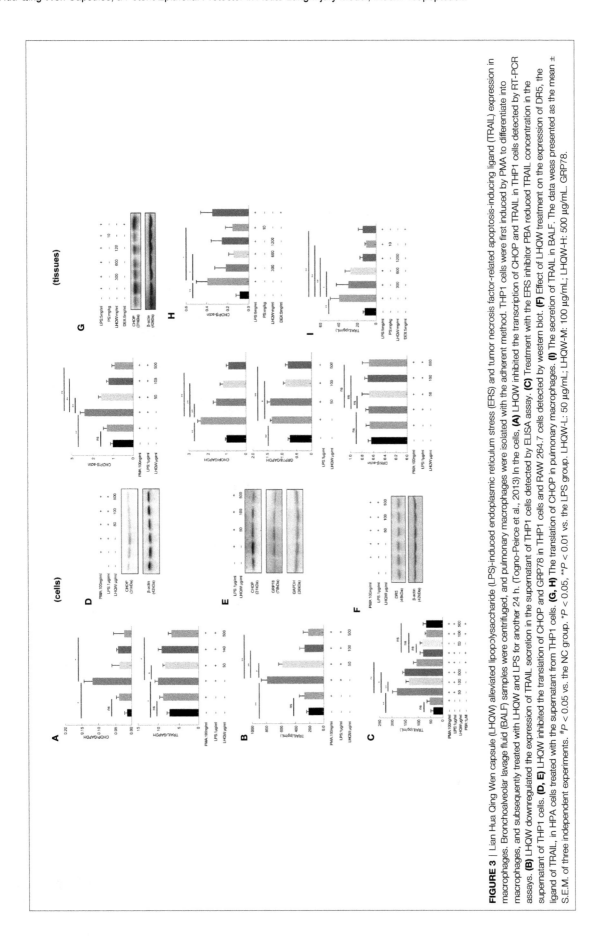

FIGURE 3 | Lian Hua Qing Wen capsule (LHQW) alleviated lipopolysaccharide (LPS)-induced endoplasmic reticulum stress (ERS) and tumor necrosis factor-related apoptosis-inducing ligand (TRAIL) expression in macrophages. Bronchoalveolar lavage fluid (BALF) samples were centrifuged, and pulmonary macrophages were isolated with the adherent method. THP1 cells were first induced by PMA to differentiate into macrophages, and subsequently treated with LHQW and LPS for another 24 h. (Togno-Peirce et al., 2013) In the cells, **(A)** LHQW inhibited the transcription of CHOP and TRAIL in THP1 cells detected by RT-PCR assays. **(B)** LHQW downregulated the expression of TRAIL secretion in the supernatant of THP1 cells detected by ELISA assay. **(C)** Treatment with the ERS inhibitor PBA reduced TRAIL concentration in the supernatant of THP1 cells. **(D, E)** LHQW inhibited the translation of CHOP and GRP78 in THP1 cells and RAW 264.7 cells detected by western blot. **(F)** Effect of LHQW treatment on the expression of DR5, the ligand of TRAIL, in HPA cells treated with the supernatant from THP1 cells. **(G, H)** The translation of CHOP in pulmonary macrophages. **(I)** The secretion of TRAIL in BALF. The data weas presented as the mean ± S.E.M. of three independent experiments. #$P < 0.05$ vs. the NC group. *$P < 0.05$, **$P < 0.01$ vs. the LPS group. LHQW-L: 50 µg/mL; LHQW-M: 100 µg/mL; LHQW-H: 500 µg/mL. GRP78.

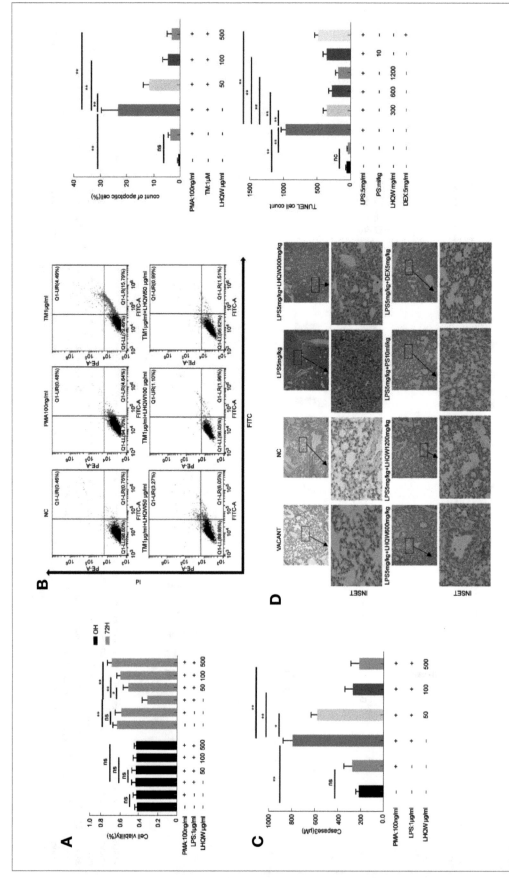

FIGURE 4 | Lian Hua Qing Wen capsule (LHQW) protected alveolar epithelial cells against TRAIL-induced apoptosis. Lung tissue come from ALI model mice were fixed in 4% PFA, then 3-5-μm sections were prepared after paraffin embedding. All sections were subjected to immunohistochemistry. In the macrophage-epithelial co-cultural model, human pulmonary alveolar epithelial cells (HPA cells) in 6-well plates were incubated with supernatant from THP1 cells that were treated with LHQW, tunicamycin (TM), and lipopolysaccharide (LPS). **(A)** The effect of LHQW on increasing the cell counting of HPA cells in the macrophage-epithelial co-cultural model, which was based on MTT assays. **(B, C)** LHQW alleviated apoptosis in the macrophage-epithelial co-cultural model measured by **(B)** AV-PI assay and **(C)** caspase3 activity. **(D)** The number of apoptotic cells (dark brown) in lung tissue measured by TUNEL (200×). THP1 cells in 6-well plates were first treated with PMA for 24 h, followed by LHQW and LPS for another 24 h, then the supernatant was collected. The data was presented as the mean ± S.E.M. of three independent experiments. #P < 0.05 vs. the NC group. *P < 0.05, **P < 0.01 vs. the LPS group. LHQW-L: 50 μg/ml; LHQW-M: 100 μg/ml; LHQW-H: 500 μg/ml; TM: tunicamycin.

LHQW Specifically Inhibited ERS Through JNK Pathway Activation

To determine the ability of LHQW to reverse ERS-mediated TRAIL up-regulation, we prepared a SOCS3 antibody for western blot assays in three macrophage lines: THP1 cells, RAW 264.7 cells, and alveolar macrophages. We detected increased expression in response to LHQW treatment in THP1 cells and RAW 264.7 cells (**Figures 5A, B**). Furthermore, consistent with vitro results, SOCS3 expression was upregulated nearly 1-fold in alveolar macrophages from mice treated with LHQW 1,200 mg.kg-1 (**Figure 5C**).

We finally turned our attention to the JNK pathway, which is closely associated with TRAIL transcription and translation. Western blots clearly showed that JNK expression was markedly increased in the LPS group compared to the NC group, but levels were significantly downregulated after LHQW and SP600125 treatment compared with the LPS group (**Figure 5D**). Together, these findings indicate that LHQW attenuated the increase in SOCS3 expression, with the ultimate result of restricting TRAIL production.

DISCUSSION

Here, we investigated how LHQW affects epithelial cells apoptosis and ERS. By targeting its regulatory effects in the JNK pathway, we revealed that LHQW could decrease SOCS3 expression and as a resultant, restrict TRAIL production in macrophages. Our results provide evidence that LHQW is an effective treatment for ALI and suggests that it could be used as an adjunctive treatment to antibiotics.

Accumulating evidence indicates that ALI is not only the core pathological process of bacterial infection, but also the common pathological process of damage of various respiratory infectious diseases induced by viruses, mycoplasma, fungi and other pathogenic agents. The etiology of respiratory infectious diseases system is caused by the invasion of pathogens or foreign bodies, however, the pathogenic mechanism and damage causes of diseases are more due to the body's inflammatory imbalance and immune damage(Tabas, 2010; Alessandri et al., 2013; Condamine et al., 2014; Huang et al., 2015). Thus, treatment of respiratory infections diseases have provided insight into pathogen–host interactions, and host directed therapeutic strategies are becoming feasible adjuncts to standard antimicrobial treatment (Zumla et al., 2016).

Under the background of global outbreak of COVID-19, mortality from the most severe respiratory infections disease remains high. Subsequently, lots of drugs that have once shown promising antiviral efficacy have nearly failed in clinical trials. However, traditional Chinese medicine LHQW capsule can significantly improve the symptoms of COVID-19 suspected cases such as fever, cough, fatigue, shortness of breath, and reduce the proportion of severe cases, providing preliminary clinical evidence for the prevention and treatment of the disease. The facts remind us again that focusing on immunity is of great clinical significance to develop new strategies for the treatment of respiratory infectious

diseases, which is a good way to make up for the defects of pathogen inhibition, improve the efficiency of pathogen inhibition and reduce tissue damage. According to the theory of traditional Chinese medicine, we focus on "people" of the disease, highlight the "sick people" and "human diseases" integrated interactions. Newer approaches to improving treatment outcomes would put its insights into pathogen–host interactions, the host's innate and acquired immune responses, which are leading to identification and development of a wide range of host-directed therapies with different mechanisms of action. Host-directed therapies targeting host immune and inflammatory pathways to enhance immune responses and alleviate immunopathology could benefit treatment outcomes in a range of bacterial, viral, and parasitic diseases(Cheng et al., 2014) (Zumla et al., 2016).

Recent studies showed that the lung's response to inflammatory conditions was characterized by epithelial injury, pulmonary inflammation, formation of distinctive fibroblasts and excessive extracellular matrix accumulation (Galkina and Ley, 2009). In our study, the tracheal injection of LPS for 24 h can slightly lead to alveolar spaces shrinks and alveolar wall thickening compared to normal group. However, we can hardly observe these symptoms treated with LHQW 1,200 mg.kg-1. We could conclude that LHQW might have potential in resolving pulmonary fibrosis. In addition, some researchers said that pulmonary fibrosis has an indispensable relationship with inflammatory damage and tissue structure destruction (Seimon et al., 2010).

It is well-known that tissue damage is a common feature of many infectious diseases, specifically in ALI (Headland and Norling, 2015). (Freire and Van Dyke, 2013). The interactions between macrophages and epithelial cells, which eventually leads to disease progression, were recently revealed as the therapeutic target in ALI. Subsequently, they can reverse the pathological process of ALI and protect organs from damaging (Hogner et al., 2013; Peteranderl et al., 2016). Under the inflammatory conditions, TRAIL facilitated the inflammatory reaction that promotes unspecific tissue injury and disease severity. TRAIL is closely related to the ERS response and might activate DRs on target cell membranes or alter intracellular pathways, and the pathogen itself might exploit TRAIL-induced pathways for its own survival and replication (Tiwary et al., 2010; Liu et al., 2016). Therefore, TRAIL or its downstream signaling events might reflect ALI severity. Importantly, the regulation of TRAIL expression in the setting of ERS was accompanied by a significant decrease in SOCS3 (Kim et al., 2013; Chen et al., 2015) (Huang et al., 2015). In summary, our studies suggested that LHQW can enhance SOCS3 expression to reverse ERS-induced aberrant expression of TRAIL through JNK pathway, which is closely related with ERS-induced transcription and translation of TRAIL. Based on the analysis above, we concluded that LHQW have potential in alleviating tissue damage induced by TRAIL and it just provide new insight to infectious disease.

In conclusion, the present study demonstrated that LHQW effectively ameliorated inflammatory damage, blocking ALI progression. Furthermore, we need a systematic analysis to

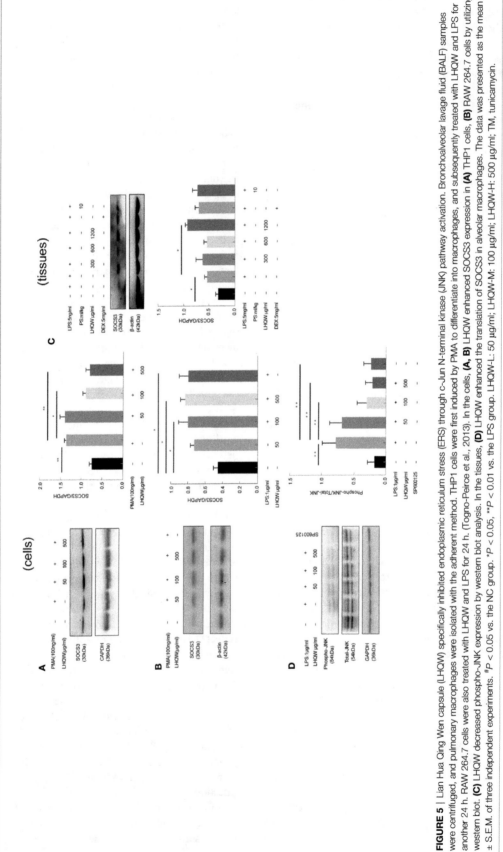

FIGURE 5 | Lian Hua Qing Wen capsule (LHQW) specifically inhibited endoplasmic reticulum stress (ERS) through c-Jun N-terminal kinase (JNK) pathway activation. Bronchoalveolar lavage fluid (BALF) samples were centrifuged, and pulmonary macrophages were isolated with the adherent method. THP1 cells were first induced by PMA to differentiate into macrophages, and subsequently treated with LHQW and LPS for another 24 h. RAW 264.7 cells were also treated with LHQW and LPS for 24 h. (Togno-Peirce et al., 2013). In the cells, **(A)** THP1 cells, **(B)** RAW 264.7 cells by utilizing western blot. **(C)** LHQW enhanced SOCS3 expression in alveolar macrophages. In the tissues, **(C)** LHQW enhanced SOCS3 expression in **(A, B)** LHQW enhanced SOCS3 expression in alveolar macrophages. **(D)** LHQW enhanced the translation of SOCS3 in alveolar macrophages. The data was presented as the mean ± S.E.M. of three independent experiments. #P < 0.05 vs. the NC group. *P < 0.05, **P < 0.01 vs. the LPS group. LHQW-L: 50 μg/ml; LHQW-M: 100 μg/ml; LHQW-H: 500 μg/ml; TM, tunicamycin.

Lian Hua Qing Wen Capsules, a Potent Epithelial Protector in Acute Lung Injury Model, Block Proapoptotic...

205

determine how LHQW regulate the immune injury and pharmacologically protect tissues from damaging.

ETHICS STATEMENT

The animal study was reviewed and approved by Laboratory Animal Ethics Committee of the Institute of basic theory of traditional Chinese medicine, of the China Academy of Chinese Medical Sciences.

AUTHOR CONTRIBUTIONS

QR and QL participated in the manuscript writing and experimental design and performed the experiments. LS, JY, TL, LL, and ZZ participated in the experiments. QY, YL, YC, XW, YW, and WC participated in the manuscript writing, manuscript editing, and data analysis. XZ participated in the manuscript writing, experimental design, and data analysis. All authors contributed to the article and approved the submitted version.

REFERENCES

Alessandri, A. L., Sousa, L. P., Lucas, C. D., Rossi, A. G., Pinho, V., and Teixeira, M. M. (2013). Resolution of inflammation: mechanisms and opportunity for drug development. *Pharmacol. Ther.* 139, 189–212. doi: 10.1016/j.pharmthera.2013.04.006

Chen, F., Li, Q., Zhang, Z., Lin, P., Lei, L., Wang, A., et al. (2015). Endoplasmic Reticulum Stress Cooperates in Zearalenone-Induced Cell Death of RAW 264.7 Macrophages. *Int. J. Mol. Sci.* 16, 19780–19795. doi: 10.3390/ijms160819780

Cheng, G., Hao, H., Xie, S., Wang, X., Dai, M., Huang, L., et al. (2014). Antibiotic alternatives: the substitution of antibiotics in animal husbandry? *Front. Microbiol.* 5:217:217. doi: 10.3389/fmicb.2014.00217

Condamine, T., Kumar, V., Ramachandran, I. R., Youn, J. I., Celis, E., Finnberg, N., et al. (2014). ER stress regulates myeloid-derived suppressor cell fate through TRAIL-R-mediated apoptosis. *J. Clin. Invest.* 124, 2626–2639. doi: 10.1172/JCI74056

Dong, L., Xia, , J.-w., Gong, Y., Chen, Z., Yang, , H.-h., Zhang, J., et al. (2014). Effect of Lianhuaqingwen Capsules on Airway Inflammation in Patients with Acute Exacerbation of Chronic Obstructive Pulmonary Disease. *Evidence-Based Complement. Altern. Med.* 2014, 1–11. doi: 10.1155/2014/637969

Freire, M. O., and Van Dyke,, T. E. (2013). Natural resolution of inflammation. *Periodontology* 2000 63, 149–164. doi: 10.1111/prd.12034

Galkina, E., and Ley, K. (2009). Immune and inflammatory mechanisms of atherosclerosis (*). *Annu. Rev. Immunol.* 27, 165–197. doi: 10.1146/annurev.immunol.021908.132620

Gordon, D., ,. R., Caldwell, E., Peabody, E., Weaver, J., Martin, D. P., Neff, M., et al. (2005). Incidence and Outcomes of Acute Lung Injury. *N. Engl. J. Med.* 353, 1685–1697. doi: 10.1056/NEJMoa050333

Hamid, T., Guo, S. Z., Kingery, J. R., Xiang, X., Dawn, B., and Prabhu, S. D. (2011). Cardiomyocyte NF-kappaB p65 promotes adverse remodelling, apoptosis, and endoplasmic reticulum stress in heart failure. *Cardiovasc. Res.* 89, 129–138. doi: 10.1093/cvr/cvq274

Headland, S. E., and Norling, L. V. (2015). The resolution of inflammation: Principles and challenges. *Semin. Immunol.* 27, 149–160. doi: 10.1016/j.smim.2015.03.014

Hogner, K., Wolff, T., Pleschka, S., Plog, S., Gruber, A. D., Kalinke, U., et al. (2013). Macrophage-expressed IFN-beta contributes to apoptotic alveolar epithelial cell injury in severe influenza virus pneumonia. *PLoS Pathog.* 9, e1003188. doi: 10.1371/journal.ppat.1003188

Huang, Q., Lu, G., Shen, H. -M., Chung, M. C. M., and Ong, C. N. (2007). Anticancer properties of anthraquinones from rhubarb. *Med. Res. Rev.* doi: 10.1002/med.20094

Huang, Y., Wang, Y., Li, X., Chen, Z., Li, X., Wang, H., et al. (2015). Molecular mechanism of ER stress-induced gene expression of tumor necrosis factor-related apoptosis-inducing ligand (TRAIL) in macrophages. *FEBS J.* 282, 2361–2378. doi: 10.1111/febs.13284

Imai, Y., Kuba, K., Neely, G. G., Yaghubian-Malhami, R., Perkmann, T., van Loo, G., et al. (2008). Identification of oxidative stress and Toll-like receptor 4 signaling as a key pathway of acute lung injury. *Cell* 133, 235–249. doi: 10.1016/j.cell.2008.02.043

Jia, W., Wang, C., Wang, Y., Pan, G., Jiang, M., Li, Z., et al. (2015). Qualitative and quantitative analysis of the major constituents in Chinese medical preparation Lianhua-Qingwen capsule by UPLC-DAD-QTOF-MS. *The Scientific World Journal* 2015, 731765. doi: 10.1155/2015/731765

Kim, H. J., Jeong, J. S., Kim, S. R., Park, S. Y., Chae, H. J., and Lee, Y. C. (2013). Inhibition of endoplasmic reticulum stress alleviates lipopolysaccharide-induced lung inflammation through modulation of NF-kappaB/HIF-1alpha signaling pathway. *Sci. Rep.* 3:1142. doi: 10.1038/srep01142

Korkina, L., Kostyuk, V., Luca, C. D., and Pastore, S. (2011). Plant phenylpropanoids as emerging anti-inflammatory agents. *Mini Rev. Med. Chem.* 11 (10). doi: 10.2174/138955711796575489

Li, G., and De Clercq, E. (2020). Therapeutic options for the 2019 novel coronaviru-nCoV. *Nat. Rev. Drug Discovery* 19, 149–150. doi: 10.1038/d41573-020-00016-0

Li, Z. (2003). Flavonoids: Promising Anticancer Agents. *Med. Res. Rev.* 23, 519–534. doi: 10.1002/med.10033

Liu, F., Cheng, W., Bi, X., Zhang, Y., Zhao, Y., and Jiang, F. (2016). Stage-dependent effects of exogenous TRAIL on atherogenesis: role of ER stress-mediated sensitization of macrophage apoptosis. *Clin. Exp. Pharmacol. Physiol.* 43, 543–551. doi: 10.1111/1440-1681.12561

Oeckinghaus, A., Hayden, M. S., and Ghosh, S. (2011). Crosstalk in NF-kappaB signaling pathways. *Nat. Immunol.* 12, 695–708. doi: 10.1038/ni.2065

Oflazoglu, E., Boursalian, T. E., Zeng, W., Edwards, A. C., Duniho, S., McEarchern, J. A., et al. (2018). (Blocking of CD27-CD70 Pathway by Anti-CD70 Antibody Ameliorates Joint Disease in Murine Collagen-Induced Arthritis. *J. Immunol.* 183, 3770–3777. doi: 10.4049/jimmunol.0901637

Peteranderl, C., Morales-Nebreda, L., Selvakumar, B., Lecuona, E., Vadasz, I., Morty, R. E., et al. (2016). Macrophage-epithelial paracrine crosstalk inhibits lung edema clearance during influenza infection. *J. Clin. Invest.* 126, 1566–1580. doi: 10.1172/JCI83931

Petronelli, A., Pannitteri, G., and Testa, U. (2009). Triterpenoids as new promising anticancer drugs. *Anticancer Drugs* 20 (10), 880–892 doi: 10.1097/CAD.0b013e328330fd90

Quartin, A. A., Campos, M. A., Maldonado, D. A., Ashkin, D., Cely, C. M., and Schein, R. M. H. (2009). Acute lung injury outside of the ICU: incidence in respiratory isolation on a general ward. *Chest* 135, 261–268. doi: 10.1378/chest.08-0280

Seimon, T. A., Nadolski, M. J., Liao, X., Magallon, J., Nguyen, M., Feric, N. T., et al. (2010). Atherogenic lipids and lipoproteins trigger CD36-TLR2-dependent apoptosis in macrophages undergoing endoplasmic reticulum stress. *Cell Mctab.* 12, 467–482. doi: 10.1016/j.cmet.2010.09.010

Tabas, I. (2010). Macrophage death and defective inflammation resolution in atherosclerosis. *Nat. Rev. Immunol.* 10, 36–46. doi: 10.1038/nri2675

Tiwary, R., Yu, W., Li, J., Park, S. K., Sanders, B. G., and Kline, K. (2010). Role of endoplasmic reticulum stress in alpha-TEA mediated TRAIL/DR5 death receptor dependent apoptosis. *PloS One* 5, e11865. doi: 10.1371/journal.pone.0011865

Togno-Peirce, C., Nava-Castro, K., Terrazas, L. I., and Morales-Montor, J. (2013). Sex-associated expression of co-stimulatory molecules CD80, CD86, and accessory molecules, PDL-1, PDL-2 and MHC-II, in F480+ macrophages during murine cysticercosis. *BioMed. Res. Int.* 2013:570158. doi: 10.1155/2013/570158

Yang, M., Liu, J., Piao, C., Shao, J., and Du, J. (2015). ICAM-1 suppresses tumor metastasis by inhibiting macrophage M2 polarization through blockade of efferocytosis. *Cell Death Dis.* 6, e1780. doi: 10.1038/cddis.2015.144

Yamazaki, M., Hirota, K., Chiba, K., Mohri, T., and Khiro, R. (1994). Promotion of neuronal differentiation of pc12h cells by natural lignans and iridoids. *Biol. Pharm. Bull.* doi: 10.1248/bpb.17.1604

Zumla, A., Rao, M., Wallis, R. S., Kaufmann, S. H. E., Rustomjee, R., Mwaba, P., et al. (2016). Host-directed therapies for infectious diseases: current status, recent progress, and future prospects. *Lancet Infect. Dis.* 16, e47–e63. doi: 10.1016/s1473-3099(16)00078-5

17

Organ-on-a-Chip: Opportunities for Assessing the Toxicity of Particulate Matter

Jia-Wei Yang [1,2†], Yu-Chih Shen [2,3†], Ko-Chih Lin [1,2], Sheng-Jen Cheng [1,2], Shiue-Luen Chen [1,2], Chong-You Chen [1,2], Priyank V. Kumar [4], Shien-Fong Lin [1,2], Huai-En Lu [5*] and Guan-Yu Chen [1,2,6*]

[1] Department of Electrical and Computer Engineering, College of Electrical and Computer Engineering National Chiao Tung University, Hsinchu, Taiwan, [2] Institute of Biomedical Engineering, College of Electrical and Computer Engineering, National Chiao Tung University, Hsinchu, Taiwan, [3] Ph.D. Degree Program of Biomedical Science and Engineering, National Chiao Tung University, Hsinchu, Taiwan, [4] School of Chemical Engineering, University of New South Wales, Sydney, NSW, Australia, [5] Bioresource Collection and Research Center, Food Industry Research and Development Institute, Hsinchu, Taiwan, [6] Department of Biological Science and Technology, National Chiao Tung University, Hsinchu, Taiwan

Correspondence:
Huai-En Lu
hel@firdi.org.tw
Guan-Yu Chen
guanyu@nctu.edu.tw

[†] These authors have contributed equally to this work

Recent developments in epidemiology have confirmed that airborne particulates are directly associated with respiratory pathology and mortality. Although clinical studies have yielded evidence of the effects of many types of fine particulates on human health, it still does not have a complete understanding of how physiological reactions are caused nor to the changes and damages associated with cellular and molecular mechanisms. Currently, most health assessment studies of particulate matter (PM) are conducted through cell culture or animal experiments. The results of such experiments often do not correlate with clinical findings or actual human reactions, and they also cause difficulty when investigating the causes of air pollution and associated human health hazards, the analysis of biomarkers, and the development of future pollution control strategies. Microfluidic-based cell culture technology has considerable potential to expand the capabilities of conventional cell culture by providing high-precision measurement, considerably increasing the potential for the parallelization of cellular assays, ensuring inexpensive automation, and improving the response of the overall cell culture in a more physiologically relevant context. This review paper focuses on integrating the important respiratory health problems caused by air pollution today, as well as the development and application of biomimetic organ-on-a-chip technology. This more precise experimental model is expected to accelerate studies elucidating the effect of PM on the human body and to reveal new opportunities for breakthroughs in disease research and drug development.

Keywords: particulate matter, air pollution, respiratory health, cardiovascular effects, organ-on-a-chip

INTRODUCTION

With the development of epidemiology in recent years, scientists have confirmed that airborne particulate matter (PM) is directly associated with respiratory pathology and mortality (Kim et al., 2018; Khaniabadi et al., 2019). For every 10 $\mu g/m^3$ increase in PM_{10} concentration, respiratory system-related mortality increases by 0.58% (Analitis et al., 2006), and for every 10 $\mu g/m^3$ increase in $PM_{2.5}$, the incidence of respiratory-system related diseases increases by 2.07% (Zanobetti et al., 2009). These studies indicate that impaired lung function also increases the incidence and mortality of cardiopulmonary disease (Zanobetti et al., 2009; de Oliveira et al., 2012). In addition to the problem of increased risk of respiratory disease caused by compromised lung function, PM may also increase the incidence of lung cancer (Raaschou-Nielsen et al., 2016). In a large-scale study conducted in the United States with a sample of 188,699 non-smokers, each 10 $\mu g/m^3$ increase in $PM_{2.5}$ concentrations increased lung cancer-related mortality by 15–27% (Turner et al., 2011). Although PM is a global concern, severe air pollution episodes are often associated with industrialization, and urbanization. As China's rapid economic growth, several recent studies paid attentions to frequent air pollution episodes (Li et al., 2016; Lin et al., 2018). The air quality statistics report of Beijing from 2013 to 2015 shows that the 2 year average $PM_{2.5}$ concentrations from 69 to 89 $\mu g/m^3$ and the daily average concentrations ranged from 3 to 437 $\mu g/m^3$ (Batterman et al., 2016). These studies have shown that it is imperative to address the harmful effects of PM on the human body, in addition to traditionally known respiratory diseases such as asthma and chronic obstructive pulmonary disease (COPD) (Hopke et al., 2019). The incidence of cardiopulmonary disease and lung cancer are also associated with a high mortality rate (Hamanaka and Mutlu, 2018). Therefore, it is essential to quickly and accurately elucidate the effects of PM on the human body, determine the causes of diseases, and formulate response strategies.

PARTICULATE MATTER AND RESPIRATORY SYSTEM

PM is one of the most important components of air pollution that affects human health and disease. It is classified based on the relative size, which is defined in terms of aerodynamic equivalent diameter (AED), not directly by the diameter of their actual particles. In other words, the size of the actual particles is converted into an equivalent diameter having the same aerodynamic properties (Raabe, 1976). PM can be divided into three AED levels based on the deposition and penetration ability of the particles in the human respiratory system: $\leq$ 10 μm, $\leq$ 2.5 μm, and $\leq 0.1\,\mu m$ (PM_{10}, $PM_{2.5}$, and $PM_{0.1}$, respectively) (**Figure 1A**). Particles with AED diameters >10 μm have a relatively small half-life in suspension and are mostly filtered by the nasal and upper respiratory tract, so researchers have classified PM >10 μm into three categories: (i) coarse PM ($PM_{2.5-10}$), (ii) fine PM ($PM_{0.1-2.5}$), and (iii) ultrafine PM ($PM_{0.1}$) (Anderson et al., 2012).

Although the effects of PM exposure depend on individual physical characteristics, such as the pattern and rate of breathing, weight, and age, the size of the particles has been identified as a direct cause of health problems (Brown et al., 2013). Generally, the smaller the particles, the faster they penetrate and deposit in the deeper levels of the respiratory system. In nasal breathing, cilia and mucous membranes are very effective in filtering most particles larger than 10 μm in diameter. Because of the rapid deposition of PM with larger particle size, they tend

to remain in the trachea or bronchi (upper respiratory tract). They initially accumulate in the nose and throat, and the body will eliminate these invasive PM through some reactive processes such as sneezing and coughing. Up to now, particles <10 μm in diameter are considered to have the greatest impact on human health, and because of their high penetration ability, they can evade the protective mechanisms of the upper respiratory tract and enter the alveoli deep in the lungs (Löndahl et al., 2006; Kim et al., 2015). Computer simulations have shown that particles with diameters between 1 and 10 μm are primarily deposited in the nasopharyngeal and laryngeal of upper airway regions, and particles with diameters between 1 and 100 nm are deposited in the lower bronchial and alveolar region, where gas exchange occurs (Tsuda et al., 2013) (**Figure 1B**). However, particles smaller than 1 μm tend to behave like gas molecules, so it is extremely easy for them to penetrate into the alveoli and affect gas exchange in the lungs and even penetrate the barrier of the lungs and enter the circulatory system, further migrating to other cells, tissues, or circulatory and metabolic systems and leading to serious health problems (**Table 1**).

Currently, there have been many studies on the biological mechanism and effects of PM on the respiratory system (Xing et al., 2016), which primarily involve the following aspects: (1) Functional injury caused by free radical peroxidation. Studies have shown that free radicals, metals, and organic components in $PM_{2.5}$ can induce the free radical formation, cause oxidation of lung cells, and also cause the production of reactive oxygen species (ROS), resulting in DNA damage and cell death (Donaldson et al., 1996; Lodovici and Bigagli, 2011). (2) Imbalance of intracellular calcium regulation (calcium homeostasis). Calcium ion is a physiological index of cell function regulation. However, free radical and ROS reactions induced by $PM_{2.5}$ can cause abnormal intracellular calcium concentrations, which lead to apoptosis and necrosis (Li et al., 2015; Al Hanai et al., 2019). (3) Inflammatory injury. This is also the most extensive part of current studies. $PM_{2.5}$ can cause significant immune responses and inflammation in lung cells (Nadeau et al., 2010; He et al., 2017). These inflammatory responses to Th1 and Th2 triggered by Toll-like receptor (TLRs) pathways can lead to activation of neutrophils, T cells, and alveolar macrophages, which is also associated with asthma and COPD (Nemmar et al., 2013) (**Figure 1C**). Although studies on PM and its biological mechanisms are currently ongoing, an important future research direction is to elucidate the inflammatory response to PM in the lungs.

PARTICULATE MATTER AND CARDIOVASCULAR EFFECTS

With the development of epidemiology in recent years, scientists have validated the effects of long-term PM exposure on the respiratory system. PM can penetrate deep into the trachea and bronchi and can even deposit in alveolar tissue. Hydroxyl radicals ($\cdot OH$) produced from reactive oxygen species (ROS) through activated metals are the main factors that cause oxidative damage to DNA. If damaged DNA is not repaired in a timely

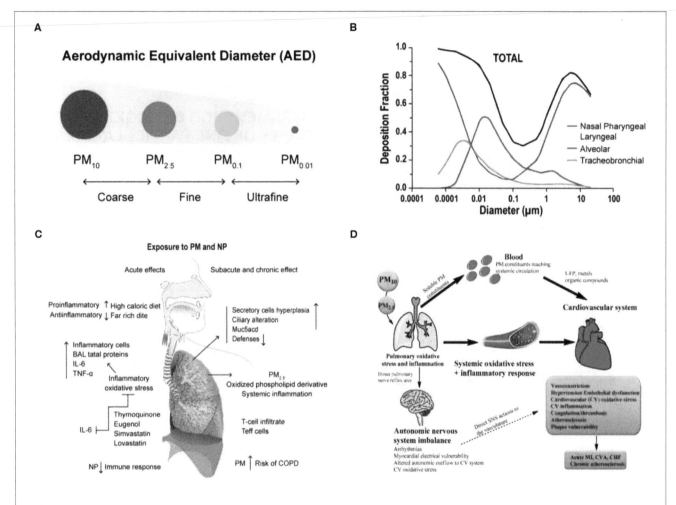

FIGURE 1 | The transport and health effects of PM in human lung and cardiovascular. **(A)** Classification of PM size by aerodynamic equivalent diameter (AED). **(B)** PM deposition curves in the extrathoracic, bronchial, and alveolar regions for adult humans. Reproduced with permission from Tsuda et al. (2013). **(C)** The schematization of the immune responses and inflammation in lung cells by inhaled PM. Reproduced with permission from Nemmar et al. (2013). **(D)** There are three main hypotheses that PM can cause biological pathways for cardiovascular impairment. Reproduced with permission from Ngoc et al. (2018).

matter, it can induce cancer or lead to other irreversible damage (Valavanidis et al., 2005). Environmental exposure to this fine PM not only causes respiratory disease but also affects heart rate, blood pressure, vascular tone, blood coagulation, and formation of atherosclerotic lesions (Suwa et al., 2002; Bennett et al., 2018; Huang et al., 2018). In addition, there is a positive correlation between fine PM and the incidence and mortality of cardiopulmonary disease. The World Health Organization (WHO) reported that 3.7 million deaths in 2012 were due to air pollution, which accounted for 6.7% of deaths worldwide. Of these, 16% were deaths due to lung cancer, 11% were due to chronic obstructive pulmonary disease and associated diseases, 29% were due to heart disease and stroke, and about 13% were due to respiratory infections. In addition, fine PM in the air that is inhaled into the lungs can translocate to the bloodstream and be transported to the blood vessels and the heart, which can induce arrhythmia and reduce myocardial contractility and coronary blood flow (Nemmar et al., 2003). The possible mechanisms for

cardiopulmonary risk following inhalation of fine PM into the lungs can be roughly classified into three groups: (1) Stimulating the production of inflammatory factors: inducing the secretion of inflammatory factors such as cytokines, activated immune cells, platelets, and endothelin, from basal cells in the lungs (Kido et al., 2011; Tsai et al., 2012). (2) Translocation of PM: toxic effects caused by translocation of PM or its components to the circulatory system (Nemmar et al., 2002). (3) Neuroendocrine disorders: the balance of the autonomic nervous system or heart rate is affected by the binding of PM to receptors located on the lungs or nerves (Ngoc et al., 2018; Snow et al., 2018) (**Figure 1D**).

Du *et al.* summarized recent research results on short- and long-term exposure to $PM_{2.5}$ (Du et al., 2016). The results show that every 10 $\mu g/m^3$ increase in short-term $PM_{2.5}$ exposure concentration increases overall mortality and cardiovascular-related mortality by 0.4–1.0%, while every 10 $\mu g/m^3$ increase in long-term exposure increases overall mortality by 10% and cardiovascular-related mortality by 3–76%. With respect to various cardiovascular diseases, $PM_{2.5}$ has the greatest impact on coronary heart disease, moderate impact on heart failure and stroke, and the smallest impact on peripheral vascular diseases and arrhythmia. Because these risk factors not only cause a sharp increase in the risk of cardiovascular disease, and the metabolic syndrome secondary to it is closely associated with some of the most significant causes of death worldwide, including increased risk of Alzheimer's disease, Parkinson disease, dementia, and stroke (Fu et al., 2019). Although the true pathogenic mechanism is currently unknown and the impairment of cardiopulmonary function due to fine PM is due to a complex series of effects, the establishment of an *in vitro* model that represents the human body in a large number

of studies is an urgent need. It is expected that establishing an *in vitro* model of cardiopulmonary function will yield new possibilities and opportunities for understanding the hazards and influencing mechanisms associated with environmental engineering and human health.

ASSESSMENT FOR BIOLOGICAL TOXICITY OF FINE PARTICULATE MATTER

Epidemiological and clinical studies have linked exposure to fine PM to adverse health outcomes, which may also be associated with increased mortality and morbidity in various cardiopulmonary diseases. Despite much evidence of the effects of PM on human health, the causes of physiological responses and the changes and damage to cellular and molecular mechanisms have not yet been fully explained. There are currently two main methods for elucidating the mechanisms of PM toxicity (Fröhlich and Salar-Behzadi, 2014; Yang et al., 2017) (**Figure 2A**). One is the use of *in vivo* animal models to evaluate the effects of fine PM on the respiratory and cardiovascular systems (**Figure 2B**). The other type is *in vitro* cell experiment models (**Figure 2C**); the use of various *in vitro* models has proven valuable for studying the molecular and cellular mechanisms behind different physiological effects more deeply.

Studies using animal models have demonstrated the effects of fine PM exposure on different organs and the incidence of different diseases. With respect to acute reactions, most studies have focused on inflammatory responses, and relatively few researchers have investigated specific responses to disease (Hong et al., 2016; Wang H. et al., 2017). Conversely, with respect to chronic reactions, a large number of disease-related findings have been reported, including DNA damage, lung parenchyma

TABLE 1 | Effects of PM on the human respiratory system.

Diameter (μm)	Distribution characteristics	Effects on human physiology
PM_{10}	Deposits in nose and throat	Can cause allergic rhinitis, cough, asthma, and other symptoms
$PM_{2.5-10}$	Deposits in upper nasal cavity and deep respiratory tract	Causes fibrous paralysis, bronchial mucus hypersecretion, and mucosal gland hyperplasia leading to reversible bronchospasm, inhibits deep breathing and spreading to bronchi
$PM_{2.5}$	Less than 10% deposits in bronchi, ~20–30% deposits in lungs	Can cause chronic bronchitis, bronchiole expansion, pulmonary edema, bronchial fibrosis, or other symptoms
$PM_{0.1}$	Deposits inside alveolar tissue	Promotes significant increase in macrophages in the lungs, causes emphysema and alveolar destruction

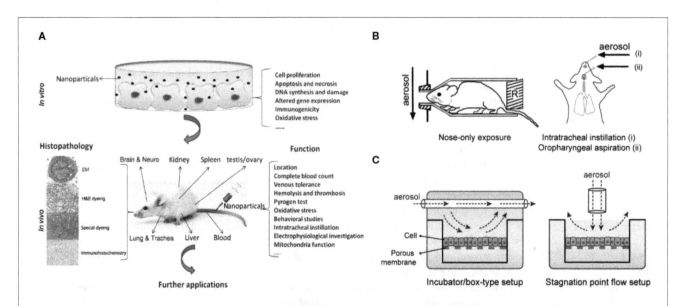

FIGURE 2 | Two main methods for elucidating the mechanisms of PM toxicity. **(A)** *In vitro* and *in vivo* toxicity assessment of PM. Reproduced with permission from Yang et al. (2017). **(B)** *In vitro* animal experiments exposed to aerosols mainly include nose exposure, intratracheal instillation, and oropharyngeal aspiration. Reproduced with permission from Fröhlich and Salar-Behzadi (2014). **(C)** Air–liquid interface (ALI) *in vitro* models for investigating respiratory research.

damage, pulmonary fibrosis, and granuloma formation (Xu et al., 2013; Shadie et al., 2014). Meanwhile, because *in vitro* models have demonstrated that cell experiments are the most suitable model for investigating mechanisms of toxicity, such as initiation events for inflammatory effects or genotoxicity, these data cannot be explained because of genetic differences in animal experiments (Wang J. et al., 2017). In view of this, the genotoxicity and biological indicators linking disease and cancer have been clearly recognized in particular, but this is still a challenge in other applications, which also includes further elucidation of the mechanism of fine PM toxicity in humans (Vawda et al., 2013).

Although current knowledge does not fully understand the health effects of PM exposure, studies over the past decade have suggested the potential cytotoxicity. It has been observed in cell studies that PM stimulation has caused cell viability decline, cell death, ultrastructural disruptions, genetic toxicity (mutagenicity and DNA damage), and oxidative stress (Peixoto et al., 2017). These mechanisms involved in the inflammatory response, including the up-regulation of cytokines downstream of the caspase cascade and the kinase pathway, the up-regulation of metal-redox sensitive transcription factors NF-κβ and AP-1 (Øvrevik et al., 2015). In addition, the PM also increases inflammatory mediator-related gene expression and protein secretion, such as TNF-α, IL-1β, IL-8, IL-6, and MCP-1 (Fuentes-Mattei et al., 2010; Ryu et al., 2019). On the other hand, similar reactions have been observed in animal experiments, showing DNA damage, oxidative stress and inflammatory mediator-related protein secretion and recruitment of inflammatory cells in many organs (de Oliveira et al., 2018). In addition, many studies have shown association between exposure to PM and chronic diseases. These adverse health effects include asthma, chronic obstructive pulmonary disease (COPD), atherosclerosis, diabetes and allergic sensitization (Guo et al., 2018; Li et al., 2018).

Mammalian cell culture studies are often used as the first step in toxicity evaluation, cell-based studies are still greatly limited with respect to the complex structures of physiological mechanisms in humans, and it is impossible to simulate the complex conditions and the interrelated physiological information of the entire organism. Animal experiments play an important role in PM research, where they allow *in vivo* toxicological testing by exposing animals to various PM environments via the oral and dermal routes. Although animals can inhale PM and develop comprehensive systemic outcomes, there is often a large difference between mechanistic and genetic indicator data and clinical outcomes. This is primarily due to differences among species and their physiological functions, such as differences in respiratory rate between experimental mice and humans (Curbani et al., 2019), as well as the problems of genetics, low throughput, high cost, and ethical concerns.

As yet, there is currently no ideal experimental model for study the toxicity of fine particulate matter since both *in vitro* and *in vivo* models have limitations. Notably, the interpretation of chronic toxicity studies is relatively lacking of information, which requires consideration of whether the information obtained from animal studies is similar to human responses. This issue may be expected to be overcome through the advancement of biotechnology and biomedical engineering technologies, thereby

obtaining a useful *in vitro* model that allow long-term cultivation of functional responses that express the human organ. In addition, due to the diversity and regional differences of PM composition, how to systematically study the toxicology of PM on the human body (including single components and the interaction between components) is also the focus of future research (Jia et al., 2017; Park et al., 2018).

ORGANS-ON-CHIPS

With respect to the effects of PM exposure on the human body, many studies have demonstrated the relationship between PM and health risk, but further understanding of the mechanisms of human toxicity is still lacking. The problems faced are derived from the major differences in genes and structures between the species used in animal experiments and humans. Although biomimetic technology experiments are the most appropriate model for investigating mechanisms of toxicity, only a complete description and definition of genotoxicity and indicators between disease and cancer have been made at present, and other aspects are still being researched. In this field, improving the representativeness of *in vitro* experiments and strengthening the reference value of data has become important issues in research. This topic has been discussed by other authors (Vanderburgh et al., 2017; Ahadian et al., 2018; Costa and Ahluwalia, 2019). Developments and progress in biomimetic technology will bring unlimited potential for breaking through the research bottlenecks faced in this field.

To resolve the great differences between animal experiments and clinical trials, techniques have been developed in recent years for construction of organs-on-chips, with the goal of replacing animal experiments and achieving more accurate and reliable preclinical data (Alépée et al., 2014; Zhang et al., 2017, 2018) (**Figure 3A**). Currently, organ-on-a-chip development mostly relies on materials with high biocompatibility for construction of a 3D microenvironment suitable for cell growth so that cells can establish cell-to-cell interactions that are not possible in most 2D cell culture environments, to observe the phenomena of simulated organs more accurately. In particular, this new organ-on-a-chip models provide unlimited potential to replicate critical tissue-tissue responses by reconstructing dynamic physiological forces, cellular microenvironments, and 3D structures of human organ. The development of organ-on-chips and in-depth descriptions have been heatedly discussed in other reviews (Rothbauer et al., 2018; Nawroth et al., 2019) (**Figure 3B**). In addition, when combined with the "induced pluripotent stem cell (iPSCs)" technique in somatic cells, it is possible to successfully differentiate individualized target tissues of interest without traumatizing the organs. Researchers have successfully integrated various iPSC-derived cells with organ-on-chips, such as blood vessels-on-chip, a blood–brain barrier-on-chip and heart-on-chip systems. The different methods for creating organ-on-chips using stem cells also have been described in depth by other groups (Geraili et al., 2018; Jodat et al., 2018; Cochrane et al., 2019).

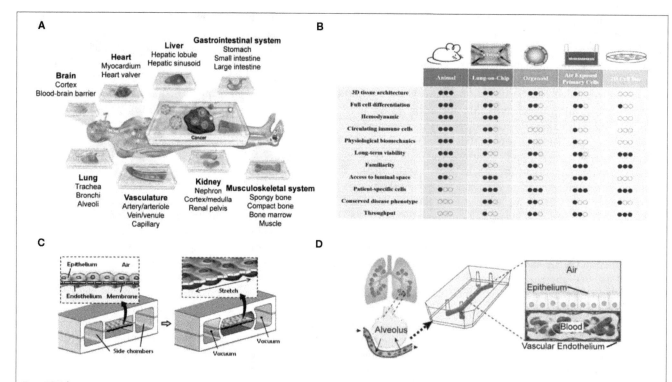

FIGURE 3 | Organs-on-chips technology for tissue model development. **(A)** Organs-on-chips platform provides an *in vitro* model of various organs. Reproduced with permission from Zhang et al. (2017). **(B)** Comparison of experimental strategies for current *in vitro*, *in vivo*, and Organs-on-chips models. Adapted with permission from Nawroth et al. (2019). **(C)** A lung-on-a-chip microdevice reproduce human physiological respiratory movements. Reproduced with permission from Huh et al. (2010). **(D)** Construction of a lung-on-a-chip with tissue/organ-level physical microstructure and microenvironment. Reproduced with permission from Jain et al. (2018).

LUNG-ON-A-CHIP

Although different organs-on-chips have their own requirements, applications associated with the respiratory tract are always very strong. For example, when the lungs are infected by fine PM, bacteria, or viruses, white blood cells accumulate, and the mucus produced block the airway. These processes are difficult to observe in animals and further highlight the importance of developing lung-on-a-chip technology. The Wyss Institute at Harvard University has been a worldwide pioneer in the development of *in vitro* organ-on-a-chip, and the lung-on-a-chip they developed was the first in the world (Huh et al., 2010) (**Figures 3C,D**). It is entirely based on polydimethylsiloxane (PDMS) material, with an upper and a lower layer of channels separated by a porous membrane coated with extracellular matrix. In its internal structure, the upper layer consists of alveolar epithelial cells that allow gases to pass through, and the lower layer consists of microvascular epithelial cells that allow white blood cells to pass through, thus simulating lung function. In 2016, Benam et al. used this technology to test smoking and non-smoking conditions, and confirmed that using the lung-on-a-chip yielded experimental results that were closer to clinical physiological and inflammatory reactions compared with those from animal experiments, and previously undiscovered biomarkers that were even more accurate were found and analyzed (Benam et al., 2016a). At the same time, other teams have developed lung chip models with different

design structures and physiological responses (Fishler et al., 2015; Fishler and Sznitman, 2016; Humayun et al., 2018; Stucki et al., 2018; Khalid et al., 2020). The lung-on-a-chip have been developed to demonstrate their importance in drug development and disease models, but still have several practical challenges must be overcome if such devices are to be used in toxicology research and application (Low and Tagle, 2017; Wu et al., 2020). The aim of overcoming these challenges is to improve the usability of these devices and to simulate metabolism in the human body more accurately.

HEART-ON-A-CHIP

In addition, evidence from animal studies has shown that nanoparticles can cross the alveolar-capillary barrier and subsequently deposit in extrapulmonary organs such as the vasculature and heart (Choi et al., 2010). Using specific organ chips, such as heart-on-a-chip to investigate the toxicity of PM may also have great potential value. The heart-on-a-chip is mainly used to study electrical stimulation (Xiao et al., 2014), cardiac electrophysiology (Sidorov et al., 2017) and disease models (Wang et al., 2014). Marsano et al. recently established heart-on-a-chip platform integrates mechanical stress and 3D matrix microenvironment, showing better differentiation and electromechanical coupling of the iPSC-derived cardiomyocyte (Marsano et al., 2016). Liu *et al.* demonstrated the latest bioelectronic heart-on-a-chip model, which can regulate the concentration of oxygen through the microfluidic channel, and integrated bioelectronic devices to successfully monitor the cardiac electrophysiology responses to acute hypoxia (Liu et al., 2020). These examples fully demonstrate that heart-on-a-chip may provide greater ability to recapitulation the cellular microenvironment and tissue function. In the future, it is expected that suitable heart-on-a-chip models can be selected to investigate the human toxicity investigation of PM deposition, penetration and metabolism, but it is necessary to consider whether to choose particles with corresponding size, composition and complex for stimulation or exposure assessment. Of particular interest are the mechanisms of PM-mediated toxicity on the systemic health effects. In recent years, with the gradual advancement of multi-organ chips technology, it is expected to provide more clues to accelerate the clarification of the human toxicity of PM deposition, penetration and metabolism (Yuancheng et al., 2018; Carvalho et al., 2019), especially for the specific examples of lung- heart- on chip model, which could be used to investigate the systemic toxicology of PM into the human body.

OPPORTUNITIES AND CHALLENGES

It is worth mentioning that the organ-on-a-chip not only shows the application value in research, but also the establishment of related companies has started to appear in the past 5 years (Mastrangeli et al., 2019), such as TissUse GmbH, Emulate, Inc., MIMETAS Inc., Nortis, Inc., AlveoliX AG., Hesperos Inc.. In addition, the U.S. Food and Drug Administration (FDA) announced in April 2017 that it had signed a multi-year cooperation agreement with Emulate Inc. (spinoff from the Wyss Institute for Biologically Inspired Engineering at Harvard University), and will begin a series of trials using organ-on-a-chip technology to develop a testing platform for toxicological safety assessment (Isoherranen et al., 2019). These results demonstrate the potential of applying organ-on-a-chip systems to human health assessments. In the future, the organ-on-a-chip technology is able to integrate stem cell technology, microenvironment and personalization parameters (e.g., breathing pattern, heart rate, substance abuse, etc.) to allow the construction of models of different genders, regions, ages, and diseases to minute minor physiological differences, thereby promoting the development of precision health (van den Berg et al., 2019).

Despite the progress made with organ-on-a-chip models, there remains a question that the organ-level functional replication is limited by the source of cells. In the case of pulmonary alveolar model, the aspect of long-term culture of primary human alveolar type I and type II epithelial cells is particularly challenging limitation (Shiraishi et al., 2019; Weiner et al., 2019). Therefore, the organ-on-a-chip technology faces limited availability and the inability to expand primary cells, requiring the establishment of cell cultures directly from donors and patients, which will increase the cost of experiments and the difficulty of popularizing the technology. On the other hand, the most organ-on-a-chip are made of PDMS due to their

high biocompatibility, oxygen permeability, and transparency. The PDMS chip devices can directly match conventional cell culture incubators and biological microscopes. However, a large amount of protein molecules will be adsorbed on the surface of PDMS (Wong and Ho, 2009; Gokaltun et al., 2017), which results in that the supplement or stimulating substance of the cell culture cannot fully interact with the cells. To avoid adsorption of non-specific proteins, some teams have used polylactic acid (PLA) (Ongaro et al., 2020), poly (methyl methacrylate) (PMMA) (Nguyen et al., 2019), polystyrene (PS) (Lee et al., 2018), and polycarbonate (PC) (Henry et al., 2017), and more advantages and limitations of PDMS materials also have been introduced in detail by other teams (Halldorsson et al., 2015; Gokaltun et al., 2017).

MULTI-ORGAN CHIPS

With the development of organs-on-chips in the past decade, the establishment of single types of organ-on-a-chip or the development of disease models on a chip has gradually matured. Although the organ-on-chips have seen great progress, it is not enough to rely on a simulation single organ model for a comprehensive understanding due to the highly complex interactions between human organs. In 2004, Dr. Shuler and colleagues first proposed the concept of reproducing human physiological functions in chip devices (Sin et al., 2004). The increasing demand for in vitro models, chips integrating multiple organs have become a major topic in recent years, and they also represent a major step forward in organ-on-a-chip technology (**Figure 4A**). Currently, chips capable of representing multiple organs in an integrated manner and fully and accurately simulating human tissue are still being developed (Skardal et al., 2017; Oleaga et al., 2018; Boos et al., 2019; Sung et al., 2019; Zhao et al., 2019). For example, a new model for physiological pharmacokinetics (PKs) and pharmacodynamics (PDs) has successfully predicted the clinical patient data of cisplatin PDs. This model is linked through fluidically coupled vascularized organ chips to investigate PK and PD parameters of oral and injectable drugs (Herland et al., 2020). It is worth noting that the experiments of this model have reached an automated system through robotic fluidic coupling of multiple organ chips, and maintained the long-term culture of organ-specific functions for 3 weeks (Novak et al., 2020). The automated multi-organ chip system integrated with high-throughput screening has the potential to improve the prediction of drugs (or other foreign substances) absorption, distribution, metabolism, excretion and toxicity for clinical trials.

As another example, the device in a recent study mainly integrates four tissues—liver, heart, muscle, and neurons (Oleaga et al., 2016). It is composed of the liver (which serves to process drug metabolites and drug processes drugs or prodrugs), heart (which is the most important organ in the human body), skeletal muscle (which is responsible for glucose storage levels in the body), and neurons (which represent a particularly sensitive cell system). After culturing this system in a continuous flow environment for 14 days, its feasibility and

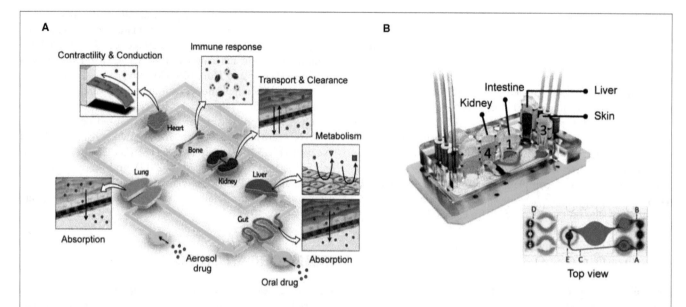

FIGURE 4 | Integrate multi-organ chip platforms to create complex interactions between human organs. **(A)** The design concept of the human body chip. One of the most promising *in vitro* system for replicating the systemic responses of human body. Reproduced with permission from Huh et al. (2011). **(B)** Four-organs-on-a-chip system employed intestine, liver, skin, and kidney tissue that proportionately simulated the physiological environment of the human body. Reproduced with permission from Maschmeyer et al. (2015).

functionality were demonstrated, and because the cells used in the system were primary cells and cells derived from iPSCs, they exhibited the exchange of metabolites and signaling molecules. In addition, by measuring heart rate, muscle contractility, neuroelectrophysiology, and production of liver albumin and urea, it served as an accurate model for predicting toxicity in multiple human organs. In another study, Maschmeyer et al. integrated pre-formed bowel and skin models into a hepatic spheroid and renal epithelial barrier tissue model, establishing a microchannel system that could support the functions of four types of organs in a co-culture over a long period of 1 month (Maschmeyer et al., 2015) (**Figure 4B**). In addition, this four-organs-on-a-chip system employed a structure that more proportionately simulated the physiological fluid and tissue environment of the human body. It simulated drug absorption and metabolism in the small intestine, metabolism by the liver, and excretion by the kidneys, which are all key factors that determine the efficacy and safety of drug treatments. These systems allow us to further understand metabolic and genetic analyses and provide an alternative to systemic toxicity testing. In addition, these examples demonstrate that integrated multi-organ chips are an important part in the ability to simulate complex reactions and interactions between tissues, whether in drug testing, toxicological screening, or construction of organ-on-a-chip models.

Therefore, integrating multi-organ chips are expected to replace the inadequacies of traditional *in vitro* models, promoting studies of the effects of air pollution on the body and the early development of drugs, as these devices are designed to mimic the physiological structure of internal organs and interactions with soluble metabolites, thereby achieving *in vitro* the interactive effects between organs. However, current multi-organ chip models are mainly used for systemic processes of oral and injectable drugs, but lacks models for PM inhalation. In a recent human inhalation study, Miller et al. investigated the transport behavior of gold nanoparticle inhaled into the lung (Miller et al., 2017). The results showed that the blood and urine of the volunteers still found gold nanoparticle after 3 months of exposure, indicating systemic retention and delayed urinary excretion. This study clearly understands the ability of inhaled nanoparticles to penetrate lung tissue, but investigating the interactions between human organs, especially for the cardiopulmonary system remains a challenge. Based on the most direct impact of PM on cardiopulmonary function, in the future, it is urgent to form an integrated platform by connecting the organ chips of the lung and heart in the future. Even PM gas can be exposed to such a platform for discussion. It is hoped that the cardiopulmonary function model established *in vitro* can be used to obtain new possibilities and opportunities for PM analysis, so that it can more effectively clarify the impact of PM on the human body *in vitro* and find out the causes of cardiopulmonary diseases.

OUTLOOK

In addition to well-known respiratory diseases such as COPD, fine PM in the air that is inhaled into the lungs are translocated to the bloodstream and transported to the blood vessels and heart, where they induce arrhythmia, reduce myocardial contractility, and reduce coronary blood flow, thereby increasing the incidence and mortality of cardiopulmonary diseases. Related studies have shown that the harmful effects of fine PM on health may reach an uncontrollable point by 2030. Therefore, it is essential to quickly and accurately elucidate their effects on the

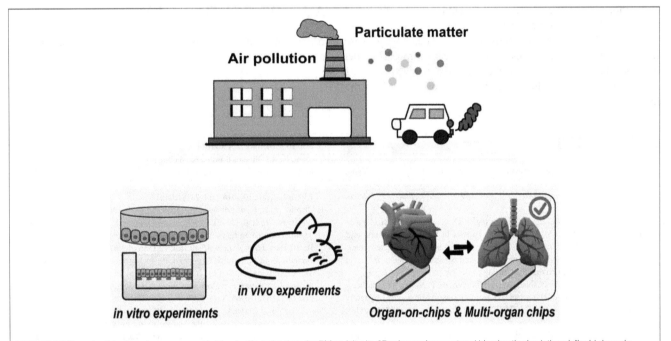

FIGURE 5 | The potential value of organ-on-a-chip biomimetic technology for PM toxicity. Its 3D microenvironment and biomimetic circulating air/liquid dynamic environment are expected to be used for PM health assessment.

human body, determine the causes of disease, and formulate response strategies.

Although epidemiological and clinical studies have produced much evidence of the effects of fine PM on human health, it has not yet been fully explained how physiological responses and cellular and molecular mechanisms of change and injury are caused. Currently, most health evaluation studies of fine PM are conducted through cell culture or animal experiments. Cell-based studies are still greatly limited compared to the complex structures of physiological mechanisms in humans, and it is impossible to simulate the complex conditions and the interrelated physiological information of the entire organism. Animal experiments play an important role in studies on fine PM, where they allow *in vivo* toxicological testing by exposing animals to various fine PM environments via the oral and dermal routes. Although animals can inhale fine PM and develop comprehensive systemic outcomes, there is often a large difference between mechanistic and genetic indicator data and clinical outcomes. This is primarily due to differences among species and their physiological functions, such as differences in respiratory rate between experimental mice and humans, as well as the problems of genetics, low throughput, high cost, and ethical concerns. These reasons have caused difficulty when investigating the causes of air pollution and associated human health hazards, the analysis of biomarkers, and the development of future pollution control strategies. Organ-on-a-chip biomimetic technology will bring unlimited potential for breaking through the bottlenecks faced in previous studies.

Reviewing the current development of organ-on-chips, most research focuses on drug development and disease models (Huh

et al., 2012; Esch et al., 2015; Benam et al., 2016b). Except for the toxicological applications of lung-on-a-chip and cigarette smoking, other integrated studies related to environmental PM have not been extensive. According to previous reviews (see the section on Particulate matter and respiratory system and Particulate matter and cardiovascular effects), there are several clues worthy of attention such as DNA damage, inflammatory injury and PM translocation. For these research topics, it is believed that there is a great opportunity to obtain more undiscovered information by applying current organ-on-chips and multi-organ chips technology. For example, DNA damage and inflammatory injury could refer to related research on drug toxicity testing, translocation of PM could refer to related research on nanoparticle drug delivery, and further research on chronic toxicology could refer to the multi-organ chips model with PKs and PDs parameters. On the other hand, organ-on-a-chip systems have been shown to be closer to clinical physiology and inflammatory response, compared to traditional experimental model approaches. It has the potential to be a useful *in vitro* model for investigating the relationship between PM and related diseases. Therefore, the successful development of *in vitro* chips for simulating organs is a necessary avenue toward modern assessment of the health effects of air pollution. Its rapid and efficient screening capabilities are expected to help governmental agencies and the clinical sector move toward the correct policy and drug development routes, reduce costs, and significantly shorten the process of drug and foreign substance toxicity testing (Ronaldson-Bouchard and Vunjak-Novakovic, 2018).

The technology is still evolving from single organ to multi-organ chips, it is expected to be realized as a long-term and highly active cardiopulmonary chip. Its 3D microenvironment and more biomimetic cyclic dynamic environment combined with fine PM are expected to be applied to health evaluation, physiological indicators, creation of cardiopulmonary disease models, and drug testing. This more precise experimental model is expected to replace existing cell culture or animal experiments and accelerate studies elucidating the effect of fine PM on the human body (**Figure 5**).

AUTHOR CONTRIBUTIONS

All authors contributed toward conceptualization, preparation, and validation of the manuscript.

REFERENCES

Ahadian, S., Civitarese, R., Bannerman, D., Mohammadi, M. H., Lu, R., Wang, E., et al. (2018). Organ-on-a-chip platforms: a convergence of advanced materials, cells, and microscale technologies. *Adv. Healthcare Mater.* 7:1700506. doi: 10.1002/adhm.201700506

Al Hanai, A. H., Antkiewicz, D. S., Hemming, J. D. C., Shafer, M. M., Lai, A. M., Arhami, M., et al. (2019). Seasonal variations in the oxidative stress and inflammatory potential of PM2.5 in Tehran using an alveolar macrophage model: the role of chemical composition and sources. *Environ. Int.* 123, 417–427. doi: 10.1016/j.envint.2018.12.023

Alépée, N., Bahinski, A., Daneshian, M., De Wever, B., Fritsche, E., Goldberg, A., et al. (2014). State-of-the-art of 3D cultures (organs-on-a-chip) in safety testing and pathophysiology. *ALTEX* 31, 441–477. doi: 10.14573/altex1406111

Analitis, A., Katsouyanni, K., Dimakopoulou, K., Samoli, E., Nikoloulopoulos, A. K., Petasakis, Y., et al. (2006). Short-term effects of ambient particles on cardiovascular and respiratory mortality. *Epidemiology* 17, 230–233. doi: 10.1097/01.ede.0000199439.57655.6b

Anderson, J. O., Thundiyil, J. G., and Stolbach, A. (2012). Clearing the air: a review of the effects of particulate matter air pollution on human health. *J. Med. Toxicol.* 8, 166–175. doi: 10.1007/s13181-011-0203-1

Batterman, S., Xu, L., Chen, F., Chen, F., and Zhong, X. (2016). Characteristics of PM(2.5) concentrations across Beijing during 2013-2015. *Atmos. Environ.* 145, 104–114. doi: 10.1016/j.atmosenv.2016.08.060

Benam, K. H., Novak, R., Nawroth, J., Hirano-Kobayashi, M., Ferrante, T. C., Choe, Y., et al. (2016a). Matched-comparative modeling of normal and diseased human airway responses using a microengineered breathing lung chip. *Cell Syst.* 3, 456–466.e454. doi: 10.1016/j.cels.2016.10.003

Benam, K. H., Villenave, R., Lucchesi, C., Varone, A., Hubeau, C., Lee, H.-H., et al. (2016b). Small airway-on-a-chip enables analysis of human lung inflammation and drug responses *in vitro*. *Nat. Methods* 13, 151–157. doi: 10.1038/nmeth.3697

Bennett, B. A., Spannhake, E. W., Rule, A. M., Breysse, P. N., and Tankersley, C. G. (2018). The acute effects of age and particulate matter exposure on heart rate and heart rate variability in Mice. *Cardiovasc. Toxicol.* 18, 507–519. doi: 10.1007/s12012-018-9461-3

Boos, J. A., Misun, P. M., Michlmayr, A., Hierlemann, A., and Frey, O. (2019). Microfluidic multitissue platform for advanced embryotoxicity testing *in vitro*. *Adv. Sci.* 6:1900294. doi: 10.1002/advs.201900294

Brown, J. S., Gordon, T., Price, O., and Asgharian, B. (2013). Thoracic and respirable particle definitions for human health risk assessment. *Part. Fibre Toxicol.* 10:12. doi: 10.1186/1743-8977-10-12

Carvalho, M. R., Barata, D., Teixeira, L. M., Giselbrecht, S., Reis, R. L., et al. (2019). Colorectal tumor-on-a-chip system: a 3D tool for precision onco-nanomedicine. *Sci. Adv.* 5:eaaw1317. doi: 10.1126/sciadv.aaw1317

Choi, H. S., Ashitate, Y., Lee, J. H., Kim, S. H., Matsui, A., Insin, N., et al. (2010). Rapid translocation of nanoparticles from the lung airspaces to the body. *Nat. Biotechnol.* 28, 1300–1303. doi: 10.1038/nbt.1696

Cochrane, A., Albers, H. J., Passier, R., Mummery, C. L., van den Berg, A., Orlova, V. V., et al. (2019). Advanced *in vitro* models of vascular biology: human induced pluripotent stem cells and organ-on-chip technology. *Adv. Drug Deliv. Rev.* 140, 68–77. doi: 10.1016/j.addr.2018.06.007

Costa, J., and Ahluwalia, A. (2019). Advances and current challenges in intestinal *in vitro* model engineering: a digest. *Front. Bioeng. Biotechnol.* 7:144.

doi: 10.3389/fbioe.2019.00144

Curbani, F., de Oliveira Busato, F., Marcarini do Nascimento, M., Olivieri, D. N., and Tadokoro, C. E. (2019). Inhale, exhale: why particulate matter exposure in animal models are so acute? Data and facts behind the history. *Data Brief.* 25:104237. doi: 10.1016/j.dib.2019.104237

de Oliveira, A. A. F., de Oliveira, T. F., Dias, M. F., Medeiros, M. H. G., Di Mascio, P., Veras, M., et al. (2018). Genotoxic and epigenotoxic effects in mice exposed to concentrated ambient fine particulate matter (PM2.5) from São Paulo city, Brazil. *Part. Fibre Toxicol.* 15:40. doi: 10.1186/s12989-018-0276-y

de Oliveira, B. F. A., Ignotti, E., Artaxo, P., do Nascimento Saldiva, P. H., Junger, W. L., and Hacon, S. (2012). Risk assessment of PM2.5 to child residents in Brazilian Amazon region with biofuel production. *Environ. Health* 11:64. doi: 10.1186/1476-069X-11-64

Donaldson, K., Beswick, P. H., and Gilmour, P. S. (1996). Free radical activity associated with the surface of particles: a unifying factor in determining biological activity? *Toxicol. Lett.* 88, 293–298. doi: 10.1016/0378-4274(96)03752-6

Du, Y., Xu, X., Chu, M., Guo, Y., and Wang, J. (2016). Air particulate matter and cardiovascular disease: the epidemiological, biomedical and clinical evidence. *J. Thorac. Dis.* 8, E8–E19. doi: 10.3978/j.issn.2072-1439.2015.11.37

Esch, E. W., Bahinski, A., and Huh, D. (2015). Organs-on-chips at the frontiers of drug discovery. *Nat. Rev. Drug Discov.* 14, 248–260. doi: 10.1038/nrd4539

Fishler, R., Hofemeier, P., Etzion, Y., Dubowski, Y., and Sznitman, J. (2015). Particle dynamics and deposition in true-scale pulmonary acinar models. *Sci. Rep.* 5:14071. doi: 10.1038/srep14071

Fishler, R., and Sznitman, J. (2016). A microfluidic model of biomimetically breathing pulmonary acinar airways. *J. Vis. Exp.* 9:53588. doi: 10.3791/53588

Fröhlich, E., and Salar-Behzadi, S. (2014). Toxicological assessment of inhaled nanoparticles: role of *in vivo, ex vivo, in vitro*, and *in silico* studies. *Int. J. Mol. Sci.* 15, 4795–4822. doi: 10.3390/ijms15034795

Fu, P., Guo, X., Cheung, F. M. H., and Yung, K. K. L. (2019). The association between PM2.5 exposure and neurological disorders: a systematic review and meta-analysis. *Sci. Total Environ.* 655, 1240–1248. doi: 10.1016/j.scitotenv.2018.11.218

Fuentes-Mattei, E., Rivera, E., Gioda, A., Sanchez-Rivera, D., Roman-Velazquez, F. R., and Jimenez-Velez, B. D. (2010). Use of human bronchial epithelial cells (BEAS-2B) to study immunological markers resulting from exposure to PM(2.5) organic extract from Puerto Rico. *Toxicol. Appl. Pharmacol.* 243, 381–389. doi: 10.1016/j.taap.2009.12.009

Geraili, A., Jafari, P., Hassani, M. S., Araghi, B. H., Mohammadi, M. H., Ghafari, A. M., et al. (2018). Controlling differentiation of stem cells for developing personalized organ-on-chip platforms. *Adv. Healthc. Mater.* 7:1700426. doi: 10.1002/adhm.201700426

Gokaltun, A., Yarmush, M. L., Asatekin, A., and Usta, O. B. (2017). Recent advances in nonbiofouling PDMS surface modification strategies applicable to microfluidic technology. *Tech. Singap. World Sci.* 5, 1–12. doi: 10.1142/S2339547817300013

Guo, C., Zhang, Z., Lau, A. K. H., Lin, C. Q., Chuang, Y. C., Chan, J., et al. (2018). Effect of long-term exposure to fine particulate matter on lung function decline and risk of chronic obstructive pulmonary disease in Taiwan: a longitudinal, cohort study. *Lancet Planet. Health* 2, e114–e125. doi: 10.1016/S2542-5196(18)30028-7

Halldorsson, S., Lucumi, E., Gómez-Sjöberg, R., and Fleming, R. M. T. (2015). Advantages and challenges of microfluidic cell culture in polydimethylsiloxane devices. *Biosens. Bioelectro.* 63, 218–231. doi: 10.1016/j.bios.2014.07.029

Hamanaka, R. B., and Mutlu, G. M. (2018). Particulate matter air pollution: effects on the cardiovascular system. *Front. Endocrinol.* 9:680.

doi: 10.3389/fendo.2018.00680

He, F., Liao, B., Pu, J., Li, C., Zheng, M., Huang, L., et al. (2017). Exposure to ambient particulate matter induced COPD in a rat model and a description of the underlying mechanism. *Sci. Rep.* 7:45666. doi: 10.1038/srep45666

Henry, O. Y. F., Villenave, R., Cronce, M. J., Leineweber, W. D., Benz, M. A., and Ingber, D. E. (2017). Organs-on-chips with integrated electrodes for trans-epithelial electrical resistance (TEER) measurements of human epithelial barrier function. *Lab Chip.* 17, 2264–2271. doi: 10.1039/C7LC00155J

Herland, A., Maoz, B. M., Das, D., Somayaji, M. R., Prantil-Baun, R., Novak, R., et al. (2020). Quantitative prediction of human pharmacokinetic responses to drugs via fluidically coupled vascularized organ chips. *Nat. Biomed. Eng.* 4, 421–436. doi: 10.1038/s41551-019-0498-9

Hong, Z., Guo, Z., Zhang, R., Xu, J., Dong, W., Zhuang, G., et al. (2016). Airborne fine particulate matter induces oxidative stress and inflammation in human nasal epithelial cells. *Tohoku J. Exp. Med.* 239, 117–125. doi: 10.1620/tjem.239.117

Hopke, P. K., Croft, D., Zhang, W., Lin, S., Masiol, M., Squizzato, S., et al. (2019). Changes in the acute response of respiratory diseases to PM2.5 in New York State from 2005 to 2016. *Sci. Total Environ.* 677, 328–339. doi: 10.1016/j.scitotenv.2019.04.357

Huang, W., Wang, L., Li, J., Liu, M., Xu, H., Liu, S., et al. (2018). Short-term blood pressure responses to ambient fine particulate matter exposures at the extremes of global air pollution concentrations. *Am. J. Hypertens.* 31, 590–599. doi: 10.1093/ajh/hpx216

Huh, D., Hamilton, G. A., and Ingber, D. E. J. T. (2011). From 3D cell culture to organs-on-chips. *Trends Cell Biol.* 21, 745–754. doi: 10.1016/j.tcb.2011.09.005

Huh, D., Leslie, D. C., Matthews, B. D., Fraser, J. P., Jurek, S., Hamilton, G. A., et al. (2012). A human disease model of drug toxicity–induced pulmonary edema in a lung-on-a-chip microdevice. *Sci. Transl. Med.* 4:159ra147. doi: 10.1126/scitranslmed.3004249

Huh, D., Matthews, B. D., Mammoto, A., Montoya-Zavala, M., Hsin, H. Y., and Ingber, D. E. (2010). Reconstituting organ-level lung functions on a chip. *Science* 328, 1662–1668. doi: 10.1126/science.1188302

Humayun, M., Chow, C.-W., and Young, E. W. K. (2018). Microfluidic lung airway-on-a-chip with arrayable suspended gels for studying epithelial and smooth muscle cell interactions. *Lab Chip.* 18, 1298–1309. doi: 10.1039/C7LC01357D

Isoherranen, N., Madabushi, R., and Huang, S.-M. (2019). Emerging role of organ-on-a-chip technologies in quantitative clinical pharmacology evaluation. *Clin. Transl. Sci.* 12, 113–121. doi: 10.1111/cts.12627

Jain, A., Barrile, R., van der Meer, A., Mammoto, A., Mammoto, T., De Ceunynck, K., et al. (2018). Primary human lung alveolus-on-a-chip model of intravascular thrombosis for assessment of therapeutics. *Clin. Pharmacol. Ther.* 103, 332–340. doi: 10.1002/cpt.742

Jia, Y.-Y., Wang, Q., and Liu, T. (2017). Toxicity Research of PM(2.5) Compositions *in vitro*. *Int. J. Environ. Res. Public Health.* 14:232. doi: 10.3390/ijerph14030232

Jodat, Y. A., Kang, M. G., Kiaee, K., Kim, G. J., Martinez, A. F. H., Rosenkranz, A., et al. (2018). Human-derived organ-on-a-chip for personalized drug development. *Curr. Pharm. Des.* 24, 5471–5486. doi: 10.2174/138161282566619030815 0055

Khalid, M. A. U., Kim, Y. S., Ali, M., Lee, B. G., Cho, Y.-J., and Choi, K. H. (2020). A lung cancer-on-chip platform with integrated biosensors for physiological monitoring and toxicity assessment. *Biochem. Eng. J.* 15:107469. doi: 10.1016/j.bej.2019.107469

Khaniabadi, Y. O., Sicard, P., Takdastan, A., Hopke, P. K., Taiwo, A. M., Khaniabadi, F. O., et al. (2019). Mortality and morbidity due to ambient air pollution in Iran. *Clin. Epidemiol. Glob. Health* 7, 222–227. doi: 10.1016/j.cegh.2018.06.006

Kido, T., Tamagawa, E., Bai, N., Suda, K., Yang, H.-H. C., Li, Y., et al. (2011). Particulate matter induces translocation of IL-6 from the lung to the systemic circulation. *Am. J. Respir. Cell Mol. Biol.* 44, 197–204. doi: 10.1165/rcmb.2009-0427OC

Kim, D., Chen, Z., Zhou, L.-F., and Huang, S.-X. (2018). Air pollutants and early origins of respiratory diseases. *Chronic Dis. Transl. Med.* 4, 75–94. doi: 10.1016/j.cdtm.2018.03.003

Kim, K.-H., Kabir, E., and Kabir, S. (2015). A review on the human

health impact of airborne particulate matter. *Environ. Int.* 74, 136–143. doi: 10.1016/j.envint.2014.10.005

Lee, Y., Choi, J. W., Yu, J., Park, D., Ha, J., Son, K., et al. (2018). Microfluidics within a well: an injection-molded plastic array 3D culture platform. *Lab Chip.* 18, 2433–2440. doi: 10.1039/C8LC00336J

Li, G., Fang, C., Wang, S., and Sun, S. (2016). The effect of economic growth, urbanization, and industrialization on fine particulate matter (PM2.5) concentrations in China. *Environ. Sci. Technol.* 50, 11452–11459. doi: 10.1021/acs.est.6b02562

Li, R., Kou, X., Geng, H., Xie, J., Yang, Z., Zhang, Y., et al. (2015). Effect of ambient PM2.5 on lung mitochondrial damage and fusion/fission gene expression in rats. *Chem. Res. Toxicol.* 28, 408–418. doi: 10.1021/tx5003723

Li, T., Hu, R., Chen, Z., Li, Q., Huang, S., Zhu, Z., et al. (2018). Fine particulate matter [PM(2.5)]: the culprit for chronic lung diseases in China. *Chronic Dis. Transl. Med.* 4, 176–186. doi: 10.1016/j.cdtm.2018.07.002

Lin, Y., Zou, J., Yang, W., and Li, C.-Q. (2018). A review of recent advances in research on PM2.5 in China. *Int. J. Environ. Res. Public Health.* 15:438. doi: 10.3390/ijerph15030438

Liu, H., Bolonduro, O. A., Hu, N., Ju, J., Rao, A. A., Duffy, B. M., et al. (2020). Heart-on-a-chip model with integrated extra- and intracellular bioelectronics for monitoring cardiac electrophysiology under acute hypoxia. *Nano Lett.* 20, 2585–2593. doi: 10.1021/acs.nanolett.0c00076

Lodovici, M., and Bigagli, E. (2011). Oxidative stress and air pollution exposure. *J. Toxicol.* 2011:487074. doi: 10.1155/2011/487074

Löndahl, J., Pagels, J., Swietlicki, E., Zhou, J., Ketzel, M., Massling, A., et al. (2006). A set-up for field studies of respiratory tract deposition of fine and ultrafine particles in humans. *J. Aerosol Sci.* 37, 1152–1163. doi: 10.1016/j.jaerosci.2005.11.004

Low, L. A., and Tagle, D. A. (2017). Organs-on-chips: progress, challenges, and future directions. *Exp. Biol. Med. (Maywood)* 242, 1573–1578. doi: 10.1177/1535370217700523

Marsano, A., Conficconi, C., Lemme, M., Occhetta, P., Gaudiello, E., Votta, E., et al. (2016). Beating heart on a chip: a novel microfluidic platform to generate functional 3D cardiac microtissues. *Lab Chip.* 16, 599–610. doi: 10.1039/C5LC01356A

Maschmeyer, I., Lorenz, A. K., Schimek, K., Hasenberg, T., Ramme, A. P., Hübner, J., et al. (2015). A four-organ-chip for interconnected long-term co-culture of human intestine, liver, skin and kidney equivalents. *Lab Chip.* 15, 2688–2699. doi: 10.1039/C5LC00392J

Mastrangeli, M., Millet, S., and van den Eijnden-van Raaij, J. (2019). Organ-on-chip in development: towards a roadmap for organs-on-chip. *ALTEX* 36, 650–668. doi: 10.14573/altex.1908271

Miller, M. R., Raftis, J. B., Langrish, J. P., McLean, S. G., Samutrtai, P., Connell, S. P., et al. (2017). Inhaled nanoparticles accumulate at sites of vascular disease. *ACS Nano.* 11, 4542–4552. doi: 10.1021/acsnano.6b08551

Nadeau, K., McDonald-Hyman, C., Noth, E. M., Pratt, B., Hammond, S. K., Balmes, J., et al. (2010). Ambient air pollution impairs regulatory T-cell function in asthma. *J. Allergy Clin. Immunol.* 126, 845–852.e810. doi: 10.1016/j.jaci.2010.08.008

Nawroth, J. C., Barrile, R., Conegliano, D., van Riet, S., Hiemstra, P. S., and Villenave, R. (2019). Stem cell-based lung-on-chips: the best of both worlds? *Adv. Drug Deliv. Rev.* 140, 12–32. doi: 10.1016/j.addr.2018.07.005

Nemmar, A., Hoet, P. H. M., Dinsdale, D., Vermylen, J., Hoylaerts, M. F., and Nemery, B. (2003). Diesel exhaust particles in lung acutely enhance experimental peripheral thrombosis. *Circulation* 107, 1202–1208. doi: 10.1161/01.CIR.0000053568.13058.67

Nemmar, A., Hoet, P. H. M., Vanquickenborne, B., Dinsdale, D., Thomeer, M., Hoylaerts, M. F., et al. (2002). Passage of inhaled particles into the blood circulation in humans. *Circulation* 105, 411–414. doi: 10.1161/hc0402.104118

Nemmar, A., Holme, J. A., Rosas, I., Schwarze, P. E., and Alfaro-Moreno, E. (2013). Recent advances in particulate matter and nanoparticle toxicology: a review of the *in vivo* and *in vitro* studies. *BioMed. Res. Int.* 2013:279371. doi: 10.1155/2013/279371

Ngoc, L. T. N., Kim, M., Bui, V. K. H., Park, D., and Lee, Y.-C. (2018). Particulate matter exposure of passengers at bus stations: a review. *Int. J. Environ. Res. Public Health.* 15:E2886. doi: 10.3390/ijerph15122886

Nguyen, T., Jung, S. H., Lee, M. S., Park, T.-E., Ahn, S. K., and Kang, J. H. (2019). Robust chemical bonding of PMMA microfluidic devices to porous PETE membranes for reliable cytotoxicity testing of drugs. *Lab Chip.* 19, 3706–3713. doi: 10.1039/C9LC00338J

Novak, R., Ingram, M., Marquez, S., Das, D., Delahanty, A., Herland, A., et al. (2020). Robotic fluidic coupling and interrogation of multiple vascularized organ chips. *Nat. Biomed. Eng.* 4, 407–420.

Oleaga, C., Bernabini, C., Smith, A. S. T., Srinivasan, B., Jackson, M., McLamb, W., et al. (2016). Multi-organ toxicity demonstration in a functional human *in vitro* system composed of four organs. *Sci. Rep.* 6:20030. doi: 10.1038/srep20030

Oleaga, C., Riu, A., Rothemund, S., Lavado, A., McAleer, C. W., Long, C. J., et al. (2018). Investigation of the effect of hepatic metabolism on off-target cardiotoxicity in a multi-organ human-on-a-chip system. *Biomaterials* 182, 176–190. doi: 10.1016/j.biomaterials.2018.07.062

Ongaro, A. E., Giuseppe, D. D., Kermanizadeh, A., Crespo, A. M., Mencatti, A., Ghibelli, L., et al. (2020). Polylactic is a sustainable, low absorption, low autofluorescence alternative to other plastics for microfluidic and organ-on-chip applications. *Anal. Chem.* 92, 6693–6701. doi: 10.1021/acs.analchem.0c00651

Øvrevik, J., Refsnes, M., Låg, M., and Holme, J. A., Schwarze, P.E. (2015). Activation of proinflammatory responses in cells of the airway mucosa by particulate matter: oxidant- and non-oxidant-mediated triggering mechanisms. *Biomolecules* 5, 1399–1440. doi: 10.3390/biom5031399

Park, M., Joo, H. S., Lee, K., Jang, M., Kim, S. D., Kim, I., et al. (2018). Differential toxicities of fine particulate matters from various sources. *Sci. Rep.* 8:17007. doi: 10.1038/s41598-018-35398-0

Peixoto, M. S., de Oliveira Galvão, M. F., and de Batistuzzo Medeiros, S. R. (2017). Cell death pathways of particulate matter toxicity. *Chemosphere* 188, 32–48. doi: 10.1016/j.chemosphere.2017.08.076

Raabe, O. G. (1976). Aerosol aerodynamic size conventions for inertial sampler calibration. *J. Air Pollut. Control Assoc.* 26, 856–860. doi: 10.1080/00022470.1976.10470329

Raaschou-Nielsen, O., Beelen, R., Wang, M., Hoek, G., Andersen, Z. J., Hoffmann, B., et al. (2016). Particulate matter air pollution components and risk for lung cancer. *Environ. Int.* 87, 66–73. doi: 10.1016/j.envint.2015.11.007

Ronaldson-Bouchard, K., and Vunjak-Novakovic, G. (2018). Organs-on-a-chip: a fast track for engineered human tissues in drug development. *Cell Stem Cell.* 22, 310–324. doi: 10.1016/j.stem.2018.02.011

Rothbauer, M., Zirath, H., and Ertl, P. (2018). Recent advances in microfluidic technologies for cell-to-cell interaction studies. *Lab Chip.* 18, 249–270. doi: 10.1039/C7LC00815E

Ryu, Y. S., Kang, K. A., Piao, M. J., Ahn, M. J., Yi, J. M., Hyun, Y.-M., et al. (2019). Particulate matter induces inflammatory cytokine production via activation of NFκB by TLR5-NOX4-ROS signaling in human skin keratinocyte and mouse skin. *Redox Biol.* 21:101080. doi: 10.1016/j.redox.2018.101080

Shadie, A. M., Herbert, C., and Kumar, R. K. (2014). Ambient particulate matter induces an exacerbation of airway inflammation in experimental asthma: role of interleukin-33. *Clin. Exp. Immunol.* 177, 491–499. doi: 10.1111/cei.12348

Shiraishi, K., Nakajima, T., Shichino, S., Deshimaru, S., Matsushima, K., and Ueha, S. (2019). *In vitro* expansion of endogenous human alveolar epithelial type II cells in fibroblast-free spheroid culture. *Biochem. Biophys. Res. Commun.* 515, 579–585. doi: 10.1016/j.bbrc.2019.05.187

Sidorov, V. Y., Samson, P. C., Sidorova, T. N., Davidson, J. M., Lim, C. C., and Wikswo, J. P. (2017). I-wire heart-on-a-chip i: three-dimensional cardiac tissue constructs for physiology and pharmacology. *Acta Biomater.* 48, 68–78. doi: 10.1016/j.actbio.2016.11.009

Sin, A., Chin, K. C., Jamil, M. F., Kostov, Y., Rao, G., and Shuler, M. L. (2004). The design and fabrication of three-chamber microscale cell culture analog devices with integrated dissolved oxygen sensors. *Nat. Rev. Mol. Cell Biol.* 20, 338–345. doi: 10.1021/bp034077d

Skardal, A., Murphy, S. V., Devarasetty, M., Mead, I., Kang, H.-W., Seol, Y.-J., et al. (2017). Multi-tissue interactions in an integrated three-tissue organ-on-a-chip platform. *Sci. Rep.* 7:8837. doi: 10.1038/s41598-017-08879-x

Snow, S. J., Henriquez, A. R., Costa, D. L., and Kodavanti, U. P. (2018). Neuroendocrine regulation of air pollution health effects: emerging insights. *Toxicol. Sci.* 164, 9–20. doi: 10.1093/toxsci/kfy129

Stucki, J. D., Hobi, N., Galimov, A., Stucki, A. O., Schneider-Daum, N., Lehr, C.-M., et al. (2018). Medium throughput breathing human primary cell alveolus-on-chip model. *Sci. Rep.* 8:14359. doi: 10.1038/s41598-018-32523-x

Sung, J. H., Wang, Y. I., Narasimhan Sriram, N., Jackson, M., Long, C., Hickman,

J. J., et al. (2019). Recent advances in body-on-a-chip systems. *Anal. Chem.* 91, 330–351. doi: 10.1021/acs.analchem.8b05293

Suwa, T., Hogg, J. C., Quinlan, K. B., Ohgami, A., Vincent, R., and van Eeden, S. F. (2002). Particulate air pollution induces progression of atherosclerosis. *J. Am. Coll. Cardiol.* 39, 935–942. doi: 10.1016/S0735-1097(02)01715-1

Tsai, D.-H., Amyai, N., Marques-Vidal, P., Wang, J.-L., Riediker, M., Mooser, V., et al. (2012). Effects of particulate matter on inflammatory markers in the general adult population. *Part. Fibre Toxicol.* 9:24. doi: 10.1186/1743-8977-9-24

Tsuda, A., Henry, F. S., and Butler, J. P. (2013). Particle transport and deposition: basic physics of particle kinetics. *Compr. Physiol.* 3, 1437–1471. doi: 10.1002/cphy.c100085

Turner, M. C., Krewski, D., C., Arden Pope, I., Chen, Y., Gapstur, S. M., et al. (2011). Long-term ambient fine particulate matter air pollution and lung cancer in a large cohort of never-smokers. *Am. J. Respir. Crit. Care Med.* 184, 1374–1381. doi: 10.1164/rccm.201106-1011OC

Valavanidis, A., Fiotakis, K., Bakeas, E., and Vlahogianni, T. (2005). Electron paramagnetic resonance study of the generation of reactive oxygen species catalysed by transition metals and quinoid redox cycling by inhalable ambient particulate matter. *Redox Rep.* 10, 37–51. doi: 10.1179/135100005X21606

van den Berg, A., Mummery, C. L., Passier, R., and van der Meer, A. D. (2019). Personalised organs-on-chips: functional testing for precision medicine. *Lab Chip.* 19, 198–205. doi: 10.1039/C8LC00827B

Vanderburgh, J., Sterling, J. A., and Guelcher, S. A. (2017). 3D printing of tissue engineered constructs for *in vitro* modeling of disease progression and drug screening. *Ann. Biomed. Eng.* 45, 164–179. doi: 10.1007/s10439-016-1640-4

Vawda, S., Mansour, R., Takeda, A., Funnell, P., Kerry, S., Mudway, I., et al. (2013). Associations between inflammatory and immune response genes and adverse respiratory outcomes following exposure to outdoor air pollution: a HuGE systematic review. *Am. J. Epidemiol.* 179, 432–442. doi: 10.1093/aje/kwt269

Wang, G., McCain, M. L., Yang, L., He, A., Pasqualini, F. S., Agarwal, A., et al. (2014). Modeling the mitochondrial cardiomyopathy of Barth syndrome with induced pluripotent stem cell and heart-on-chip technologies. *Nat. Med.* 20, 616–623. doi: 10.1038/nm.3545

Wang, H., Song, L., Ju, W., Wang, X., Dong, L., Zhang, Y., et al. (2017). The acute airway inflammation induced by PM2.5 exposure and the treatment of essential oils in Balb/c mice. *Sci. Rep.* 7:44256. doi: 10.1038/srep44256

Wang, J., Huang, J., Wang, L., Chen, C., Yang, D., Jin, M., et al. (2017). Urban particulate matter triggers lung inflammation via the ROS-MAPK-NF-κB signaling pathway. *J. Thorac. Dis.* 9, 4398–4412. doi: 10.21037/jtd.2017.09.135

Weiner, A. I., Jackson, S. R., Zhao, G., Quansah, K. K., Farshchian, J. N., Neupauer, K. M., et al. (2019). Mesenchyme-free expansion and transplantation of adult alveolar progenitor cells: steps toward cell-based regenerative therapies. *NPJ Regen. Med.* 4:17. doi: 10.1038/s41536-019-0080-9

Wong, I., and Ho, C.-M. (2009). Surface molecular property modifications for poly(dimethylsiloxane) (PDMS) based microfluidic devices. *Microfluid. Nanofluidics.* 7, 291–306. doi: 10.1007/s10404-009-0443-4

Wu, Q., Liu, J., Wang, X., Feng, L., Wu, J., Zhu, X., et al. (2020). Organ-on-a-chip: recent breakthroughs and future prospects. *Biomed. Eng. Online* 19:9. doi: 10.1186/s12938-020-0752-0

Xiao, Y., Zhang, B., Liu, H., Miklas, J. W., Gagliardi, M., Pahnke, A., et al. (2014). Microfabricated perfusable cardiac biowire: a platform that mimics native cardiac bundle. *Lab Chip.* 14, 869–882. doi: 10.1039/C3LC51123E

Xing, Y. F., Xu, Y. H., Shi, M. H., and Lian, Y. X. (2016). The impact of PM2.5 on the human respiratory system. *J. Thorac. Dis.* 8, E69–E74. doi: 10.3978/j.issn.2072-1439.2016.01.19

Xu, X., Jiang, S. Y., Wang, T.-Y., Bai, Y., Zhong, M., Wang, A., et al. (2013). Inflammatory response to fine particulate air pollution exposure: neutrophil versus monocyte. *PLoS ONE* 8:e71414. doi: 10.1371/journal.pone.0071414

Yang, Y., Qin, Z., Zeng, W., Yang, T., Cao, Y., Mei, C., et al. (2017). Toxicity assessment of nanoparticles in various systems and organs. *Nanotechnol. Rev.* 6:279. doi: 10.1515/ntrev-2016-0047

Yuancheng, L., Kai, Z., Xiao, L., and Yu Shrike, Z. (2018). Blood-vessel-on-a-chip platforms for evaluating nanoparticle drug delivery systems. *Curr. Drug Metab.* 19, 100–109. doi: 10.2174/1389200218666170925114636

Zanobetti, A., Franklin, M., Koutrakis, P., and Schwartz, J. (2009). Fine particulate air pollution and its components in association with cause-specific emergency admissions. *Environ. Health* 8:58. doi: 10.1186/1476-069X-8-58

Zhang, B., Korolj, A., Lai, B. F. L., and Radisic, M. (2018). Advances in organ-on-a-chip engineering. *Nat. Rev. Mater.* 3, 257–278. doi: 10.1038/s41578-018-0034-7

Zhang, Y. S., Zhang, Y.-N., and Zhang, W. (2017). Cancer-on-a-chip systems at the frontier of nanomedicine. *Drug Discov. Today* 22, 1392–1399. doi: 10.1016/j.drudis.2017.03.011

Zhao, Y., Kankala, R. K., Wang, S.-B., and Chen, A.-Z. (2019). Multi-organs-on-chips: towards long-term biomedical investigations. *Molecules* 24:675. doi: 10.3390/molecules24040675

18

Glycated Albumin Triggers an Inflammatory Response in the Human Airway Epithelium and Causes an Increase in Ciliary Beat Frequency

Moira L. Aitken[1]*, Ranjani Somayaji[1], Thomas R. Hinds[2], Maricela Pier[1], Karla Droguett[3], Mariana Rios[3], Shawn J. Skerrett[1,3] and Manuel Villalon[3]

[1] Department of Medicine, School of Medicine, University of Washington, Seattle, WA, United States, [2] Department of Pharmacy, School of Medicine, University of Washington, Seattle, WA, United States, [3] Department of Physiology, Faculty of Biological Sciences, Pontificia Universidad Católica de Chile, Santiago, Chile

*Correspondence:
Moira L. Aitken
moira@uw.edu

The role of inflammation in airway epithelial cells and its regulation are important in several respiratory diseases. When disease is present, the barrier between the pulmonary circulation and the airway epithelium is damaged, allowing serum proteins to enter the airways. We identified that human glycated albumin (GA) is a molecule in human serum that triggers an inflammatory response in human airway epithelial cultures. We observed that single-donor human serum induced IL-8 secretion from primary human airway epithelial cells and from a cystic fibrosis airway cell line (CF1-16) in a dose-dependent manner. IL-8 secretion from airway epithelial cells was time dependent and rapidly increased in the first 4 h of incubation. Stimulation with GA promoted epithelial cells to secrete IL-8, and this increase was blocked by the anti-GA antibody. The IL-8 secretion induced by serum GA was 10–50-fold more potent than TNF$_\alpha$ or LPS stimulation. GA also has a functional effect on airway epithelial cells in vitro, increasing ciliary beat frequency. Our results demonstrate that the serum molecule GA is pro-inflammatory and triggers host defense responses including increases in IL-8 secretion and ciliary beat frequency in the human airway epithelium. Although the binding site of GA has not yet been described, it is possible that GA could bind to the receptor for advanced glycated end products (RAGE), known to be expressed in the airway epithelium; however, further experiments are needed to identify the mechanism involved. We highlight a possible role for GA in airway inflammation.

Keywords: airways, airway disease, glycated albumin, inflammation, cytokine, human, ciliary beat frequency

Abbreviations: BAL, Bronchial alveolar lavage; COPD, Chronic obstructive pulmonary disease; CBF, Ciliary beat frequency; CF, Cystic fibrosis; GA, Glycated albumin; HBSS, Hank's balanced salt solution; HRP, Horseradish peroxidase; IL-8, Interleukin 8; IEF, Isoelectric focusing; KSFM, Keratinocyte serum-free medium; PMNs, Polymorphonuclear granulocytes; PVDF, Polyvinylidene difluoride; SEM, Standard error of the mean; TCA, Trichloroacetic acid; UP, Unknown protein.

INTRODUCTION

Airway epithelial cells participate in host defense by generating a wide variety of cytokines and chemokines that initiate or amplify acute and chronic inflammation by mediating the recruitment, activation, and survival of inflammatory cells within the airway (Standiford et al., 1990; Marini et al., 1992; Levine, 1995). Interleukin 8 (IL-8) is a pro-inflammatory molecule that is found in high concentration in the bronchial alveolar lavage (BAL) of patients with airway inflammatory diseases like cystic fibrosis (CF) (Konstan et al., 1994; O'Sullivan and Fredman, 2009), asthma (Lamblin et al., 1998), and chronic obstructive pulmonary disease (COPD) (Keatings et al., 1996; Hollander et al., 2007) and in the nasal mucosa of patients with allergic rhinitis (Cui et al., 2015). Respiratory epithelial cells (or cell lines) produce IL-8 in response to stimulation with IL-1α or TNFα or with other stimuli including neutrophil elastase, viruses, bacteria, and bacterial products (Standiford et al., 1990; Nakamura et al., 1992; Kwon et al., 1994; Levine, 1995). IL-8 is thought to play a major regulatory role in the airways as a potent chemo-attractant of polymorphonuclear granulocytes (PMNs) (Nakamura et al., 1991).

In airway diseases such as CF, asthma, and respiratory infections including viral infections notably SARS-CoV-2, the epithelial barrier is injured causing increased permeability and markedly greater plasma and serum protein movement across this barrier (McElvaney et al., 1992), a possible mechanism leading to a worse outcome in COVID-19 patients. Macromolecules of very different size and charge (i.e., 60-kDa albumin and the 700-kDa α_2-macroglobulin) have been demonstrated to move equally across all barriers that exist between the venular compartment and the mucosal surface of airways (Svenson et al., 1995). The airway epithelium also participates in host defense through mucociliary clearance (MCC) which is designed to remove bacteria and contaminant particles from entering the lung parenchyma (Knowles and Boucher, 2002). MCC is determined by the frequency of ciliated cells and the rheological properties of the mucus released by secretory cells (van der Baan, 2000). The efficiency of MCC is affected by airway inflammation, which in turn induces the release of local pro-inflammatory molecules resulting in mucus hypersecretion or ciliary dysfunction (Seybold et al., 1990; Cowley et al., 1997; Waugh and Wilson, 2008; Schmid et al., 2010; Koblizek et al., 2011).

Limited understanding exists regarding the precise roles of serum molecules in the inflammatory response of the airway epithelium affecting MCC. We conducted the study herein to identify the protein in serum leading to this pro-inflammatory effect. We hypothesized that this protein induces increased airway inflammation and will cause functional effects such as on ciliary function, which plays an important role in chronic airway diseases.

MATERIALS AND METHODS

Human Airway Epithelial Cells

We obtained nasal mucosa samples of 22 non-CF patients (mean age 47 years, range: 19–71 years); bronchial mucosa sample from one CF patient (33 years, cystic fibrosis genotype F508del homozygous); and adenoid tissue from non-CF patients (mean age 7 years, range: 3–12 years) who had undergone surgery for adenoid hypertrophy.

We also used an immortalized cell line from CF nasal polyp airway epithelial cells (CF 1-16 cells) with a homozygous F508del genotype, a gift from Dr. Christine Halbert, Fred Hutchinson Cancer Research Center, Seattle, WA, United States (Halbert et al., 1996). Tissue acquisition was approved by the ethic committee of the Pontificia Universidad Católica de Chile and the Human Subjects Review Committee of the University of Washington.

Nasal and Bronchial Mucosa Samples

Nasal epithelial cells were isolated from the mucosa by methodologies previously described (Standiford et al., 1990; Nakamura et al., 1991; McElvaney et al., 1992; Levine, 1995). Primary cultures from adenoid explant epithelial cells were prepared in Rose chambers as previously described (Gonzalez et al., 2013).

Human epithelial cells were isolated from the mucosa by methodologies previously described (Nakamura et al., 1991; McElvaney et al., 1992; Aitken et al., 1993, 1995; Levine, 1995; Gras et al., 2010; Gonzalez et al., 2013). Briefly, cells were rinsed and plated onto Vitrogen (Collagen Biomedical, Palo Alto, CA, United States)-coated 12-well plates (Costar, Cambridge, MA, United States) and cultured in 3.0 mL keratinocyte serum-free medium (KSFM) (Gibco BRL, Grand Island, NY, United States) with 5% fetal calf serum (FCS) (HyClone, Logan, UT, United States). After 12–24 h, the medium was changed to KSFM with 5 ng/mL epidermal growth factor (Gibco BRL, Grand Island, NY, United States) and 50 μg/mL bovine pituitary extract (Gibco BRL) until confluent (4–14 days). Experiments were performed on confluent cells. The monolayers were rinsed three times with either Hank's balanced salt solution (HBSS) (H9269, Sigma, St Louis, MO, United States) or KSFM and incubated with KSFM under various experimental conditions.

Adenoid Tissue

Primary cultures were prepared to obtain explants of epithelial cells in Rose chambers as previously described (Gonzalez et al., 2013). Briefly, small pieces of adenoid tissue (2–4 mm) were washed with HBSS and rinsed in NHS media (137 mM NaCl, 5.09 mM KCl, 1.14 mM Na_2HPO_4, × 2 H_2O, 0.18 mM KH_2PO_4, 0.923 mM $MgCl_2$ × 6H_2O, 0.91 mM $CaCl_2$ × 2H_2O, 4.07 mM $NaHCO_3$, 21.5 mM glucose, pH 7.4) supplemented with 1% vitamins, 1% essential amino acids, 1% non-essential amino acids, and 1% pyruvate and antibiotics (neomycin 0.2 mg/mL and penicillin 0.12 mg/mL) (all these reagents: Invitrogen Corp, NY, United States). Small pieces of epithelium were placed on a cover glass pretreated with 0.1% gelatin (G9391, VWR Scientific, Radnor, PA, United States) and then placed in Rose chambers. Explants were covered with a sterile dialysis membrane pretreated with the NHS culture medium. The Rose chambers were filled with 2 mL of NHS medium, which contain 10% of horse inactivated serum (Biological Industries, Israel) (pH 7.2–7.4), and the explants were incubated at 37°C. The culture media within the Rose chambers were renewed every 48 h.

After approximately 7 days, patches of epithelial cells with synchronized activity were obtained.

Stimulation of Human Airway Epithelial Cells

Nasal human epithelial cell cultures were incubated in KSFM supplemented with commercial pooled serum (AB-Human Serum from Life Technologies, Biocompare, South San Francisco, CA, United States), single-donor serum, or plasma-derived serum, at concentrations ranging from 0.1 to 50%. In the stimulation experiments, after specified time intervals, supernatants were harvested and stored at −70°C. In some experiments, cells were incubated with single-donor serum in the presence of a neutralizing human monoclonal antibody against GA (A717, Exocell, Inc., Philadelphia, PA, United States. RRID:AB_2225805) at a concentration of 10 pg/mL.

The different serums were prepared as follows: single-donor serum was prepared from blood from a healthy subject. Blood was allowed to clot at room temperature, spun at 1,000 × g for 15 min, and subsequently the serum fraction was stored at −70°C. For plasma-derived serum, whole blood (50 mL) from a single donor was collected into a chilled syringe (4°C) containing 5 mL of 3.8% sodium citrate. The citrated blood was then centrifuged at 30,000 × g for 20 min at 4°C. The plasma was removed and mixed with 1.0 M CaCl$_2$ (1:50) and then incubated at 37°C for 2 h and centrifuged at 25,000 × g for 20 min at room temperature. Serum was collected and stored at −70°C.

IL-8 ELISA in the Monolayer Cells

Measurement of IL-8 was performed using "sandwich" enzyme-linked immunosorbent assay (ELISA). A 96-well plate was coated overnight with 100 μL of monoclonal antibody against human IL-8 (I2519, Sigma, RRID:AB_260157) at a concentration of 0.5 μg/mL, rinsed with PBS-Tween 20, and blocked with 2% BSA. The samples were then diluted, run in triplicate, and allowed to incubate at room temperature for 2 h. The plates were washed three times with PBS-Tween 20. A polyclonal antibody conjugated to horseradish peroxidase (HRP) was added to the plate, incubated, and washed. The chromogenic substrate 3,3′,5,5′-tetramethylbenzidine was added, and the absorbance was read at 450 nm. Unknowns were compared to serial dilution standards (0–2,000 pg/mL). IL-8 measurements are expressed in ng/mL considering 1×10^6 cells per culture well.

IL-8 ELISA in Rose Chamber Adenoid Cells

IL-8 production was measured from supernatants which were stored at −20°C until used. We used ELISA KIT Quantikine® (minimum detectable dose: 3.5 pg/mL, D8000C, R&D Systems, Minneapolis, MN, United States). IL-8 measurements are expressed in ng/mL/mg of total protein with approximately 3×10^6 cells per culture/mL.

Identification of the Serum Factor (Glycated Albumin) That Increased IL-8 Secretion

Chromatography of Human Serum on DEAE Cellulose, pH 7: Ion exchange chromatography of human serum was performed on a 12-mL DEAE cellulose column (Whatman Specialty Products, Fairfield, NJ, United States) equilibrated in 50 mM NaCl, 10 mM phosphate, pH 7.5. Three milliliter of human serum dialyzed in equilibration buffer was added to the column, washed with seven column volumes of buffer, and collected in four equal fractions (zero absorbance in fourth fraction). A linear 50-mL salt gradient of 50–1,000 mM NaCl (in 10 mM phosphate, pH 7.5) was used to elute proteins from the column, and 0.6-mL fractions were collected. The salt concentration was monitored with an osmometer. The protein concentration was measured at 280 nm with a Beckman DU/64 spectrophotometer with a micro cuvette. Between 85 and 90 percent of the IL-8 secretory activity of primary non-CF nasal epithelial cells was found in the pre-gradient wash buffer fractions; these fractions were pooled and concentrated.

Protein G Column

Immunoglobulins were removed from the pooled active fractions with a protein G Sepharose column (P3296, Sigma). A 5.0-mL column was washed in buffer containing 137 mM NaCl, 10 mM phosphate, pH 6.5. Serum or DEAE flow-through was dialyzed against the column buffer and applied to the column. The flow-through was collected along with 10 column volumes of wash buffer. Bound IgG was eluted with 100 mM of glycine, pH 2.5, and immediately neutralized with 0.5 N NaOH to pH 6.5. The flow-through and the eluted immunoglobulins were concentrated to their original volume with Millipore Ultrafree-15 centrifugal filters and dialyzed against 137 mM NaCl, 10 mM phosphate buffer, pH 7.5 (PBS). The majority of the IL-8 secretory activity of primary non-CF nasal epithelial cells was found in the flow-through and wash buffer fraction. No IL-8 secretion was found associated with the eluted immunoglobulin.

Gel Filtration

The molecular size of the active protein from the previous steps was determined with a 12-mL S-200 Sephacryl gel column (GE17-0584-10, Sigma). The column was run with PBS. Two hundred microliters of concentrated protein was layered onto the gel, and 150-μL fractions were collected. The protein concentration was measured at 280 nm with a Beckman DU/64 spectrophotometer with a micro cuvette.

Sequencing of IL-8-Stimulating Protein

The identity of the unknown protein (UP) was determined by sequencing. The most active protein fraction in stimulating IL-8 secretion (fraction 38, **Figure 1B**) was electrophoresed on a native 7.5% acrylamide gel. Following electrophoresis, the gel was equilibrated for 5 min in a blotting buffer consisting of 100 mL of 10 mM CAPS buffer and 10% methanol, pH 11.0. The gel and a polyvinylidene difluoride (PVDF) membrane (Millipore, Bedford, MA, United States) were sandwiched and blotted for

45 min at 4°C. The membrane was washed and stained with Coomassie Blue R-250 for 5 min. Then, the membrane was destained in 50% methanol until the bands were clearly visible. The blotted membrane was rinsed in water and stored wet in a saran wrap at –20°C. The protein band of interest was sequenced from a trypsin digest of protein excised out of the PVDF and chromatographed by HPLC on a C18 column. Three peptides were separated out and sequenced using mass spectroscopy. The sequences obtained were used in a BLAST (RRID:SCR_004870)[1] search of human proteins as a means to identify the protein.

IEF (Isoelectric Focusing) Gel Electrophoresis

To further compare the UP with commercial human albumin (A1887, Sigma) and commercial glycated human albumin (A8301, Sigma), the iso-electro point of the three proteins was determined (**Figure 1C**). Equal amounts (6.9 μg) of the three proteins were run along with standards on a precast Bio-Rad IEF gel pH 3–10 (Bio-Rad, Hercules, CA, United States). The IEF standards were soybean trypsin inhibitor, 4.6 pI (10109886001, Sigma), and bovine milk β-lactoglobulin A, 5.1 pI (L3908, Sigma). The protein bands of interest were flanked on both sides by the standards in the gel. The gel was run for 3 h at various voltages; 1 h at 100 V, 1 h at 250 V, and 30 min at 500 V. The gel was fixed in 10% trichloroacetic acid (TCA) for 10 min. Excess ampholytes were removed by an additional overnight 1% TCA soak. To detect the protein bands, the gel was washed in water three times and stained with GELCODE Blue Stain Reagent (Pierce, Rockville, IL, United States).

Western Blot With the Anti-GA Antibody

Human albumin (HA, A3782, Sigma), GA, and the UP were electrophoresed on a 4–20% native gradient gel (**Figure 1D**). Each lane contained 20 μg of protein. After electrophoresis, the proteins were transferred onto polyvinylidene difluoride (PVDF) membranes (Millipore, Bedford, MA, United States) and blocked with 2% gelatin in PBS pH 7.4 overnight. The blot was probed with a human monoclonal antibody against GA (A717, Exocell, Inc., Philadelphia, PA, United States. RRID: AB 2225805) diluted 1:500. It was then incubated with a secondary polyclonal antibody rabbit anti-mouse conjugated to HRP diluted 1:2,000 and visualized with ECL substrate (Amersham Biosciences Corp, Piscataway, NY, United States).

Stimulation of CF1-16 Cells With GA, TNFα, and LPS

The levels of production measured through ligand stimulation with GA, TNFα, and LPS on epithelial cells were determined. CF1-16 cells were cultured with increasing concentrations of TNFα (0.2–20 ng/mL, T6674, Sigma), LPS (1–1,000 ng/mL, L3137 Sigma), and GA (0.2 μg/mL–2.0 mg/mL, A8301, Sigma). After a 5 h incubation at 5% CO_2, 37°C, the supernatants were harvested and stored at –70°C until analyzed for IL-8 secretion by ELISA. Samples were run in triplicate and compared to a standard

curve in the same methods described above. To calculate the EC50 and the extrapolated value for Vmax (maximum response), we used a standard model for fitting the data (non-cooperative activity). GraphPad Prism (RRID:SCR_002798)[2].

Ciliary Beat Frequency (CBF) Measurements

CBF was measured by microphotodensitometry as previously described (Hermoso et al., 2001; Barrera et al., 2004). Light fluctuations produced by the ciliary beat were sensed by a photodiode (FDS015, Thorlabs Inc., Newton, NJ, United States) placed on a phase microscope (Nikon 300 Diaphot Inverted Microscope). Signal was processed and displayed by a spectral analyzer (SAI-51C Honeywell, Charlotte, North Caroline, United States). Human adenoid epithelial cells in Rose chambers with spontaneous ciliary activity were washed with HBSS. Cultures were left with 2 mL of HBSS as supernatants. CBF was tested in monolayers of human epithelial cells in Rose Chambers. CBF was measured from 2 to 3 cells in each culture, and a CBF baseline was established for 30 min prior to adding a substrate. CBF was then measured every 15 min for up to 4 h. From each adenoid sample, we obtained around five cultures, each one with four or five explants surrounded by a monolayer of ciliated cells. In this study, we used 34 cultures of ciliated cells, obtained from seven patients. Each time course on CBF effect or Il-8 measurements was performed in 4–5 cultures.

Statistical Analysis

Data were expressed as means ± standard error of the mean (SEM). Correlations between groups were calculated using the Spearman's rank test. We used Student t-tests for mean comparisons between experimental groups, and linear regression was conducted to compare trends over time between groups. Dose–response curves on Il-8 secretion for GA, TNFα, and LPS were analyzed by one-way ANOVA followed by Holm–Sidak's multiple-comparison test, using a square-root transformation of the original data. Graphics were performed using GraphPad Prism (see text footnote 2, RRID:SCR_002798). CBF data were analyzed following arcsin transformation. A $p < 0.05$ was considered statistically significant.

RESULTS

Identification of the Serum Component Responsible for Stimulation of IL-8 Secretion

Serum from four healthy donors and commercial pooled AB serum all stimulated IL-8 secretion from primary airway epithelial cells at a range of 0.4–1.3 ng/mL/10^5 cells.

We did not use pooled samples; rather, the individual whose serum had caused consistently the higher IL-8 response (1.7 ng/mL/10^5 cells). Human nasal epithelial cells were incubated for 6 h at concentrations from 0.1 to 50% of the volume, and the level

---

[1] http://blast.ncbi.nlm.nih.gov/Blast.cgi

[2] http://www.graphpad.com/

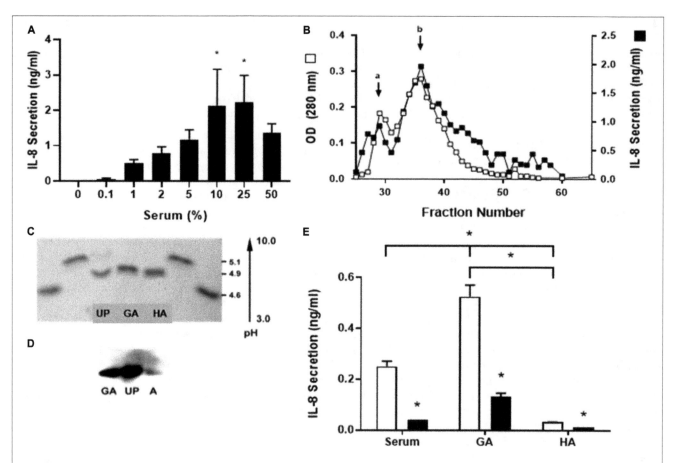

FIGURE 1 | Identification of the serum component responsible for stimulation of IL-8 secretion. Human single-dose serum induced IL-8 secretion in a dose-dependent manner. **(A)** Nasal epithelial cells were incubated for 5 h with a different percentage of human single-dose serum, and IL-8 secretion was measured. Serum induced a dose-dependent IL-8 secretion with a maximum at 25%. * Indicates a statistically significant increase ($p < 0.05$) in IL-8 compared to control. **(B)** Different serum fractions obtained from an S-200 Sephacryl gel column were assayed for IL-8 secretion, and the optical densities at 280 nm were compared. Two peaks were obtained (a and b); the major peak (b) seems to be a dimmer of the active protein. These peptides from a trypsin digest of the peak protein were analyzed by MS and used in a BLAST search of human proteins to identify the unknown protein (UP). **(C)** UP was isoelectric focused with glycated albumin (GA) and human albumin (HA) to determine their isoelectric point (pI). Two standards used soybean trypsin inhibitor (4.6 pI) and bovine β-lactoglobulin A (5.1 pI) loaded at both sides from the bands of interest. UP has the same pI as GA and HA. **(D)** A Western blot with anti-glycated albumin antibody was carried out. GA, UP, and HA were recognized with the same molecular weight. **(E)** IL-8 secretion induced by serum and glycated albumin (GA) in CF1-16 cells was reduced with an anti-human GA antibody. The CF epithelial cell line was incubated for 5 h with commercial pooled human serum (serum), GA (2 mg/mL), or albumin (HA, 2 mg/mL) and an anti-human GA antibody (black bar). Open bars have no antibody. Serum and GA increased IL-8 secretion, which was blocked when cells were coincubated with the GA antibody. * Indicates a statistically significant ($p < 0.05$) reduction in IL-8 secretion in the presence of the antibody in all groups (open vs. black bar) or higher IL-8 secretion in cell cultures incubated with GA compared to serum or HA and serum compared to HA. $n = 3$ for experiments included in **(A,E)**. Experiments for **(B–D)** were repeated three times.

of IL-8 secretion was measured. Serum induced a dose-dependent IL-8 secretion with a maximum of 25% (**Figure 1A**).

To identify the serum component responsible for stimulating IL-8 secretion, an ion exchange chromatography of human serum was performed to identify the unknown protein (UP) (**Figure 1B**). When fractionated, two distinct peaks were identified: a major peak with a molecular weight of about 65 kDa (non-glycated albumin) and a minor peak at approximately 130 kDa (glycated albumin). In subsequent purifications, we noticed that the minor peak quantity was variable. It was postulated that the IL-8 released was associated with both peaks and that the minor peak could be a dimer or aggregate of the active UP. The most active fraction (fraction 38) was sent for sequencing, and the resultant sequence was used in a BLAST search against human

proteins as a mean to identify the UP. The BLAST result indicated with a high probability that the UP was human serum albumin which has a molecular weight of ~69 kDa which was similar to the UP weight (**Figure 1C**).

UP was isoelectric focused with glycated albumin (GA) and human albumin (HA) to determine their isoelectric point (pI). Two standards, soybean trypsin inhibitor (4.6 pI) and bovine β-lactoglobulin A (5.1 pI), were loaded at both sides from the bands of interest. UP have the same pI as GA and HA (**Figure 1D**).

A Western blot with equal amounts of anti-glycated albumin antibody was carried out. The results demonstrated that the UP and GA had a strong signal while HA had a very small response as expected, as the monoclonal antibody used targeted GA and thus may not react with non-glycated albumin. Further, all three proteins had equivalent electrophoretic mobility on the 7.7% SDS PAGE gel with a molecular weight of about 67 kDa (**Figure 1E**).

IL-8 secretion induced by serum and glycated albumin (GA) in CF1-16 cells was reduced significantly with an anti-human GA antibody ($p = 0.01$). CF1-16 epithelial cells were incubated for 5 h with commercial pooled human serum, GA (2 mg/mL) or human albumin (HA, 2 mg/mL), and with an anti-human GA antibody. Open bars have no antibody; black bars have an anti-human GA antibody. Serum and GA increased IL-8 secretion, which was blocked when cells were incubated with a GA antibody. HA was unable to increase IL-8 secretion supporting the need for glycation of albumin for this to occur ($p = 0.24$).

Human Upper and Lower Airway Epithelial Cells Had Varying Responses in Il-8 Production With Human Serum Stimulation

We wished to determine if the IL-8 secretion response was similar using the immortalized human CF cell line and the bronchial CF cells (**Figure 2A**). Cells were incubated for 6 h at concentrations from 0.1 to 50%, and the level of IL-8 secretion was measured. A dose response was demonstrated in all three cell types shown in human nasal cells (**Figure 1A**) and immortalized CF1-16 and CF bronchial cells (**Figure 2A**) with a maximal serum concentration of 25% (**Figures 1A, 2A**), and a maximum IL-8 secretion of 22.30 ng/mL in the CF bronchial cells.

Further, we wished to determine if immortalized CF 1-16 cells incubated with 5% of single-donor serum or medium over 4–24 h would show an IL-8 response (**Figure 2B**).

In the three epithelial cell types (human nasal epithelial cells, immortalized CF1-16 cell line, and CF bronchial epithelial cells), the ED_{50} for serum was 5, 5, and 3% with extrapolated maximums of 2.3, 2.8, and 24 ng/mL of IL-8, respectively. The magnitude of the IL-8 response in CF-bronchial cells was 10-fold higher compared to immortalized CF 1–16 airway epithelial cells ($p = 0.02$) (**Figure 2A**). A parallel experiment using plasma-derived serum free of platelet factor contamination demonstrated a similar IL-8 dose–response relationship (to a maximum of 10%) in airway epithelial cells (data not shown).

The time dependence of IL-8 secretion was determined using CF1-16 cell cultures (**Figure 2B**). CF1-16 cells were incubated with 5% of single-donor serum in KSFM, or with KSFM alone, and the supernatants were harvested at 4, 8, 12, 16, 20, and 24 h. By 4 h of incubation, human serum induced a significant increase of IL-8 secretion compared to the control group (**Figure 2B**). No significant changes were observed for IL-8 secretion after a longer incubation period in either group.

IL-8 Secretion Induced by Glycated Albumin Compared to TNFα and LPS

The efficacy of GA to stimulate the airway epithelium to secrete IL-8 was comparatively assessed in CF 1–16 cells with other two pro-inflammatory molecules, TNFα and LPS. The concentrations of TNFα and LPS used were selected based on their pathological concentrations described in the literature (Demling et al., 2005;

Kakazu et al., 2011). All induced a dose-dependent IL-8 secretion, with a maximum effect on Il-8 production for LPS and TNF of 0.419 and 0.471 ng/mL, respectively, but GA was over four times more effective, reaching a maximum effect of 2.0 ng/mL. The EC_{50} for LPS was 0.071 and 0.00193 µg/mL for TNF compared to 424 µg/mL for GA (**Figure 3**).

Glycated Albumin Increased IL-8 Secretion and CBF in Human Adenoid Cell Cultures

Next, human primary adenoid epithelial ciliated cell cultures were used to measure IL-8 secretion following 3 h of incubation with culture medium (control), HA, and GA. An elevated level of IL-8 secretion only occurred in the cultures stimulated with GA, while there was no difference between control and HA treated cultures ($p = 0.12$) (**Figure 4A**). When ciliary beat frequency was assessed, a progressive increment was detected in response to GA incubation, compared to control or HA groups ($p < 0.001$ for GA group). Furthermore, the most significant effect upon CBF was observed following 2–4 h of incubation with GA (**Figure 4B**). CBF, expressed as area under the curve (AUC, background was subtracted), was significantly greater in the GA-treated cultures compared to HA and culture medium cultures (GA 139.40 ± 4.54; HA 66.58 ± 1.99; medium 79.67 ± 2.87, $p < 0.05$).

The temporal relationship between the effect of GA and IL-8 secretion on CBF was examined by comparing the time changes in CBF induced by GA (2 mg/mL) and IL-8 (10 nM). GA and IL-8 both induced an increase in CBF in the first 30 min of exposure, but only the increase of CBF induced by GA remained elevated. In contrast, no changes were observed in CBF in cultures incubated with HA (2 mg/mL) or medium alone (**Figures 5A,B**).

DISCUSSION

We purified a human serum factor that increases IL-8 secretion from airway epithelial cells and, using molecular and mass spectrometric methods, identified it as human serum (glycated) albumin. Through comparative assessment, we demonstrated human serum glycated albumin (GA) to be a potent pro-inflammatory molecule with functional effects on the ciliary airway. GA was able to stimulate IL-8 secretion in different epithelial respiratory cell models, including primary cultures of human epithelial nasal cells, adenoid epithelial cells, CF bronchial cells, and an immortalized CF airway epithelial cell line. GA had a greater effect on IL-8 secretion compared with conventional pro-inflammatory molecules of TNF-α and LPS. Furthermore, both GA and IL-8 increased CBF in non-CF human adenoid epithelial cells.

GA is an advanced glycation end product (AGE) considered a pro-inflammatory molecule. AGEs are formed from condensation and oxidation processed between proteins and sugars (Sorci et al., 1833). Clinically, serum GA levels, used to detect early glycemic changes (Hoonhorst et al., 2016), may be twice the normal range in diabetes (Dolhofer and Wieland, 1980;

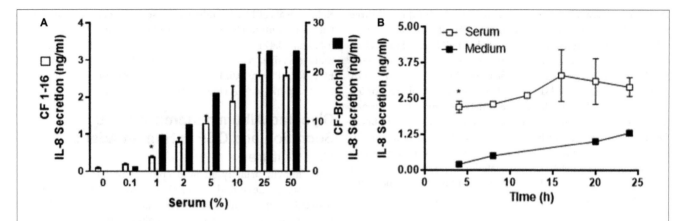

FIGURE 2 | Human serum induced IL-8 secretion from a cystic fibrosis (CF) epithelial cell line. **(A)** Immortalized CF nasal epithelial cell line (CF 1–16) (open bars, $n = 3$) and CF bronchial epithelial cells (black bars, $n = 2$) were incubated for 6 h with increasing percentages of human serum, and IL-8 secretion was measured. Human serum induced a dose-dependent IL-8 secretion in both CF cell line and the CF bronchial cells. **(A)** * indicates the lowest % of serum capable of producing a significant increase in IL-8 production. CF bronchial epithelial cells' response to serum to produce IL-8 secretion is almost one order of magnitude higher compared to the cystic fibrosis epithelial cell line. **(B)** CF 1–16 cells were incubated with 5% of single-donor serum (□, $n = 3$) or medium (■, $n = 2$), and IL-8 secretion ($n = 3$–4) was determined at 4, 8, 12, 16, 20, and 24 h. At 4 h of incubation, human serum induced a significant increase in IL-8 secretion compared to the control group. **(B)** * indicates a statistically significant ($p < 0.05$) increase in IL-8 secretion after 4 h of incubation with serum compared to the control group. No significant changes were observed for IL-8 secretion after longer period of incubation.

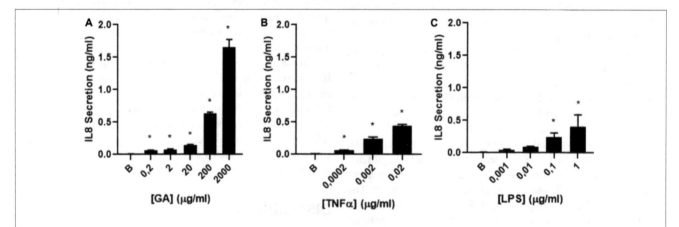

FIGURE 3 | IL-8 secretion by glycated albumin (GA) compared to TNFα and LPS. **(A)** dose–response curve of IL-8 secretion was determined in CF1-16 cells induced by **(A)** GA ($n = 3$), **(B)** TNFα ($n = 3$), and **(C)** LPS ($n = 3$). All induced a dose-dependent IL-8 secretion, with a maximum effect on Il-8 production for TNF and LPS of 477.6 and 424 ng/mL, respectively, but GA was 4–5 times more effective, reaching a max effect of 2.0 ng/mL. The EC_{50} for LPS was 0.071 and 0.00193 μg/mL for TNF compared to 424 μg/mL for GA. * indicates a significant increase ($p < 0.05$) in IL-8 secretion compared to the background **(B)**.

Jones et al., 1983). IL-8 expression is significantly elevated in patients with type II diabetes (Herder et al., 2005). These higher levels of GA are recognized as a major cause of diabetes complications such as atherosclerosis, cardiovascular disorders, nephropathy, and chronic inflammation (Sorci et al., 1833). In addition, GA has been identified as important in the induction of inflammation in retinal epithelial cells and monoclonal antibodies against GA ameliorate diabetic nephropathy in a mouse model (Cohen et al., 1994). In endothelial cells, the presence of GA is deleterious, making cells more procoagulant and promoting inflammatory responses (Rubenstein et al., 2011). Using enzyme-linked immunoassay, GA-treated human retinal pigment epithelial cells secrete levels of IL-8 detectable within 4 h (Bian et al., 1996). In human retinal pigment epithelial cells and in vascular smooth muscle cells, GA induces the expression

of IL-8 by a mechanism that involves activation of kinases, including PKC, and transcription factors such as NF-κβ (Chen et al., 2000; Bian et al., 2001; Dahrouj et al., 2015). NF-kβ induces the expression of inflammatory response-related mRNAs, such as TNFα (tumor necrosis factor α) and IL-6 (interleukin-6) (Svenson et al., 1995), inflammatory mediators that have been related with functional changes in cilia activity (Chen et al., 2000; Papathanasiou et al., 2008). Furthermore, kinases like PKC also modify the mechanism associated with cilia activity regulation by ATP (Barrera et al., 2004; Gonzalez et al., 2013).

In human primary airway epithelial ciliated cell cultures, we observed that GA induced an increase in IL-8 and CBF. Previous studies have shown that macromolecules, such as soluble hyaluronic acid, can increase CBF of tracheal ovine epithelial cells through an unknown membrane receptor (Lieb et al., 2000).

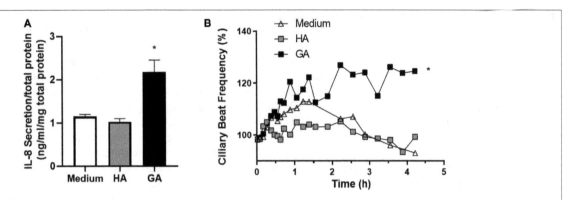

FIGURE 4 | GA increased IL-8 secretion and CBF in human adenoid epithelial cell cultures. (A) Human primary adenoid epithelial ciliated cell cultures were incubated with culture medium, HA (2 mg/mL), or GA (2 mg/mL) for 3 h. GA increased the statistical significance of IL-8 secretion with respect to HA and medium. Values are expressed as ng/mL of IL-8 corrected by mg of protein in primary culture. *$p < 0.05$. (B) Time-course changes in CBF of non-CF human adenoid ciliated cell culture treated with GA (■, 2 mg/mL), HA (□, 2 mg/mL), and control solution (△, medium). The most significant effect upon CBF was observed after 2–4 h of incubation with GA. $n = 4$–5 cultures were used for each experimental point included in the Il-8 secretion experiments and the time course changes on CBF exposed to medium, HA, and GA.

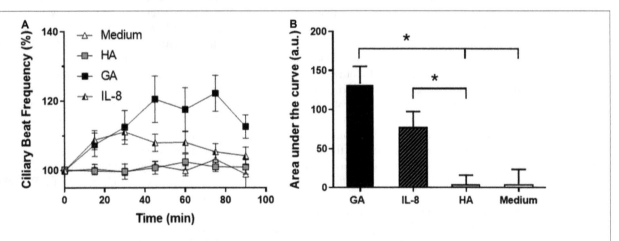

FIGURE 5 | Effect of glycated albumin (GA) and IL-8 in CBF. (A) Time-course changes in CBF of human adenoid epithelial ciliated cells cultures treated with GA (■, 2 mg/mL), IL-8 (□, 10 nM), albumin (HA, ∘, 2 mg/mL), and culture medium (△). GA and IL-8 induced an increase in CBF in the first 30 min of exposure, but only the increase of CBF induced by GA was sustained. (B) Time course of CBF in (A) expressed as area under the curve (AUC). GA induced a statistically significant increase in CBF with respect to HA and medium, and IL-8 with respect to HA. *$p < 0.05$. $n = 4$–5 cultures were used for each experimental point included in the time-course changes on CBF exposed to medium, HA, Il-8, and GA.

Non-glycated HA was unable to modify CBF. Although the binding site of GA has not yet been described, it is possible that GA could bind to the receptor for advanced glycated end products (RAGE), known to be expressed in the airway epithelium (Milutinovic et al., 2012). RAGE regulates a number of cellular processes such as inflammation, regulation of cell mass, and cell mobility (Xie et al., 2013; Whitsett and Alenghat, 2014). Studies in retinal pigment epithelial cell cultures indicate that glycated albumin-induced breakdown of RPE function is mediated by RAGE and vascular endothelial growth factor (VEGF) receptor (del Campo et al., 2011). RAGE has been shown to be present in epithelial cells and contribute to allergic airway disease, as it can act as a mediator in one or more pro-inflammatory pathways that eventuate in the altered physiology seen in allergic airways disease (Milutinovic et al., 2012). RAGE knockout mice present a lower production of IL-8 and NF-kβ

activation when they are exposed to pulmonary ischemia and reperfusion (Sternberg et al., 2008). In addition to binding AGEs, RAGE also is a signal transduction receptor for amyloid-β (Aβ) and S100/calgranulins, suggesting that RAGE could be involved in the recognition of a variety of macromolecules associated with the respiratory innate immunity response of the airway epithelium (Ma et al., 2007).

The CF 1-16 cell line in the study responded to human serum, increasing IL-8 secretion after 4 h of incubation. CF bronchial epithelial cells also responded to human serum, increasing IL-8 secretion, but CF bronchial cells appeared to be more responsive releasing 10 times more IL-8. Patients with CF suffer from chronic infections and severe inflammation and present high levels of pro-inflammatory molecules such as IL-8, IL-6, TNF$_\alpha$, and arachidonic acid metabolites (Nakamura et al., 1992; Khan et al., 1995; O'Sullivan and Fredman, 2009), indicating a possible pro-inflammatory state of these cells. In addition, CF patients with CF-related diabetes mellitus have a more rapid decline in lung function and an increased mortality rate (Milla et al., 2000). It is possible that increased GA in the airways of these patients enhances the inflammatory response in their lungs.

Previous studies have shown that TNFα induces IL-8 expression in cultured human airway epithelial cells (Kwon et al., 1994). Furthermore, LPS, a TLR4 agonist, increases IL-8 production through phosphorylation of p38 (Mizunoe et al., 2012). When we compared the effectiveness of GA to induce IL-8 secretion with TNFα and LPS, GA was 10 times more effective to induce IL-8 secretion, suggesting a critical role of GA to initiate an inflammatory response.

IL-8 induced an increase in CBF in adenoid epithelial cultures showing a correlation with the effect of GA in the first 30 min. The CXC chemokine receptor (CXCR-1/IL-8) has been found to be expressed in human small airway epithelial cells and to induce the release of IL-6 (Gras et al., 2010). Although the specific mechanism of Il-8 stimulation of CBF has not been identified, it has been reported that Il-8 can increase PLC and intracellular calcium levels, both well-known ciliary beat activators (Barrera et al., 2004). Murine primary sino-nasal cultures treated with the mouse homologue of IL-8 increased basal CBF at 24 and 48 h (Shen et al., 2012). However, IL-8 inhibits beta-agonist ciliary stimulation in bovine bronchial epithelial cells (Allen-Gipson et al., 2004). It is possible that GA and IL-8 affect CBF directly or, alternately, that IL-8 secretion induced by GA enhances CBF (Choi et al., 2010). Furthermore, it is possible that the initial activation of CBF induced by Il-8 could be reverted after longer periods of inflammation, with a deleterious effect upon mucociliary clearance.

Our results suggest that plasma exudation of serum molecules such as GA onto the airway epithelium could induce an inflammatory response, initially producing IL-8 secretion and modifying mucociliary transport by the effect on ciliary activity. A progression of this inflammatory response could involve the release of other chemotactic cytokines, an influx of polymorphonuclear neutrophils, and contribute to airway inflammation observed in chronic airway diseases (Reutershan and Ley, 2004). Future directions may include measurement of GA in several airway diseases, including SARS-CoV-2, and correlate GA levels with patient clinical outcomes. Recent studies have contributed to identifying the location of the receptor of advanced glycation end products (RAGE) in the airways, as a mediator of GA effects on the systemic inflammatory response (Hoonhorst et al., 2016). A study reported by Demling et al. (2005) reported that the RAGE receptor on alveolar epithelial type 1 cells (AT 1) was localized in the basolateral membrane, suggesting a morphological role for the receptor by strengthening the adherence of ATI cells to the alveolar basement membrane. In our study, we used different cellular epithelial cell types, including polarized and non-polarized cells, but we did not identify the specific location of the RAGE receptor. Future studies using double chambers to produce polarized cell cultures will be necessary to identify the RAGE receptor location and activation on the apical or basal membrane by GA inducing

an inflammatory response, helping to identify potential blockers to prevent the deleterious effect of AGE, including GA, on the airway epithelium.

In our study, we used different epithelial cell types including polarized and non-polarized cells. However, we did not identify the specific location of the RAGE receptor. Future studies using double chambers to produced polarized cell culture will be necessary to identify the RAGE receptor location and activation on the apical or basal membrane using GA to induce an inflammatory response to assist in identifying potential blockers to prevent the deleterious effects of AGE including GA, on the airway epithelium.

In summary, our results suggest that plasma exudation of serum molecules such as GA onto the airway epithelium can induce an inflammatory response, initially producing IL-8 secretion and modifying mucociliary transport by the effect on ciliary activity. A progression of this inflammatory response could involve the release of other chemotactic cytokines, an influx of polymorphonuclear neutrophils, and contribute to airway inflammation observed in chronic airway diseases. Future directions may include measurement of GA in several airway diseases, including SARS-CoV-2, and correlate GA levels with patient clinical outcomes. Recent studies have contributed to our understanding by identifying the location of the receptor of advanced glycation end products (RAGE) in the airways, as a mediator of GA effects on the inflammatory response (Buckley and Ehrhardt, 2010; Hoonhorst et al., 2016). However, a study by Demling et al. (2005) reported that the RAGE receptor on the alveolar epithelial type I cells (AT I) was localized in the basolateral membrane, suggesting a morphological role for the receptor by strengthening the adherence of AT I cells to the alveolar basal membrane.

CONCLUSION

In conclusion, our findings suggest that a serum protein, GA, may have an important role in the airway inflammatory response.

ETHICS STATEMENT

The studies involving human participants were reviewed and approved by the University of Washington IRB. Written informed consent for participation was not required for this study in accordance with the national legislation and the institutional requirements.

AUTHOR CONTRIBUTIONS

MA, TH, SS, and MV planned the experimental designs. MA, RS, TH, MP, KD, MR, SS, and MV wrote the manuscript. MA and SS identified a serum factor that induced inflammation. TH and MP identified glycated albumin as the inflammatory protein. MP performed the dose escalation experiments. KD, MR, and MV performed the experiments on CBF. All authors contributed to the revision and final draft of the manuscript.

ACKNOWLEDGMENTS

We thank Dr. Ernest Weymueller from the Department of Otolaryngology, University of Washington, Seattle, WA; Dr. Claudia Gonzalez and Dr. Claudio Callejas, from the Department of Otolaryngology, Faculty of Medicine, Pontificia Universidad Católica de Chile; Carmen Llados and Llilian Arzola PhD from the Department of Physiology, Faculty of Biological Science, Pontificia Universidad Católica de Chile for tissue; Christine Halbert PhD, Research Scientist, Fred Hutchinson Cancer Research Center, Seattle, WA, for the CF cell line; and Marissa Anne Lopez Pier PhD U Arizona and Wen Yu Wong PhD U Arizona for their detailed review of the manuscript.

REFERENCES

Aitken, M., Villalon, M., Pier, M., Verdugo, P., and Nameroff, M. (1995). Characterization of a marker for tracheal basal cells. *Exp. Lung. Res.* 21, 1–16. doi: 10.3109/01902149509031741

Aitken, M., Villalon, M., Pier, M., Verdugo, P., and Nameroff, M. (1993). Characterization of a marker of differentiation for tracheal ciliated cells independent of ciliation. *Am. J. Respir. Cell Mol. Biol.* 9, 26–32. doi: 10.1165/ajrcmb/9.1.26

Allen-Gipson, D., Romberger, D. J., Forget, M. A., May, K. L., Sisson, J. H., and Wyatt, T. A. (2004). IL-8 inhibits isoproterenol-stimulated ciliary beat frequency in bovine bronchial epithelial cells. *J. Aerosol. Med.* 17, 107–115. doi: 10.1089/0894268041457138

Barrera, N., Morales, B., and Villalón, M. (2004). Plasma and intracellular membrane inositol 1, 4, 5-trisphosphate receptors mediate the Ca(2+) increase associated with the ATP-induced increase in ciliary beat frequency. *Am. J. Physiol. Cell Physiol.* 287, C1114–C1124.

Bian, Z., Elner, S. G., Strieter, R. M., Glass, M. B., Lukacs, N. W., Kunkel, S. L., et al. (1996). Glycated serum albumin induces chemokine gene expression in human retinal pigment epithelial cells. *J. Leukoc. Biol.* 60, 405–414. doi: 10.1002/jlb.60.3.405

Bian, Z., Elner, V. M., Yoshida, A., Kunkel, S. L., and Elner, S. G. (2001). Signaling pathways for glycated human serum albumin-induced IL-8 and MCP-1 secretion in human RPE cells. *Invest. Ophthalmol. Vis. Sci.* 42, 1660–1668.

Buckley, S. T., and Ehrhardt, C. (2010). The Receptor for advanced glycation end products (RAGE) and the Lung. *J. Biomed. Biotechnol.* 2010:917108. doi: 10.1155/2010/917108

Chen, J., Takeno, S., Osada, R., Ueda, T., and Yayin, K. (2000). Modulation of ciliary activity by tumor necrosis factor-alpha in cultured sinus epithelial cells. Possible roles of nitric oxide. *Hiroshima J. Med. Sci.* 49, 49–55.

Choi, K., Park, J. W., Kim, H. Y., Kim, Y. H., Kim, S. M., Son, Y. H., et al. (2010). Cellular factors involved in CXCL8 expression induced by glycated serum albumin in vascular smooth muscle cells. *Atherosclerosis* 209, 58–65. doi: 10.1016/j.atherosclerosis.2009.08.030

Cohen, M., Hud, E., and Wu, V. Y. (1994). Amelioration of diabetic nephropathy by treatment with monoclonal antibodies against glycated albumin. *Kidney Int.* 45, 1673–1679. doi: 10.1038/ki.1994.219

Cowley, E., Wang, C. G., Gosselin, D., Radzioch, D., and Eidelman, D. H. (1997). Mucociliary clearance in cystic fibrosis knockout mice infected with *Pseudomonas aeruginosa*. *Eur. Respir. J.* 10, 2312–2318. doi: 10.1183/09031936.97.10102312

Cui, X., Chen, X., Yu, C. J., Yang, J., Lin, Z. P., Yin, M., et al. (2015). Increased expression of toll-like receptors 2 and 4 and related cytokines in persistent allergic rhinitis. *Otolaryngol. Head Neck Surg.* 152, 233–238. doi: 10.1177/0194599814562173

Dahrouj, M., Desjardins, D. M., Liu, Y., Crosson, C. E., and Ablonczy, Z. (2015). Receptor mediated disruption of retinal pigment epithelium function in acute glycated-albumin exposure. *Exp. Eye Res.* 137, 50–56. doi: 10.1016/j.exer.2015.06.004

del Campo, R., Martinez, E., del Fresno, C., Alenda, R., Gómez-Piña, V., Fernández-Ruíz, I., et al. (2011). Translocated LPS might cause endotoxin tolerance in circulating monocytes of cystic fibrosis patients. *PLoS One* 6:e295777. doi: 10.1371/journal.pone.0029577

Demling, N., Ehrhardt, C., Kasper, M., Laue, M., Knels, L., and Rieber, E. P. (2005). Promotion of cell adherence and spreading: a novel function of RAGE, the highly selective differentiation marker of human alveolar epithelial type I cells. *Cell Tissue Res.* 323, 475–488. doi: 10.1007/s00441-005-0069-0

Dolhofer, R., and Wieland, O. H. (1980). Increased glycosylation of serum albumin in diabetes mellitus. *Diabetes* 29, 417–422. doi: 10.2337/diabetes.29.6.417

Gonzalez, C., Espinosa, M., Sanchez, M. T., Droguett, K., Rios, M., Fonseca, X., et al. (2013). Epithelial cell culture from human adenoids: a funcional study model for ciliated and secretory cells. *Biomed. Res. Int.* 2013:478713.

Gras, D., Tiers, L., Vachier, I., de Senneville, L. D., Bourdin, A., Godard, P., et al. (2010). Regulation of CXCR/IL-8 in human airway epithelial cells. *Int. Arch. Allergy Immunol.* 152, 140–150. doi: 10.1159/000265535

Halbert, C., Aitken, M. L., and Miller, A. D. (1996). Retroviral vectors efficiently transduce basal and secretory airway epithelial cells *in vitro* resulting in persistent gene expression in organotypic culture. *Hum. Gene. Ther.* 7, 1871–1881. doi: 10.1089/hum.1996.7.15-1871

Herder, C., Haastert, B., Muller-Scholze, S., Koenig, W., Thorand, B., Holle, R., et al. (2005). Association of systemic chemokine concentrations with impaired glucose tolerance and type 2 diabetes: results from the Cooperative Health Research in the Region of Augsburg Survey S4 (KORA S4). *Diabetes* 54, S11–S17.

Hermoso, M., Barrera, N., Morales, B., Perez, S., and Villalon, M. (2001). Platelet activating factor increases ciliary activity in the hamster oviduct through epithelial production of prostaglandin E2. *Pflugers Arch.* 442, 336–345. doi: 10.1007/s004240100550

Hollander, C., Sitkauskiene, B., Sakalauskas, R., Westin, U., and Janciauskiene, S. M. (2007). Serum and bronchial lavage fluid concentrations of IL-8, SLPI, sCD14 and sICAM-1 in patients with COPD and asthma. *Respir. Med.* 101, 1947–1953. doi: 10.1016/j.rmed.2007.04.010

Hoonhorst, S. J. M., Lo Tam Loi, A. T., Pouwels, S. D., Faiz, A., Telenga, E. D., van den Burge, M., et al. (2016). Advanced glycation endproducts and their receptor in different body compartments in COPD. *Respir. Res.* 17:46. doi: 10.1186/s12931-016-0363-2

Jones, I., Owens, D. R., Williams, S., Ryder, R. E., Birtwell, A. J., Jones, M. K., et al. (1983). Glycosylated serum albumin: an intermediate index of diabetic control. *Diabetes Care* 6, 501–503. doi: 10.2337/diacare.6.5.501

Kakazu, E., Ueno, Y., Kondo, Y., Inoue, J., Ninomiya, M., Kimura, O., et al. (2011). Plasma L-Cystine/L-Glutamate imbalance increases tumor necrosis factor-Alpha from CD14+ circulating monocytes in patients with advanced cirrhosis. *PLoS One* 6:e23402. doi: 10.1371/journal.pone.0023402

Keatings, V., Collins, P. D., Scott, D. M., and Barnes, P. J. (1996). Differences in interleukin-8 and tumor necrosis factor-alpha in induced sputum from patients with chronic obstructive pulmonary disease or asthma. *Am. J. Respir. Crit. Care Med.* 153, 530–534. doi: 10.1164/ajrccm.153.2.8564092

Khan, T., Wagener, J. S., Bost, T., Martinez, J., Accurso, F. J., and Riches, D. W. (1995). Early pulmonary inflammation in infants with cystic fibrosis. *Am. J. Respir. Care Med.* 151, 1075–1082.

Knowles, M. R., and Boucher, R. C. (2002). Mucus clearance as a primary innate defense mechanism for mammalian airways. *J. Clin. Invest.* 109, 571–577. doi: 10.1172/jci0215217

Koblizek, V., Tomsova, M., Cermakova, E., Papousek, P., Pracharova, S., Mandalia, R. A., et al. (2011). Impairment of nasal mucociliary clearance in former smokers with stable chronic obstructive pulmonary disease relates to the presence of a chronic bronchitis phenotype. *Rhinology* 49, 397–406.

Konstan, M., Hilliard, K. A., Norvell, T. M., and Berger, M. (1994). Bronchoalveolar lavage findings in cystic fibrosis patients with stable, clinically mild lung disease suggest ongoing infection and inflammation. *Am. J. Respir. Crit. Care Med.* 150, 448–454. doi: 10.1164/ajrccm.150.2.8049828

Kwon, O., Au, B. T., Collins, P. D., Adcock, I. M., Mak, J. C., Robbins, R. R., et al. (1994). Tumor necrosis factor-induced interleukin-8 expression in cultured human airway epithelial cells. *Am. J. Physiol.* 267, L398–L405.

Lamblin, C., Gosset, P., Tillie-Leblond, I., Saulnier, F., Marquette, C. H., Wallaert, B., et al. (1998). Bronchial neutrophilia in patients with noninfectious status asthmaticus. *Am. J. Respir. Crit. Care Med.* 157, 394–402. doi: 10.1164/ajrccm. 157.2.97-02099

Levine, S. (1995). Bronchial epithelial cell-cytokine interactions in airway inflammation. *J. Invest. Med.* 43, 241–249.

Lieb, T., Forteza, R., and Salathe, M. (2000). Hyaluronic acid in cultures ovine tracheal cells and its effect on ciliary beat frequency *in vitro. J. Aerosol. Med.* 13, 231–237. doi: 10.1089/jam.2000.13.231

Ma, W., Lee, S. E., Guo, J., Qu, W., Hudson, B. I., Schmidt, A. M., et al. (2007). RAGE ligand upregulation of VEGF secretion in ARPE-19 cells. *Invest. Ophthalmol. Vis. Sci.* 48, 1355–1361. doi: 10.1167/iovs.06-0738

Marini, M., Vittori, E., Hollemborg, J., and Mattoli, S. (1992). Expression of the potent inflammatory cytokines, granulocyte-macrophage-colony-stimulating factor and interleukin-6 and interleukin-8, in bronchial epithelial cells of patients with asthma. *J. Allergy Clin. Immunol.* 89, 1001–1009. doi: 10.1016/ 0091-6749(92)90223-o

McElvaney, N., Nakamura, H., Birrer, P., Hébert, C. A., Wong, W. L., Alphonso, M., et al. (1992). Modulation of airway inflammation in cystic fibrosis. In vivo suppression of interleukin-8 levels on the respiratory epithelial surface by aerosolization of recombinant secretory leukoprotease inhibitor. *J. Clin. Invest.* 90, 1296–1301. doi: 10.1172/jci115994

Milla, C., Warwick, W. J., and Moran, A. (2000). Trends in pulmonary function in patients with cystic fibrosis correlate with the degree of glucose intolerance at baseline. *Am. J. Respir. Crit. Care Med.* 162, 891–895. doi: 10.1164/ajrccm.162. 3.9904075

Milutinovic, P., Alcorn, J. F., Englert, J. M., Crum, L. T., and Oury, T. D. (2012). The receptor for advanced glycation end products is a central mediator of asthma. *Am. J. Pathol.* 181, 1215–1225. doi: 10.1016/j.ajpath.2012.06.031

Mizunoe, S., Shuto, T., Suzuki, S., Matsumoto, C., Watanabe, K., Ueno-Shuto, K., et al. (2012). Synergism between interleukin (IL)-17 and Toll-like receptor 2 and 4 signals to induce IL-8 expression in cystic fibrosis airway epithelial cell. *J. Pharmacol. Sci.* 118, 512–520. doi: 10.1254/jphs.11240fp

Nakamura, H., Yoshimura, K., Jaffe, H. A., and Crystal, R. G. (1991). Interleukin-8 gene expression in human bronchial epithelial cells. *J. Biol. Chem.* 266, 19611–19617. doi: 10.1016/s0021-9258(18)55037-7

Nakamura, H., Yoshimura, K., McElvaney, N. G., and Crystal, R. G. (1992). Neutrophil elastase in respiratory epithelial lining fluid of individuals with cystic fibrosis induces interleukin-8 gene expression in a human bronchial epithelial cell line. *J. Clin. Invest.* 89, 1478–1484. doi: 10.1172/jci115738

O'Sullivan, B., and Fredman, S. D. (2009). Cystic fibrosis. *Lancet* 373, 1891–1904.

Papathanasiou, A., Djahanbakhch, O., Saridogan, E., and Lyons, R. A. (2008). The effect of interleukin-6 on ciliary beat frequency in the human fallopian tube. *Fertil Steril* 90, 391–394. doi: 10.1016/j.fertnstert.2007.07.1379

Reutershan, J., and Ley, K. (2004). Bench-to-bedside review: acute respiratory distress syndrome - how neutrophils migrate into the lung. *Crit. Care* 8, 453–461.

Rubenstein, D., Maria, Z., and Yin, W. (2011). Glycated albumin modulates endothelial cell thrombogenic and inflammatory responses. *J. Diabetes Sci. Technol.* 5, 703–713. doi: 10.1177/193229681100500325

Schmid, A., Sutto, Z., Schmid, N., Novak, L., Ivonnet, P., Horvath, G., et al. (2010). Decreased soluble adenylyl cyclase activity in cystic fibrosis is related to defective apical bicarbonate exchange and affects ciliary beat frequency regulation. *J. Biol. Chem.* 285, 29998–30007. doi: 10.1074/jbc.m110.113621

Seybold, Z., Mariassy, A. T., Stroh, D., Kim, C. S., Gazeroglu, H., and Wanner, A. (1990). Mucociliary interaction *in vitro*: effects of physiological and inflammatory stimuli. *J. Appl. Physiol.* 68, 1421–1426. doi: 10.1152/jappl.1990. 68.4.1421

Shen, J., Chen, B., and Cohen, N. A. (2012). Keratinocyte chemoattractant (interleukin-8) regulation of sinonasal cilia function in a murine model. *Int. Forum. Allergy Rhinol.* 2, 75–79. doi: 10.1002/alr.20087

Sorci, G., Riuzzi, F., Giambanco, I., and Donato, R. (1833). RAGE in tissue homeostasis, repair and regeneration. *Biochim. Biophys. Acta* 10:2013.

Standiford, T., Kunkel, S. L., Basha, M. A., Chensue, S. W., Lynch, J. P., Toews, G. B., et al. (1990). Interleukin-8 gene expression by a pulmonary epithelial cell line. A model for cytokine networks in the lung. *J. Clin. Invest.* 86, 1945–1953. doi: 10.1172/jci114928

Sternberg, D., Gowda, R., Mehra, D., Qu, W., Weinberg, A., Twaddell, W., et al. (2008). Blockade of receptor for advanced glycation end product attenuates pulmonary reperfusion injury in mice. *J. Thorac. Cardiovasc. Surg.* 136, 1576–1585. doi: 10.1016/j.jtcvs.2008.05.032

Svenson, C., Gronneberg, R., Andersson, M., Alkner, U., Andersson, O., Billing, B., et al. (1995). Allergen challenge-induced entry of alpha-2-macroglobulin and trystase into human nasal and bronhial airways. *J. Allergy Clin. Immunol.* 96, 239–246. doi: 10.1016/s0091-6749(95)70013-7

van der Baan, B. (2000). Ciliary function. *Acta Otorhinolaryngol. Belg.* 54, 293–298.

Waugh, D. J. J., and Wilson, C. (2008). The interleukin-8 pathway in cancer. *Clin. Cancer Res.* 14, 6735–6741. doi: 10.1158/1078-0432.ccr-07-4843

Whitsett, J., and Alenghat, T. (2014). Respiratory epithelial cells orchestrate pulmonary innate immunity. *Nat. Immunol.* 16, 27–37. doi: 10.1038/ni. 3045

Xie, J., Méndez, J. D., Méndez-Valenzuela, V., and Aguilar-Hernández, M. M. (2013). Cellular signaling of the receptor for advanced glycation end products (RAGE). *Cell. Signal.* 25, 2185–2197. doi: 10.1016/j.cellsig.2013. 06.013

19

Where we Stand: Lung Organotypic Living Systems that Emulate Human-Relevant Host–Environment/Pathogen Interactions

Rocio J. Jimenez-Valdes[1], Uryan I. Can[1], Brian F. Niemeyer[1] and Kambez H. Benam[1,2,3]*

[1] Division of Pulmonary Sciences and Critical Care Medicine, Department of Medicine, University of Colorado Anschutz Medical Campus, Aurora, CO, United States, [2] Department of Bioengineering, University of Colorado Denver, Aurora, CO, United States, [3] Linda Crnic Institute for Down Syndrome, University of Colorado Anschutz Medical Campus, Aurora, CO, United States

*Correspondence:
Kambez H. Benam
kambez.benam@cuanschutz.edu

Lung disorders such as chronic obstructive pulmonary disease (COPD) and lower respiratory tract infections (LRTIs) are leading causes of death in humans globally. Cigarette smoking is the principal risk factor for the development of COPD, and LRTIs are caused by inhaling respiratory pathogens. Thus, a thorough understanding of host–environment/pathogen interactions is crucial to developing effective preventive and therapeutic modalities against these disorders. While animal models of human pulmonary conditions have been widely utilized, they suffer major drawbacks due to inter-species differences, hindering clinical translation. Here we summarize recent advances in generating complex 3D culture systems that emulate the microarchitecture and pathophysiology of the human lung, and how these platforms have been implemented for studying exposure to environmental factors, airborne pathogens, and therapeutic agents.

Keywords: spheroids, organoids, bio-scaffolds, precision cut lung slices, bronchial biopsies, 3D bioprinting, lung-on-a-chip, inhalation models

INTRODUCTION

Lung disorders represent a great socioeconomic challenge and a major burden on health care systems worldwide; chronic obstructive pulmonary disease (COPD) and lower respiratory tract infections (LRTIs) are the third and fourth leading causes of death globally, respectively (World Health Organization [WHO], 2018). Cigarette smoke exposure is the principal risk factor for COPD development and exacerbation, and LRTIs are consequent to inhalation of airborne pathogens. Therefore, a better understanding of the pulmonary system at health and disease and recreation of respiratory host–environment/pathogen interactions are crucial if we are to prevent and treat lung disorders. While animal models of human respiratory conditions have been instrumental in advancing our knowledge, they suffer major drawbacks due to inter-species (e.g., genetic, homeostatic physiology, pathology, and respiratory tree anatomy, airway histology, etc.) differences hindering clinical translation. Rodent animal models, for instance, which have widely been applied to shed light on signaling networks and lung development, are fundamentally different from humans in terms of lung cellular composition, airway branching, and immune system function (Rackley and Stripp, 2012). Besides, rodents are obligate nose breathers with intricate and highly developed nasal turbinates that lead to different particulate deposition patterns compared to humans during breathing (Hecht, 2005). Due to these factors, rodents at best are passive inhalers and, unlike humans, are unable to actively inhale therapeutic candidates or cigarette smoke.

To circumvent some of these shortcomings with animal models, simple two-dimensional (2D) cell culture models that emulate naturally present lung air–liquid interface (ALI) have been developed to study human lung pathophysiology *in vitro* (Prunieras et al., 1983). Recently, these systems have been used in combination with cell exposure systems that mimic the natural route of exposure of lung epithelium to environmental factors in order to measure the risks of potentially damaging inhaled nanoparticles (Lenz et al., 2009) or cigarette smoke (Thorne and Adamson, 2013). However, despite their use of primary human lung airway epithelial cells (hAECs) and recapitulation of mucociliated histology, they have several limitations in recreating organ-level functionalities of the human lung. For example, they do not enable (1) real-time analysis of dynamic intercellular (e.g., leukocyte-endothelial cell) interactions under physiological flow, (2) study of inhalation exposure to whole cigarette smoke, as a representative inhaled material, under physiological breathing airflow without disturbing ALI, (3) recreation of blood-like vascular perfusion to continually supply nutrients and growth factors, (4) introduction and perturbation of vascular and airflow shear stress to simulate different pathophysiological conditions, and (5) high-resolution kinetic analysis of biological responses (e.g., the time-course release of secreted factors, like cytokines/chemokines, in response to pathogenic challenge) (Fang and Eglen, 2017; Ainslie et al., 2019). In addition, these platforms are commonly used in the absence of sub-epithelial extracellular matrix (ECM; Yamaya et al., 1992; Gray et al., 1996).

Recent advances in tissue engineering and microfabrication have led to the development and application of more complex 3D culture systems and biomimetic microfluidic platforms to capture the structural and functional complexity of the human lung (Miller and Spence, 2017). In this review, we assess these state-of-the-art complex *in vitro* lung models, and the efforts made to expose these models to environmental factors, pathogens, and therapeutic agents. Finally, we discuss future directions on tackling the challenges of *in vitro* lung models that were observed over the past decade and share our vision on how to further enhance these models for more accurate and better clinical translation.

RECENT ADVANCES IN CREATING COMPLEX 3D *IN VITRO* MODELS OF HUMAN LUNG

Spheroids and Organoids

Among the simplest of the 3D lung models are spheroids. Spheroids are multicellular sphere-like culture systems that enable recapitulation of cell–cell interactions; they are either utilized as freely floating cell aggregates or get seeded onto 3D bio-scaffolds (Ainslie et al., 2019). Spheroids utilize tumor-derived cells, patient-derived xenograft cells, and immortalized cell lines, and have been applied to study intercellular interactions and response to therapies in the context of cancer (Ekert et al., 2014; Meenach et al., 2016; Klameth et al., 2017; Lewis et al., 2018), lung progenitor cells differentiation (Chimenti et al., 2017), and pulmonary fibrosis (Surolia et al., 2017). However, spheroid culture systems still suffer deficiencies such as a lack of vasculature and ALI, hard to control cell ratios and aggregate size, as well as a failure to mimic organ function (Fang and Eglen, 2017); therefore, spheroids do not represent good *in vitro* lung models to study host–environment/pathogen interactions. Another similar yet distinct preclinical system is organoids; these are cultured organ-specific cell types, which are derived from a population of stem cells (adult or pluripotent), and are capable of maintaining stem cells during *in vitro* culture. During formation, organoids develop into 3D tissues that recreate *in vivo*-observed microanatomy through self-organization (Fang and Eglen, 2017; Ainslie et al., 2019). Compared to spheroids, organoids exhibit long-term viability and rely on internal developmental processes (rather than cell–cell adhesions) to drive tissue/organ-like microarchitecture formation. Human lung organoids have been generated to replicate bronchi/bronchioles (Konishi et al., 2016; Mccauley et al., 2017; Miller et al., 2018), alveoli (Zacharias et al., 2018), and even multi-lineage structures (Dye et al., 2016). While helpful in advancing our understanding of the respiratory system, particularly from a developmental perspective, this models lack several of key organ features such as vascularization, and mechanical forces associated with breathing, and it is difficult to obtain fully differentiated lung cell types (Barkauskas et al., 2017). Lung organoids have been sparsely used for host-environment/pathogen exposure studies, since the organoid lumen, which represents the apical surface of the lungs through which a natural exposure would occur *in vivo*, is difficult to access, thus treatments or stimuli are applied in the environment in which the organoids are embedded. In this scenario, murine organoids have been infected with influenza virus (Quantius et al., 2016), and human organoids have been infected with respiratory syncytial virus (RSV; Sachs et al., 2019). Some attempts have been made to microinject pathogens or their by-products into organoids using custom made tools, primarily in gastrointestinal organoids (Williamson et al., 2018); however, in lung organoids, this technique has only been applied to propagate Cryptosporidium, a protozoan parasite (Heo et al., 2018).

Precision Cut Lung Slices

To address the disconnection that often exists in spheroids and organoids in including both cellular and organ-level complexities *in vitro*, some groups have turned to an *ex vivo* system called precision cut lung slices (PCLS), which maintain the cellular structure and the biological processes of the lung (Ainslie et al., 2019). Importantly, PCLS generation from healthy explants and diseased tissue can reveal differences in the cellular and molecular interactions within the microenvironment of the lung. Disease modeling of healthy tissue can be achieved *ex vivo* through mimicking disease characteristics and used for exploring therapeutic treatments (Alsafadi et al., 2020). Precision cut lung slices have been applied for cytotoxicity assessment to low-molecular-weight (LMW) chemicals (Lauenstein et al., 2014), evaluation of biological responses to inflammatory stimuli such as lipopolysaccharide endotoxin (LPS), macrophage-activating lipopeptide-2 (MALP-2), interferon gamma (IFNgamma) (Henjakovic et al., 2008), and recreation of pathologies such as pulmonary fibrosis, through the use of a combination of profibrotic growth factors and signaling molecules (Alsafadi et al., 2017) and COPD models induced with 1-(3-Hydroxy-5-(thiophen-2-yl)phenyl)-3-(naphthalen-2-yl)urea (FzM1) (Skronska-Wasek et al., 2017). However, PCLS are often cultivated only for short periods of time (they are very challenging to maintain viable and functional for weeks), their use is impacted by the limited availability of whole/resected organ for slicing, and they only represent a brief snapshot of the cell populations in the tissue. Besides, the PCLS cannot fully recapitulate all attributes seen *in vivo*; for instance, there are major challenges with preserving arteriole morphology and localization of lung airway smooth muscle cells (Sanderson, 2011). Precision cut lung slices can reproduce the initial interactions and inflammatory responses to industrial chemicals (Lauenstein et al., 2014) and pathogens [e.g., influenza viruses (Liu et al., 2015), rhinovirus (Beale et al., 2014), *Yersinia pestis* (Banerjee et al., 2019), and *Coxiella burnetiid* (Graham et al., 2016)] in the human respiratory system; however, the extent to which the immune response can replicate the *in vivo* situation is limited, as demonstrated by Neuhaus et al. (2017), who observed that LPS-induced tumor necrosis factor-alpha (TNF-α) secretion decreased significantly over a period of 15 days, and it is not possible to recruit non-resident immune cells. Moreover, while murine-derived PCLS models have been adapted to study the effects of cigarette smoke (Donovan et al., 2016), the PCLS per se have not been utilized for inhalation exposure studies *in vitro*, principally because the route of administration represents a challenge (e.g., physiological ALI cannot be established in this model system), and often the entire slice is bathed in the compound or stimulant of interest (Liu et al., 2019). Changing from ALI conditions to liquid-submerged conditions represents a drawback, as it impacts epithelial cells' glycoprotein secretion profile, tight junction integrity, and permeability (Grainger et al., 2006). In addition, the physio-chemical properties of pulmonary stimuli such as airborne pollutants, gaseous substances, novel medications, and therapeutic agents can alter when in liquid suspension (Upadhyay and Palmberg, 2018). In addition to this, PCLS become static systems, lacking the shear flows associated with air and blood flow in the ALI and vascular endothelium, respectively, which could impact cell–cell/ECM responses and interactions in tissues.

Bronchial Biopses

Bronchial biopsies are samples of airway tissue obtained from the carinae of large and small cartilaginous airways. These samples are often fixed and used to measure airway remodeling by morphometric analyses of airway epithelial mucin stores, measurements of reticular basement membrane thickness, quantification of the number and size of globlet cells, the analysis of the content and density of the smooth muscle of the airways, as well as quantification and characterization of inflammatory cells (Woodruff and Innes, 2006). In addition, some effort have been made to culture the bronchial biopsies for short-term exposure studies *in vitro*. For instance, this culture model has been used to study the effects of chemotherapeutic treatments on non-small cell lung cancer (Lang et al., 2007), to evaluate cellular responses by exposing asthmatic lung tissue to allergen *Dermatophagoides pteronyssinus* (Jaffar et al., 1999; Lordan et al., 2001; Vijayanand et al., 2010), and to test the antiviral efficacy of therapeutic drugs against influenza virus infection (Nicholas et al., 2015). The advantages of bronchial biopsies include retaining the three-dimensional structure of the lungs if the extraction procedure is successful, which requires a trained bronchoscopist, allowing sampling from healthy subjects as well as patients with lung diseases, and the minimally invasive nature of the sampling procedure. However, this system has similar drawbacks as the PCLS, and is impacted by scarcity of donor tissue availability, small sample size (usually 1–3 mm) and number of biopsies that can be obtained at any given time (∼4–10). In addition the *in vitro* viability in often low, therefore exposure studies on bronchial biopsies usually do not last more than a single day.

Cellularized Bio-Scaffolds

Extracellular matrix is the 3D network of extracellular macromolecules that provide structural integrity and biochemical support to tissue-resident cells. Extracellular matrix both serves as a scaffold and modulates cellular responses such as self-renewal, quiescence, migration, proliferation, phenotype maintenance, differentiation, and apoptosis (Akhmanova et al., 2015). Hydrogels can mimic ECM *in vitro* using natural products (like collagen, hyaluronic acid, chitosan, alginate, or Matrigel) or synthetic polymers [such as polyethylene glycol (PEG) or polyacrylamide (PAA)] (Zhou et al., 2018). Natural hydrogels have been predominantly used to culture lung cells and organoids (Sato et al., 2017; Zacharias et al., 2018); however, artificial matrices have been demonstrated as a viable alternative (Miller et al., 2019), since their components are biologically inert, and can be functionalized by the addition of proteins, peptides, and/or polysaccharides (Akhmanova et al., 2015).

Besides hydrogels, lung ECM can be generated via decellularization of the whole/resected lung through perfusion with detergents, which allows considerable preservation of the micro- and macro-architecture of the organ, and the ECM composition (Gilpin and Wagner, 2018). Extracellular matrix has been recognized as a bioactive medium that modulates cellular responses in its surroundings. By using cellularized bio-scaffolds it will therefore be possible to mimic some pathological alterations, and the consequent functional changes that occur in lung diseases, especially those with a chronic nature (Burgess et al., 2016). Decellularized lung scaffolds have enabled studying cell–ECM interactions in tissues of healthy people and patients with chronic lung diseases, such as lung cancer (Stratmann et al., 2014), idiopathic pulmonary fibrosis

(IPF; Van Der Velden et al., 2018), and scleroderma (Sun et al., 2016). These matrices are instrumental in evaluating lung repair and regeneration and have been recellularized with different types of human cells, including fibroblasts, endothelial cells, epithelial cells, stem cells from multiple organ sources, and organoids (Porzionato et al., 2018; Giobbe et al., 2019). However, it has not been possible to completely recellularize these matrices to allow recreation of lung physiology and function, their application has been partly hindered due to the limited number of whole/resected human lungs, and to our knowledge, their utilization [beyond regenerative medicine and orthotopic transplantation (Guenthart et al., 2019)] for studying host–environment/pathogen interactions has not been demonstrated.

3D Bioprinting

To more faithfully replicate tissue microarchitectures of the human lung, 3D bioprinting has emerged as a great technological platform ideally positioned to create finely defined and controlled biological structures and living systems by utilizing a wide array of materials (natural, synthetic, or even hybrid hydrogels) and cell types. This technology can achieve a high degree of precision in cell positioning and can be scalable for automation (Gungor-Ozkerim et al., 2018). However, 3D bioprinting has been predominantly applied for the development of vascularized tissues (Kolesky et al., 2014), rather than generating functional whole organ or organ-like mimicries. To our knowledge, only a few studies have focused on the lungs. Horvath et al. (2015) biofabricated a three-part mimetic (composed of an endothelial cell layer, basement membrane, and an epithelial cell layer) of air–blood barrier analog of the human lung alveoli within a transwell insert. While a great initiative, the study utilized cell lines, rather than primary human-derived cells, and the authors only focused on model validation (viability, cellular proliferation, and barrier function) and no data were presented on the application of the platform for the analysis of host-environment/pathogen interactions. More recently, a new method for 3D bioprinting of tissues by stereolithography was reported, whereby it was possible to make a model inspired by alveolar morphology, capable of withstanding mechanical strain for cyclical ventilation and oxygen transport (Grigoryan et al., 2019). While successful in creating entangled vascular networks of the lung alveoli, the bioprinted tissue lacked alveolar epithelial cells, and the platform was applied neither for toxicological studies nor for inhaled exposure to a respiratory pathogen or therapeutic agents. Altogether, 3D bioprinting offers the possibility of developing biologically inspired lung organotypic models; however, despite the advantages of 3D bioprinting, wide spread utilization of these techniques has been limited by the requirement of expensive and complex technologies as well as a steep learning curve.

Lung-on-a-Chip Models

Organ-on-a-Chips are biomimetic, microfluidic, cell culture devices created with microchip manufacturing methods that contain continuously perfused hollow microchannels inhabited by living tissue cells arranged to simulate organ-level physiology (Bhatia and Ingber, 2014; Benam et al., 2015). By recapitulating the multicellular architectures, tissue–tissue interfaces, chemical gradients, mechanical cues, and vascular perfusion of the body, these devices produce levels of tissue and organ functionality with well-defined structures and highly controlled microenvironments that would not be possible with conventional 2D or 3D culture systems. They also enable high-resolution, real-time imaging and *in vitro* analysis of biochemical, genetic and metabolic activities of living human cells in a functional human tissue and organ context. Adaptation of Organ-on-a-Chip technology by pulmonary scientists has led to the development of model systems that emulate human lung pathophysiology *in vitro*.

Lung-on-a-Chip devices have been developed to model different regions of the respiratory system and recapitulate *in vivo*-observed multicellular architecture and physicochemical environment of the lung (airway and alveoli). The use of this technology (Alveolus-on-a-Chip) has enabled a better understanding of different aspects of human alveolar pathologies; such as evaluating the influence of breathing-associated mechanical cues on the growth and migration pattern of Non-Small Cell Lung Cancer tumor cells (NSCLC; Hassell et al., 2017), reproducing interleukin-2 (IL-2) induced alveolar edema observed in human cancer patients at similar doses and over the same time frame, and its pharmacological inhibition (Huh et al., 2012), mimicking pulmonary thrombosis by treatment with inflammatory stimuli (TNF-α) and bacterial products (LPS) corroborated in murine models (Jain et al., 2018), studying inhaled exposure of the alveolar epithelium to aerosolized LPS and its immune-modulatory impact (Artzy-Schnirman et al., 2019), and recreating recruitment of circulating leukocytes and inflammation induction after treatment of epithelial cells with TNF-a, *Escherichia coli*, and silica nanoparticles (Huh et al., 2010). In these microphysiological systems primary, cancerous or immortalized cell line of human alveolar epithelial origin have been co-cultured with human lung microvascular endothelial cells (Huh et al., 2010, 2012; Hassell et al., 2017) or human umbilical vascular endothelial cells (HUVECs; Jain et al., 2018).

In the context of conducting airways, we have developed and applied Lung-on-a-Chip devices (Airway-on-a-Chip) for culture and differentiation of primary human epithelial cells in co-culture with primary human lung microvascular endothelial cells, to model small airways, reproduce the mechanical forces associated with inhalation-exhalation respiration cycles (airflow shear), mimic the shear forces across endothelial cell layers (via vascular flow), and recreate the ALI barrier of human airways (Benam et al., 2015, 2016a,b, 2017, 2018, 2019, 2015; Benam and Ingber, 2016; Niemeyer et al., 2018). This technology has been adapted to allow first-in-kind studies that reproduce and characterize tissue–tissue crosstalk between pulmonary epithelium and airway smooth muscle (Humayun et al., 2018) and enable better understanding infectious disease biogenesis processes through analysis of the production of inflammatory cytokines and immune cell recruitment (neutrophils) following exposure to respiratory fungi (e.g., *Aspergillus fumigatus*) and the bacteria (e.g., *Pseudomonas aeruginosa*) (Barkal et al.,

2017) by other investigators. Similay utilizing Airway-on-a-Chip we have been able to dissect inflammatory processes involved in the pathobiology of chronic lung conditions such as asthma induced by the exposure of ephitelium to IL-13 and COPD by recreating terminally differentiated mucociliated airway epithelia on-chip, and exposing cells to the viral mimic polyinosinic–polycytidylic acid (poly(I:C)) or to LPS (Benam et al., 2016b), and identify novel biomarkers of human lung diseases and test efficacy of lead therapeutic compounds (Benam et al., 2016b).

We developed a Breathing-Smoking Lung-on-a-Chip platform that recreates smoke-induced pathologies in humans (Benam et al., 2016b). The system consisted of a Lung Small Airway-on-a-Chip (Benam et al., 2016b) that reproduces the living bronchiolar tissue for exposure to inhaled whole cigarette smoke (WCS), a "microrespirator" that emulates diaphragm and rib cage function and reproduces inhalation-exhalation airflow at physiological rhythms and patterns, a "biomimetic smoking robot" (Benam et al., 2020) that mimics human mouth and generates fresh WCS

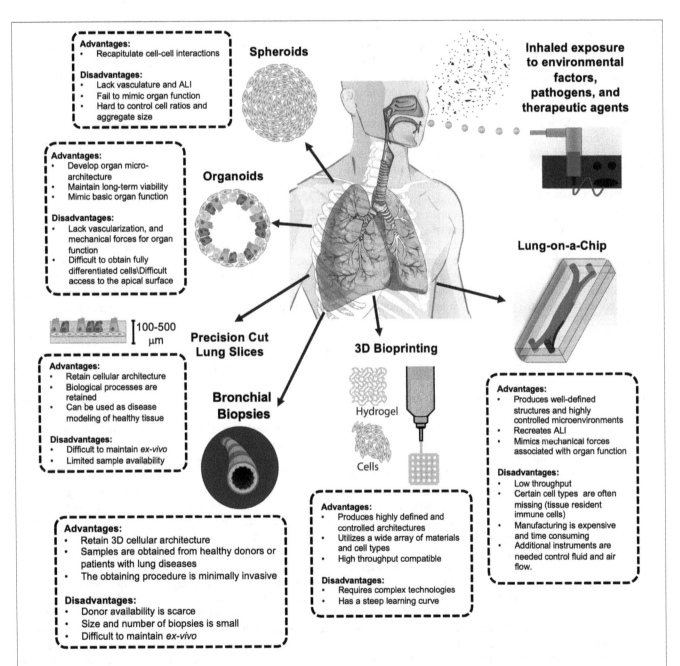

FIGURE 1 | Advantages and disadvantages of complex 3D *in vitro* culture models of the human lung for inhalation exposure studies. Each model presented has unique benefits and challenges. Improved airway modeling can be achieved through incorporating inhalation exposure systems. The digital images of human lung at the center and bronchus near the bottom left were acquired from Shutterstock and Biorender, respectively.

and regulates the passage of inhale/exhale air/smoke, and software that represents the brain of human smoker and controls "smoking topography" and "breathing" behavior. Using this platform, we flowed WCS horizontally across the apical surface of differentiated human bronchiolar epithelia (as occurs in the lungs of human smokers), from normal subjects and COPD patients, at representative smoking topography parameters for puff time, puff volume and inter-puff interval under clinically relevant breathing conditions. We found that inhaled smoke exposure transformed ciliary beat frequency (CBF) pattern, range, and variability and induced oxidative stress. Importantly, it was observed that submerging the ciliated airway epithelia with cell culture medium alone was sufficient to mask the impact of inhaled WCS on ciliary micro-pathologies. In addition, we discovered new smoke-mounted biological markers that distinguish COPD epithelia from those from healthy individuals (Benam et al., 2016a).

Recently, Elias-Kirma et al. (2020) developed an interesting model of branching Airway-on-a-Chip for toxicological evaluation of inhaled particulate matter. The authors utilized primary human bronchial epithelial cells for culture, and exposed the epithelium on-chip to anti-vanilloid receptor 1 (VR1) antibody-coated polystyrene microparticles. The microparticles were generated using a commercial aerosolizing machine and brought into contact with the cells through a pinch valve-controlled antistatic tube. While the device design in this study was unique, the exposure did not mimic what naturally occurs during rhythmic breathing cycles and the authors did not study biological impact of exposure to environmental pollutants, tobacco products or therapeutic agents.

These study implies that Lung-on-a-Chip platforms have the potential for recreation of in vivo-like inhaled exposure to pathogens, environmental threats, and drug treatments. However, for such platforms to be more applicable and physiologically relevant, it is important to enhance their multicellularity and complexity, for instance by the addition of parenchymal cells, such as fibroblasts, tissue-resident and circulating immune cells, muscle cells, and/or ECM. One of the drawbacks of microfluidics is that manufacturing is often expensive and time consuming; in addition, instruments such as syringe pumps or air pressure systems are required to control fluid flow within the chips. Furthermore, the devices need to become more user friendly (particularly for biologists with little/no engineering expertise) and be amenable for increased throughput. On the other hand, although microphysiological systems have great flexibility with respect to the experimental design, there are important challenges due to miniaturization, such as reduced media volumes, different media exchange rates and methods, and lower number of cells tested; finally, and an additional challenge in conducting host-pathogen/environment studies is the stimulus dose. Therefore, it is necessary to carefully evaluate these differences when comparing cell behavior and viability in microfluidic devices versus macroscopic cultures, and especially when comparing against in vivo results to validate the systems. Moreover,

from a high-level perspective investigators utilizing Organ-on-Chip devices must consider as accurate and as feaible as possible validating and qualifying these models against tissues that they are aiming to replicate – i.e., human samples and clinical data. Lastly, we would like to mention that multiple factors have contributed to popularity and quick and widespread adaptation of PDMS for fabrication of Lung-on-a-Chip microfluidic devices. These include ability for rapid prototyping and multilayer device fabrication, optical transparency from 240 to 1100 nm (enabling utilization by various optical detection schemes), flexibility (allowing axial stretch), gas-permeablity (so that oxygen can feasibly penetrate the device and reach the cells embedded within the chip), being non-toxic, inexpensive and not breaking (like glass). However, a drawback of PDMS has been its absorption of small, hydrophobic molecules from flowing solution (Toepke and Beebe, 2006). To mitigate this, we apply either of these two approaches: (1) correcting for absorption of small hydrophobic molecules by quantifying the loss (e.g., via mass spectrometry) and (2) saturating the chips prior to cell culture or experimentation to minimize loss.

CONCLUSION AND FUTURE DIRECTIONS

In this article, we reviewed the most recent advances in creating preclinical 3D model systems that reproduce human lung pathophysiology in vitro and discussed their respective merits and drawbacks in the context of host-environment/pathogen interactions (**Figure 1**). It has been a long road for the transition from 2D to 3D cell culture systems; however, 3D models are gaining popularity in use and adaptation due to their critical advantages over static cell cultures. Spheroids, organoids, and PCLS have proven to be invaluable tools for studying lung development and pathologies, but they lack natural ALI and are unable to reproduce breathing-associated airflow, thus it is not possible to perform inhalation exposure studies using these platforms. Cellularized scaffolds have been widely used to study cell–ECM interactions at health and disease, and for regenerative purposes; however, these have not yet been used to assess host–environment/pathogen interactions. Recently, 3D bioprinting has emerged as a promising technique for developing more intricate lung living systems with great potential for high throughput yield; but numerous technical challenges need to be tackled and complex-system building to integrate multiple organ-specific cells and tissue (beyond generating vascularized constructs) must become a priority. In contrast, microfluidic Lung-on-a-Chip microdevices have emerged as an attractive alternative to mimic lung function and biology as seen in vivo. In the particular case of lung models, and more specifically in the study of the host–environment/pathogen interaction, it is important how the treatments and/or stimuli are delivered, in this sense, the microfluidic platforms have demonstrated to be very robust and physiologically relevant in vitro tools that can incorporate biochemical, physical and mechanical cues. We envision considerable improvement and adaption of Lung-on-a-Chip platforms for the study of host–environment/pathogen interactions. The improvements include allowing higher throughput analysis, and integration of ECM and additional cellular complexity. These microdevices will be utilized for the study of nebulized and dry powder treatments and recreation of clinically relevant exposure to airborne respiratory pathogens (instead of lung cells being exposed submerged to the infective agents). We also anticipate the *in vitro* cell culture of cellularized matrices and potentially PCLS within the Lung-on-a-Chip system to provide dynamism and enhanced viability *ex vivo*. In line with this, 3D bioprinting techniques could revolutionize the way microfluidic devices are currently manufactured, allowing for increased production and reproducibility.

AUTHOR CONTRIBUTIONS

KB conceptualized and critically revised the manuscript. RJ-V, UC, and BN drafted the manuscript. All authors contributed to the article and approved the submitted version.

REFERENCES

Ainslie, G. R., Davis, M., Ewart, L., Lieberman, L. A., Rowlands, D. J., Thorley, A. J., et al. (2019). Microphysiological lung models to evaluate the safety of new pharmaceutical modalities: a biopharmaceutical perspective. *Lab Chip* 19, 3152–3161.

Akhmanova, M., Osidak, E., Domogatsky, S., Rodin, S., and Domogatskaya, A. (2015). Physical, spatial, and molecular aspects of extracellular matrix of *in vivo* niches and artificial scaffolds relevant to stem cells research. *Stem Cells Int.* 2015:167025.

Alsafadi, H. N., Staab-Weijnitz, C. A., Lehmann, M., Lindner, M., Peschel, B., Konigshoff, M., et al. (2017). An *ex vivo* model to induce early fibrosis-like changes in human precision-cut lung slices. *Am. J. Physiol. Lung Cell. Mol. Physiol.* 312, L896–L902.

Alsafadi, H. N., Uhl, F. E., Pineda, R. H., Bailey, K. E., Rojas, M., Wagner, D. E., et al. (2020). Applications and approaches for three-dimensional precision-cut lung slices. Disease modeling and drug discovery. *Am. J. Respir. Cell Mol. Biol.* 62, 681–691. doi: 10.1165/rcmb.2019-0276tr

Artzy-Schnirman, A., Zidan, H., Elias-Kirma, S., Ben-Porat, L., Tenenbaum-Katan, J., Carius, P., et al. (2019). Capturing the onset of bacterial pulmonary infection in acini-on-chips. *Advan. Biosys.* 3:e1900026.

Banerjee, S. K., Huckuntod, S. D., Mills, S. D., Kurten, R. C., and Pechous, R. D. (2019). Modeling pneumonic plague in human precision-cut lung slices highlights a role for the plasminogen activator protease in facilitating type 3 secretion. *Infect. Immun.* 87:e00175-19.

Barkal, L. J., Procknow, C. L., Alvarez-Garcia, Y. R., Niu, M., Jimenez-Torres, J. A., Brockman-Schneider, R. A., et al. (2017). Microbial volatile communication in human organotypic lung models. *Nat. Commun.* 8:1770.

Barkauskas, C. E., Chung, M. I., Fioret, B., Gao, X., Katsura, H., and Hogan, B. L. (2017). Lung organoids: current uses and future promise. *Development* 144, 986–997. doi: 10.1242/dev.140103

Beale, J., Jayaraman, A., Jackson, D. J., Macintyre, J. D. R., Edwards, M. R., and Walton, R. P. (2014). Rhinovirus-induced IL-25 in asthma exacerbation drives type 2 immunity and allergic pulmonary inflammation. *Sci. Transl. Med.* 6:256ra134. doi: 10.1126/scitranslmed.3009124

Benam, K. H., Dauth, S., Hassell, B., Herland, A., Jain, A., and Jang, K. J. (2015). Engineered in vitro disease models. *Annu. Rev. Pathol.* 10, 195–262.

Benam, K. H., Gilchrist, S., Kleensang, A., Satz, A. B., Willett, C., and Zhang, Q. (2019). Exploring new technologies in biomedical research. *Drug Discov. Today* 24, 1242–1247. doi: 10.1016/j.drudis.2019.04.001

Benam, K. H., and Ingber, D. E. (2016). Commendation for exposing key advantage of organ chip approach. *Cell Syst.* 3:411. doi: 10.1016/j.cels.2016.11.009

Benam, K. H., Konigshoff, M., and Eickelberg, O. (2018). Breaking the in vitro barrier in respiratory medicine. engineered microphysiological systems for chronic obstructive pulmonary disease and beyond. *Am. J. Respir. Crit. Care Med.* 197, 869–875. doi: 10.1164/rccm.201709-1795pp

Benam, K. H., Mazur, M., Choe, Y., Ferrante, T. C., Novak, R., and Ingber, D. E. (2017). Human lung small airway-on-a-chip protocol. *Methods Mol. Biol.* 1612, 345–365. doi: 10.1007/978-1-4939-7021-6_25

Benam, K. H., Novak, R., Ferrante, T. C., Choe, Y., and Ingber, D. E. (2020). Biomimetic smoking robot for in vitro inhalation exposure compatible with microfluidic organ chips. *Nat. Protoc.* 15, 183–206. doi: 10.1038/s41596-019-0230-y

Benam, K. H., Novak, R., Nawroth, J., Hirano-Kobayashi, M., Ferrante, T. C., Choe, Y., et al. (2016a). Matched-comparative modeling of normal and diseased human airway responses using a microengineered breathing lung chip. *Cell Syst.* 3, 456–466.e4. doi: 10.1016/j.cels.2016.10.003

Benam, K. H., Villenave, R., Lucchesi, C., Varone, A., Hubeau, C., Lee, H. H., et al. (2016b). Small airway-on-a-chip enables analysis of human lung inflammation and drug responses *in vitro. Nat. Methods* 13, 151–157. doi: 10.1038/nmeth.3697

Bhatia, S. N., and Ingber, D. E. (2014). Microfluidic organs-on-chips. *Nat. Biotechnol.* 32, 760–772. doi: 10.1038/nbt.2989

Burgess, J. K., Mauad, T., Tjin, G., Karlsson, J. C., and Westergren-Thorsson, G. (2016). The extracellular matrix - the under-recognized element in lung disease? *J. Pathol.* 240, 397–409. doi: 10.1002/path.4808

Chimenti, I., Pagano, F., Angelini, F., Siciliano, C., Mangino, G., Picchio, V., et al. (2017). Human lung spheroids as *in vitro* niches of lung progenitor cells with distinctive paracrine and plasticity properties. *Stem Cells Transl. Med.* 6, 767–777. doi: 10.5966/sctm.2015-0374

Donovan, C., Seow, H. J., Bourke, J. E., and Vlahos, R. (2016). Influenza A virus infection and cigarette smoke impair bronchodilator responsiveness to beta-adrenoceptor agonists in mouse lung. *Clin. Sci.* 130, 829–837. doi: 10.1042/cs20160093

Dye, B. R., Dedhia, P. H., Miller, A. J., Nagy, M. S., White, E. S., Shea, L. D., et al. (2016). A bioengineered niche promotes *in vivo* engraftment and maturation of pluripotent stem cell derived human lung organoids. *eLife* 5:e19732.

Ekert, J. E., Johnson, K., Strake, B., Pardinas, J., Jarantow, S., Perkinson, R., et al. (2014). Three-dimensional lung tumor microenvironment modulates therapeutic compound responsiveness *in vitro*–implication for drug development. *PLoS One* 9:e92248. doi: 10.1371/journal.pone.0092248

Elias-Kirma, S., Artzy-Schnirman, A., Das, P., Heller-Algazi, M., Korin, N., and Sznitman, J. (2020). *In situ*-like aerosol inhalation exposure for cytotoxicity assessment using airway-on-chips platforms. *Front. Bioeng. Biotechnol.* 8:91. doi: 10.3389/fbioe.2020.00091

Fang, Y., and Eglen, R. M. (2017). Three-dimensional cell cultures in drug discovery and development. *SLAS Discov.* 22, 456–472. doi: 10.1177/1087057117696795

Gilpin, S. E., and Wagner, D. E. (2018). Acellular human lung scaffolds to model lung disease and tissue regeneration. *Eur. Respir. Rev.* 27:180021. doi: 10.1183/16000617.0021-2018

Giobbe, G. G., Crowley, C., Luni, C., Campinoti, S., Khedr, M., Kretzschmar, K., et al. (2019). Extracellular matrix hydrogel derived from decellularized tissues enables endodermal organoid culture. *Nat. Commun.* 10:5658.

Graham, J. G., Winchell, C. G., Kurten, R. C., and Voth, D. E. (2016). Development of an ex vivo tissue platform to study the human lung response to *Coxiella burnetii. Infect. Immun.* 84, 1438–1445. doi: 10.1128/iai.00012-16

Grainger, C. I., Greenwell, L. L., Lockley, D. J., Martin, G. P., and Forbes, B. (2006). Culture of Calu-3 cells at the air interface provides a representative model of the airway epithelial barrier. *Pharm. Res.* 23, 1482–1490. doi: 10.1007/s11095-006-0255-0

Gray, T. E., Guzman, K., Davis, C. W., Abdullah, L. H., and Nettesheim, P. (1996). Mucociliary differentiation of serially passaged normal human tracheobronchial epithelial cells. *Am. J. Respir. Cell Mol. Biol.* 14, 104–112. doi: 10.1165/ajrcmb.14.1.8534481

Grigoryan, B., Paulsen, S. J., Corbett, D. C., Sazer, D. W., Fortin, C. L., Zaita, A. J., et al. (2019). Multivascular networks and functional intravascular topologies within biocompatible hydrogels. *Science* 364, 458–464. doi: 10.1126/science. aav9750

Guenthart, B. A., O'neill, J. D., Kim, J., Fung, K., Vunjak-Novakovic, G., and Bacchetta, M. (2019). Cell replacement in human lung bioengineering. *J. Heart Lung Transplant.* 38, 215–224. doi: 10.1016/j.healun.2018.11.007

Gungor-Ozkerim, P. S., Inci, I., Zhang, Y. S., Khademhosseini, A., and Dokmeci, M. R. (2018). Bioinks for 3D bioprinting: an overview. *Biomater. Sci.* 6, 915–946.

Hassell, B. A., Goyal, G., Lee, E., Sontheimer-Phelps, A., Levy, O., Chen, C. S., et al. (2017). Human organ chip models recapitulate orthotopic lung cancer growth, therapeutic responses, and tumor dormancy *in vitro. Cell Rep.* 21, 508–516. doi: 10.1016/j.celrep.2017.09.043

Hecht, S. S. (2005). Carcinogenicity studies of inhaled cigarette smoke in laboratory animals: old and new. *Carcinogenesis* 26, 1488–1492. doi: 10.1093/carcin/bgi148

Henjakovic, M., Sewald, K., Switalla, S., Kaiser, D., Muller, M., Veres, T. Z., et al. (2008). *Ex vivo* testing of immune responses in precision-cut lung slices. *Toxicol. Appl. Pharmacol.* 231, 68–76. doi: 10.1016/j.taap.2008.04.003

Heo, I., Dutta, D., Schaefer, D. A., Iakobachvili, N., Artegiani, B., Sachs, N., et al. (2018). Modelling cryptosporidium infection in human small intestinal and lung organoids. *Nat. Microbiol.* 3, 814–823. doi: 10.1038/s41564-018-0177-8

Horvath, L., Umehara, Y., Jud, C., Blank, F., Petri-Fink, A., and Rothen-Rutishauser, B. (2015). Engineering an in vitro air-blood barrier by 3D bioprinting. *Sci. Rep.* 5:7974.

Huh, D., Leslie, D. C., Matthews, B. D., Fraser, J. P., Jurek, S., Hamilton, G. A., et al. (2012). A human disease model of drug toxicity-induced pulmonary edema in a lung-on-a-chip microdevice. *Sci. Transl. Med.* 4:159ra147. doi: 10.1126/scitranslmed.3004249

Huh, D., Matthews, B. D., Mammoto, A., Montoya-Zavala, M., Hsin, H. Y., and Ingber, D. E. (2010). Reconstituting organ-level lung functions on a chip. *Science* 328, 1662–1668. doi: 10.1126/science.1188302

Humayun, M., Chow, C. W., and Young, E. W. K. (2018). Microfluidic lung airway-on-a-chip with arrayable suspended gels for studying epithelial and smooth muscle cell interactions. *Lab Chip* 18, 1298–1309. doi: 10.1039/c7lc01357d

Jaffar, Z., Roberts, K., Pandit, A., Linsley, P., Djukanovic, R., and Holgate, S. (1999). B7 costimulation is required for IL-5 and IL-13 secretion by bronchial biopsy tissue of atopic asthmatic subjects in response to allergen stimulation. *Am. J. Respir. Cell Mol. Biol.* 20, 153–162. doi: 10.1165/ajrcmb.20.1.3255

Jain, A., Barrile, R., Van Der Meer, A. D., Mammoto, A., Mammoto, T., De Ceunynck, K., et al. (2018). Primary human lung alveolus-on-a-chip model of intravascular thrombosis for assessment of therapeutics. *Clin. Pharmacol. Ther.* 103, 332–340. doi: 10.1002/cpt.742

Klameth, L., Rath, B., Hochmaier, M., Moser, D., Redl, M., Mungenast, F., et al. (2017). Small cell lung cancer: model of circulating tumor cell tumorospheres in chemoresistance. *Sci. Rep.* 7:5337.

Kolesky, D. B., Truby, R. L., Gladman, A. S., Busbee, T. A., Homan, K. A., and Lewis, J. A. (2014). 3D bioprinting of vascularized, heterogeneous cell-laden tissue constructs. *Adv. Mater.* 26, 3124–3130. doi: 10.1002/adma.201305506

Konishi, S., Gotoh, S., Tateishi, K., Yamamoto, Y., Korogi, Y., Nagasaki, T., et al. (2016). Directed induction of functional multi-ciliated cells in proximal airway epithelial spheroids from human pluripotent stem cells. *Stem Cell Rep.* 6, 18–25. doi: 10.1016/j.stemcr.2015.11.010

Lang, D. S., Droemann, D., Schultz, H., Branscheid, D., Martin, C., Ressmeyer, A. R., et al. (2007). A novel human ex vivo model for the analysis of molecular events during lung cancer chemotherapy. *Respir. Res.* 8:43.

Lauenstein, L., Switalla, S., Prenzler, F., Seehase, S., Pfennig, O., Forster, C., et al. (2014). Assessment of immunotoxicity induced by chemicals in human precision-cut lung slices (PCLS). *Toxicol. In Vitro* 28, 588–599. doi: 10.1016/j.tiv.2013.12.016

Lenz, A. G., Karg, E., Lentner, B., Dittrich, V., Brandenberger, C., Rothen-Rutishauser, B., et al. (2009). A dose-controlled system for air-liquid interface cell exposure and application to zinc oxide nanoparticles. *Part. Fibre Toxicol.* 6:32. doi: 10.1186/1743-8977-6-32

Lewis, K. J. R., Hall, J. K., Kiyotake, E. A., Christensen, T., Balasubramaniam, V., and Anseth, K. S. (2018). Epithelial-mesenchymal crosstalk influences cellular behavior in a 3D alveolus-fibroblast model system. *Biomaterials* 155, 124–134. doi: 10.1016/j.biomaterials.2017.11.008

Liu, G., Betts, C., Cunoosamy, D. M., Aberg, P. M., Hornberg, J. J., Sivars, K. B., et al. (2019). Use of precision cut lung slices as a translational model for the study of lung biology. *Respir. Res.* 20:162.

Liu, R., An, L., Liu, G., Li, X., Tang, W., and Chen, X. (2015). Mouse lung slices: an *ex vivo* model for the evaluation of antiviral and anti-inflammatory agents against influenza viruses. *Antiviral Res.* 120, 101–111. doi: 10.1016/j.antiviral.2015.05.008

Lordan, J. L., Davies, D. E., Wilson, S. J., Dent, G., Corkhill, A., Jaffar, Z., et al. (2001). The role of CD28-B7 costimulation in allergen-induced cytokine release by bronchial mucosa from patients with moderately severe asthma. *J. Allergy Clin. Immunol.* 108, 976–981. doi: 10.1067/mai.2001.119740

Mccauley, K. B., Hawkins, F., Serra, M., Thomas, D. C., Jacob, A., and Kotton, D. N. (2017). Efficient derivation of functional human airway epithelium from pluripotent stem cells via temporal regulation of Wnt signaling. *Cell Stem Cell* 20, 844–857.e6. doi: 10.1016/j.stem.2017.03.001

Meenach, S. A., Tsoras, A. N., Mcgarry, R. C., Mansour, H. M., Hilt, J. Z., and Anderson, K. W. (2016). Development of three-dimensional lung multicellular spheroids in air- and liquid-interface culture for the evaluation of anticancer therapeutics. *Int. J. Oncol.* 48, 1701–1709. doi: 10.3892/ijo.2016.3376

Miller, A. J., Dye, B. R., Ferrer-Torres, D., Hill, D. R., Overeem, A. W., Shea, L. D., et al. (2019). Generation of lung organoids from human pluripotent stem cells *in vitro. Nat. Protoc.* 14, 518–540.

Miller, A. J., Hill, D. R., Nagy, M. S., Aoki, Y., Dye, B. R., Chin, A. M., et al. (2018). *In vitro* induction and *in vivo* engraftment of lung bud tip progenitor cells derived from human pluripotent stem cells. *Stem Cell Rep.* 10, 101–119. doi: 10.1016/j.stemcr.2017.11.012

Miller, A. J., and Spence, J. R. (2017). *In vitro* models to study human lung development, disease and homeostasis. *Physiology* 32, 246–260. doi: 10.1152/physiol.00041.2016

Neuhaus, V., Schaudien, D., Golovina, T., Temann, U. A., Thompson, C., Lippmann, T., et al. (2017). Assessment of long-term cultivated human precision-cut lung slices as an ex vivo system for evaluation of chronic cytotoxicity and functionality. *J. Occup. Med. Toxicol.* 12:13.

Nicholas, B., Staples, K. J., Moese, S., Meldrum, E., Ward, J., Dennison, P., et al. (2015). A novel lung explant model for the ex vivo study of efficacy and mechanisms of anti-influenza drugs. *J. Immunol.* 194, 6144–6154. doi: 10.4049/jimmunol.1402283

Niemeyer, B. F., Zhao, P., Tuder, R. M., and Benam, K. H. (2018). Advanced microengineered lung models for translational drug discovery. *SLAS Discov.* 23, 777–789. doi: 10.1177/2472555218760217

Porzionato, A., Stocco, E., Barbon, S., Grandi, F., Macchi, V., and De Caro, R. (2018). Tissue-engineered grafts from human decellularized extracellular matrices: a systematic review and future perspectives. *Int. J. Mol. Sci.* 19:4117. doi: 10.3390/ijms19124117

Prunieras, M., Regnier, M., and Woodley, D. (1983). Methods for cultivation of keratinocytes with an air-liquid interface. *J. Invest. Dermatol.* 81, 28s–33s.

Quantius, J., Schmoldt, C., Vazquez-Armendariz, A. I., Becker, C., El Agha, E., Wilhelm, J., et al. (2016). Influenza virus infects epithelial stem/progenitor cells of the distal lung: impact on fgfr2b-driven epithelial repair. *PLoS Pathog.* 12:e1005544. doi: 10.1371/journal.ppat.1005544

Rackley, C. R., and Stripp, B. R. (2012). Building and maintaining the epithelium of the lung. *J. Clin. Invest.* 122, 2724–2730. doi: 10.1172/jci60519

Sachs, N., Papaspyropoulos, A., Zomer-Van Ommen, D. D., Heo, I., Bottinger, L., Klay, D., et al. (2019). Long-term expanding human airway organoids for disease modeling. *EMBO J.* 38:e100300.

Sanderson, M. J. (2011). Exploring lung physiology in health and disease with lung slices. *Pulm. Pharmacol. Ther.* 24, 452–465. doi: 10.1016/j.pupt.2011.05.001

Sato, T., Morita, M., Tanaka, R., Inoue, Y., Nomura, M., Sakamoto, Y., et al. (2017). Ex vivo model of non-small cell lung cancer using mouse lung epithelial cells. *Oncol. Lett.* 63–6868.

Skronska-Wasek, W., Mutze, K., Baarsma, H. A., Bracke, K. R., Alsafadi, H. N., Lehmann, M., et al. (2017). Reduced frizzled receptor 4 expression prevents WNT/beta-catenin-driven alveolar lung repair in chronic obstructive pulmonary disease. *Am. J. Respir. Crit. Care Med.* 1.96, 172–185. doi: 10.1164/rccm.201605-0904oc

Stratmann, A. T., Fecher, D., Wangorsch, G., Gottlich, C., Walles, T., Walles, H., et al. (2014). Establishment of a human 3D lung cancer model based on a biological tissue matrix combined with a Boolean in silico model. *Mol. Oncol.* 8, 351–365. doi: 10.1016/j.molonc.2013.11.009

Sun, H., Zhu, Y., Pan, H., Chen, X., Balestrini, J. L., Lam, T. T., et al. (2016). Netrin-1 regulates fibrocyte accumulation in the decellularized fibrotic sclerodermatous lung microenvironment and in bleomycin-induced pulmonary fibrosis. *Arthritis Rheumatol.* 68, 1251–1261.

Surolia, R., Li, F. J., Wang, Z., Li, H., Liu, G., Zhou, Y., et al. (2017). 3D pulmospheres serve as a personalized and predictive multicellular model for assessment of antifibrotic drugs. *JCI Insight* 2:e91377.

Thorne, D., and Adamson, J. (2013). A review of *in vitro* cigarette smoke exposure systems. *Exp. Toxicol. Pathol.* 65, 1183–1193. doi: 10.1016/j.etp.2013.06.001

Toepke, M. W., and Beebe, D. J. (2006). PDMS absorption of small molecules and consequences in microfluidic applications. *Lab Chip* 6, 1484–1486.

Upadhyay, S., and Palmberg, L. (2018). Air-liquid interface: relevant in vitro models for investigating air pollutant-induced pulmonary toxicity. *Toxicol. Sci.* 164, 21–30. doi: 10.1093/toxsci/kfy053

Van Der Velden, J. L., Wagner, D. E., Lahue, K. G., Abdalla, S. T., Lam, Y. W., Weiss, D. J., et al. (2018). TGF-beta1-induced deposition of provisional extracellular matrix by tracheal basal cells promotes epithelial-to-mesenchymal transition in a c-Jun NH2-terminal kinase-1-dependent manner. *Am. J. Physiol. Lung Cell. Mol. Physiol.* 314, L984–L997.

Vijayanand, P., Durkin, K., Hartmann, G., Morjaria, J., Seumois, G., Staples, K. J., et al. (2010). Chemokine receptor 4 plays a key role in T cell recruitment into the airways of asthmatic patients. *J. Immunol.* 184, 4568–4574. doi: 10.4049/jimmunol.0901342

Williamson, I. A., Arnold, J. W., Samsa, L. A., Gaynor, L., Disalvo, M., Cocchiaro, J. L., et al. (2018). A high-throughput organoid microinjection platform to study gastrointestinal microbiota and luminal physiology. *Cell. Mol. Gastroenterol. Hepatol.* 6, 301–319. doi: 10.1016/j.jcmgh.2018.05.004

Woodruff, P. G., and Innes, A. L. (2006). Quantitative morphology using bronchial biopsies. *Eur. Respir. Rev.* 15, 157–161. doi: 10.1183/09059180.00010106

World Health Organization [WHO] (2018). *The Top 10 Causes of Death.* Available online at: https://www.who.int/news-room/fact-sheets/detail/the-top-10-causes-of-death (accessed March 31, 2020).

Yamaya, M., Finkbeiner, W., Chun, S., and Widdicombe, J. (1992). Differentiated structure and function of cultures from human tracheal epithelium. *Am. J. Physiol. Lung Cell. Mol. Physiol.* 262, L713–L724.

Zacharias, W. J., Frank, D. B., Zepp, J. A., Morley, M. P., Alkhaleel, F. A., Kong, J., et al. (2018). Regeneration of the lung alveolus by an evolutionarily conserved epithelial progenitor. *Nature* 555, 251–255. doi: 10.1038/nature25786

Zhou, Y., Horowitz, J. C., Naba, A., Ambalavanan, N., Atabai, K., Balestrini, J., et al. (2018). Extracellular matrix in lung development, homeostasis and disease. *Matrix Biol.* 73, 77–104.

Permissions

All chapters in this book were first published by Frontiers; hereby published with permission under the Creative Commons Attribution License or equivalent. Every chapter published in this book has been scrutinized by our experts. Their significance has been extensively debated. The topics covered herein carry significant findings which will fuel the growth of the discipline. They may even be implemented as practical applications or may be referred to as a beginning point for another development.

The contributors of this book come from diverse backgrounds, making this book a truly international effort. This book will bring forth new frontiers with its revolutionizing research information and detailed analysis of the nascent developments around the world.

We would like to thank all the contributing authors for lending their expertise to make the book truly unique. They have played a crucial role in the development of this book. Without their invaluable contributions this book wouldn't have been possible. They have made vital efforts to compile up to date information on the varied aspects of this subject to make this book a valuable addition to the collection of many professionals and students.

This book was conceptualized with the vision of imparting up-to-date information and advanced data in this field. To ensure the same, a matchless editorial board was set up. Every individual on the board went through rigorous rounds of assessment to prove their worth. After which they invested a large part of their time researching and compiling the most relevant data for our readers.

The editorial board has been involved in producing this book since its inception. They have spent rigorous hours researching and exploring the diverse topics which have resulted in the successful publishing of this book. They have passed on their knowledge of decades through this book. To expedite this challenging task, the publisher supported the team at every step. A small team of assistant editors was also appointed to further simplify the editing procedure and attain best results for the readers.

Apart from the editorial board, the designing team has also invested a significant amount of their time in understanding the subject and creating the most relevant covers. They scrutinized every image to scout for the most suitable representation of the subject and create an appropriate cover for the book.

The publishing team has been an ardent support to the editorial, designing and production team. Their endless efforts to recruit the best for this project, has resulted in the accomplishment of this book. They are a veteran in the field of academics and their pool of knowledge is as vast as their experience in printing. Their expertise and guidance has proved useful at every step. Their uncompromising quality standards have made this book an exceptional effort. Their encouragement from time to time has been an inspiration for everyone.

The publisher and the editorial board hope that this book will prove to be a valuable piece of knowledge for researchers, students, practitioners and scholars across the globe.

List of Contributors

Mohammed Ali Selo
School of Pharmacy and Pharmaceutical Sciences and Trinity Biomedical Sciences Institute, Trinity College Dublin, Dublin, Ireland
Faculty of Pharmacy, University of Kufa, Al-Najaf, Iraq

Anne-Sophie Delmas, Lisa Springer, Johannes A. Sake, Caoimhe G. Clerkin, Sabrina Nickel and Carsten Ehrhardt
School of Pharmacy and Pharmaceutical Sciences and Trinity Biomedical Sciences Institute, Trinity College Dublin, Dublin, Ireland

Viktoria Zoufal
School of Pharmacy and Pharmaceutical Sciences and Trinity Biomedical Sciences Institute, Trinity College Dublin, Dublin, Ireland
Preclinical Molecular Imaging, AIT Austrian Institute of Technology GmbH, Seibersdorf, Austria

Hanno Huwer
Department of Cardiothoracic Surgery, Völklingen Heart Centre, Völklingen, Germany

Nicole Schneider-Daum
Helmholtz Institute for Pharmaceutical Research Saarland, Helmholtz Centre for Infection Research, Saarbrücken, Germany

Claus-Michael Lehr
Helmholtz Institute for Pharmaceutical Research Saarland, Helmholtz Centre for Infection Research, Saarbrücken, Germany
Department of Pharmacy, Saarland University, Saarbrücken, Germany

Oliver Langer
Preclinical Molecular Imaging, AIT Austrian Institute of Technology GmbH, Seibersdorf, Austria
Department of Clinical Pharmacology, Medical University of Vienna, Vienna, Austria
Division of Nuclear Medicine, Department of Biomedical Imaging and Image-guided Therapy, Medical University of Vienna, Vienna, Austria

Cristina García-Mouton, Alberto Hidalgo, Raquel Arroyo, Mercedes Echaide, Antonio Cruz and Jesús Pérez-Gil
Department of Biochemistry and Molecular Biology, Faculty of Biology, Research Institute "Hospital 12 de Octubre (imas12)," Complutense University, Madrid, Spain

Justus C. Horstmann, Claus-Michael Lehr and Patrick Carius
Helmholtz Institute for Pharmaceutical Research Saarland (HIPS), Saarbrücken, Germany
Department of Pharmacy, Saarland University, Saarbrücken, Germany

Chelsea R. Thorn
Clinical and Health Science, University of South Australia, Adelaide, SA, Australia

Florian Graef, Xabier Murgia and Cristiane de Souza Carvalho-Wodarz
Helmholtz Institute for Pharmaceutical Research Saarland (HIPS), Saarbrücken, Germany
Department of Pharmacy, Saarland University, Saarbrücken, Germany

Shani Elias-Kirma, Arbel Artzy-Schnirman, Prashant Das, Metar Heller-Algazi, Netanel Korin and Josué Sznitman
Department of Biomedical Engineering, Technion – Israel Institute of Technology, Haifa, Israel

Caroline Majoral, Alain Le Pape and Laurent Vecellio
INSERM, Research Center for Respiratory Diseases, Tours, France
Université de Tours, Tours, France

Allan L. Coates
Hospital for Sick Children, Toronto, ON, Canada

Patrick Carius, Claus-Michael Lehr and Morvarid Ajdarirad
Department of Drug Delivery (DDEL), Helmholtz-Institute for Pharmaceutical Research Saarland (HIPS), Helmholtz Centre for Infection Research (HZI), Saarbrücken, Germany
Department of Pharmacy, Biopharmaceutics and Pharmaceutical Technology, Saarland University, Saarbrücken, Germany

Aurélie Dubois and Nicole Schneider-Daum
Department of Drug Delivery (DDEL), Helmholtz-Institute for Pharmaceutical Research Saarland (HIPS), Helmholtz Centre for Infection Research (HZI), Saarbrücken, Germany

Arbel Artzy-Schnirman and Josué Sznitman
Department of Biomedical Engineering, Technion–Israel Institute of Technology, Haifa, Israel

Xinhui Wu, John-Poul Ng-Blichfeldt, Ana Matias and Reinoud Gosens
Department of Molecular Pharmacology, Faculty of Science and Engineering, University of Groningen, Groningen, Netherlands
Groningen Research Institute for Asthma and COPD, University Medical Center Groningen, University of Groningen, Groningen, Netherlands

Vicky Verschut
AQUILO BV, Groningen, Netherlands

Manon E. Woest and Loes E. M. Kistemaker
Department of Molecular Pharmacology, Faculty of Science and Engineering, University of Groningen, Groningen, Netherlands
Groningen Research Institute for Asthma and COPD, University Medical Center Groningen, University of Groningen, Groningen, Netherlands
AQUILO BV, Groningen, Netherlands

Gino Villetti, Alessandro Accetta and Fabrizio Facchinetti
Corporate Pre-Clinical R and D, Chiesi Farmaceutici S.p.A., Parma, Italy

Jarred R. Mondoñedo
Department of Biomedical Engineering, College of Engineering, Boston University, Boston, MA, United States
Boston University School of Medicine, Boston, MA, United States

Elizabeth Bartolák-Suki, Samer Bou Jawde, Kara Nelson, Kun Cao, Walter Patrick Obrochta, Jasmin Imsirovic and Béla Suki
Department of Biomedical Engineering, College of Engineering, Boston University, Boston, MA, United States

Adam Sonnenberg
Department of Systems Engineering, College of Engineering, Boston University, Boston, MA, United States

Sumati Ram-Mohan and Ramaswamy Krishnan
Department of Emergency Medicine, Beth Israel Deaconess Medical Center, Harvard Medical School, Boston, MA, United States

Julia Nemeth, Annika Schundner, Veronika E. Winkelmann and Manfred Frick
Institute of General Physiology, Ulm University, Ulm, Germany

Karsten Quast
Boehringer Ingelheim Pharma GmbH & Co. KG, Biberach, Germany

Ali Doryab, Andreas Schröppel, Sezer Orak, Carola Voss, Markus Rehberg, Tobias Stöger and Otmar Schmid
Comprehensive Pneumology Center Munich, Member of the German Center for Lung Research, Munich, Germany
Helmholtz Zentrum München—German Research Center for Environmental Health, Institute of Lung Biology and Disease, Munich, Germany

Mehmet Berat Taskin and Philipp Stahlhut
Department of Functional Materials in Medicine and Dentistry, Bavarian Polymer Institute, University of Würzburg, Würzburg, Germany

Arti Ahluwalia
Research Center "E. Piaggio", University of Pisa, Pisa, Italy
Department of Information Engineering, University of Pisa, Pisa, Italy

Anne Hilgendorff
Comprehensive Pneumology Center Munich, Member of the German Center for Lung Research, Munich, Germany
Helmholtz Zentrum München—German Research Center for Environmental Health, Institute of Lung Biology and Disease, Munich, Germany
Center for Comprehensive Developmental Care (CDeCLMU), Dr. von Haunersches Children's Hospital University, Hospital of the Ludwig-Maximilians University, Munich, Germany

Jürgen Groll
Department of Functional Materials in Medicine and Dentistry, Bavarian Polymer Institute, University of Würzburg, Würzburg, Germany

Barbara Drasler, Bedia Begum Karakocak, Esma Bahar Tankus, Hana Barosova, Mauro Sousa de Almeida and Barbara Rothen-Rutishauser
Institut Adolphe Merkle, Faculté des Sciences et de Médecine, Université de Fribourg, Fribourg, Switzerland

Jun Abe
Department of Oncology, Microbiology and Immunology, Faculty of Science and Medicine, University of Fribourg, Fribourg, Switzerland

Alke Petri-Fink
Institut Adolphe Merkle, Faculté des Sciences et de Médecine, Université de Fribourg, Fribourg, Switzerland
Département de Chimie, Faculté des Sciences et de Médecine, Université de Fribourg, Fribourg, Switzerland

Shih-En Tang and Kun-Lun Huang
Institute of Aerospace and Undersea Medicine, National Defense Medical Center, Taipei, Taiwan
Department of Internal Medicine, Tri-Service General Hospital, National Defense Medical Center, Taipei, Taiwan

Wen-I Liao
Department of Emergency Medicine, Tri-Service General Hospital, National Defense Medical Center, Taipei, Taiwan

Hsin-Ping Pao
The Graduate Institute of Medical Sciences, National Defense Medical Center, Taipei, Taiwan

Chin-Wang Hsu
Department of Emergency and Critical Medicine, Wan Fang Hospital, Taipei Medical University, Taipei, Taiwan

Shu-Yu Wu
Institute of Aerospace and Undersea Medicine, National Defense Medical Center, Taipei, Taiwan

Shi-Jye Chu
Department of Internal Medicine, Tri-Service General Hospital, National Defense Medical Center, Taipei, Taiwan

Cameron Yamanishi, Eric Parigoris and Shuichi Takayama
Wallace H. Coulter Department of Biomedical Engineering, Georgia Institute of Technology, Atlanta, GA, United States
The Parker H. Petit Institute of Bioengineering and Bioscience, Georgia Institute of Technology, Atlanta, GA, United States

Weiwei Yu, Yi Huang, Yang Peng, Qin Xia and Zhang Cuntai
Department of Geriatric Medicine, Tongji Hospital, Tongji Medical College, Huazhong University of Science and Technology, Wuhan, China

Ting Ye
Department of Clinical Nutrition, Tongji Hospital, Tongji Medical College, Huazhong University of Science and Technology, Wuhan, China

Jie Ding
Urology Department of Xin Hua Hospital, Xin Hua Hospital Affliated to Shanghai Jiao Tong University, Shanghai, China

Qi Li, Qingsen Ran, Lidong Sun, Ting Luo, Li Liu, Zheng Zhao, Qing Yang, Yujie Li, Ying Chen, Xiaogang Weng, Yajie Wang, Weiyan Cai and Xiaoxin Zhu
Institute of Chinese Materia Medica, China Academy of Chinese Medical Sciences, Beijing, China

Jie Yin
School of Chinese Materia Medica, Capital Medical University, Beijing, China

Jia-Wei Yang, Ko-Chih Lin, Sheng-Jen Cheng, Shiue-Luen Chen, Chong-You Chen and Shien-Fong Lin
Department of Electrical and Computer Engineering, College of Electrical and Computer Engineering National Chiao Tung University, Hsinchu, Taiwan
Institute of Biomedical Engineering, College of Electrical and Computer Engineering, National Chiao Tung University, Hsinchu, Taiwan

Yu-Chih Shen
Institute of Biomedical Engineering, College of Electrical and Computer Engineering, National Chiao Tung University, Hsinchu, Taiwan
Ph.D. Degree Program of Biomedical Science and Engineering, National Chiao Tung University, Hsinchu, Taiwan

Priyank V. Kumar
School of Chemical Engineering, University of New South Wales, Sydney, NSW, Australia

Huai-En Lu
Bioresource Collection and Research Center, Food Industry Research and Development Institute, Hsinchu, Taiwan

Guan-Yu Chen
Department of Electrical and Computer Engineering, College of Electrical and Computer Engineering National Chiao Tung University, Hsinchu, Taiwan
Institute of Biomedical Engineering, College of Electrical and Computer Engineering, National Chiao Tung University, Hsinchu, Taiwan
Department of Biological Science and Technology, National Chiao Tung University, Hsinchu, Taiwan

Moira L. Aitken, Ranjani Somayaji and Maricela Pier
Department of Medicine, School of Medicine, University of Washington, Seattle, WA, United States

Thomas R. Hinds
Department of Pharmacy, School of Medicine, University of Washington, Seattle, WA, United States

Karla Droguett, Mariana Rios and Manuel Villalon
Department of Physiology, Faculty of Biological Sciences, Pontificia Universidad Católica de Chile, Santiago, Chile

Shawn J. Skerrett
Department of Medicine, School of Medicine, University of Washington, Seattle, WA, United States
Department of Physiology, Faculty of Biological Sciences, Pontificia Universidad Católica de Chile, Santiago, Chile

Rocio J. Jimenez-Valdes, Uryan I. Can and Brian F. Niemeyer
Division of Pulmonary Sciences and Critical Care Medicine, Department of Medicine, University of Colorado Anschutz Medical Campus, Aurora, CO, United States

Kambez H. Benam
Division of Pulmonary Sciences and Critical Care Medicine, Department of Medicine, University of Colorado Anschutz Medical Campus, Aurora, CO, United States
Department of Bioengineering, University of Colorado Denver, Aurora, CO, United States
Linda Crnic Institute for Down Syndrome, University of Colorado Anschutz Medical Campus, Aurora, CO, United States

Index